I0057362

Concepts, Theories and Applications of Genetics

Concepts, Theories and Applications of Genetics

Edited by **Luke Stanton**

hayle
medical

New York

Published by Hayle Medical,
30 West, 37th Street, Suite 612,
New York, NY 10018, USA
www.haylemedical.com

Concepts, Theories and Applications of Genetics
Edited by Luke Stanton

© 2016 Hayle Medical

International Standard Book Number: 978-1-63241-423-6 (Hardback)

This book contains information obtained from authentic and highly regarded sources. Copyright for all individual chapters remain with the respective authors as indicated. All chapters are published with permission under the Creative Commons Attribution License or equivalent. A wide variety of references are listed. Permission and sources are indicated; for detailed attributions, please refer to the permissions page and list of contributors. Reasonable efforts have been made to publish reliable data and information, but the authors, editors and publisher cannot assume any responsibility for the validity of all materials or the consequences of their use.

The publisher's policy is to use permanent paper from mills that operate a sustainable forestry policy. Furthermore, the publisher ensures that the text paper and cover boards used have met acceptable environmental accreditation standards.

Trademark Notice: Registered trademark of products or corporate names are used only for explanation and identification without intent to infringe.

Printed in the United States of America.

Contents

Preface

Genetics is a field of study which generally comes under the field of biology but sometimes it is closely related to information systems and life sciences. It refers to the study of genes, genetic variation and heredity in living beings. It has many branches namely evolutionary genetics, ecological genetics, human genetics, microbial, molecular and medical genetics, etc. This book traces the progress of this field and highlights some of its key concepts, theories and applications. It contains some path-breaking studies in this field. It includes the topics which are of utmost significance and are bound to provide incredible insights to the readers. Coherent flow of topics, reader-friendly language and extensive use of case studies make this book an invaluable source of knowledge and a beneficial guide of reference for both academicians and students.

This book is a comprehensive compilation of works of different researchers from varied parts of the world. It includes valuable experiences of the researchers with the sole objective of providing the readers (learners) with a proper knowledge of the concerned field. This book will be beneficial in evoking inspiration and enhancing the knowledge of the interested readers.

In the end, I would like to extend my heartiest thanks to the authors who worked with great determination on their chapters. I also appreciate the publisher's support in the course of the book. I would also like to deeply acknowledge my family who stood by me as a source of inspiration during the project.

Editor

Deletion of 7q33-q35 in a Patient with Intellectual Disability and Dysmorphic Features: Further Characterization of 7q Interstitial Deletion Syndrome

Kristen Dilzell,[1] Diana Darcy,[2] John Sum,[3] and Robert Wallerstein[2]

[1]*Department of Medical Genetics, University of Pennsylvania, Philadelphia, PA 19104, USA*
[2]*Silicon Valley Genetics Center, Santa Clara Valley Medical Center, San Jose, CA 95128, USA*
[3]*Pediatric Neurology, Santa Clara Valley Medical Center, San Jose, CA 95120, USA*

Correspondence should be addressed to Robert Wallerstein; robert.wallerstein@hhs.sccgov.org

Academic Editor: Silvia Paracchini

This case report concerns a 16-year-old girl with a 9.92 Mb, heterozygous interstitial chromosome deletion at 7q33-q35, identified using array comparative genomic hybridization. The patient has dysmorphic facial features, intellectual disability, recurrent infections, self-injurious behavior, obesity, and recent onset of hemihypertrophy. This patient has overlapping features with previously reported individuals who have similar deletions spanning the 7q32-q36 region. It has been difficult to describe an interstitial 7q deletion syndrome due to variations in the sizes and regions in the few patients reported in the literature. This case contributes to the further characterization of an interstitial distal 7q deletion syndrome.

1. Introduction

While a syndrome due to a terminal deletion of 7q has been described [1, 2], interstitial deletions in 7q have been less well categorized. Previously reported 7q interstitial deletions have spanned different chromosomal segments of varying sizes, making it difficult to define a 7q interstitial deletion syndrome. Furthermore, many of these patients were reported prior to the implementation of genome-wide array comparative genomic hybridization (array CGH) and knowledge of many gene locations and functions.

We report on a patient with a 9.92 Mb interstitial chromosome deletion of 7q33-q35 and summarize the clinical features seen in this patient, other patients with 7q33-q35 deletions, and patients with other 7q interstitial and terminal deletions, to help understand the range of phenotypes seen in patients with interstitial 7q deletions. We also review the known genes in this region to assess relevant genotype-phenotype correlations.

2. Case Presentation

The patient, now 16 years old, was born to a 23-year-old G4, P3 → 4 mother and 30-year-old father. During the pregnancy there was concern for decreased fetal movement. Labor was induced due to fetal distress at 36 weeks' gestation. Birth weight was 2614 g (<3%) and birth length was 44.5 cm (<3%). She had a positive toxicology screen for barbiturates and was noted to have large open fontanels. The patient remained in the hospital for 5 days after birth due to feeding difficulties.

The patient came to attention again around 6 months of age due to developmental delay and was evaluated by neurology. At around one year of age, the patient also began having seizure activity. EEG results were normal; a brain MRI at 14 months of age showed prominent CSF space posterior to cerebellar vermis, most likely representing large cisterna magna. A karyotype revealed abnormal results, 46,XX,del (7)(q32-q34). The patient's mother had a normal karyotype and her father remains unavailable for testing but is not known to have any features similar to the patient; her deletion is presumed to be de novo based on its large size. Her seizures resolved by 2.5 years of age.

The patient has had multiple recurrent infections throughout her life; by 28 months of age, she had been hospitalized for pneumonia 3 times. The patient has continued to experience multiple upper respiratory infections, recurrent otitis media, and urinary tract infections. Immunology work-up was normal; therefore the patient is not suspected of having a primary immunodeficiency. The patient has a history of chronic otitis media and abnormal tympanometry and audiology examinations; she had ear tubes placed at 30 months of age. An audiogram performed at age 8 showed right moderate conductive hearing loss and left borderline to mild hearing loss, and hearing aids were recommended. The patient was first evaluated by ophthalmology at 33 months and noted to have hyperopia and bilateral astigmatism but no evidence of optic atrophy, as reported in some patients with 7q interstitial deletions.

At age 7 the patient was diagnosed with likely obstructive sleep apnea syndrome. She has a history of snoring and insomnia. In the same year the patient was noted to have elevated ALT and AST levels, which have progressively increased; suspected etiology is nonalcoholic steatohepatitis. A liver biopsy revealed macrovesicular steatosis and a modest number of lymphocytes in a few portal triads. The patient has also been followed up by endocrinology since age 10 due to abnormal weight gain, acanthosis nigricans, and insulin resistance. She was diagnosed with type II diabetes at age 11 and started on metformin. Additionally, the patient is reported to have large, foul smelling stools since 12 years of age.

At age 14, the patient developed hemihypertrophy on her right side and swelling of the right side of her face in the morning that regresses during the day. The hypertrophy interferes with walking and causes pain in her right foot. Genetic testing for Beckwith-Wiedemann syndrome was negative. A CT scan of the lower extremities showed increased diameter of the right leg in relation to the left, with a relative increase in both subcutaneous fat and muscle size. The increased musculature may represent compensatory hypertrophy secondary to the increased overall mass of the right lower extremity, but idiopathic or genetic reasons for hemihypertrophy cannot be excluded. There is no visible mass to account for the apparent disparity in size. An abdominal ultrasound showed a diffusely echogenic liver, compatible with fatty infiltration. Previous echocardiograms and EKGs have been normal. At age 15, the patient's lower left leg also appeared to be growing in size. The patient currently has menstrual cycles two times per month. She developed a hyperpigmented spot on her forehead at age 15.

The patient has a history of significant developmental delay and intellectual disability. She sat at one year and walked at two years. At 28 months she had one or two understandable words but was mostly nonverbal. At age 7 her vocabulary was 15 words, but she did not yet put words together in phrases or sentences. At age 13 she was in a special education class in the 7th grade, assessed to be at a 3-year-old level. Currently at age 16, she is not able to name colors or count, but she can write her name, speak in simple sentences, and name some body parts. She has not lost any skills over time. The patient has a history of violent behaviors towards others and self-injurious behavior, including skin picking which began around 3 years of age and continues to present. Methylation analysis for Prader-Willi syndrome (due to features of obesity, intellectual disability, and skin-picking behaviors) and testing for cystic fibrosis (due to bowel concerns) were both normal.

The patient has dysmorphic features including small ears, a right preauricular ear pit, a large mouth with downturned corners, a smooth philtrum, a thin upper lip, hypertelorism, bulbous nose, a low posterior hairline, and a short neck. Lumbar lordosis was first noted around 3 years of age and continues to present. The patient also has a small umbilical hernia.

The patient's family history is not significant for chromosome abnormalities, developmental delay, or intellectual disability. She has six maternal half-siblings who all reportedly have ADD and several paternal half-siblings who have no known medical or developmental concerns and are not available for testing. She has no full siblings. She is of African American and Northern European descent.

SNP microarray was performed by Integrated Genetics using the Affymetrix Cytoscan HD platform, using 743,000 SNP probes and 1,953,000 NPCN probes. A 9.22 Mb interstitial deletion of 7q33-7q35 was identified, arr 7q33-q35 (133,297,307–143,218,955) × 1.

3. Discussion

Table 1 reports on the clinical features of other patients with 7q interstitial deletions overlapping the same region as our patient. Malmgren et al. reported on a family with an interchromosomal insertion of 7q33-q34 into 6p25, resulting in some family members who were balanced carriers giving rise to three offspring with a 7q33-q34 deletion of 7.6 Mb [3]. All three individuals with the deletion are reported to have intellectual disability, a long philtrum, a thin upper lip, a bulbous nose, a large mouth, and hypertelorism, as does our patient. Two of those three patients described by Malmgren had ear abnormalities and recurrent infections, and two patients had growth retardation or short stature. As shown in Table 1, these features have also been reported in other patients with interstitial deletions of varying sizes between 7q31-7q35. Our patient's facial appearance is quite similar to the patients described by Malmgren, particularly individuals IV: 6 and III: 3.

In addition to the features described in previous patients, our patient presents with additional findings of sleep apnea and insomnia, type 2 diabetes, obesity, echogenic liver, frequent menstruation, aggressive and self-mutilating behaviors, and her most recent concern of hemihypertrophy. Currently it is unclear which of these features can be explained by the patient's deletion. However, Rossi et al. describe a patient with a 7q33-q35 deletion who also presents with obesity and sleep disturbances, as well as mood shifts [4].

The patients currently reported with interstitial 7q deletions show some phenotypic differences from patients with 7q34-ter or 7q35-ter deletions. Holoprosencephaly and Currarino triad have been reported in terminal deletions [5]; these conditions are attributed to the loss of *MNX1* and *SHH*. Additional features reported in 7q terminal deletions include microcephaly, cleft lip and palate, large ears, abnormal genitalia, and cardiac anomalies [6]. However, patients with both interstitial and terminal deletions in this region have had intellectual disability, similar dysmorphic facial features, and growth abnormalities [6, 7].

TABLE 1: Clinical features of individuals with interstitial 7q33-q35 deletions.

Patient demographics	Present case	Malmgren et al. [3] IV:6	Malmgren et al. [3] III:1	Malmgren et al. [3] III:3	Nielsen et al. [10] III:11	Nielsen et al. [10] III:10	Nielsen et al. [10] III:8	Stallard and Juberg [2]	Verma et al. [11]	Petrin et al. [8]	Rossi et al. [4]	Fagan et al. [12]
Patient												
Deletion region	q33-q34	q33-q34	q33-q34	q33-q34	q32-q34	q32-q34	q32q34	q31-q34	q33-q35	q33-q35	q33-q35	q35
Gender/age	F/15	M/15	M/40	F/25	F/6	M/6	F/13.5	F/1	F/4	M/22	F/adult	F/11
Neurological/development												
Intellectual disability	+	−	+	+	+	+	+	NA	+	−	+	+
Developmental delay	+	+	+	+	+	+		+	+	+	+	+
Speech delay/disorder	+	+						NA	+	+	+	+
Abnormal brain MRI	+	+						+		+	+	
Mood shifts	+										+	
Self-mutilating behaviors	+											
Seizures	+						+		+		+	
Sleep difficulty	+										+	
Diparesis/truncal ataxia											+	
Craniofacial												
Microcephaly								+	+			
Hypertelorism	+	+	+	+	+	+	+	+	+		+	+
Epicanthal folds	+	+					+	+				
Broad/depressed nasal bridge	+	+	+	+	+	+	+	+		+	+	+
Bulbous nose	+	+	+	+	+	+	+				+	
Large mouth	+	+	+	+	+	+	+				+	
Long philtrum	+	+	+	+	+	+						
Thin upper lip	+	+			+	+		+				
Micrognathia	+	+										
Low set ears/ear	+	+	+		+	+		+			+	+
Preauricular ear pits	+											+
Growth												
Slow growth/short stature	+	−	+	+	−	+	+	+	−		+	
Truncal obesity	+											
Hemihypertrophy	+											
Hand and feet differences		+					+			+	+	
Other												
Ophthalmologic abnormality	+						+		−			
Hearing deficit	+	+							+	−		
Repeated infections	+	+						+	+			
Primary amenorrhea	−	N/A	N/A			N/A	N/A			N/A	+	
Frequent menses	+	N/A	N/A							N/A	+	
Umbilical hernia	+										−	

Rush et al. recently reported on a patient with a 7q34-q36.1 interstitial deletion and reviewed patients with similar deletions in overlapping q34-q36 regions [7]. Although this is a slightly different location than our patient's, these patients also show some phenotypic overlap with our case and others with q32-q35 deletions, including facial characteristics such as bulbous nasal tip and broad nasal root, intellectual disability, impulsive behavior, hearing loss, and seizures. The shared phenotypic characteristic of these bordering deleted segments may help further narrow down the 7q34-q35 region as the responsible area for these shared features.

There are 64 OMIM-described genes known to be located in the particular area of 7q deleted in our patient (Table 2). None of these genes are known to be imprinted. Like the patients previously described with similar deletions, our patient's deleted region includes the genes *CNOT4*, *MTPN*, *CHRM2*, and *PTN*, which are of special interest given their involvement in nervous system development [3, 8]. Deletions of these genes could cause differences in nervous system development that could explain the intellectual disability and behavioral concerns seen in our patient and individuals with similar 7q deletions. Several deleted genes have also been implicated in autosomal dominant movement disorders including *CLCN1* (Thomson dominant myotonia) and *DHMN1* (distal hereditary motor neuronopathy). While our patient does not carry a label of either of these diagnoses, she does have increasing difficulty with walking and movement.

The gene *TBXAS1*, which encodes thromboxane synthase involved in platelet aggregation and clotting, may be of interest given that our patient has two menstrual cycles a month, and two other patients with deletions spanning the 7q33 to 7q36 region have had the opposite phenotype of primary amenorrhea [4, 9]. However, while homozygous and compound heterozygous mutations are known to cause Ghosal hematodiaphyseal syndrome, the significance of haploinsufficiency is unclear. The patient also has several deleted genes that encode the T-cell receptor beta chain, and while interesting given her immunological concerns, no phenotype has been reported with alterations to these genes to date.

Mutations in *BRAF* have been associated with RASopathies, most commonly cardiofaciocutaneous syndrome (CFC) but also Noonan and LEOPARD syndrome. Mutations causing these syndromes lead to activation of the RAS-MAPK pathway. *BRAF* haploinsufficiency is not expected to be a causative mechanism of CFC; however it is interesting to note that our patient's course facial features overlap with many course facial features of CFC, including bulbous nasal tip and depressed nasal bridge, hypertelorism, downslanting palpebral fissures, and prominent philtrum.

OTCS2 has been implicated in otosclerosis, resulting in conductive hearing loss, which is of interest given our patient's history of conductive hearing loss and hearing loss seen in other patients with similar deletions. Other genes in the deleted region have shown associations with other diseases not currently seen in our patient, including *HIPK2* with leukemia, *ATP6V0A4* with renal tubular acidosis, *TRIM24* with papillary thyroid carcinoma, *PRSS1* with pancreatitis, and *GPDS1* with glaucoma and optic nerve degeneration.

TABLE 2: Known deleted genes in 7q33-q35 region in OMIM.

Known deleted genes in OMIM		
AGK	HIPK2	TAS2R3
AKR1B1	KEL	TAS2R4
AKR1B10	KIAA1549	TAS2R5
AKR1D1	LUC7L2	TAS2R38
ATP6V0A4	LUZP6	TAS2R40
BPGM	MGAM	TAS2R41
BRAF	MTPN	TAS2R60
CALD1	MRPS33	TBXAS1
CASP2	NUP205	TRIM24
CHRM2	OTSC2	TRBC1
CLCN1	PARP12	TRBC2
CLEC5A	PIP	TRBD1
CNOT4	PTN	TRBD2
CREB3L2	PRSS1	TRBJ@
D7S437	PRSS2	TRBV@
DFNB13	SLC13A4	TRPV5
DGKI	SLC35B4	TRPV6
DHMN1	SLI4	UBN2
EPHA1	SSBP1	WEE2
EPHB6	STRA8	ZC3HAV1
GPDS1	SVOPL	ZYX
GSTK1		

4. Conclusion

The patient presented exhibits similar features to other individuals with similar deletions, particularly intellectual disability and similar dysmorphic facial features, further helping to characterize a 7q interstitial deletion syndrome encompassing the q33-q35 region. This patient also exhibits unique features including recent onset of hemihypertrophy, frequent menses, and self-mutilation behaviors. There are many known genes in this region that play important roles in brain development and organ function whose haploinsufficiency could contribute to the features seen in our patient and others with similar deletions.

Ethical Approval

This report was approved by the Santa Clara Valley Medical Center Institutional Review Board.

Conflict of Interests

The authors declare that there is no conflict of interests regarding the publication of this paper.

Acknowledgment

The authors would like to thank the patient and her family for their contribution to this report.

References

[1] E. L. Harris, R. S. Wappner, C. G. Palmer et al., "7q deletion syndrome (7q32 → 7qter)," *Clinical Genetics*, vol. 12, no. 4, pp. 233–238, 1977.

[2] R. Stallard and R. C. Juberg, "Partial monosomy 7q syndrome due to distal interstitial deletion," *Human Genetics*, vol. 57, no. 2, pp. 210–213, 1981.

[3] H. Malmgren, G. Malm, S. Sahlén, M. Karlsson, and E. Blennow, "Molecular cytogenetic characterization of an insertional translocation, ins(6;7)(p25;q33q34): deletion/duplication of 7q33-34 and clinical correlations," *The American Journal of Medical Genetics*, vol. 139, no. 1, pp. 25–31, 2005.

[4] E. Rossi, A. P. Verri, M. G. Patricelli et al., "A 12 Mb deletion at 7q33-q35 associated with autism spectrum disorders and primary amenorrhea," *European Journal of Medical Genetics*, vol. 51, no. 6, pp. 631–638, 2008.

[5] M. Masuno, K. Imaizumi, N. Aida et al., "Currarino triad with a terminal deletion 7q35 → qter," *Journal of Medical Genetics*, vol. 33, no. 10, pp. 877–878, 1996.

[6] C.-P. Chen, S.-R. Chern, T.-Y. Chang et al., "Prenatal diagnosis of *de novo* terminal deletion of chromosome 7q," *Prenatal Diagnosis*, vol. 23, no. 5, pp. 375–379, 2003.

[7] E. T. Rush, J. M. Stevens, W. G. Sanger, and A. H. Olney, "Report of a patient with developmental delay, hearing loss, growth retardation, and cleft lip and palate and a deletion of 7q34-36.1: review of distal 7q deletions," *The American Journal of Medical Genetics, Part A*, vol. 161, no. 7, pp. 1726–1732, 2013.

[8] A. L. Petrin, C. M. Giacheti, L. P. Maximino et al., "Identification of a microdeletion at the 7q33-q35 disrupting the CNTNAP2 gene in a Brazilian stuttering case," *American Journal of Medical Genetics, Part A*, vol. 152, no. 12, pp. 3164–3172, 2010.

[9] L. T. Sehested, R. S. Møller, I. Bache et al., "Deletion of 7q34-q36.2 in two siblings with mental retardation, language delay, primary amenorrhea, and dysmorphic features," *The American Journal of Medical Genetics. Part A*, vol. 152, no. 12, pp. 3115–3119, 2010.

[10] K. B. Nielsen, F. Egede, I. Mouridsen, and J. Mohr, "Familial partial 7q monosomy resulting from segregation of an insertional chromosome rearrangement," *Journal of Medical Genetics*, vol. 16, no. 6, pp. 461–466, 1979.

[11] R. S. Verma, R. A. Conte, S. E. Sayegh, and D. Kanjilal, "The interstitial deletion of bands q33-q35 of long arm of chromosome 7: a review with a new case report," *Clinical Genetics*, vol. 41, pp. 82–86, 1992.

[12] K. Fagan, C. Kennedy, L. Roddick, and A. Colley, "An interstitial deletion of chromosome 7(q35)," *Journal of Medical Genetics*, vol. 31, no. 9, pp. 738–739, 1994.

Case of 7p22.1 Microduplication Detected by Whole Genome Microarray (REVEAL) in Workup of Child Diagnosed with Autism

Veronica Goitia,[1] **Marcial Oquendo,**[1] **and Robert Stratton**[2]

[1]*Department of Pediatrics, Driscoll Children's Hospital, Corpus Christi, TX 78411, USA*
[2]*Department of Medical Genetics, Driscoll Children's Hospital, Corpus Christi, TX 78411, USA*

Correspondence should be addressed to Veronica Goitia; veronica.goitia@dchstx.org

Academic Editor: Mohnish Suri

Introduction. More than 60 cases of 7p22 duplications and deletions have been reported with over 16 of them occurring without concomitant chromosomal abnormalities. *Patient and Methods.* We report a 29-month-old male diagnosed with autism. Whole genome chromosome SNP microarray (REVEAL) demonstrated a 1.3 Mb interstitial duplication of 7p22.1 ->p22.1 arr 7p22.1 (5,436,367–6,762,394), the second smallest interstitial 7p duplication reported to date. This interval included 14 OMIM annotated genes (*FBXL18, ACTB, FSCN1, RNF216, OCM, EIF2AK1, AIMP2, PMS2, CYTH3, RAC1, DAGLB, KDELR2, GRID2IP, and ZNF12*). *Results.* Our patient presented features similar to previously reported cases with 7p22 duplication, including brachycephaly, prominent ears, cryptorchidism, speech delay, poor eye contact, and outburst of aggressive behavior with autism-like features. Among the genes located in the duplicated segment, *ACTB* gene has been proposed as a candidate gene for the alteration of craniofacial development. Overexpression of *RNF216L* has been linked to autism. *FSCN1* may play a role in neurodevelopmental disease. *Conclusion.* Characterization of a possible 7p22.1 Duplication Syndrome has yet to be made. Recognition of the clinical spectrum in patients with a smaller duplication of 7p should prove valuable for determining the minimal critical region, helping delineate a better prediction of outcome and genetic counseling

1. Introduction

More than 60 cases of 7p22 duplications and deletions have been reported in [1] with over 16 of them occurring without concomitant chromosomal abnormalities [2]. Several cases of de novo 7p duplications have been reported in recent years [2–4]; however, familial cases due to malsegregation of a parental balanced translocation or abnormal recombination caused by a parental inversion seem to be the most common cause of 7p duplications [5, 6]. These patients often include findings such as developmental delay, intellectual disability, behavioral problems, abnormal speech development, autism spectrum disorder (ASD), hypotonia, craniofacial dysmorphism with large anterior fontanel, broad forehead, hypertelorism, downslanting palpebral fissures, low-set and/or malformed ears, abnormal palate, micrognathia and/or retrognathia, pegged teeth, abnormal palmar creases, broad thumbs, cardiovascular abnormalities, skeletal abnormalities, joint dislocations and/or contractures, and undescended testes [1, 2, 4, 7, 8].

Recently, translocations in the 7p22 region were proposed as a candidate for autism [9]. A case of a boy diagnosed with autism, no dysmorphic features, and a de novo balanced translocation 46, XY,t(7;16)(p22.1;p11.2) suggests that overexpression of gene *RNF216* (localized to 7p22.1 by the Mammalian Gene Collection) resulting in abnormalities in E3 ubiquitin ligase may be linked to autism as well as other developmental and psychiatric conditions [9, 10].

We report a 29-month-old patient, recently diagnosed by his pediatrician with autism spectrum disorder, who was sent for genetic evaluation. He was found to have significant speech delay, poor eye contact, and several facial anomalies including brachycephaly and prominent ears. Whole genome microarray demonstrated a 1.3 Mb interstitial duplication of 7p22.1, the second smallest interstitial 7p duplication reported in the literature to date.

2. Clinical Report

The patient was a 29-month-old Hispanic male, referred for evaluation of developmental delay. The patient was born at 39 weeks gestation by normal spontaneous vaginal delivery after an uncomplicated pregnancy; birth weight was 3.528 (51–75th centile), head circumference was 34.3 cm (26–50th centile), and length was 52.1 cm (51–75th centile). At birth physical exam he was noted to have wide-spaced eyes, febrile, coarse, and decreased breath sounds, tachypnea, subcostal retractions, umbilical hernia, right undescended testes, and rocker bottom feet as per medical record. The patient was transferred to neonatal intensive care unit (NICU) for progressive respiratory distress and suspected sepsis and was placed on high flow nasal cannula and antibiotic therapy. Karyotype done 46XY. Patient has no siblings and parents were nonconsanguineous. Family history was remarkable for maternal grandmother having three miscarriages.

Echocardiogram at birth showed a large patent ductus arteriosus (PDA) (4 mm) with left to right shunt, mild tricuspid regurgitation (PG 33 mmHg), and patent foramen ovale (3 mm) with left to right shunt, no coarctation of the aorta, otherwise normal. Repeat echocardiogram on day 18 of life showed no PDA and showed mild tricuspid regurgitation (PSG 29 mHg) revealing mildly elevated pulmonary systolic pressure, otherwise normal. Other testing in medical record consist of X-ray of right foot with no congenital abnormality appreciated, unremarkable renal ultrasound, head ultrasound negative for IVH and testicular US that showed right testicle located at right external inguinal ring.

The review of systems was positive for brachycephaly, no eye contact, rolling his head side to side before going to sleep, unilateral right cryptorchidism, feet deformity which resolved spontaneously, and developmental delay. The patient walked at 16 months of age and did not use any words and did not point for what he wanted. Though diagnosed with ASD, no typical ritualistic behaviors were described. Despite not being able to speak, he attempted to communicate with family.

On physical exam, weight was 15.8 kg (90–95th centile) and OFC was 49 cm (50th centile). The head was brachycephalic and the anterior fontanel was closed. Hair was straight and black and of normal distribution and density. There were two posterior whorls and bifrontal upsweeps with a widow's peak. The palpebral fissures were horizontal, inner canthal distance was 31 mm (90th centile), and lower face was prominent. Nasal width was 31 mm (90–95th centile). His mouth was 50 mm (90–95th centile) wide with normal vermillion. Both ears measured 62 mm (90–95th centile), the right ear protruded more than the left ear, and both have a flat posterior helix (Figure 1). Right testicle was not palpable in scrotum. The right distal palmar crease extends to the 2-3 interspace with a small bridged proximal crease. The left palmar creases bridged to form one (Figure 2). There was dorsally placed second toes and flat arches; the toenails were

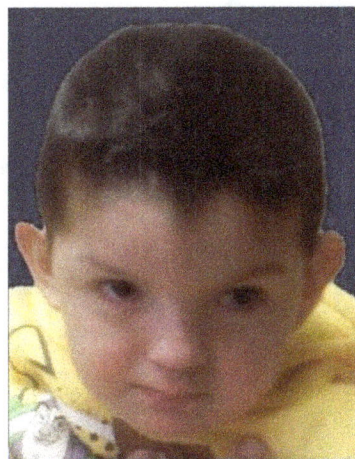

(a)

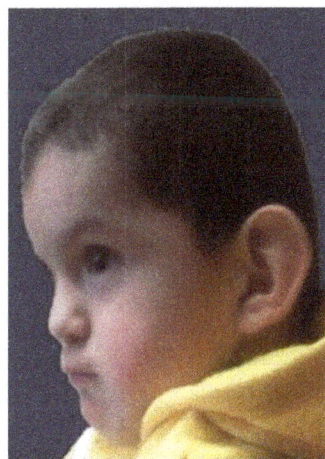

(b)

FIGURE 1: Phenotypic facial features of our patient at the first evaluation in the Driscoll Children's Hospital McAllen Genetics Clinic at 29 months of age. Notable findings include brachycephaly, inner canthal distance of 31 mm (90th centile for age), and prominent lower face and right ear protruded more than left ear.

convex. The patient cooperated poorly with examiner and muscle tone was difficult to assess.

Genetic testing included a fragile X PCR DNA analysis, with 31 CGG repeats. Whole genome chromosome SNP microarray (REVEAL) analysis showed a 1.326 Mb interstitial duplication of 7p22.1 >p22.1 arr 7p22.1 (5,436,367–6,762,394) × 3. This interval includes 14 OMIM annotated genes (*FBXL18, ACTB, FSCN1, RNF216, OCM, EIF2 K1, AIMP2, PMS2, CYTH3, RAC1, DAGLB, KDELR2, GRID2IP, and ZNF12*) (Figure 3). Test was interpreted as "possible familial variant" per report.

A duplication variant at Xp22.31 (6,455,151 to 8,135,644) × 2 was also detected. Although deletion of this region spanning the STS gene is associated with ichthyosis in males, familial passage of duplications of this region to normal males has been well documented. Females are unaffected by either deletion or duplication. No extended contiguous regions

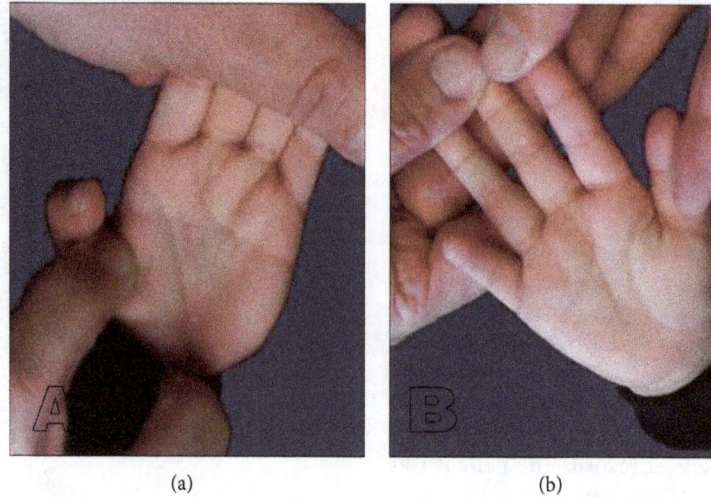

(a)   (b)

FIGURE 2: Palmar features. (a) The left palmar creases bridged to form one and distal extends to 2-3 interspace. (b) The right distal palmar crease extends to the 2-3 interspace.

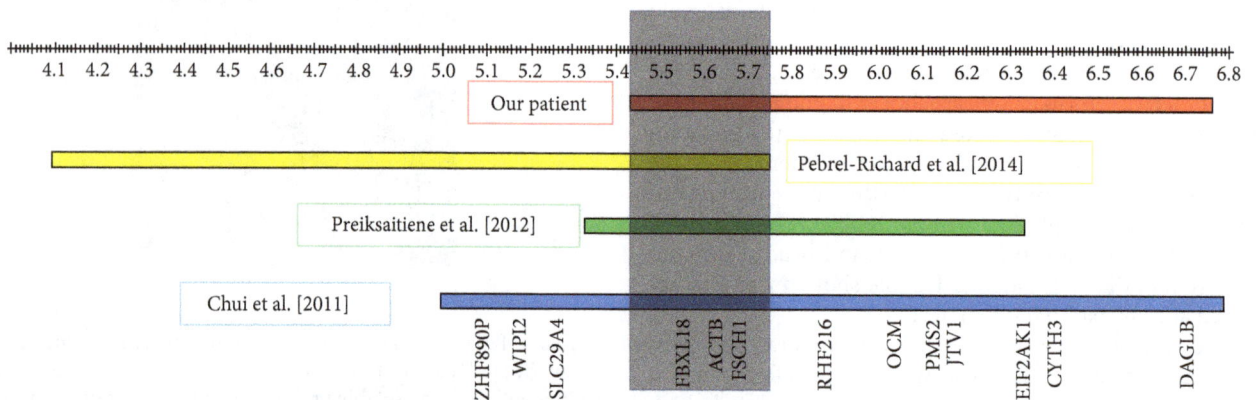

FIGURE 3: Graphic representation of chromosome 7 with array CGH results Arr 7p22.1 (5,436,367–6,762,394) × 3 in our patient as well as in the patients reported by Chui et al. [4], Preiksaitiene et al. [1], and Pebrel-Richard et al. [11].

of homozygotic alleles associated with UPD (single chromosome) or consanguinity (multiple chromosomes) were observed.

Because both anomalies were considered "normal variants," parental samples were not able to be studied due to healthcare insurance refusing to cover genetic testing at this time.

The patient continued to follow up in the Genetic Clinics at Driscoll Children's Hospital. He was subsequently placed on Guanfacine by his pediatrician for aggressive behavior and outbursts of screaming and walking out of the house during a tantrum. During his last visit in 2013, the patient was 3 years and 9 months old and had a 6-single-word vocabulary. Though still diagnosed with ASD, no typical ritualistic behavior was described by parents and despite his speech delay, he attempted to communicate with family through gestures. During examination, he would at times establish eye contact and share his toy truck with examiner.

3. Discussion

Chui et al. [4] reported a case of a 28-month-old Hispanic male with features of a 7p21 duplication syndrome that included developmental and speech delay and craniofacial abnormalities similar to our patient, such as prominent forehead and hypertelorism, as well as cryptorchidism and bridged palmar creases; other abnormalities not seen in our patient included anteverted nares and anterior fontanel closure delay. The duplication was 1.7 Mb in size and located at 7p22.1 region (arr7 p22.1 (5,092,748–6797,449) × 3 (hg18)). Preiksaitiene et al. [1] reported a case of a 14.5-year-old female

TABLE 1: Comparison of patients with 7p22.1 patients*.

	Chui et al. [4]	Preiksaitiene et al. [1]	Pebrel-Richard et a.. [11]	Our patient
Duplication region	7p22.1 (5,092,748–6,797,449) 1.7 Mb in size.	7p22.1 (5,337,072–6,316,915) 1 Mb in size.	7p22.1 (4,207,513–5,766,245) 1.5 Mb in size.	7p22.1 (5,436,367–6,762,394) 1.3 Mb in size.
Facial characteristics	Open anterior fontanel (20 mm), frontal bossing with a flat, broad, nasal bridge, anteverted nares, ocular hypertelorism, low-set and posteriorly rotated ears with a left preauricular pit, and wide-spaced and pegged teeth.	Low-set and protruding ears, downslanting palpebral fissures, ocular hypertelorism, short nose, anteverted nares, midface hypoplasia, facial asymmetry, severe microretrognathia, high and narrow palate, microstomia, thin vermilion of the lips, and midline pseudocleft upper lip.	Prominent forehead, widely spaced eyes, high-arched eyebrows, downslanted palpebral fissures, anteverted nares, large mouth with thin vermilion, and low-set and small ears with narrow external auditory canals.	Brachycephaly, hypertelorism, prominent lower face, and right ear protruded more than left ear.
Presence of developmental delay	Speech delay. No intelligible words at 33 months.	Difficulty in walking and spastic diplegic cerebral palsy. No mention of verbal abilities.	Few words at 3 years of age. Expressive language impairment was apparently more severe than was receptive language. Could not jump or run and showed slow execution of movements and drawing difficulties.	Poor eye contact and speech delay. Diagnosed with autism spectrum disorder.
Other malformations	Mild kyphosis, bilateral bridged palmar creases, broad thumbs, and an undescended left testis.	Tapering fingers, abnormal palmar dermatoglyphic patterns, contractures of the Achilles tendons, scoliosis, short 5th toes.	Undescended testes, joint hypermobility, and flat arches of feet. Gait was unstable.	Undescended right testicle. The right distal palmar crease extends to the 2-3 interspace with a small bridged proximal crease. The left palmar creases bridged to form one.
Other tests	Normal head UA, normal thyroid function, bone age of left wrist of 16 months at 24 months; echocardiogram: small patent foramen ovale versus a small and hemodynamically insignificant secundum atrial septal defect (ASD); head CT: asymmetry of the anterior fontanel and slight prominence of the right frontal and left occipital bones with no hydrocephalus.	EEG showed diffuse changes in brain electrical activity and increased stimulation in deep brain structures, predominantly in frontal, temporal, and parietal regions. A CT scan of the brain was remarkable for moderate internal hydrocephalus. Electrocardiogram showed signs of vegetodystonia.	Cranial MRI confirmed suspected moderate hydrocephalus and showed a small corpus callosum. Echoencephalogram showed no abnormalities. Ophthalmic examination identified hypermetropia and astigmatism. Hematological, endocrinology, and metabolic tests were normal. Normal thyroid function.	Echocardiogram at birth: large patent ductus arteriosus (PDA) with left to right shunt, mild tricuspid regurgitation, and patent foramen ovale with left to right shunt. Right testicle located at right external inguinal ring on US. Normal head and renal US.

* In previously reported cases of 7p22.1 duplication has arisen de novo. In our patient, parental testing was not available.

with a smaller size duplication, a 979.8 Kb located at 7p22.1 region (position 5,337,072–6,316,915 × 3), who had developmental and speech delay, low-set and protruding ears, slanting down palpebral fissures, ocular hypertelorism, midface hypoplasia, microretrognathia, tapering fingers, abnormal palmar dermatoglyphic patterns, and short 5th toes. In both cases, it was found that the duplication was absent in the parents and therefore occurred *de novo*. The duplication in our patient does overlap completely with the patient reported by Chui et al. [4] and partially with the patient reported by Preiksaitiene et al. [1].

A more recent article by Pebrel-Richard et al. [11] presented a 3-year-old boy with a 1,559 Mb microduplication (4,207,513 Mb–5,766,245 Mb) located at the 7p22.2p22.1 region. Their patient presented with psychomotor developmental delay and unusual facial features. He had expressive and receptive language impairment. Physical examination showed prominent forehead, widely spaced eyes, high-arched eyebrows, downslanted palpebral fissures, anteverted nares, large mouth with thin vermilion, and low-set and small ears with narrow external auditory canals, as well as undescended testes, joint hypermobility, and flat arches of feet [11]. Authors attempt to refine a critical region by describing a 430 Kb region of overlap between their patient and Bousman et al. [12]. Our patient further refines this section to 330 Kb region, between 5,436,367 and 5,766,245, which encompasses four RefSeq genes: *FBXL18, ACTB, FSCN1, and RNF216*, where only *RNF216* (OMIM 6609948) and *ACTB* (OMIM 102630) are known to cause diseases in humans (Figure 3).

Papadopoulou et al. [2] and Zahed et al. [3] presented a list of abnormalities described in the literature as an attempt to establish a phenotype or clinical spectrum in patients with 7p duplication. Among these abnormalities, there were described craniofacial dysmorphism, brachycephaly, macrognathia, cryptorchid testes, mental retardation, and one case of autism. Our patient's previous medical records did not include information regarding delayed closure/large fontanels, often described as a common physical finding in reported cases of 7p duplications. When comparing the cases described by Chui et al., Preiksaitiene et al., and Pebrel-Richard et al. with ours, our patient presented many significant similarities but only some of the craniofacial dysmorphic features (Table 1), even though a significant overlap of genes exists when compared to their reported cases, including the *ACTB* gene which has been proposed as a strong candidate gene for the alteration of craniofacial development [1]. This could be due to incomplete penetrance and/or variable expressivity of microduplications/deletions of the same region with resulting different clinical phenotypes [11].

Due to microarray testing of patients with intellectual disability and/or congenital anomalies becoming readily available, there are stronger links between 7p microduplications and developmental disorders, such as autism, speech delay, and mental retardation. The role of other genes in this region such as *RNF216L (Q6NUR6)*, which encodes an E3 ubiquitin-protein ligase and is expressed in a variety of human tissues (brain) at all developmental stages [9], is associated with protein quality control as well as regulation of transcription factors such as p53 and androgen receptors [12]. Ubiquitin-ligase complexes have been linked to a number of psychiatric diseases such as bipolar disorder and schizophrenia, as well as developmental disorders including autism (with higher blood levels of E3 ubiquitin in comparison to controls), intellectual disability, Angelman syndrome, and recessive juvenile Parkinson's disease [9]. The *ACTB* gene, encoding b-actin, an essential component of the cytoskeleton, as mentioned before has been suggested as a candidate gene for craniofacial dysmorphism associated with 7p22.1 duplication.

FSCN1, which codes for fascin, a protein involved in nerve growth and development, is expressed in mature dendritic cells, epithelial cells, glia, and neurons and plays a critical role in dendritic cell functions and with the accurate establishment of neuronal circuits [13, 14]. Studies on prenatally stressed rats, characterized by an anxious/depressive phenotype associated with neuroadaptive changes in the hippocampus, showed significant changes in the expression of this protein, which may be related to early life stress triggered developmental programming [15]. Similarly, studies have correlated the reduction in dendritic arborizations with intellectual disability, showing a decreased neuronal size and a major cell packing density in patients with a defined neurological disorder. Dendritic abnormalities could lead to a cognitive deficit by reducing the synaptic density or by arresting the synaptic development [15]. Furthermore, microarray assays revealed a significant downexpression of the FSCN1 gene in CREB binding protein-depleted cells found in Rubinstein–Taybi syndrome that is characterized by intellectual disability and growth restriction, multiple congenital malformations such as broad thumbs and big toes, heart defects, cryptorchidism, and increased tumor risk [16]; some of these features are also present in 7p22 patients.

Further investigation is needed in order to determine the relation between these genes which are poorly understood and the characterization of a 7p22.1 duplication syndrome. Recognition of the clinical spectrum in patients with a smaller duplication of 7p should prove valuable for determining the minimal critical region, helping delineate a better prediction of outcome and genetic counselling in patients with duplications in this region [3].

Conflict of Interests

The authors declare that there is no conflict of interests regarding the publication of this paper.

References

[1] E. Preiksaitiene, J. Kasnauskiene, Z. Ciuladaite, B. Tumiene, P. C. Patsalis, and V. Kučinskas, "Clinical and molecular characterization of a second case of 7p22.1 microduplication," *American Journal of Medical Genetics, Part A*, vol. 158, no. 5, pp. 1200–1203, 2012.

[2] E. Papadopoulou, S. Sifakis, C. Sarri et al., "A report of pure 7p duplication syndrome and review of the literature," *The American Journal of Medical Genetics Part A*, vol. 140, no. 24, pp. 2802–2806, 2006.

[3] L. Zahed, T. Pramparo, C. Farra, M. Mikati, and O. Zuffardi, "A patient with duplication (7)(p22.1pter) characterized by array-CGH," *American Journal of Medical Genetics, Part A*, vol. 143, no. 2, pp. 168–171, 2007.

[4] J. V. Chui, J. D. Weisfeld-Adams, J. Tepperberg, and L. Mehta, "Clinical and molecular characterization of chromosome 7p22.1 microduplication detected by array CGH," *American Journal of Medical Genetics, Part A*, vol. 155, no. 10, pp. 2508–2511, 2011.

[5] O. Reish, S. A. Berry, G. Dewald, and R. A. King, "Duplication of 7p: further delineation of the phenotype and restriction of the critical region to the distal part of the short arm," *The American Journal of Medical Genetics*, vol. 61, no. 1, pp. 21–25, 1996.

[6] T. Cai, P. Yu, D. A. Tagle, and J. Xia, "Duplication of 7p21.2 → pter due to maternal 7p;21q translocation: implications for critical segment assignment in the 7p duplication syndrome," *American Journal of Medical Genetics*, vol. 86, no. 4, pp. 305–311, 1999.

[7] C. Kozma, B. R. Haddad, and J. M. Meck, "Trisomy 7p resulting from 7p15;9p24 translocation: report of a new case and review of associated medical complications," *American Journal of Medical Genetics*, vol. 91, no. 4, pp. 286–290, 2000.

[8] A. Mégarbané, M. Le Lorc'h, H. Elghezal et al., "Pure partial 7p trisomy including the TWIST, HOXA, and GLI3 genes," *Journal of Medical Genetics*, vol. 38, no. 3, pp. 178–182, 2001.

[9] R. M'Rad, N. Bayou, A. Belhadj et al., "Exploring the 7p22.1 chromosome as a candidate region for autism," *Journal of Biomedicine and Biotechnology*, vol. 2010, Article ID 423894, 4 pages, 2010.

[10] S. Y. Lee, J. Ramirez, M. Franco et al., "Ube3a, the E3 ubiquitin ligase causing Angelman syndrome and linked to autism, regulates protein homeostasis through the proteasomal shuttle Rpn10," *Cellular and Molecular Life Sciences*, vol. 71, no. 14, pp. 2747–2758, 2014.

[11] C. Pebrel-Richard, C. Rouzade, S. Kemeny et al., "Refinement of the critical region in a new 7p22.1 microduplication syndrome including craniofacial dysmorphism and speech delay," *American Journal of Medical Genetics Part A*, vol. 164, no. 11, pp. 2964–2967, 2014.

[12] C. A. Bousman, G. Chana, S. J. Glatt et al., "Preliminary evidence of ubiquitin proteasome system dysregulation in schizophrenia and bipolar disorder: convergent pathway analysis findings from two independent samples," *The American Journal of Medical Genetics Part B: Neuropsychiatric Genetics*, vol. 153, no. 2, pp. 494–502, 2010.

[13] S. Yamashiro, "Functions of fascin in dendritic cells," *Critical Reviews in Immunology*, vol. 32, no. 1, pp. 11–22, 2012.

[14] J. Nagel, C. Delandre, Y. Zhang, F. Förstner, A. W. Moore, and G. Tavosanis, "Fascin controls neuronal class-specific dendrite arbor morphology," *Development*, vol. 139, no. 16, pp. 2999–3009, 2012.

[15] J. Mairesse, A. S. Vercoutter-Edouart, J. Marrocco et al., "Proteomic characterization in the hippocampus of prenatally stressed rats," *Journal of Proteomics*, vol. 75, no. 6, pp. 1764–1770, 2012.

[16] F. Megiorni, P. Indovina, B. Mora, and M. C. Mazzilli, "Minor expression of fascin-1 gene (FSCN1) in NTera2 cells depleted of CREB-binding protein," *Neuroscience Letters*, vol. 381, no. 1-2, pp. 169–174, 2005.

3

A Novel *PHEX* Mutation in Japanese Patients with X-Linked Hypophosphatemic Rickets

Tetsuya Kawahara,[1] **Hiromi Watanabe,**[2] **Risa Omae,**[3]
Toshiyuki Yamamoto,[4] **and Tetsuya Inazu**[3,5]

[1]*Division of Endocrinology and Metabolism, Department of Internal Medicine, Niigata Rosai Hospital, Niigata 9428502, Japan*
[2]*Department of Clinical Laboratory, Niigata National Hospital, Niigata 9458585, Japan*
[3]*Department of Pharmacy, College of Pharmaceutical Sciences, Ritsumeikan University, Shiga 5258577, Japan*
[4]*Tokyo Women's Medical University, Institute of Integrated Medical Sciences, Tokyo 1620054, Japan*
[5]*Department of Clinical Research, Saigata National Hospital, Niigata 9493193, Japan*

Correspondence should be addressed to Tetsuya Kawahara; k-tetsuy@med.uoeh-u.ac.jp and Tetsuya Inazu; tinazu@fc.ritsumei.ac.jp

Academic Editor: Mohnish Suri

X-linked hypophosphatemic rickets (XLH) is a dominant inherited disorder characterized by renal phosphate wasting, aberrant vitamin D metabolism, and abnormal bone mineralization. Inactivating mutations in the gene encoding phosphate-regulating gene with homologies to endopeptidases on the X chromosome (*PHEX*) have been found to be associated with XLH. Here, we report a 16-year-old female patient affected by hypophosphatemic rickets. We evaluated her serum fibroblast growth factor 23 (FGF23) levels and conducted sequence analysis of the disease-associated genes of FGF23-related hypophosphatemic rickets: *PHEX*, *FGF23*, dentin matrix protein 1, and ectonucleotide pyrophosphatase/phosphodiesterase 1. She was diagnosed with XLH based on her clinical features and family history. Additionally, we observed elevated FGF23 levels and a novel *PHEX* exon 9 mutation (c.947G>T; p.Gly316Val) inherited from her father. Although bioinformatics showed that the mutation was neutral, Gly316 is perfectly conserved among humans, mice, and rats, and there were no mutations in other FGF23-related rickets genes, suggesting that *in silico* analysis is limited in determining mutation pathogenicity. In summary, we present a female patient and her father with XLH harboring a novel *PHEX* mutation that appears to be causative of disease. Measurement of FGF23 for hypophosphatemic patients is therefore useful for the diagnosis of FGF23-dependent hypophosphatemia.

1. Introduction

X-linked hypophosphatemic rickets (XLH; OMIM number 307800) is the most common genetic disorder of renal phosphate wasting, with an approximate prevalence of 1 in 20,000 [1]. The clinical features of this X-linked dominant disease include short stature, bone pain, enthesopathy, and lower extremity deformities from rickets and osteomalacia. The disease is only partially corrected by treatment with high doses of phosphate and 1,25-dihydroxyvitamin D_3 (25-$(OH)_2D_3$) [2, 3].

XLH results from mutations in the phosphate-regulating gene with homologies to endopeptidases on the X chromosome (*PHEX*) [4]. Plasma concentrations of the phosphaturic hormone fibroblast growth factor 23 (FGF23)

are reported to be elevated in most affected individuals [5, 6]. Furthermore, FGF23 is overexpressed in the bone of the Hyp mouse, an animal model of XLH, suggesting that increased FGF23 expression is the likely cause of the clinical XLH phenotype [7]. Hypophosphatemic rickets and elevated serum FGF23 levels including XLH [6, 8], autosomal dominant hypophosphatemic rickets (ADHR) [6, 9], and autosomal recessive hypophosphatemic rickets 1 and 2 (ARHR1 [10, 11] and ARHR2 [12, 13]) are caused by mutations in *PHEX*, *FGF23*, dentin matrix protein 1 (*DMP1*), and ectonucleotide pyrophosphatase/phosphodiesterase 1 (*ENPP1*) genes, respectively.

The aim of this study was to investigate the etiology of patients with hypophosphatemic rickets who exhibited serum FGF23 elevation and harbored a novel *PHEX* mutation.

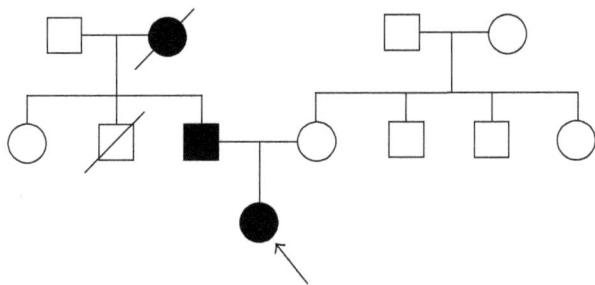

FIGURE 1: Family pedigree showing that the proband and her father have hypophosphatemic rickets and that the grandmother might have had the same disease. The death of the father's brother was unrelated to the disease. The remaining family members are healthy.

2. Case Presentation

The proband was a 16-year-old Japanese girl, born at full term with a normal delivery. Her father showed short stature (−2 SD smaller than the average height for male individuals of the same age) and had a history of treatment for short stature in childhood. Her grandmother (paternal side) also exhibited short stature; however, no detailed information was available because she died 10 years previously (Figure 1). At 3 years of age, the patient was evaluated for height retardation and slight mental retardation. She was diagnosed with hypophosphatemic rickets at 4 years of age based on her clinical features, such as short stature, dental abscess, osteopenia, genu valgum, and low serum phosphate levels. At this age, her height was 90 cm (−2.24 SD) and her weight was 17 kg (+0.9 SD). Treatment with 0.5–1.5 g/day of phosphate and 0.05–0.2 μg/kg/day of 1,25-(OH)$_2$D$_3$ was initiated to compensate for her lack of serum phosphate and vitamin D.

We measured the levels of serum minerals, FGF23, intact-parathyroid hormone (PTH), and kidney function of the patient and her parents using blood and urine samples. Ultrasound screening of the kidney was also conducted and X-rays were taken of the lower limbs. Serum FGF23 measurement was performed using the FGF-23 ELISA kit, which is a two-site enzyme-linked immunosorbent assay to measure full-length FGF23 (KAINOS Laboratories Inc., Tokyo, Japan), as described previously [6]. The institutional review board and the ethics committee of each organization approved the study. Informed written consent was obtained from all participants and volunteers.

Table 1 shows the mean laboratory data of the patient undergoing medical treatment, which included phosphate (P) 2.0 mg/dL (normal range, 3.0–4.5 mg/dL), calcium (Ca) 9.2 mg/dL (normal range, 8.7–10.2 mg/dL), alkaline phosphatase (ALP) 2374 IU/L (normal range, 100–325 IU/L), intact PTH 68.5 pg/mL (normal range, 12–72 pg/mL), 25-hydroxyvitamin D$_3$ (25-(OH)D$_3$) 11.0 ng/mL (normal range, 9.7–41.7 ng/mL), 1,25-(OH)$_2$D$_3$ 37.5 pg/mL (normal range, 20–60 pg/mL), and FGF23 400 pg/mL (normal range, 13.7–40.5 pg/mL). Urine P was 3.8 g/day (normal range, 0.4–1.2 g/day), the tubular maximum phosphate reabsorption per glomerular filtration rate was 2.1 mg/dL (normal range, 2.5–4.5 mg/dL), and the urine Ca/creatinine ratio was 0.09

(normal range, 0.05–0.25), which met the diagnostic criteria of XLH. FGF23 levels of the patient's father and mother were 68 and 29 pg/mL, respectively. Ultrasound showed normal kidney findings, while lower limb X-rays revealed a widening of the proximal tibial metaphysis with medial bowing.

To confirm the diagnosis, we conducted molecular studies, which included the direct sequencing analysis of PCR products. Genomic DNA was obtained and extracted from whole blood samples using the blood and cell genomic DNA extraction kit (Qiagen, Venlo, Netherlands). PCR amplified all 22 exons and exon-intron boundaries of PHEX and also all exons and exon-intron boundaries of FGF23, DMP1, and ENPP1 to exclude ADHR, ARHR1, and ARHR2, respectively, using previously described primer pairs [1, 11, 14, 15]. Additionally, for PHEX, we analyzed the approximately 2 kb promoter region upstream the start codon.

We identified a mutation in exon 9 (c.947G>T; p.Gly316Val) of PHEX in the patient (Figure 2(a)). Additionally, we sequenced PHEX from her parents and showed that the mutation was inherited from her father, who also exhibited short stature (Figure 2(a)). To determine the frequency of this mutation, we carried out restriction fragment length polymorphism analysis of genomic DNA from unrelated Japanese volunteers (100 were male and 100 were female; a total of 300 X chromosomes). DNA was amplified by PCR using primers on either side of the mutation in exon 9. Amplified products were digested using Acc I and separated on a 4% agarose gel. Digestion of the 233 bp fragment with Acc I would generate fragments of 177 plus 56 bp in the presence of the mutation (Figure 2(b)). This analysis showed that only one chromosome harbored the mutation (0.33%). We further analyzed the exons and exon-intron boundaries of FGF23, DMP-1, and ENPP1 and found no additional mutations.

When the PHEX mutation (Gly316Val) was identified, we conducted SIFT (http://sift.jcvi.org/) [16], PolyPhen-2 (http://genetics.bwh.harvard.edu/pph/) [17], and PROVEAN (http://provean.jcvi.org/index.php) [18] in online in silico analyses of Gly316 and Tyr317, which is an amino acid adjacent to Gly316. It was previously reported that the Tyr317Phe mutant protein exhibits 50–60% of PHEX activity [19]. SHIFT, PolyPhen-2, and PROVEN analyses predicted both variants (Gly316Val and Tyr317Phe) to be tolerated, benign, and neutral, respectively (data not shown). However, residues Gly316 and Tyr317 were shown to be perfectly conserved among humans, mice, and rats.

3. Discussion

The present study identified a novel heterozygous mutation in exon 9 (c. 947G>T; p.Gly316Val) of PHEX, which was inherited from the patient's father who exhibited short stature, so it appears to be etiological. The biochemical parameters of the female patient were more severe than those of her father, even though she had received treatment involving supplementary phosphate and 1,25-(OH)$_2$D$_3$. This could be explained by the required amount of phosphate decreasing with the reduction of the growth plate in her father, causing the symptoms of

---

TABLE 1: Laboratory data of the patient, her father, and her mother.

		Patient	Father	Mother
P	(3.0–4.5 mg/dL)	**2.0**	**2.9**	3.8
Ca	(8.7–10.2 mg/dL)	9.2	9.4	9.5
ALP	(100–325 IU/L)	**2347**	**1085**	320
Intact PTH	(12–72 pg/mL)	68.5	60.8	55.1
25-(OH)D$_3$	(9.7–41.7 ng/mL)	11.0	14.5	22.6
1,25-(OH)$_2$D$_3$	(20–60 pg/mL)	37.5	24.1	54.0
FGF23	(10–50 pg/mL)	**400**	**68**	29
TmP/GFR	(2.5–4.5 mg/dL)	**2.1**	2.8	4.4
Urine Ca/Cre ratio	(0.05–0.25)	0.09	0.08	0.11

Values within parentheses are the normal ranges of the variant.

P, phosphate; Ca, calcium; ALP, alkaline phosphatase; intact PTH, intact parathyroid hormone; 25-(OH)D$_3$, 25-hydroxyvitamin D$_3$; 1,25-dihydroxyvitamin D$_3$, 1,25-(OH)$_2$D$_3$; FGF23, fibroblast growth factor 23; TmP/GFR, tubular maximum phosphate reabsorption per glomerular filtration rate; urine Ca/Cre ratio, urine calcium/creatinine ratio.

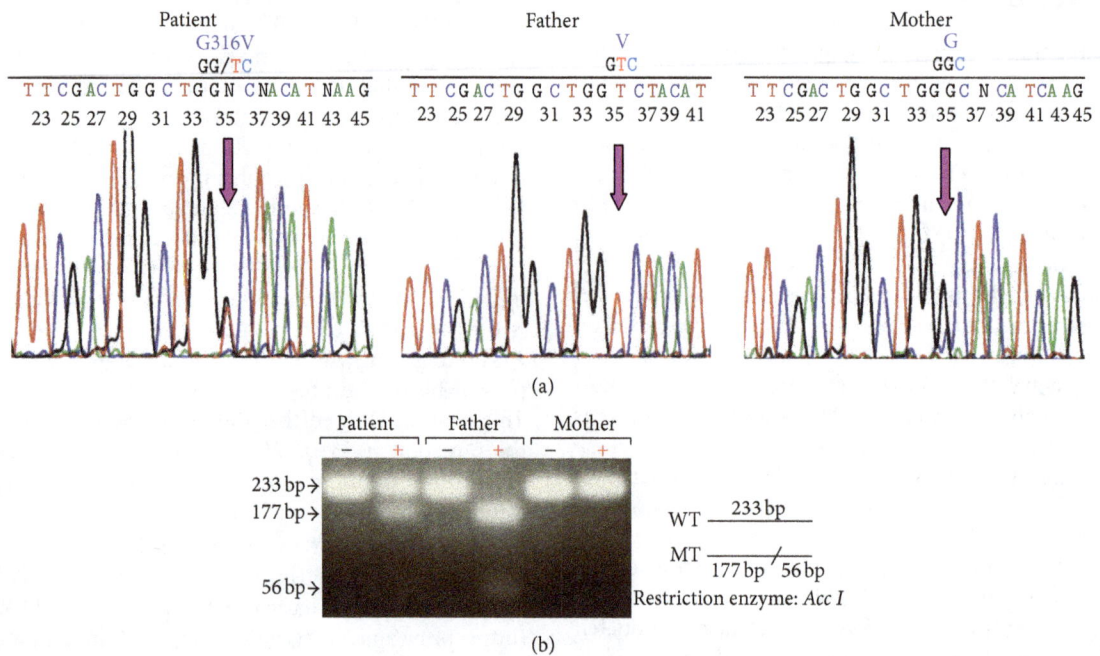

FIGURE 2: Mutation analyses. (a) *PHEX* mutation analysis in the patient's family. A missense mutation in exon 9 (c.947G>T; p.Gly316Val) of the patient was heterozygous. Her father, who exhibited short stature, carried the same mutation. Her mother has no mutation. (b) Restriction enzyme analysis. PCR products of *PHEX* exon 9 were digested with *Acc I* and separated on a 4% agarose gel. The wild-type PCR product (233 bp) lacks the restriction site, but the c.947G>T mutation introduces an *Acc I* site enabling the digestion of the product into 177 and 56 bp fragments. This analysis confirmed that the patient was heterozygous for the mutant and normal alleles and that her father also carried the mutant allele. The frequency of the mutation in 200 unrelated Japanese volunteers (100 were male and 100 were female; a total of 300 X chromosomes) was shown to be 0.33% (1/300).

rickets to improve by themselves, as previously shown in adults [20]. Alternatively, some patients who responded well to treatment were able to stop receiving medication after initial therapy [21]. Therefore, the patient's father may not show such severe symptoms of rickets as the patient herself.

We identified the frequency of the mutation as 1/300 (less than 1%) in the normal Japanese population, so it was not considered to be a single nucleotide polymorphism. Although the p.Gly316Val mutation did not show pathogenicity in *in silico* analysis, Gly316 is perfectly conserved among humans, mice, and rats, so it appears to be an indispensable amino acid. Similarly, the adjacent missense mutation of p.Tyr317Phe did not show pathogenicity in *in silico* analysis, and Try317 is also perfectly conserved among these same species. In addition, the Tyr317Phe mutant protein exhibits 50–60% of the endopeptidase activity of wild-type PHEX *in vitro*, indicating that this missense mutation interferes with catalytic function [19]. Therefore, *in silico* analysis is limited in its ability to determine whether a mutation shows pathogenicity. However, because we could not investigate whether the p.Gly316Val mutant protein interferes with catalytic function and influences its activity, it remains a possibility that the mutation does not show pathogenicity. Therefore, we performed mutational screening of the *PHEX* promoter region and other genes responsible for FGF23-related rickets; this analysis identified no mutations, so we concluded that the p.Gly316Val mutation is likely to be causative of XLH.

In this study, we used the KAINOS intact assay to measure serum FGF23 levels. This is the most sensitive of all FGF23 measurement assays, which also include the Immunotopics C-terminal assay and Immunotopics intact assay [22]. The absence of a lower limit for the reference range in the C-terminal assay (≤150 RU/mL) means that we cannot distinguish between this range and lower levels. However, the KAINOS intact assay has a reference range (10–50 pg/mL), and Endo et al. proposed that its measurement of serum FGF23 levels >30 pg/mL should typically be used as a diagnostic criterion for the presence of disease caused by excess FGF23 action, such as FGF23-dependent hypophosphatemia, irrespective of medical treatment [23]. The FGF23 levels of our patient and her father were 400 and 68 pg/mL, respectively, so the data also matched the criteria, which added weight to their usefulness. Further studies examining the function of the p.Gly316Val mutation are required to extend our findings.

Conflict of Interests

The authors declare that there is no conflict of interests regarding the publication of this paper.

Acknowledgment

The authors thank Ms. Saori Tsujimoto for her technical assistance.

References

[1] K. M. Roetzer, F. Varga, E. Zwettler et al., "Novel PHEX mutation associated with hypophosphatemic rickets," *Nephron: Physiology*, vol. 106, no. 1, pp. 8–12, 2007.

[2] R. V. Thakker and J. L. H. O'Riordan, "7 Inherited forms of rickets and osteomalacia," *Bailliere's Clinical Endocrinology and Metabolism*, vol. 2, no. 1, pp. 157–191, 1988.

[3] P. S. N. Rowe, "The role of the PHEX gene (PEX) in families with X-linked hypophosphataemic rickets," *Current Opinion in Nephrology and Hypertension*, vol. 7, no. 4, pp. 367–376, 1998.

[4] F. Francis, S. Hennig, B. Korn et al., "A gene (*PEX*) with homologies to endopeptidases is mutated in patients with X-linked hypophosphatemic rickets," *Nature Genetics*, vol. 11, pp. 130–136, 1995.

[5] K. B. Jonsson, R. Zahradnik, T. Larsson et al., "Fibroblast growth factor 23 in oncogenic osteomalacia and X-linked hypophosphatemia," *The New England Journal of Medicine*, vol. 348, no. 17, pp. 1656–1663, 2003.

[6] Y. Yamazaki, R. Okazaki, M. Shibata et al., "Increased circulatory level of biologically active full-length FGF-23 in patients with hypophosphatemic rickets/osteomalacia," *Journal of Clinical Endocrinology and Metabolism*, vol. 87, no. 11, pp. 4957–4960, 2002.

[7] S. Liu, R. T. Premont, C. D. Kontos, J. Huang, and D. C. Rockey, "Endothelin-1 activates endothelial cell nitric-oxide synthase via heterotrimeric G-protein $\beta\gamma$ subunit signaling to protein kinase B/Akt," *The Journal of Biological Chemistry*, vol. 278, no. 50, pp. 49929–49935, 2003.

[8] S. Liu, R. Guo, L. G. Simpson, Z.-S. Xiao, C. E. Burnham, and L. D. Quarles, "Regulation of fibroblastic growth factor 23 expression but not degradation by PHEX," *The Journal of Biological Chemistry*, vol. 278, no. 39, pp. 37419–37426, 2003.

[9] K. E. White, W. E. Evans, J. L. H. O'Riordan et al., "Autosomal dominant hypophosphataemic rickets is associated with mutations in FGF23," *Nature Genetics*, vol. 26, no. 3, pp. 345–348, 2000.

[10] J. Q. Feng, L. M. Ward, S. Liu et al., "Loss of DMP1 causes rickets and osteomalacia and identifies a role for osteocytes in mineral metabolism," *Nature Genetics*, vol. 38, no. 11, pp. 1310–1315, 2006.

[11] B. Lorenz-Depiereux, M. Bastepe, A. Benet-Pagès et al., "DMP1 mutations in autosomal recessive hypophosphatemia implicate a bone matrix protein in the regulation of phosphate homeostasis," *Nature Genetics*, vol. 38, no. 11, pp. 1248–1250, 2006.

[12] B. Lorenz-Depiereux, D. Schnabel, D. Tiosano, G. Häusler, and T. M. Strom, "Loss-of-function ENPP1 mutations cause both generalized arterial calcification of infancy and autosomal-recessive hypophosphatemic rickets," *American Journal of Human Genetics*, vol. 86, no. 2, pp. 267–272, 2010.

[13] V. Levy-Litan, E. Hershkovitz, L. Avizov et al., "Autosomal-recessive hypophosphatemic rickets is associated with an inactivation mutation in the ENPP1 gene," *The American Journal of Human Genetics*, vol. 86, no. 2, pp. 273–278, 2010.

[14] T. Larsson, X. Yu, S. I. Davis et al., "A novel recessive mutation in fibroblast growth factor-23 causes familial tumoral calcinosis," *Journal of Clinical Endocrinology and Metabolism*, vol. 90, no. 4, pp. 2424–2427, 2005.

[15] K. Goji, K. Ozaki, A. H. Sadewa, H. Nishio, and M. Matsuo, "Clinical case seminar: somatic and germline mosaicism for a mutation of the *PHEX* gene can lead to genetic transmission of X-linked hypophosphatemic rickets that mimics an autosomal dominant trait," *The Journal of Clinical Endocrinology and Metabolism*, vol. 91, no. 2, pp. 365–370, 2006.

[16] P. Kumar, S. Henikoff, and P. C. Ng, "Predicting the effects of coding non-synonymous variants on protein function using the SIFT algorithm," *Nature Protocols*, vol. 4, no. 7, pp. 1073–1082, 2009.

[17] I. A. Adzhubei, S. Schmidt, L. Peshkin et al., "A method and server for predicting damaging missense mutations," *Nature Methods*, vol. 7, no. 4, pp. 248–249, 2010.

[18] Y. Choi, G. E. Sims, S. Murphy, J. R. Miller, and A. P. Chan, "Predicting the functional effect of amino acid substitutions and indels," *PLoS ONE*, vol. 7, no. 10, Article ID e46688, 2012.

[19] Y. Sabbagh, G. Boileau, M. Campos, A. K. Carmona, and H. S. Tenenhouse, "Structure and function of disease-causing missense mutations in the PHEX gene," *Journal of Clinical Endocrinology and Metabolism*, vol. 88, no. 5, pp. 2213–2222, 2003.

[20] M. Sahay and R. Sahay, "Rickets-vitamin D deficiency and dependency," *Indian Journal of Endocrinology and Metabolism*, vol. 16, pp. 164–176, 2012.

[21] T. O. Carpenter, E. A. Imel, I. A. Holm, S. M. Jan de Beur, and K. L. Insogna, "A clinician's guide to X-linked hypophosphatemia," *Journal of Bone and Mineral Research*, vol. 26, no. 7, pp. 1381–1388, 2011.

[22] E. A. Imel, M. Peacock, P. Pitukcheewanont et al., "Sensitivity of fibroblast growth factor 23 measurements in tumor-
induced osteomalacia," *Journal of Clinical Endocrinology and
Metabolism*, vol. 91, no. 6, pp. 2055–2061, 2006.

[23] I. Endo, S. Fukumoto, K. Ozono et al., "Clinical usefulness
of measurement of fibroblast growth factor 23 (FGF23) in
hypophosphatemic patients: proposal of diagnostic criteria
using FGF23 measurement," *Bone*, vol. 42, no. 6, pp. 1235–1239,
2008.

4

12q14 Microdeletions: Additional Case Series with Confirmation of a Macrocephaly Region

Adrian Mc Cormack,[1] **Cynthia Sharpe,**[2] **Nerine Gregersen,**[3] **Warwick Smith,**[4]
Ian Hayes,[3] **Alice M. George,**[1] **and Donald R. Love**[1]

[1]*Diagnostic Genetics, LabPLUS, Auckland City Hospital, P.O. Box 110031, Auckland 1148, New Zealand*
[2]*Department of Neuroservices, Starship Children's Health, Private Bag 92024, Auckland 1142, New Zealand*
[3]*Genetic Health Service New Zealand-Northern Hub, Auckland City Hospital, Private Bag 92024, Auckland 1142, New Zealand*
[4]*Middlemore Hospital, Private Bag 93311, Otahuhu, Auckland 1640, New Zealand*

Correspondence should be addressed to Donald R. Love; donaldl@adhb.govt.nz

Academic Editor: Patrick Morrison

To date, there have been only a few reports of patients carrying a microdeletion in chromosome 12q14. These patients usually present with pre- and postnatal growth retardation, and developmental delay. Here we report on two additional patients with both genotype and phenotype differences. Similar to previously published cases, one patient has haploinsufficiency of the *HMGA2* gene and shows severe short stature and developmental delay. The second patient is only one of a handful without the loss of the *HMGA2* gene and shows a much better growth profile, but with absolute macrocephaly. This patient's deletion is unique and hence defines a likely macrocephaly locus that contributes to the general phenotype characterising the 12q14 syndrome.

1. Introduction

Microarray technology has revolutionised the detection of human chromosomal abnormalities within cytogenetics by discovering new, as well as refining, existing syndromes. The technology has recently revealed the existence of a previously unknown deletion syndrome at 12q14. Initial case series have helped categorise and partially refine the genotype and phenotype correlations of this emerging syndrome [1–5], Table 1.

Menten et al. [2] investigated the causative gene for Osteopoikilosis using microarray technology and were the first to report three unrelated patients with *de novo* deletions of 12q14. Patients carrying heterozygous deletions in this region exhibited a common phenotype that included failure to thrive, short stature, and learning difficulties, which was noted to be phenotypically similar to Silver-Russell Syndrome (SRS). SRS is characterized by a variable clinical spectrum of pre- and postnatal growth retardation, relative macrocephaly, body asymmetry, and triangle facial gestalt [6, 7]. It is mainly caused by two mechanisms: maternal UPD chromosome 7 or hypomethylation at the imprinting centre region 1 (ICR1) on 11p15 [6, 7]. Generally, patients who fulfil specific clinical criteria can be reliably diagnosed with SRS; however, for 50% of patients the etiology is unknown and these patients are often referred to as having an "SRS-like" phenotype [7]. Of these patients, those with deletions in the 12q14 region form a subgroup.

The 12q14 interstitial deletions found in these initial cases encompassed two critical genes: *LEMD3* and *HMGA2*. Mutations in the former gene are implicated in Osteopoikilosis, while mutations in the latter gene in mice have a strong influence on height [8, 9]. Mari et al. [5] confirmed the role of *HMGA2* haploinsufficiency in the etiology of short stature and failure to thrive in reporting patients with deletions of this gene. A further case series reported by Buysse et al. [1] described patients without Osteopoikilosis, despite the loss of *LEMD3* gene, and confirmed that heterozygous intragenic deletions of *HMGA2* have a significant effect on human height. They proposed a minimum region of overlap

TABLE 1: Comparison of the main clinical indications of Patients 1 and 2 and six previously reported patients carrying 12q14 microdeletions.

	Patient 1	Patient 2	Spengler et al. (2010) [3]	Takenouchi et al. (2012) [4]	Mari et al. (2009) [5]	Menten et al. (2007) [2] #D0502619	Menten et al. (2007) [2] #4818	Buysse et al. (2009) [1] #03g1858
Hg[19] coordinates	63,169,460–66,983,229	60,220,054–65,843,601	~66,200,000–67,550,000	66,080,229–70,062,135	~66,173,733–68,023,733	~61,800,000–66,800,000	~65,100,000–68,500,000	~61,500,000–67,600,000
Deletion size (Mb)	3.8	5.6	1.35	4	1.8	5	~3.4	~6
Pregnancy	IUGR	Uncomplicated	IUGR	Severe IUGR	Severe IUGR	Oligohydramnios	Hyperemesis	Uncomplicated
Birth measurements	Wgt: 2550 g, Lgt: 48 cm, HC: 35 cm	Wgt: 2600 g (75th centile), HC: 33 cm (75th–91th centile)	Wgt: 2700 g (−1.83 SD), Lgt: 46 cm (−2.59 SD), HC: not noted	Wgt: 527 g (−3.78 SD), Lgt: 30.5 cm, HC: 22 cm	Wgt: 1730 g (<10th centile), Lgt: 43 cm (−4 SD), OFC: 29 cm (−3.66 SD)	Wt: 2300 g (<P3), Lgt: not noted, OFC: not noted	Wgt: at 3rd centile, Lgt: at 10th centile	Wgt: 2060 g (<P3), Lgt. & HC not noted
Growth parameters	3 years: Wgt: 11 kg (0.5 kg <3rd centile), Hgt: 82.6 cm (−3.5 SD), HC: 49.5 cm (40th percentile)	3 years 8 months: Wgt: 17.4 Kg, HC: 54 cm, Hgt: 102.2 cm	1 year 9 months: Wgt: 6.8 Kg (−5.4 SD), Hgt: 70.8 cm (−4.5 SD), OFC: 43.7 (−3.3 SD)	29 months: Wgt: 10.5 kg (−0.75 SD), Hgt: 76 cm (−3.13 SD), HC: 42.5 cm (−3.53 SD)	3 years: Wgt: 6.5 Kg (−5 SD), Hgt: 77 cm (−4.85 SD), OFC: 44.5 cm (−5.1SD)	14 years: Wgt: 51.3 kg (mean for age), Hgt: 142.3 cm (−3.5 SD), HC: 53.3 cm (−0.66 SD)	18 years, Wgt: 41 kg, Hgt: 152 cm (both below 3rd centile)	16 years: Hgt 131.5 cm (−6.2SD), HC: 49 cm (−4.4 SD)
Clinical presentation	Severe SS, relative macrocephaly	Absolute macrocephaly	SS, FTT, relative macrocephaly	SS, severe FTT	Severe proportionate SS, FTT	SS	SS, FTT	Proportionate SS, FTT
Developmental delay	Mild	Yes	Mild	Not noted	Yes	Yes	Mild	Yes
Dysmorphic features	Alternating esotropia, severe myopia	Strabismus, prominent brow, large and slightly low set eyes	Prominent head, slight triangle face, dysplastic ears, clinodactyly of 5th finger	Cleft lip with alveolar cleft on the right, atrial septal defect	Triangle face with prominent forehead, low set ears, vaulted palate, micrognathia	Scoliosis, deep set eyes, bushy eyebrows, thin lips	Triangle face with wide spaced eyes	Synophrys, mild hypertelorism, broad & high nasal bridge, micrognathia & maxillary overbite
Behavioural issues	Possible ADHD, mild ASD	ASD	Not noted	No	Not noted	Not noted	Not noted	Not noted

HC: head circumference, OFC: Occipital Frontal Circumference, IUGR: Intrauterine Growth Retardation, ASD: Autism Spectrum Disorder, ADHD: Attention Deficit Hyperactivity Disorder, FTT: failure to thrive, and SS: short stature.

encompassing approximately 11 genes that were thought to play a role in patients manifesting 12q14 microdeletion syndrome. Finally Takenouchi et al. [4] examined the correlation between the location (and extent) of deletions in 12q14 and clinical phenotype and proposed that relative macrocephaly may involve deletions upstream of the *HMGA2* gene.

The study described here comprises an additional two patients with interstitial 12q14 microdeletions. Patient 1 carries a 3.8 Mb heterozygous deletion involving the interstitial region 12q14.2q14.3, and Patient 2 carries a 5.6 Mb heterozygous deletion involving the interstitial region 12q14.1q14.3.

2. Clinical Report

2.1. Patient 1. A healthy male was born at 41-week gestation with asymmetrical growth restriction weighing 2550 g (<3rd centile), with length 48 cm (20th centile) and head circumference 35 cm (50th centile). The mother is a hyperactive, verbally aggressive and difficult individual who drank excessively during the pregnancy. She is also relatively short with a height of approximately 153 cm and has a strabismus. The father is approximately 183 cm tall, cannot read or write, and is socially reclusive. There were no concerns about the child's motor skills and achieved expected milestones. He was noted to be a behaviourally difficult child, always on the go, demanding attention, and seemingly always talking. He understood language and could talk well although at times his speech was unclear and he spoke in an unusual voice.

Paediatric assessment of the proband at three years of age noted that he was short, with height 82.6 cm (3.5 SD below the mean), weight 11 kg (0.5 kg less than the 3rd percentile), and head circumference 49.5 cm (on the 40th percentile). He had deep set eyes and a thin upper lip but normal philtrum and palpebral fissures each 22 mm (−2 SD). He wore glasses suggesting severe myopia and manifested alternating esotropia. He had no clear features of Fetal Alcohol Syndrome, but there were concerns over possible mild dysmorphic features. It was noted that social communication was poor and that he talked in unusual voice prosody, with reasonable receptive and expressive language. He was diagnosed with mild Autism Spectrum Disorder (ASD), was hyperactive and aggressive, and had many features of ADHD. A final genetics consultation at four years of age confirmed previous findings and his guardians stated that he had problems with fine motor skills. Head circumference was near the 50th centile and height below the 3rd centile. He had the appearance of relative macrocephaly but little else to see from a dysmorphology perspective. The child never had X-rays so we cannot say if there were skeletal changes consistent with a diagnosis of Osteopoikilosis.

2.2. Patient 2. A female was delivered at 35-week gestation following a breech presentation. Family medical history was unremarkable. Birth head circumference was 33 cm (75th–91st percentile for 35-week gestation), birth weight was 2.6 kg (75th percentile), and she had some issues with poor feeding. By 2 months of age her head had grown to 38.5 cm on the 98th percentile for her corrected gestational age and accelerated further to the 99th percentile by 6 months of age.

She passed her developmental screen at one year of age but a further assessment at 19 months revealed developmental delay. Macrocephaly was also first noted at this visit. Her head circumference has been stable 1-2 cm above the 98th percentile since then. Her motor skills were delayed and speech was also delayed and she met the criteria for ASD. She received speech therapy for six months, but this was stopped because at three years of age she had hundreds of words, was speaking in 2-3-word phrases, and understood most of what was said.

An MRI was performed at 27 months of age showing mild hyperintensity in the deep white matter in the periventricular regions of the occipital area bilaterally, more so on the right. There was no mass effect and the brain was normally formed, with no hydrocephalus noted.

Further paediatric examination at 3 years 8 months of age showed height of 102.2 cm (75th centile), weight of 17.4 kg (75-90th centile), and head circumference of 54 cm (13.5 SD). There were no obvious dysmorphic features or neuro-cutaneous stigmata and she was undergoing treatment for a strabismus. She had evidence of both gross motor/fine motor and language delay but was showing excellent catching up of her development with appropriate inputs. Her last review at 4 years 5 months showed that her head circumference continued to track above the centiles at 55 cm; she was 108 cm tall (75–90th centile) and weighed 20 kg (90th centile). She still met the criteria for a diagnosis of ASD and had global gross motor/fine motor and language delay but was showing very encouraging improvements in all aspects of her development. It was noted that she had mild plagiocephaly, a prominent brow, and mild hypertelorism (Figure 1(b)). The patient does not exhibit Osteopoikilosis, but she may be too young to manifest symptoms. The patient proved negative for mutations in the *PTEN* gene (by both dosage and sequencing), which was performed in light of macrocephaly and the diagnosis of autism.

2.3. Molecular Studies. DNA was extracted from both Patients 1 and 2 with genome-wide copy number analysis determined using an Affymetrix Cytogenetics Whole-Genome 2.7M array and CytoScan 750K Array, respectively, according to the manufacturer's instructions. Regions of copy number change were determined using the Affymetrix Chromosome Analysis Suite software (ChAS) either v.1.0.1 or v.1.2.2 and interpreted with the aid of the UCSC genome browser (http://genome.ucsc.edu/; Human March 2006 (hg18) assembly or February 2009 GRCh37/hg19 assembly), Figure 2.

Patient 1 carried a 3.8 Mb heterozygous deletion involving the interstitial chromosome region 12q14.2q14.3 (hg19 coordinates 63,169,460–66,983,229) encompassing 16 OMIM genes (*AVPR1A, DPY19L2, TMEM5, SRGAP1, XPOT, TBK1, RASSF3, GNS, TBC13D0, WIF1, LEMD3, MSRB3, HMGA2, IRAK3, HELB,* and part of *GRIP1*). Patient 2 carried a 5.6 Mb heterozygous deletion involving the interstitial chromosome region 12q14.1q14.3 (hg19 coordinates 60,220,054–65,843,601)

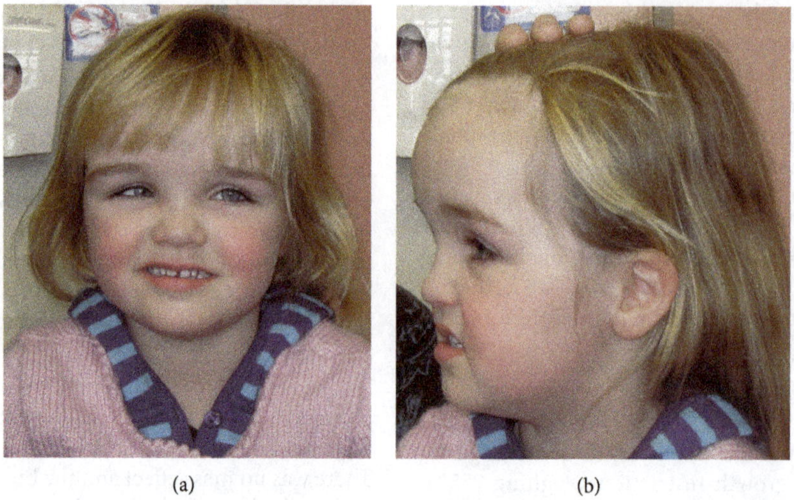

FIGURE 1: (a) Image of Patient 2. (b) Patient 2 exhibits frontal bossing and macrocephaly.

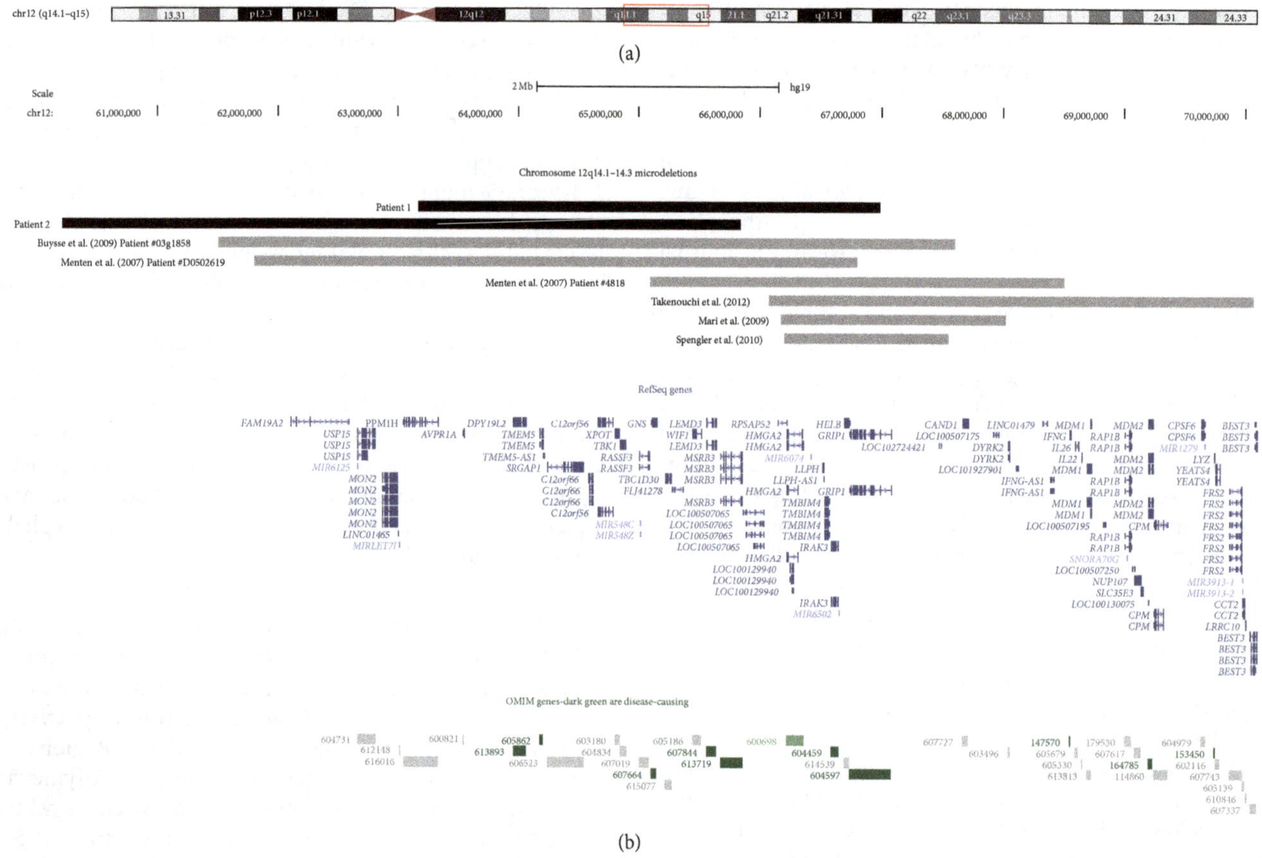

(a)

(b)

FIGURE 2: Schematic of chromosome 12q14 containing microdeletions. (a) shows an ideogram of chromosome 12. (b) shows the location and extent of the deletions detected in the patients described here and other cases reported in the literature, as well as RefSeq and OMIM genes that lie within 12q14. These graphics were taken from the UCSC genome browser (http://genome.ucsc.edu/).

encompassing 14 OMIM genes (*USP15, MIRLET7I, AVPR1A, DPY19L2, TMEM5, SRGAP1, XPOT, TBK1, RASSF3, GNS, TBC1D30, WIF1, LEMD3,* and part of *MSRB3*). The parents of Patient 1 were unavailable for follow-up analysis while the parents of Patient 2 showed normal molecular karyotypes.

3. Discussion

In the study described here, we report two patients with overlapping deletions in 12q14: a 3.8 Mb deletion in Patient 1 with extreme short stature, mild autism, behavioural problems,

TABLE 2: OMIM genes that lie in the 12q14 interval bounded by *USP15* and *MSRB3*.

Gene	OMIM	Description
USP15	604731	USP15 is required for TGFB and BMP responses in both mammalian cells and frog embryos. The *USP15* gene encodes for a deubiquitinating enzyme. Animal models have shown that it regulates bone morphogenetic signalling during embryogenesis [10].
PPM1H	616016	Knockdown of PPM1H significantly increases proliferation in BT474 breast cancer cells [11].
AVPR1A	600821	The *AVPR1A* gene encodes for a receptor that is involved in vasopressin signalling, which is involved in behavioural responses, including stress management and territorial aggression as well as social bonding and recognition [12].
DPY19L2	613893	*DPY19L2* represents the major gene causing globozoospermia [13].
TMEM5	605862	The *TMEM5* gene encodes for a type II membrane protein of unknown function, but mutations have been associated with gonadal dysgenesis, neural tube defects, and most recently being a cause of severe cobblestone lissencephaly [14].
SRGAP1	606523	SRGAP1 interacts with Roundabout transmembrane receptors, together with SLIT proteins, which guide neuronal and leukocyte migration [15].
XPOT	603180	Exportin-t is a specific mediator of tRNA export [16, 17].
TBK1	604834	TBK1 is a binding partner for optineurin [18].
RASSF3	607019	The *RASSF3* gene encodes for a putative tumor suppressor [19].
GNS	607664	The *GNS* gene encodes for N-acetylglucosamine-6-sulfatase, which is required for degradation of heparin sulphate. Homozygous mutations in this gene have been shown to be the cause of mucopolysaccharidosis type IIID [20].
TBC1D30	615077	TBC1D30 protein is predicted to be involved in cell signalling [21].
WIF1	605186	WIF1 binds to WNT proteins and inhibits their extracellular signaling involved in the control of embryonic development [22].
LEMD3	607844	*LEMD3* is involved in both BMP and TGF-beta signalling. Heterozygous loss-of-function mutations in the *LEMD3* gene are implicated in Osteopoikilosis and the associated Buschke-Ollendorff syndrome [8].
MRSB3	613719	The *MSRB3* gene encodes for methioinine sulfoxide reductase. Homozygous mutations in this gene are associated with a form of autosomal recessive, nonsyndromic deafness [23].

Those genes in bold italics are implicated in bone morphogenesis.
TGFB: Transforming Growth Factor Beta.
BMP: Bone Morphogenetic Protein.

severe myopia, and esotropia and a 5.6 Mb deletion in Patient 2 with absolute macrocephaly, developmental delay, learning difficulties, and autism. The deletion in Patient 1 includes both the *LEMD3* and *HMGA2* genes, while the deletion in Patient 2 includes the *LEMD3* gene but not the *HMGA2* gene. The mother of Patient 1, who has short stature, behavioural issues, and a convergent strabismus, may also harbour a deletion, but unfortunately she was not available for testing to confirm this. Patient 2 had a *de novo* deletion.

Of the reported 12q14 interstitial deletion cases, only 5 (including one of the cases presented here) have not included the *HMGA2* gene. The deleted region detected in Patient 1 includes the *HMGA2* gene and this patient shows prenatal IUGR and severe short stature but critically the deleted region in Patient 2 does not encompass the *HMGA2* gene and they exhibit no pre- or postnatal growth issues. Both cases reinforce the importance of the *HMGA2* gene's influence on growth.

The *HMGA2* gene (OMIM 600698) encodes a mammalian high mobility group (HMG) protein which is implicated in transcriptional regulation [24]. Ligon et al. [25] described a *de novo* pericentric inversion in an 8-year-old boy causing an intragenic rearrangement which truncated the *HMGA2* gene, altering its expression and causing a

phenotype which included overgrowth and lipomas. Interestingly, *hmga2* −/− mice show a "pygmy" phenotype with short stature and reduction in body fat [9]. Buysse et al. [1] reported a small intragenic deletion of the *HMGA2* gene in a boy with proportionate short stature, segregating within a larger pedigree with reduced adult height. In addition, Mari et al. [5] described a patient with a 1.84 Mb deletion encompassing six genes including the *HMGA2* gene in which the phenotype comprised pre- and postnatal growth restrictions and short stature.

Critically, Spengler et al. [3] proposed a separate locus distinct from *HMGA2* as being partially responsible for the SRS-like phenotype. Takenouchi et al. [4] reviewed deletions at 12q14 and showed that only a small group of patients had relative macrocephaly and short stature. They proposed two discernible groups of phenotypes of 12q14 microdeletions: a group of patients with short stature with relative macrocephaly and a group with an SRS-like phenotype and short stature without macrocephaly. They suggested a presumptive interval for relative macrocephaly spanning 0.5 Mb–2 Mb, but not including the *HMGA2* gene.

Patient 1, whose deletion includes the *HMGA2* gene, appears to have an SRS-like phenotype. Interestingly, Patient 2 lacks a growth retardation phenotype but has absolute macrocephaly confirming the suggestion made by Take-nouchi et al. [4] of a macrocephaly locus that contributes to the SRS-like phenotype for patients with deletions in 12q14. At this time, the function of only some of the genes located in the deleted interval detected in Patient 2 has been characterised, Table 2.

Our cases, together with those reported earlier, suggest that the SRS-like phenotype of patients with deletions in 12q14 can be refined to the following:

(1) Deletions that include (all or some of) the *HMGA2* gene correlate with a growth-based phenotype.

(2) A macrocephaly region (~2 MB in length) proximal and independent of the *HMGA2* gene correlates with an absolute macrocephaly phenotype (see Patient 2).

(3) Deletions involving both of these regions combine to form an SRS-like phenotype (see Patient 1).

In the future, smaller deletions within 12q14 may be uncovered in order to narrow down a macrocephaly locus. Of the genes described above, the most likely candidate gene appears to be *USP15* (see Table 2) because of its involvement in bone morphogenesis.

Conflict of Interests

The authors declare that there is no conflict of interests regarding the publication of this paper.

References

[1] K. Buysse, W. Reardon, L. Mehta et al., "The 12q14 microdeletion syndrome: additional patients and further evidence that HMGA2 is an important genetic determinant for human height," *European Journal of Medical Genetics*, vol. 52, no. 2-3, pp. 101–107, 2009.

[2] B. Menten, K. Buysse, F. Zahir et al., "Osteopoikilosis, short stature and mental retardation as key features of a new microdeletion syndrome on 12q14," *Journal of Medical Genetics*, vol. 44, no. 4, pp. 264–268, 2007.

[3] S. Spengler, N. Schönherr, G. Binder et al., "Submicroscopic chromosomal imbalances in idiopathic Silver-Russell syndrome (SRS): the SRS phenotype overlaps with the 12q14 microdeletion syndrome," *Journal of Medical Genetics*, vol. 47, no. 5, pp. 356–360, 2010.

[4] T. Takenouchi, K. Enomoto, T. Nishida et al., "12q14 microdeletion syndrome and short stature with or without relative macrocephaly," *The American Journal of Medical Genetics. Part A*, vol. 158, no. 10, pp. 2542–2544, 2012.

[5] F. Mari, P. Hermanns, M. L. Giovannucci-Uzielli et al., "Refinement of the 12q14 microdeletion syndrome: primordial dwarfism and developmental delay with or without osteopoikilosis," *European Journal of Human Genetics*, vol. 17, no. 9, pp. 1141–1147, 2009.

[6] T. Eggermann, D. Gonzalez, S. Spengler, M. Arslan-Kirchner, G. Binder, and N. Schönherr, "Broad clinical spectrum in Silver-Russell syndrome and consequences for genetic testing in growth retardation," *Pediatrics*, vol. 123, no. 5, pp. e929–e931, 2009.

[7] S. Fokstuen and D. Kotzot, "Chromosomal rearrangements in patients with clinical features of Silver-Russell syndrome," *American Journal of Medical Genetics, Part A*, vol. 164, no. 6, pp. 1595–1605, 2014.

[8] J. Hellemans, O. Preobrazhenska, A. Willaert et al., "Loss-of-function mutations in LEMD3 result in osteopoikilosis, Buschke-Ollendorff syndrome and melorheostosis," *Nature Genetics*, vol. 36, no. 11, pp. 1213–1218, 2004.

[9] X. Zhou, K. F. Benson, H. R. Ashar, and K. Chada, "Mutation responsible for the mouse pygmy phenotype in the developmentally regulated factor HMGI-C," *Nature*, vol. 376, no. 6543, pp. 771–774, 1995.

[10] L. Herhaus, M. A. Al-Salihi, K. S. Dingwell et al., "USP15 targets ALK3/BMPR1A for deubiquitylation to enhance bone morphogenetic protein signalling," *Open Biology*, vol. 4, no. 5, Article ID 140065, 2014.

[11] S. T. Lee-Hoeflich, T. Q. Pham, D. Dowbenko et al., "PPM1H Is a p27 phosphatase implicated in trastuzumab resistance," *Cancer Discovery*, vol. 1, no. 4, pp. 326–337, 2011.

[12] R. Charles, T. Sakurai, N. Takahashi et al., "Introduction of the human AVPR1A gene substantially alters brain receptor expression patterns and enhances aspects of social behavior in transgenic mice," *Disease Models & Mechanisms*, vol. 7, no. 8, pp. 1013–1022, 2014.

[13] E. Elinati, P. Kuentz, C. Redin et al., "Globozoospermia is mainly due to dpy19l2 deletion via non-allelic homologous recombination involving two recombination hotspots," *Human Molecular Genetics*, vol. 21, no. 16, pp. 3695–3702, 2012.

[14] S. Vuillaumier-Barrot, C. Bouchet-Séraphin, M. Chelbi et al., "Identification of mutations in TMEM5 and ISPD as a cause of severe cobblestone lissencephaly," *American Journal of Human Genetics*, vol. 91, no. 6, pp. 1135–1143, 2012.

[15] K. Wong, X.-R. Ren, Y.-Z. Huang et al., "Signal transduction in neuronal migration: roles of GTPase activating proteins and the small GTPase Cdc42 in the Slit-Robo pathway," *Cell*, vol. 107, no. 2, pp. 209–221, 2001.

[16] U. Kutay, G. Lipowsky, E. Izaurralde et al., "Identification of a tRNA-specific nuclear export receptor," *Molecular Cell*, vol. 1, no. 3, pp. 359–369, 1998.

[17] G.-J. Arts, M. Fornerod, and I. W. Mattaj, "Identification of a nuclear export receptor for tRNA," *Current Biology*, vol. 8, no. 6, pp. 305–314, 1998.

[18] S. Morton, L. Hesson, M. Peggie, and P. Cohen, "Enhanced binding of TBK1 by an optineurin mutant that causes a familial form of primary open angle glaucoma," *FEBS Letters*, vol. 582, no. 6, pp. 997–1002, 2008.

[19] S. Tommasi, R. Dammann, S.-G. Jin, X.-F. Zhang, J. Avruch, and G. P. Pfeifer, "RASSF3 and NORE1: identification and cloning of two human homologues of the putative tumor suppressor gene RASSF1," *Oncogene*, vol. 21, no. 17, pp. 2713–2720, 2002.

[20] A. Mok, H. Cao, and R. A. Hegele, "Genomic basis of mucopolysaccharidosis type IIID (MIM 252940) revealed by sequencing of GNS encoding N-acetylglucosamine-6-sulfatase," *Genomics*, vol. 81, no. 1, pp. 1–5, 2003.

[21] K. Ishibashi, E. Kanno, T. Itoh, and M. Fukuda, "Identification and characterization of a novel Tre-2/Bub2/Cdc16 (TBC) protein that possesses Rab3A-GAP activity," *Genes to Cells*, vol. 14, no. 1, pp. 41–52, 2009.

[22] J.-C. Hsieh, L. Kodjabachian, M. L. Rebbert et al., "A new secreted protein that binds to Wnt proteins and inhibits their activites," *Nature*, vol. 398, no. 6726, pp. 431–436, 1999.

[23] Z. M. Ahmed, R. Yousaf, B. C. Lee et al., "Functional null mutations of MSRB3 encoding methionine sulfoxide reductase are associated with human deafness DFNB74," *The American Journal of Human Genetics*, vol. 88, no. 1, pp. 19–29, 2011.

[24] K.-Y. Chau, U. A. Patel, K.-L. D. Lee, H.-Y. P. Lam, and C. Crane-Robinson, "The gene for the human architectural transcription factor HMGI-C consists of five exons each coding for a distinct functional element," *Nucleic Acids Research*, vol. 23, no. 21, pp. 4262–4266, 1995.

[25] A. H. Ligon, S. D. P. Moore, M. A. Parisi et al., "Constitutional rearrangement of the architectural factor HMGA2: a novel human phenotype including overgrowth and lipomas," *American Journal of Human Genetics*, vol. 76, no. 2, pp. 340–348, 2005.

5

A Prenatally Ascertained *De Novo* Terminal Deletion of Chromosomal Bands 1q43q44 Associated with Multiple Congenital Abnormalities in a Female Fetus

Carolina Sismani,[1] Georgia Christopoulou,[2] Angelos Alexandrou,[1] Paola Evangelidou,[1] Jacqueline Donoghue,[2] Anastasia E. Konstantinidou,[3] and Voula Velissariou[2]

[1]*Department of Cytogenetics and Genomics, The Cyprus Institute of Neurology and Genetics, 6 International Airport Avenue, Ayios Dometios, 2370 Nicosia, Cyprus*

[2]*Department of Genetics and Molecular Biology, General, Maternity, and Pediatric Clinic Mitera, Erythrou Stavrou 6, 15123 Athens, Greece*

[3]*Department of Pathology, Medical School, University of Athens, Mikras Assias 75, 11527 Athens, Greece*

Correspondence should be addressed to Voula Velissariou; voulavel@leto.gr

Academic Editor: Maria Descartes

Terminal deletions in the long arm of chromosome 1 result in a postnatally recognizable disorder described as 1q43q44 deletion syndrome. The size of the deletions and the resulting phenotype varies among patients. However, some features are common among patients as the chromosomal regions included in the deletions. In the present case, ultrasonography at 22 weeks of gestation revealed choroid plexus cysts (CPCs) and a single umbilical artery (SUA) and therefore amniocentesis was performed. Chromosomal analysis revealed a possible terminal deletion in 1q and high resolution array CGH confirmed the terminal 1q43q44 deletion and estimated the size to be approximately 8 Mb. Following termination of pregnancy, performance of fetopsy allowed further clinical characterization. We report here a prenatal case with the smallest pure terminal 1q43q44 deletion, that has been molecularly and phenotypically characterized. In addition, to our knowledge this is the first prenatal case reported with 1q13q44 terminal deletion and Pierre-Robin sequence (PRS). Our findings combined with review data from the literature show the complexity of the genetic basis of the associated syndrome.

1. Introduction

Pure deletions of distal chromosome 1q result in a recognizable disorder described as 1q43q44 deletion syndrome (OMIM-612337, http://www.omim.org). Although clinical manifestations vary, most patients share characteristic features such as moderate-to-severe intellectual disability, limited to no speech, dysmorphic facial features including round face, prominent forehead, flat nasal bridge, hypertelorism, epicanthal folds, and low set ears. Hypotonia, poor growth, microcephaly, corpus callosum abnormalities (CCA), and seizures are also commonly present in these patients. The case we present in the current study is, to our knowledge, the first prenatal case with the smallest pure 1q43q44 deletion in

a female fetus molecularly and phenotypically characterized and the first reported case with an association with PRS. The detailed autopsy and genetic analysis results allow further characterization, clinical correlation, and/or genotype-phenotype correlation, as well as comparison with previously described prenatal and postnatal cases.

2. Case Report

A 32-year-old pregnant woman was referred to our lab at 22 weeks of gestation for chromosomal investigation by karyotype analysis after amniocentesis, requested due to abnormal ultrasound findings. The prospective parents are both of Greek origin and apparently healthy. This was their

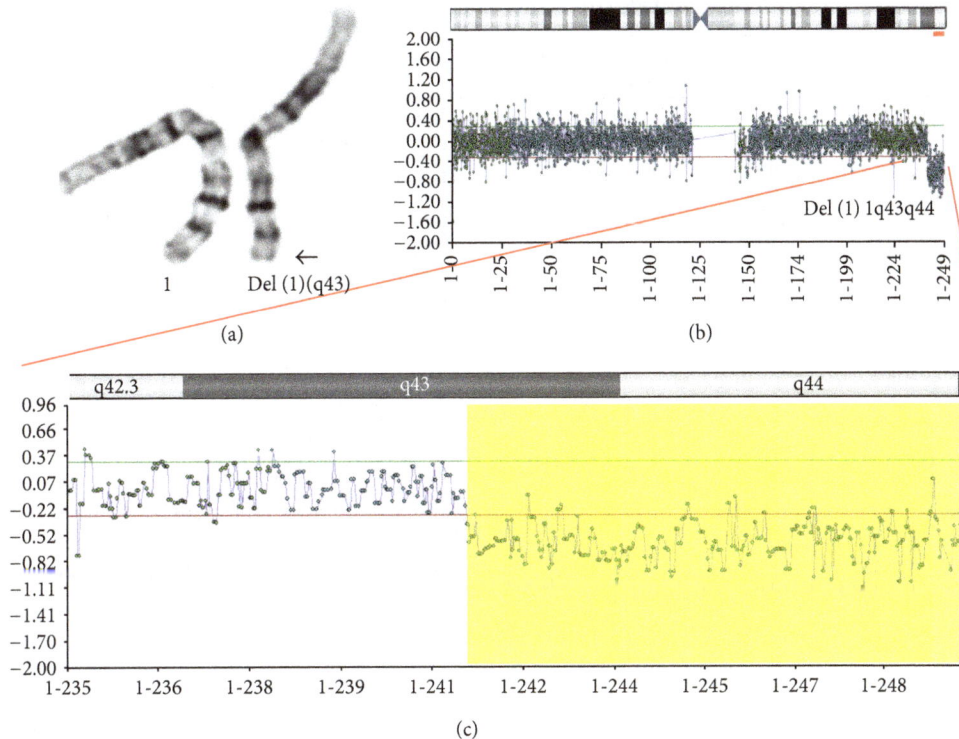

FIGURE 1: (a) Prenatal fetal karyotype. The prenatal fetal karyotype revealed a 1q43 deletion most probably terminal. Arrow points to the deleted region of the long arm of chromosome 1. (b) Array-CGH results indicating the terminal deletion chromosome 1. (c) Array-CGH analysis illustrating in depth the *de novo* terminal deletion (highlighted) of approximately 8 Mb in size on the long arm of chromosome 1 at chromosomal band 1q43 extending to band 1q44 (location: 241,178,091–249,224,121 using build GRCh37 (hg19)).

first pregnancy (gravida 1, para 0) and no previous medical or obstetrical history was recorded. The pregnancy had been conceived spontaneously and was unremarkable until this point. Routine ultrasound examination at 22 weeks of gestation revealed choroid plexus cysts (CPCs) and a single umbilical artery (SUA). Chromosomal analysis was performed on amniotic fluid cells. Conventional GTG-banding at 550 band level was applied and revealed a female fetus with a borderline visible deletion on distal 1q, most likely terminal (46,XX,del(1)(q43), Figure 1(a)). Parental karyotypes revealed that the deletion was *de novo*. MLPA was subsequently performed using the P036 and P069 subtelomeric probe mixes (MRC-Holland) on DNA isolated from cultured amniotic fluid cells and confirmed the telomeric nature of the 1q deletion (data not shown). To further delineate the breakpoint of the deletion array-CGH (Comparative Genomic Hybridization) was carried out using the Cytochip Oligo array (BlueGnome-version 1.1) with 105,000 oligos according to the recommendations of the manufacturer. Array-CGH analysis confirmed the results, revealing a female profile with a deletion of approximately 8 Mb in size on the long arm of chromosome 1 from chromosomal band 1q43 extending to 1q44 (location: 241,178,091–249,224,121 using build GRCh37 (hg19), Figures 1(b) and 1(c)). No other copy number changes were detected by array-CGH indicating a pure deletion of the region. The deleted region contains 23 OMIM genes listed in Table 1.

Genetic counseling was offered to the couple and termination of the pregnancy was decided at 28 weeks of gestation. The female fetus was sent for autopsy (a written consent was also obtained from the couple for the publication including fetopsy photos).

At autopsy the fetus was found to be symmetrically growth restricted, weighing 838 g (below the 10th centile for 28 weeks-gestation) and measuring 33.5 cm in crown-heel length, 22.5 cm in crown-rump length, and 46.5 cm in foot length, the body measurements being more appropriate for 25-week gestation. The head circumference (22.8 cm) fell below the 1st centile for 28-week gestation. External craniofacial features included microcephaly and microretrognathia with U-shaped clefting of the hard and soft palate (Pierre-Robin sequence) (Figure 2). The tip of the tongue was noted to be mildly bifid. The clitoris appeared large, with normally formed and sized labia while the anogenital distance appeared shortened. Internally, dissection of the heart revealed an atrial septal defect (ASD) secundum type. The brain weight was low (84 g; ref. for 28/40 weeks 147 g) corresponding to 23-week gestation, and the brain-to-liver-weight ratio was reduced (1.69; ref. 2.5–4), altogether indicating micrencephaly. The cerebellar vermis appeared small. Choroid plexus cysts seen at prenatal ultrasound at 22-week gestation were not confirmed, likely to have resolved in the meantime. Microscopy showed neuroglial migration defects in the periventricular and subcortical cerebral white matter.

TABLE 1: Genes included in the deleted region and associated phenotypes.

Gene/locus name	Gene/locus MIM number	Phenotype/gene function
RGS7	602517	Inhibits signal transduction by increasing the GTPase activity of G protein alpha subunits
FH, HLRCC, MCUL1	136850	Leiomyomatosis and renal cell cancer. Fumarase deficiency
KMO	603538	Catalyzes the hydroxylation of L-kynurenine (L-Kyn) to form 3-hydroxy-L-kynurenine for synthesis of quinolinic acid
OPN3, ECPN	606695	Opsins are members of the guanine nucleotide-binding protein (G protein)-coupled receptors that are expressed in extraocular tissues
CHML, REP2	118825	Binds unprenylated Rab proteins
EXO1, HEX1	606063	5′->3′ double-stranded DNA exonuclease activity
CEP170, KIAA0470	613023	Plays a role in microtubule organization
SDCCAG8, CCCAP, SLSN7	613524	Senior-Loken syndrome 7
AKT3, PKBG, MPPH	611223	Megalencephaly-polymicrogyria-polydactyly-hydrocephalus syndrome
ZBTB18, ZNF238, RP58, MRD22	608433	Mental retardation, autosomal dominant 22
ADSS	103060	Has an important role in the de novo and salvage pathway of purine nucleotide biosynthesis
DESI2, PPPDE1	614638	Protease which may deconjugate SUMO from some substrate proteins
COX20, FAM36A	614698	Protect as-yet-unassembled Cox2 from degradation
HNRNPU	602869	Component of the CRD-mediated complex that promotes MYC mRNA stabilization. Binds to pre-mRNA.
KIF26B	614026	Essential for embryonic kidney development
SMYD3	608783	Histone methyltransferase
TFB2M	607055	Required for basal transcription of mitochondrial DNA, probably via its interaction with POLRMT and TFAM
CNST	613439	Required for targeting of connexins to the plasma membrane
AHCTF1, ELYS	610853	Required for the assembly of a functional nuclear pore complex on the surface of chromosomes as nuclei form at the end of mitosis
ZNF124	194631	Affiliated with the lncRNA class and may be involved in transcriptional regulation
ZNF496, NIZP1, ZFP496	613911	DNA-binding transcription factor that can both act as an activator and a repressor
NLRP3, CIAS1, FCU, FCAS, NALP3, PYPAF1	606416	CINCA syndrome, Cold-induced autoinflammatory syndrome, familial Muckle-Wells syndrome
OR13G1	611677	Odorant receptor (potential)

The placenta weighed 169 g (around the 25th centile for 28/40 weeks) and the fetoplacental ratio was within normal range. Histology showed abnormal development of the placental parenchyma, with uneven villous maturation and features of fetal obstructive vasculopathy. The umbilical cord had 3 vessels, but one umbilical artery was seen to be collapsed, showing luminal occlusion and no evidence of blood flow at the fetal edge.

3. Discussion

The prenatal case presented in this study involves a terminal 1q43q44 deletion which in postnatal cases has been associated with a syndrome with specific clinical features (OMIM-612337, http://www.omim.org). Although manifestations may vary, our fetus had features overlapping the 1q43q44 deletion phenotype, as expected. Such characteristics are microcephaly, microretrognathia, cleft palate, cardiac defect, and small cerebellar vermis. Only three cases of terminal 1q deletions have been described during prenatal diagnosis. The first was detected in a fetus at 19 weeks with omphalocele, cerebral ventriculomegaly, and increased nuchal fold with a breakpoint at 1q41 [1]. The second was detected in a fetus at 21 weeks with hydrocephalus, ventriculomegaly, and corpus callosum agenesis with a breakpoint at 1q42.3 [2]. The third, with a breakpoint at 1q43, was detected by chorionic villous sampling (CVS) in a 12-week fetus with severe

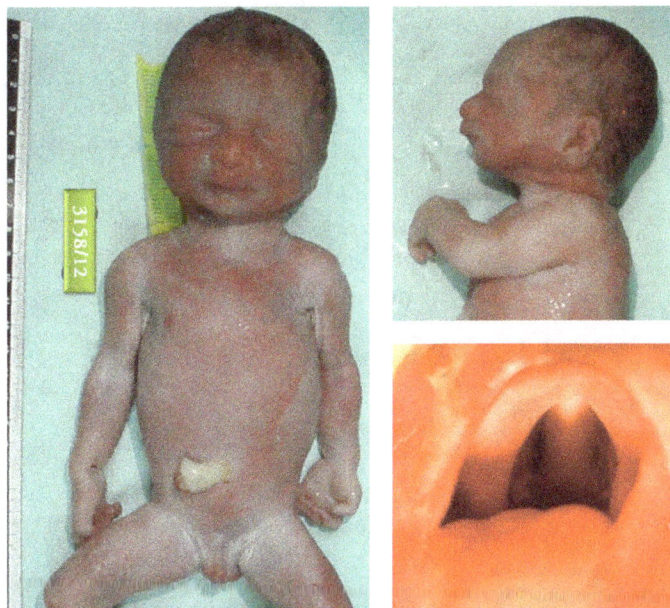

FIGURE 2: Autopsy findings revealed multiple congenital malformations. The figure shows microretrognathia and U-shaped cleft palate (Pierre-Robin sequence) as well as a large clitoris with normally formed labia.

microgenia, nasal bone aplasia, SUA, cardiac anomaly, and hyperechogenic bowel. At 16 weeks, the suspected structural abnormalities were confirmed and in addition intrauterine growth retardation (IUGR) and microcephaly were observed [3]. In the first two cases the deletions were considerably larger than in our case and easily detected during cytogenetic analysis. In the third case, although there are common clinical findings with our case such as microcephaly, SUA, and IUGR, autopsy was not performed and a detailed comparison of the phenotype between the two cases is not possible. For example, the authors report severe microgenia, which at autopsy could prove to be microretrognathia with clefting of the hard and soft palate (PRS), also present in our case. Furthermore, the breakpoint of the deletion was only determined by chromosomal analysis and it appears that the deletion is again significantly larger than ours. Finally, array CGH studies were performed only in the second case where the size of the deletion was estimated at 13.4 Mb, which is significantly larger than that in our case (8 Mb). The antenatal features of the previously three reported del(1q) syndrome prenatal cases and of our present case are summarized in Table 2.

Two recent studies [5, 6] in patients with 1q43q44 microdeletion clarified the phenotype/genotype correlation and proposed three distinct critical regions. The first encompassing ZNF238 was associated with corpus callosum anomalies (CCA) and the second includes AKT3 with microcephaly (MIC), while the third contains the two coding genes FAM36A, HNRNPU and the noncoding gene NCRNA00201 with seizures. The implication of ZNF238 in CCA has also been supported by the study of a patient with 1q44 microdeletion and dysmorphic features, seizures, hypotonia, marked developmental delay, and dysgenesis of the corpus callosum [7]. In the case presented here, AKT3, ZNF238, FAM36A, and HNRNPU are all included in the deletion. Fetoscopy showed

evidence of microcephaly which is in agreement with the implication of AKT3 in MIC as has already been proposed by others [5, 6, 8]. However, although ZNF238 is absent, CCA was not observed, demonstrating the complexity of CCA genetics. Incomplete penetrance associated with deletion of ZNF238 could be an explanation. This has also been proposed in a study in which two patients with moderate-to-severe intellectual disability, craniofacial anomalies, and seizures carrying 1q44 microdeletion including both ZNF238 and AKT3 both had MIC, but only the one presented with CCA [8].

The size of the deletion in our case is comparable to that of a boy with intellectual disability and multiple anomalies where the 1qter deletion was not microscopically visible [4]. At 20-week gestational age a cystic structure in the gastric region was seen on ultrasound which subsequently disappeared, while from 30 weeks IUGR was present. After birth major anomalies were detected and at the age of 5 years severe intellectual disability was also observed. Common features with our case are IUGR, microretrognathia, microcephaly, hypoplastic vermis, and genital abnormalities. However, the mapping of the deletion was performed by microsatellite marker analysis and not array CGH and consequently the exact comparison cannot be made, although the two cases appear to be very similar (Table 2).

The postmortem examination in our case also revealed the presence of PRS, that is, the combination of microretrognathia and posterior soft palate cleft. To date this has been strongly associated with SOX9 either directly or by position effect [9, 10]. It has also been associated with specific gene mutations and various chromosomal abnormalities including deletions, translocations, and duplications [11]. Recently, it has been associated with microdeletion 4q21, microdeletion 5q23, and microduplication 16p13.3 [12–14].

TABLE 2: Clinical features and genetic findings in one postnatal with a very similar deletion size and three prenatal reported cases with deletions spanning chromosomal region 1q41 to 1q44 and comparison with our case.

	Rotmensch et al. [1] prenatal	Chen et al. [2] prenatal	Wagner et al. [3] prenatal	van Bever et al. [4] postnatal	Our case prenatal
Karyotype	46,XY, del(1)(q41)	46,XX, del(1)(q42.3)	46, XX, del(1)(q43)	46, XY	46, XX, del(1)(q43q44)
Light microscope	Detected	Detected	Detected	Not detected	Detected
Array CGH	Not performed	13.4 Mb	Not performed	7.7–8.1 Mb§	8 Mb
Parental karyotypes	Normal	Normal	Normal	Normal	Normal
Gestational age	2nd trimester	2nd and 3rd trimester	1st and 2nd trimester	2nd and 3rd trimester	2nd and 3rd trimester
IUGR	−	+	+	+	+
Increased nuchal translucency/fold	+	−	−	−	−
Nasal bone absence/hypoplasia	−	−	+	+	−
Hyperechogenic bowel	−	−	+	−	−
Single umbilical artery	−	−	+	−	+
Omphalocele	+	−	−	−	−
Microcephaly/micrencephaly	*	−	+	*	*
Micrognathia/microgenia	−	−	+	*	*
Microretrognathia	−	−	−	*	*
Cleft palate	−	−	−	−	*
Hydrocephalus	−	+	−	−	−
Cerebral anomalies	+	−	−	*	*
Corpus callosum agenesis/hypoplasia	−	+	−	*	−
Hypoplastic vermis	−	−	−	*	*
Choroid plexus cysts	−	−	−	−	+
Urogenital anomalies	−	−	−	*	*
Cardiac anomaly	−	+	+	*	*
Fetopsy	−	−	−	**	+

§Performed by microsatellite marker analysis; IUGR: intrauterine growth retardation.
—: not specifically mentioned or undetected; *: initially detected at birth or after termination of pregnancy by observation only or fetopsy; **: born; +: present.

To our knowledge, this is the first reported case with pure 1q43q44 deletion and PRS. There is a single report on a family with cerebellar hypoplasia and PRS, partially resembling our case clinically; however array CGH and subtelomeric FISH revealed no chromosomal imbalances [9]. Our case further supports the fact that PRS conceals considerable etiological heterogeneity and that various chromosomal regions harbor genes responsible for the PRS phenotype, including 1q43q44.

In addition to PRS, the present case is the first in which neuroglial migration defects were detected in the brain, whereas in previous deletion 1q43q44 cases brain abnormalities included delayed myelination, cerebral atrophy, and hydrocephalus [2, 8].

Our findings are in agreement with most reports, the main disagreement with previous reports relates to gene *ZNF238* which although is included in the deleted region no corpus callosum abnormalities were identified. The possibility of identifying specific ultrasonographic markers for 1q43q44 deletion during pregnancy is not clear at the moment because of the limited number of cases described prenatally.

All the above findings highlight the complexity of gene implication/interaction, reflected in the difficulty of genotype-phenotype correlations, and the fact that probable additional mechanisms such as incomplete penetrance, variable expressivity, or multigenic factors may also influence phenotypic expression. Reporting such cases may contribute to better understanding of these issues.

Conflict of Interests

The authors declare that there is no conflict of interests regarding the publication of this paper.

Authors' Contribution

Carolina Sismani and Georgia Christopoulou equally contributed to this paper.

References

[1] S. Rotmensch, M. Liberati, J. S. Luo, G. Tallini, M. J. Mahoney, and J. C. Hobbins, "Prenatal diagnosis of a fetus with terminal deletion of chromosome 1 (q41)," *Prenatal Diagnosis*, vol. 11, no. 11, pp. 867–873, 1991.

[2] C. P. Chen, S. R. Chern, F. J. Tsai et al., "Prenatal diagnosis of partial monosomy 1q (1q42.3 → qter) associated with hydrocephalus and corpus callosum agenesis," *Genetic Counseling*, vol. 21, no. 4, pp. 451–455, 2010.

[3] N. Wagner, E. Guengoer, U. A. Mau-Holzmann et al., "Prenatal diagnosis of a fetus with terminal deletion of chromosome 1 (q43) in first-trimester screening: is there a characteristic antenatal 1q deletion phenotype? A case report and review of the literature," *Fetal Diagnosis and Therapy*, vol. 29, no. 3, pp. 253–256, 2011.

[4] Y. van Bever, L. Rooms, A. Laridon et al., "Clinical report of a pure subtelomeric 1qter deletion in a boy with mental retardation and multiple anomalies adds further evidence for a specific phenotype," *American Journal of Medical Genetics Part A*, vol. 135A, no. 1, pp. 91–95, 2005.

[5] B. C. Ballif, J. A. Rosenfeld, R. Traylor et al., "High-resolution array CGH defines critical regions and candidate genes for microcephaly, abnormalities of the corpus callosum, and seizure phenotypes in patients with microdeletions of 1q43q44," *Human Genetics*, vol. 131, no. 1, pp. 145–156, 2012.

[6] S. C. S. Nagamani, A. Erez, C. Bay et al., "Delineation of a deletion region critical for corpus callosal abnormalities in chromosome 1q43-q44," *European Journal of Human Genetics*, vol. 20, no. 2, pp. 176–179, 2012.

[7] S. J. Perlman, S. Kulkarni, L. Manwaring, and M. Shinawi, "Haploinsufficiency of ZNF238 is associated with corpus callosum abnormalities in 1q44 deletions," *The American Journal of Medical Genetics, Part A*, vol. 161, no. 4, pp. 711–716, 2013.

[8] G. Thierry, C. Bénéteau, O. Pichon et al., "Molecular characterization of 1q44 microdeletion in 11 patients reveals three candidate genes for intellectual disability and seizures," *American Journal of Medical Genetics, Part A*, vol. 158, no. 7, pp. 1633–1640, 2012.

[9] J. K. Rainger, S. Bhatia, H. Bengani et al., "Disruption of SATB2 or its long-range cis-regulation by SOX9 causes a syndromic form of Pierre Robin sequence," *Human Molecular Genetics*, vol. 23, no. 10, Article ID ddt647, pp. 2569–2579, 2014.

[10] S. Benko, J. A. Fantes, J. Amiel et al., "Highly conserved non-coding elements on either side of SOX9 associated with Pierre Robin sequence," *Nature Genetics*, vol. 41, no. 3, pp. 359–364, 2009.

[11] K. Izumi, L. L. Konczal, A. L. Mitchell, and M. C. Jones, "Underlying genetic diagnosis of pierre robin sequence: retrospective chart review at two children's Hospitals and a systematic literature review," *Journal of Pediatrics*, vol. 160, no. 4, pp. 645.e2–650.e2, 2012.

[12] E. Bhoj, S. Halbach, D. Mcdonald-Mcginn et al., "Expanding the spectrum of microdeletion 4q21 syndrome: a partial phenotype with incomplete deletion of the minimal critical region and a new association with cleft palate and pierre robin sequence," *The American Journal of Medical Genetics—Part A*, vol. 161, no. 9, pp. 2327–2333, 2013.

[13] M. Ansari, J. K. Rainger, J. E. Murray et al., "A syndromic form of Pierre Robin sequence is caused by 5q23 deletions encompassing FBN2 and PHAX," *European Journal of Human Genetics*, vol. 57, no. 10, pp. 587–595, 2014.

[14] M. Sun, H. Zhang, G. Li et al., "16p13.3 duplication associated with non-syndromic pierre robin sequence with incomplete penetrance," *Molecular Cytogenetics*, vol. 7, no. 1, article 76, 2014.

6

Absence of Substantial Copy Number Differences in a Pair of Monozygotic Twins Discordant for Features of Autism Spectrum Disorder

Marina Laplana,[1,2] **José Luis Royo,**[1,2] **Anton Aluja,**[3] **Ricard López,**[1,4]
Damià Heine-Sunyer,[5] **and Joan Fibla**[1,2]

[1] *Human Genetic Unit, Department of Basic Medical Sciences, University of Lleida, 25198 Lleida, Catalonia, Spain*
[2] *Genetics of Complex Diseases Research Group, Biomedical Research Institute of Lleida (IRBLleida), 25198 Lleida, Catalonia, Spain*
[3] *Biological-Factorial Models of Personality, Department of Psychology, University of Lleida, 25001 Lleida, Catalonia, Spain*
[4] *Clinical Analysis Service, Universitari Arnau de Vilanova University Hospital, 25198 Lleida, Catalonia, Spain*
[5] *Department of Genetics, Son Espases University Hospital, 07120 Palma de Mallorca, Spain*

Correspondence should be addressed to Joan Fibla; joan.fibla@cmb.udl.cat

Academic Editors: M. G. Kibriya and T. Kubota

Autism spectrum disorder (ASD) is a highly heritable disease (~0.9) with a complex genetic etiology. It is initially characterized by altered cognitive ability which commonly includes impaired language and communication skills as well as fundamental deficits in social interaction. Despite the large amount of studies described so far, the high clinical diversity affecting the autism phenotype remains poorly explained. Recent studies suggest that rare genomic variations, in particular copy number variation (CNV), may account for a significant proportion of the genetic basis of ASD. The use of disease-discordant monozygotic twins represents a powerful strategy to identify *de novo* and inherited CNV in the disorder. Here we present the results of a comparative genome hybridization (CGH) analysis with a pair of monozygotic twins affected of ASD with significant differences in their clinical manifestations that specially affect speech language impairment and communication skills. Array CGH was performed in three different tissues: blood, saliva, and hair follicle, in an attempt to identify germinal and somatic CNV regions that may explain these differences. Our results argue against a role of large CNV rearrangements as a molecular etiology of the observed differences. This forwards future research to explore *de novo* point mutation and epigenomic alterations as potential explanations of the observed clinical differences.

1. Introduction

Autism spectrum disorder (ASD) is characterized by deficits in social interaction and social communication, as well as by the presence of repetitive behaviors, restricted interests, and particular speech impairments. Studies performed in siblings indicate that 85–90% of the ASD variability can be attributed to a genetic basis with a strong genotype-to-phenotype correlation. To date, whole genome association studies and exon sequencing in sporadic patients have revealed a plethora of candidate genes that explain a limited proportion of ASD heritability [1–4]. Copy number variants (CNVs) have been found to cause or predispose to ASDs [5, 6]. Previous works have identified multiple sporadic or recurrent

CNVs, the majority of which occurred to be inherited from asymptomatic parents. Although highly penetrant CNVs or variants inherited in an autosomal recessive manner were detected in rare cases, previous results support the hypothesis that CNVs contribute to ASDs in association with other CNVs or point variants located elsewhere in the genome [5]. Several family history studies have demonstrated a strong familial background on language impairment [7]; however, their association as an endophenotype of ASD has not been systematically explored. Classical studies using a "broader autism phenotype" show a concordance rate of 92% for monozygotic twins and 10% for dizygotic twins [8]. In a more narrow ASD definition, concordance downs to 36%

TABLE 1: Comparative evaluation of TWO and TWX according to Autism Diagnostic Interview-Revised (ADI-R).

	Threshold	TWO		TWX	
		Score	Observation	Score	Observation
Social reciprocal interaction	10	29	Significant	11	Significant
Communication skills	8	13	Significant	11	Significant
Behavior patterns restricted, repetitive, and stereotyped	3	7	Significant	1	Nonsignificant
Developmental difficulties observed before 36 months or less	1	5	Significant	3	Significant

TABLE 2: Comparative evaluation of TWO and TWX according to Vineland adaptive behavior scale (VABS).

Dimensions	TWO		TWX	
	Score	Equivalent age (years old)	Score	Equivalent age (years old)
Adaptive behavior composite	46		84	
Communication	20	1.6	65	3 to 11
Daily living	20	1.4	102	9 to 18
Socialization	20	0.8	96	9 to 18

on monozygotic twins and 0% on dizygotic twins [9]. This later phenotypic discordance corresponds to twin pairs in which autism phenotype shows different degrees of the ASD manifestation. On a common genetic background predisposing to ASD, de novo germline and somatic mutations can differentially affect each twin and modify the ASD clinical manifestation. Newly developed strategies on genetic analysis such as the array comparative genomic hybridization (CGH) allow an in-depth exploration of the genomic structure of discordant siblings. In this work, we have taken advantage of array CGH to compare genomic DNA in three tissues: blood, saliva, and hair follicle, on a pair of discordant monozygotic twins with the aim to identify potential CNVs that could be associated with their differential ASD clinical outcomes.

2. Case Report

Subjects enrolled in the study were both 24-year-old male monozygotic twins denoted by TWO and TWX that were diagnosed with ASD at the age of 4. Parent consent and child assent were obtained prior to participating in this study. Their monozygosity was confirmed by concordance at SNP genotyping giving a probability of concordance by chance $<10^{-20}$. Significant behavior differences were observed between both siblings since their childhood. TWO is entirely dependent on parental care and has serious mental retardation, serious deficiencies in language, and poor social interaction. In contrast, TWX completed basic education studies and professional training that allow workforce participation through social inclusion programs. While maintaining a parental support, this twin's capacity for interaction, including both language and social skills, is great. An in-depth characterization of the twins is presented in Tables 1–3. Autism spectrum diagnosis was assessed by the Autism Diagnostic Interview-Revised (ADI-R) [11] conducted with the parents of the referred twins and covers the subject's full developmental history (Table 1). Due to TWO's language limitations, the accompanying diagnostic test Autism Diagnostic Observation Schedule (ADOS) [12] could only be applied to TWX diagnoses. In spite of

this, the Peabody Picture Vocabulary Test (PPVT-III) [13] was used to assess language capabilities on TWO. This test provides a quick estimate of verbal ability and scholastic aptitude of people who had mental retardation and reading or speech problems. Adaptive functioning was evaluated using the Vineland adaptive behavior scale (VABS) [14], a reliable test to measure a person's adaptive level of functioning at three domain structures: communication, daily living, and socialization (Table 2). The intelligence profile of the twins was assessed by two different tests: the Leiter International Performance Scale-Revised (Leiter-R) [15] applied to TWO and the Wechsler Adult Intelligence Scale (WAIS) [16] applied to TWX. Leiter-R test was devised to assess the intelligence of those with hearing or speech impairment being administered completely without the use of oral language, not even for instructions. All tests were performed by trained professional psychologist of the Institut de Diagnòstic i Atenció Psiquiàtrica i Psicològica (IDAPP) (Barcelona, Spain) and supervised by one of the coauthors (A. Aluja). A summary of the most relevant results obtained in the comparison of the twins' behaviour profile is presented in Table 3. Differences between twins on the communication and language dimension were evidenced. In addition, adaptive behavior course was clearly differentiable as reflected by twin's VABS scores.

According to the Diagnostic and Statistical Manual of Mental Disorders (4th edition) (DSM-IV) [17], TWO meets all criteria for a diagnosis of autistic disorder with moderate mental retardation. In contrast, the lack of stereotyped or repetitive behavior conducted to a diagnosis of pervasive developmental disorder not otherwise specified on TWX. Such clinical presentation contained significant differences that sustained a detailed genetic analysis. Our hypothesis was to consider that somatic mutations affecting CNVs would explain clinical differences. As somatic changes can arise randomly affecting different tissues, we tested three tissues with different embryological origins such as blood, coming from mesoderm, epidermal cells from saliva that has ectodermal origin, and hair follicle cells with ectodermal and neural crest origin [18]. Assuming that clinical difference

TABLE 3: Summary results of the comparative behavioral evaluation of TWO and TWX.

Subject	Tests and measures	Evaluated dimensions				Diagnosis
		Communication and language	Socialization	Behavior patterns and interests	Intellectual ability[1]	
TWO	(i) Parents/ subject interview (ii) PPVT-III (iii) Leiter-R (iv) ADI-R	(i) Strong limitations on communication and language (ii) Great degree of echolalia, repeating everything he says, even playing the same tone of voice (iii) Immediate echolalia of phrases that tell others, as well as echolalia of movie dialogues. Not maintaining reciprocal conversations with others (iv) Not manifesting through language and communicating his moods (v) Spontaneous verbal language not observed	(i) Enjoying verbal positive reinforcement ("good!," "fantastic!," "you are a champion!") and physical (hitting hand or touching his back) (ii) Able to imitate descriptive gestures such as "hello," "throw a kiss," "ok," and "water" and facial expressions and actions like cry, laugh, and "be happy" (iii) Able to recognize and pair "happy" and "sad" emotions in pictures and images	(i) Some stereotyped patterns of behavior (ii) Compulsive behavior by placing well and cleaning up his stuff (iii) Repetitive behavior to remove dirt from under his nails when talking or listening to others (iv) Compulsively cleaning drops that fall to the floor after showering	PPVT-III score: (i) IQ = 55 (ii) mental age equivalency = 3 years Leiter-R scores: (i) fluid reasoning scale: IQ = 48 (ii) spatial visual scale: IQ = 51	DSM-IV: autistic disorder with moderate mental retardation
TWX	(i) Parents/ subject interview (ii) WAIS (iii) ADI-R (iv) ADOS	(i) No echolalia in language (ii) Good level of language that allows good communication skills (iii) Grammatical mistakes that sometimes require clarifications of their explanations (iv) Intonation is rather drab and accompanies his explanations by some stereotype words (v) Conversation with him is hardly mutual, providing information spontaneously but showing little interest in the interlocutor (vi) Nonverbal communication level is adequate, so their explanations are accompanied by gestures appropriately varied and integrated	(i) Social and responsible with their obligations (ii) Sympathetic to the people closest to him (iii) Poorly identifying his own difficulties and how these will interfere in his relations (iv) Eye contact is seen but rather intermittent (v) Facial expressions conveying emotions, some difficulty in identifying and describing by himself.	(i) No repetitive behavior observed	WAIS scores: (i) verbal IQ = 61 (ii) performance IQ = 82 (iii) full scale IQ = 69	DSM-IV: pervasive developmental disorder, not otherwise specified

[1] Range of normal scores = 80–120; average score population = 100.
PPVT-III: Peabody Picture Vocabulary Test. Leiter-R: Leiter International Performance Scale-Revised. ADI-R: Autism Diagnostic Interview-Revised. DSM-IV: Diagnostic and Statistical Manual of Mental Disorders, Fourth Edition. WAIS: Wechsler Adult Intelligence Scale. ADOS: Autism Diagnostic Observation Schedule.

TABLE 4: CNV regions (CNVR) distribution after array CGH comparisons of twin-to-twin (blood) and twin-to-reference (blood, saliva, and hair follicle).

Chr.	Start	End	Size	Number of probes	Twin-to-twin	Twin-to-reference						Number of CNVs at DBGV[1]	Genes contained in CNV region
						Blood		Saliva		Hair follicle			
						TWO	TWX	TWO	TWX	TWO	TWX		
chr1	67955965	68093815	16	16		DEL	DEL	DEL	DEL	DEL	DEL	2	
chr1	72768855	72795480	26625	5		AMP	AMP	AMP	AMP	AMP	AMP	28	
chr1	152556449	152581944	25495	6		DEL	DEL	DEL	DEL	DEL	DEL	25	*LCE3C*
chr2	34697718	34738236	40518	8		AMP	AMP	AMP	AMP	AMP	AMP	12	
chr3	195421860	195444214	22354	9		AMP	AMP	AMP	AMP	AMP	AMP	28	*MIR570*
chr4	69387056	69483277	96221	12		AMP	AMP	AMP	AMP	AMP	AMP	23	*UGT2B17, UGT2B15*
chr6	32455274	32521929	66655	10		DEL	DEL	DEL	DEL	DEL	DEL	52	*HLA-DRB5, HLA-DRB6*
chr6	32611013	32654142	43129	9		DEL	DEL	DEL	DEL	DEL	DEL	40	*HLA-DQA1, HLA-DQB1*
chr8	39234992	39386158	151166	28		AMP	AMP	AMP	AMP	AMP	AMP	25	*ADAM5P, ADAM3A*
chr10	56448627	56468820	20193	5		AMP	AMP	AMP	AMP	AMP	AMP	9	***PCDH15***
chr12	9637323	9698517	61194	8		DEL	DEL	DEL	DEL	DEL	DEL	19	
chr14	19435611	20420849	985238	34		DEL	DEL	DEL	DEL	DEL	DEL	130	*POTEG, P704P, OR4Q3, OR4M1, OR4N2, OR4K2, OR4K5, OR4K1*
chr14	22499836	22968425	468589	102	TWO > TWX	DEL	DEL	—	—	—	—	31	*TCR alpha region*
chr14	105401140	105431289	30149	8		AMP	AMP	AMP	AMP	AMP	AMP	4	*AHNAK2*
chr15	20172544	22835945	2663401	110		AMP	AMP	AMP	AMP	AMP	AMP	282	*GOLGA6L6, GOLGA8C, BCL8, POTEB, NFIP1, LOC646214, CXADRP2, LOC727924, OR4M2, OR4N4, OR4N3P, GOLGA8D, GOLGA6L1,* ***TUBGCP5***
chr20	1563715	1580958	17243	5		DEL	DEL	DEL	DEL	DEL	DEL	27	***SIRPB1***
chr22	24347959	24409603	61644	13		AMP	AMP	AMP	AMP	AMP	AMP	33	*LOC391322, GSTT1, GSTTP2, CABIN1*
chrX (chrY)	70397	2431564	2361167	683	TWO > TWX[2]	DEL	DEL	DEL	DEL	AMP	AMP	106	*PLCXD1, GTPBP6, NCRNA00107, PPP2R3B, SHOX, CRLF2, CSF2RA, IL3RA, SLC25A6, NCRNA00105, ASMTL, P2RY8, SFRSI7A,* ***ASMT,*** *DHRSX, ZBED1*
chrX	53501375	53672366	170991	41		DEL	DEL	DEL	DEL	DEL	DEL	2	***HUWE1,*** *MIR98, MIRLET7F2*

[1] Number of CNVs at Database of Genomic Variants (DBGV, [21]) overlapping CNVR detected.
[2] Amplified in TWO blood.
Highlighted in bold-italics genes previously associated with ASD according to AUTDB [20].

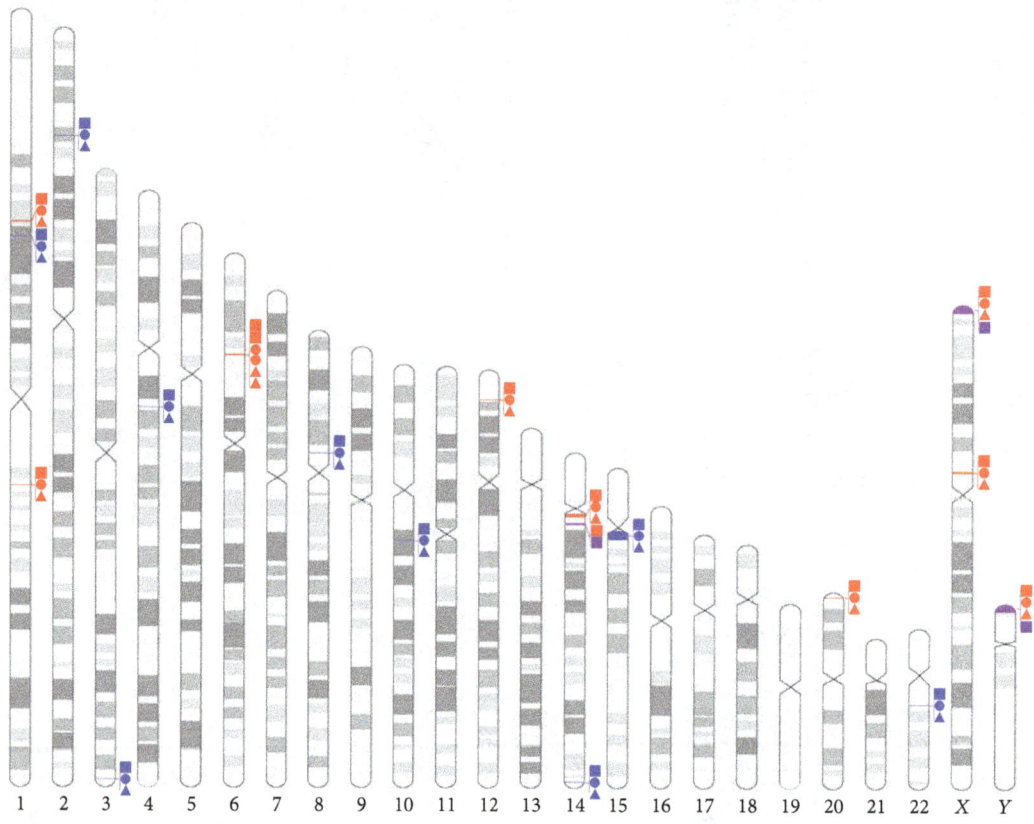

(a)

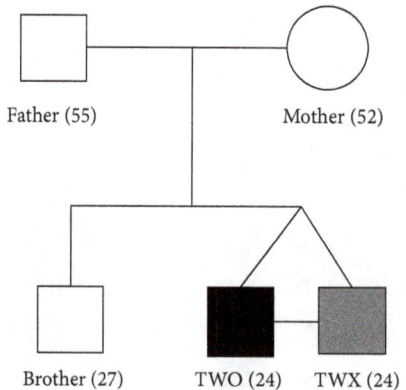

(b)

FIGURE 1: (a) Summary of copy number variant regions identified in this study plotted using *Idiographica* web server [10]. (b) Family pedigree of cases reported.

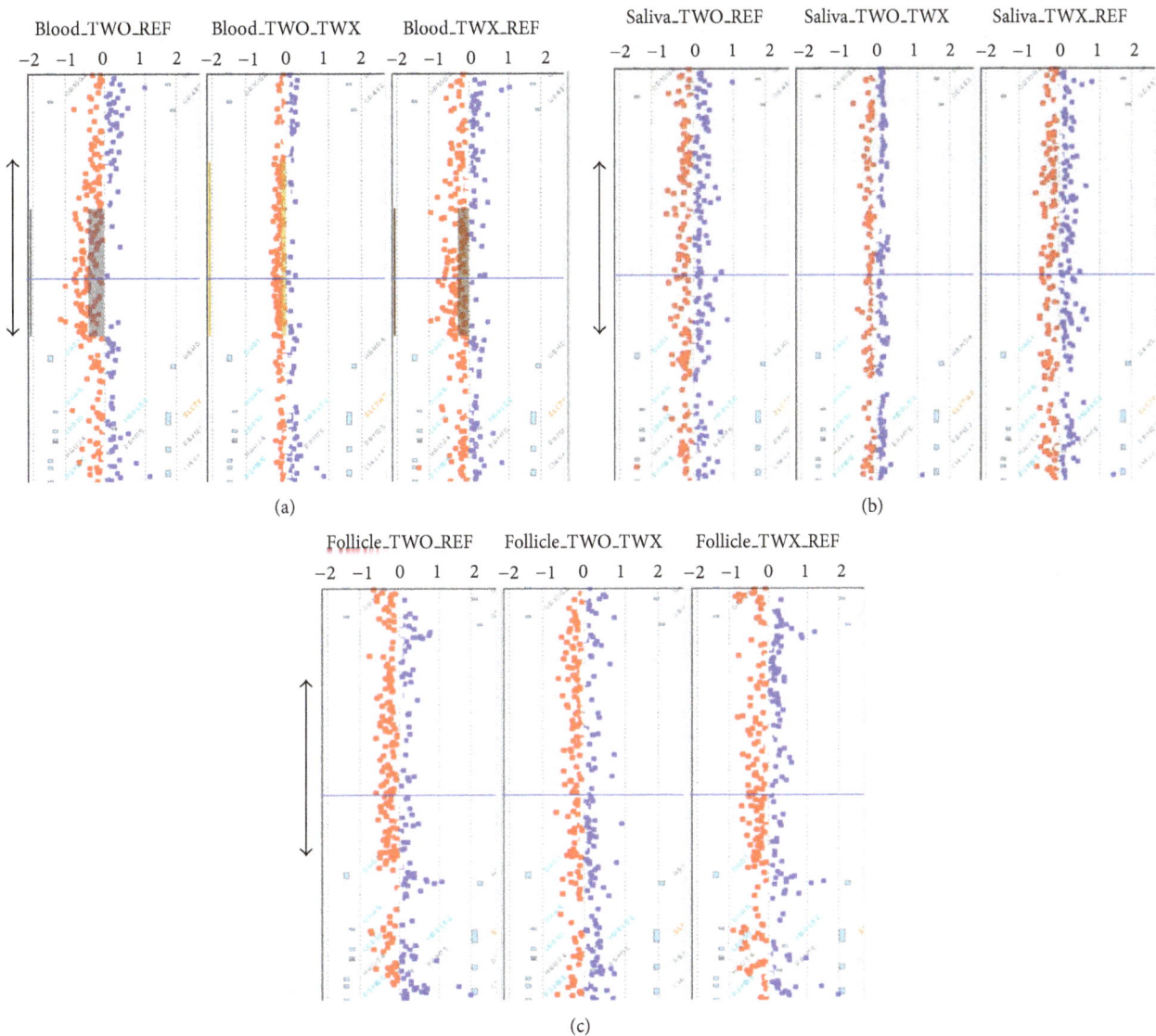

FIGURE 2: Screenshot of Agilent CytoGenomics software corresponding to chr14:22000000-23500000 region. (a) Blood, (b) saliva, and (c) hair follicle. On each panel (left to right) we present the CGH results from TWO-to-reference, twin-to-twin, and TWX-to-reference, respectively. Double arrows delimit the T-cell receptor alpha *locus*.

arises from somatic CNV mutations that affect twin's neural development, the analyses of ectodermal/neural crest derived tissues are of interest.

Samples from blood, saliva, and hair follicle were used to perform a CGH analysis with the Agilent 400 K CGH array (Agilent Technologies, CA, USA) at Oxford Gene Technology facilities (Oxford, UK) according to the manufacturer's instructions. Genomic DNAs from each twin was compared to a reference obtained from a pool of DNAs from five healthy control males matched by age. In addition, a set of twin-to-twin comparisons was also performed. Copy number variation detection was conducted using CytoGenomics software (Agilent Technologies, CA, USA) adjusted at ADM2 algorithm threshold of 4.5 for the twin-to-twin comparisons and ADM2 algorithm threshold of 8 for the twin-to-reference comparisons. CNV regions (CNVR) were those including

a minimum of 4 probes with significant *P* values. All genomic intervals are referred to as hg19. Graphical representation of data was done by Idiographica web server [10] and the Integrative Genome Viewer (IGV) [19]. DataBase of Genomic Variants (DBGV) was used as a source of the literature of described CNVs [21].

3. Results and Discussion

Pedigree examination did not reveal any family history of developmental delay (Figure 1). Normal karyotype analysis was observed in both twins and abnormalities at chromosome X affecting FMR1 *locus* methylation were discarded as an etiology for ASD. Results obtained from array CGH analyses are summarized in Figure 1 and Table 4. When twin's samples were compared to the reference pool a total

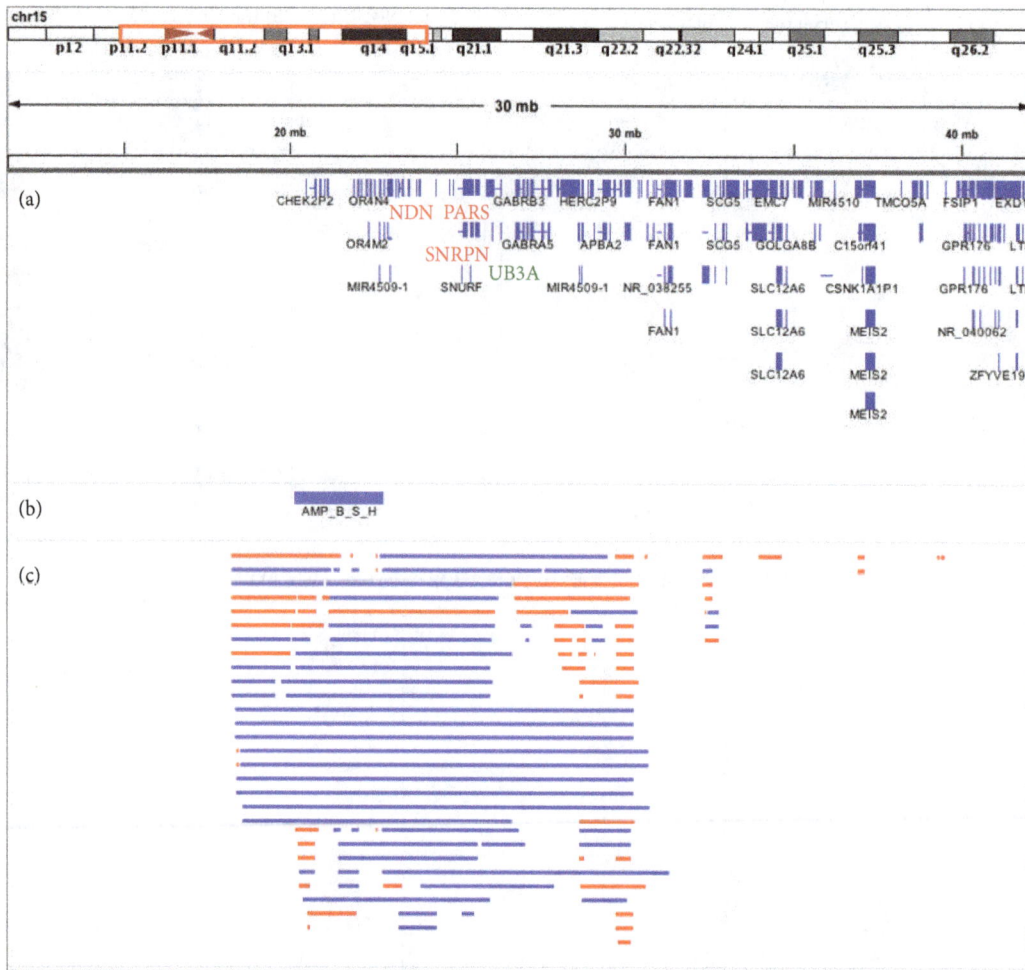

FIGURE 3: Screenshot of IGV [19] showing the 15q pericentromeric region. (a) Representation of the genes found in the vicinity. Those associated with Prader-Willi/Angelman Syndrome are highlighted in red/green, respectively. (b) Illustration of the duplicated region found in TWO and TWX. (c) Representation of the CNVRs from AUTDB previously associated with ASD (amplifications in blue and deletions in red) [20].

of 19 CNVRs were identified. All but two were concordant regardless of the tissue analyzed. The first CNVR affecting chr14:22499836-22968425 shows a complex behavior. This CNVR was observed in both twin-to-twin and twin-to-reference comparisons of blood-derived DNA but neither in saliva nor in hair-follicle-derived DNA, evidencing the existence of somatic mosaicism within twins (Figure 2). A detailed analysis revealed that this region contains the T-cell receptor alpha *locus*, which has been associated with behavioral disturbances [22]. However, the fact that T-cell receptor alpha *locus* is subjected to V(D)J recombination and reported as a commonly *de novo* rearranged region among lymphoblastic cells leads us to be cautious about proposing the involvement of this region in the observed ASD differential outcomes.

The second CNVR with a differential behavior affected chrX:70397-2431564, which corresponds to the pseudoautosomal region of the X-Y chromosomes. This region contains an amplification detected in hair follicle DNA while deleted in blood and saliva tissues. Twin-to-twin comparison revealed amplification in TWO's blood but not in saliva nor in hair. On the other hand, twin-to-reference comparison showed a deletion in blood and saliva, while in hair follicle this region appears amplified. Given these unreliable results we considered the signal at this region not to be trustworthy and discarded it from further characterizations. Therefore, we could conclude that no significant differences in CNVRs between both twins could explain the observed differences on clinical profiles.

Although this is beyond the scope of the present study, we have explored CNV regions that may enlighten about twin's ASD etiology. All 19 regions detected overlap with previously described CNVRs at the DBGV [21]. From a total of 59 genes overlapping CNVRs, four (*HUWE1, TUBGCP5, ASMT,* and *PCDH15*) were found in AUTDB database [20] and to some extent were previously associated with ASD. Nevertheless, the most consistent CNVR with potential association with ASD was observed at chr15:20172544-22835945. This region of chromosome 15q11 was amplified in both twins when compared to reference (Figure 3). It should be noted that deletions but not amplifications on 15q11-q13 have been associated with Prader-Willi Syndrome. On the other hand, amplification affecting 15q11-q13 region has been associated with developmental disorders including autistic behavior [23]. However, our critical region is narrowed to 15q11 and does not include classical Prader-Willi Syndrome associated genes. In addition, CNVs that map within the 15q11.2 *locus* have been identified in autistic individuals in a number of reports. From genes mapping in this region, *NDN* (necdin, melanoma antigen (MAGE) family member), which is thought to be involved in the regulation of neuronal growth, and *CYFIP1* (cytoplasmic FMR1 interacting protein 1) are among the candidate genes proposed by the literature [24, 25]. *NDN* is distal to our critical region, while *CYFIP1* 5′ region is close to the CNVR breakpoint, running the possibility that *CYFIP1* regulatory landscape might be affected. Further analyses will be needed to explore this possibility.

Here we describe the CGH analysis on monozygotic twins affected with ASD but presenting significant clinical differences. Global analysis discarded the role of CNVs to explain these differences, since no variations have been found between both twins beyond the ones observed in the T-cell receptor region. CNV analysis of TWO>TWX in this region rather suggests lack of V(D)J recombination in TWO that should be explored in depth. Negative results should be viewed with caution until methodological limitations are ruled out as a possible explanation. In our case, the followed approach based on array CGH technology has demonstrated enough capability to detect genomic rearrangements affecting specific tissues such as the one we observe at the T-cell receptor alpha *locus*. This reflects that the approach followed in this study has enough sensibility to detect slight somatic differences between both twins. In addition, the detection of this tissue-specific mosaicism highlights the specificity and sensitivity of the array CGH methodology, ruling out methodological limitations as plausible explanation of our negative results. To date, different results can be found in the literature regarding the role of CNV in the etiological basis of disease discordance in monozygotic twins [26–28]. Results here presented are in line with previous works showing a lack of involvement of CNV in the discordant phenotype of monozygotic twins.

The characterization of the genetic etiology underlying the observed clinical differences between TWO and TWX must be addressed to explore *de novo* mutation events not detectable by CGH such as point mutations, as well as epigenomic alterations. Significant correlations between DNA methylation pattern and quantitatively measured autistic trait scores in concordant and discordant twin pairs have been found [29]. Further characterizations of TWO and TWX cases should be necessary to identify the causative genetic/epigenetic component to explain their discordant presentation of ASD.

Conflict of Interests

The authors declare that they have no conflict of interests.

Acknowledgments

The authors wish to acknowledge the patients and their families for their willingness to participate in this study. This project was founded by "*Fundació Marató de TV3*" to Joan Fibla.

References

[1] L. Shi, X. Zhang, R. Golhar et al., "Whole-genome sequencing in an autism multiplex family," *Molecular Autism*, vol. 4, no. 1, article 8, 2013.

[2] L. Liu, A. Sabo, B. M. Neale et al., "Analysis of rare, exonic variation amongst subjects with autism spectrum disorders and population controls," *PLoS Genetics*, vol. 9, no. 4, Article ID e1003443, 2013.

[3] J. J. Michaelson, Y. Shi, M. Gujral et al., "Whole-genome sequencing in autism identifies hot spots for de novo germline mutation," *Cell*, vol. 151, no. 7, pp. 1431–1442, 2012.

[4] M. M. Ghahramani Seno, B. Y. M. Kwan, K. K. M. Lee-Ng et al., "Human PTCHD3 nulls: rare copy number and sequence variants suggest a non-essential gene," *BMC Medical Genetics*, vol. 12, article 45, 2011.

[5] C. Nava, B. Keren, C. Mignot et al., "Prospective diagnostic analysis of copy number variants using SNP microarrays in individuals with autism spectrum disorders," *European Journal of Human Genetics*, 2013.

[6] H. J. Noh, C. P. Ponting, H. C. Boulding et al., "Network topologies and convergent aetiologies arising from deletions and duplications observed in individuals with autism," *PLoS Genetics*, vol. 9, no. 6, Article ID e1003523, 2013.

[7] J. P. H. van Santen, R. W. Sproat, and A. P. Hill, "Quantifying repetitive speech in autism spectrum disorders and language impairment," *Autism Research*, vol. 6, no. 5, pp. 372–383, 2013.

[8] A. Le Couteur, A. Bailey, S. Goode et al., "A broader phenotype of autism: the clinical spectrum in twins," *Journal of Child Psychology and Psychiatry and Allied Disciplines*, vol. 37, no. 7, pp. 785–801, 1996.

[9] S. Folstein and M. Rutter, "Genetic influences and infantile autism," *Nature*, vol. 265, no. 5596, pp. 726–728, 1977.

[10] T. Kin and Y. Ono, "Idiographica: a general-purpose web application to build idiograms on-demand for human, mouse and rat," *Bioinformatics*, vol. 23, no. 21, pp. 2945–2946, 2007.

[11] C. Lord, M. Rutter, and A. L. Couteur, "Autism diagnostic interview-revised: a revised version of a diagnostic interview for caregivers of individuals with possible pervasive developmental disorders," *Journal of Autism and Developmental Disorders*, vol. 24, no. 5, pp. 659–685, 1994.

[12] C. Lord, M. Rutter, S. Goode et al., "Autism diagnostic observation schedule: a standardized observation of communicative and social behavior," *Journal of Autism and Developmental Disorders*, vol. 19, no. 2, pp. 185–212, 1989.

[13] L. M. Dunn and M. D. Douglas, *Peabody Picture Vocabulary Test*, Pearson Education, San Antonio, Tex, USA, 4th edition, 2007.

[14] S. S. Sparrow, D. V. Cicchetti, and D. A. Balla, *Vineland Adaptive Behavior Scales*, AGS, Circle Pines, Minn, USA, 2nd edition, 2005.

[15] G. H. Roid and L. J. Miller, "Leiter international performance scale—revised: examiner's manual," in *Leiter International Performance Scale-Revised*, G. H. Roid and L. J. Miller, Eds., Stoelting Co., Wood Dale, Ill, USA, 1997.

[16] D. Wechler, *Wechsler Adult Intelligence Scale (WAIS)*, Pearson Education, San Antonio, Tex, USA, 4th edition, 2008.

[17] American Psychiatric Association, *Diagnostic and Statistical Manual of Mental Disorders*, American Psychiatric Association, Washington, DC, USA, 4th edition, 2000.

[18] F. G. Scott, R. S. Susan, S. T. Mary, and N. K. Ronald, *Developmental Biology*, Sinauer Associates, Sunderland, Mass, USA, 6th edition, 2000.

[19] J. T. Robinson, H. Thorvaldsdóttir, W. Winckler et al., "Integrative genomics viewer," *Nature Biotechnology*, vol. 29, no. 1, pp. 24–26, 2011.

[20] S. N. Basu, R. Kollu, and S. Banerjee-Basu, "AutDB: a gene reference resource for autism research," *Nucleic Acids Research*, vol. 37, supplement 1, pp. D832–D836, 2009.

[21] A. J. Iafrate, L. Feuk, M. N. Rivera et al., "Detection of large-scale variation in the human genome," *Nature Genetics*, vol. 36, no. 9, pp. 949–951, 2004.

[22] J. Hallmayer, J. Faraco, L. Lin et al., "Narcolepsy is strongly associated with the T-cell receptor alpha locus," *Nature Genetics*, vol. 41, no. 6, pp. 708–711, 2009.

[23] C. C. Swanwick, E. C. Larsen, and S. Banerjee-Basu, "Genetic heterogeneity of autism spectrum disorders," in *Autism Spectrum Disorders: The Role of Genetics in Diagnosis and Treatment*, S. Deutsch, Ed., pp. 65–82, InTech Open Access Publisher, 2011.

[24] T. K. Chibuk, J. M. Bischof, and R. Wevrick, "A necdin/MAGE-like gene in the chromosome 15 autism susceptibility region: expression, imprinting, and mapping of the human and mouse orthologues," *BMC Genetics*, vol. 2, article 22, 2001.

[25] S. de Rubeis and C. Bagni, "Regulation of molecular pathways in the fragile X syndrome: insights into autism spectrum disorders," *Journal of Neurodevelopmental Disorders*, vol. 3, no. 3, pp. 257–269, 2011.

[26] R. J. Bloom, A. K. Kähler, A. L. Collins et al., "Comprehensive analysis of copy number variation in monozygotic twins discordant for bipolar disorder or schizophrenia," *Schizophrenia Research*, vol. 146, no. 1–3, pp. 289–290, 2013.

[27] E. A. Ehli, A. Abdellaoui, Y. Hu et al., "De novo and inherited CNVs in MZ twin pairs selected for discordance and concordance on attention problems," *European Journal of Human Genetics*, vol. 20, no. 10, pp. 1037–1043, 2012.

[28] S. Ono, A. Imamura, S. Tasaki et al., "Failure to confirm CNVs as of aetiological significance in twin pairs discordant for schizophrenia," *Twin Research and Human Genetics*, vol. 13, no. 5, pp. 455–460, 2010.

[29] C. Y. Wong, E. L. Meaburn, A. Ronald et al., "Methylomic analysis of monozygotic twins discordant for autism spectrum disorder and related behavioural traits," *Molecular Psychiatry*, 2013.

7

Novel Mutation in a Patient with Cholesterol Ester Storage Disease

Patrick Lin,[1,2] **Sheela Raikar,**[1,2,3] **Jennifer Jimenez,**[1,2,3]
Katrina Conard,[4] **and Katryn N. Furuya**[1,2,3]

[1]*Department of Pediatrics, Nemours/Alfred I. duPont Hospital for Children, Wilmington, DE 19803, USA*
[2]*Thomas Jefferson University, Philadelphia, PA 19107, USA*
[3]*Division of Pediatric Gastroenterology, Hepatology, and Nutrition, Nemours/Alfred I. duPont Hospital for Children, Wilmington, DE 19803, USA*
[4]*Department of Clinical and Anatomic Pathology, Nemours/Alfred I. duPont Hospital for Children, Wilmington, DE 19803, USA*

Correspondence should be addressed to Katryn N. Furuya; kfuruya@nemours.org

Academic Editor: Yoshiyuki Ban

Cholesterol ester storage disease (CESD) is a chronic liver disease that typically presents with hepatomegaly. It is characterized by hypercholesterolemia, hypertriglyceridemia, high-density lipoprotein deficiency, and abnormal lipid deposition within multiple organs. It is an autosomal recessive disease that is due to a deficiency in lysosomal acid lipase (LAL) activity, which is coded by the lysosomal acid lipase gene (LIPA). We describe the case of a 5-year-old south Asian female incidentally found to have hepatomegaly, and subsequent workup confirmed the diagnosis of CESD. DNA sequencing confirmed the presence of a novel hepatic mutation. It is a four-nucleotide deletion c.57_60delTGAG in exon 2 of the LIPA gene. This mutation is predicted to result in a premature translation stop downstream of the deletion (p.E20fs) and, therefore, is felt to be a disease-causing mutation.

1. Introduction

Cholesterol ester storage disease (CESD) is a chronic liver disease that typically presents with hepatomegaly. It is associated with hypercholesterolemia, hypertriglyceridemia, high-density lipoprotein (HDL) deficiency, and abnormal lipid deposition within multiple organs [1]. It is an autosomal recessive disease that is due to a deficiency in lysosomal acid lipase (LAL) activity. LAL hydrolyzes cholesterol esters and triglycerides within the lysosomes of hepatocytes. In the absence of LAL, lipid builds up in the endoplasmic reticulum of hepatocytes. This leads to the development of hepatic steatosis with the eventual development of fibrosis and micronodular cirrhosis [2, 3].

Disease-causing mutations in the LAL gene (lysosomal acid lipase gene [LIPA]) may result in the clinical presentation of CESD or Wolman disease (WD). Wolman disease is a severe, early-onset presentation caused by a mutation in the LIPA gene that results in the absence of LAL activity [2]. It

is typically fatal within the first few months of life. On the other hand, CESD is more prevalent than WD and typically presents later in life. We present a patient with CESD who has a novel disease-causing mutation in the LIPA gene.

2. Case Presentation

A 5-year-old south Asian female was incidentally found to have hepatomegaly on a trip to India, where she became acutely ill with fever, vomiting, and abdominal pain. Blood work done at that time demonstrated mildly elevated liver function tests (AST 48 U/L, ALT 80 U/L), and an abdominal ultrasound revealed hepatomegaly without biliary or splenic abnormalities. She was prescribed an antibiotic and her symptoms gradually resolved.

A month after her return to the United States, her pediatrician noted persistent hepatomegaly and the new development of fever. She was referred to the emergency department because of suspicion of a tropical infectious

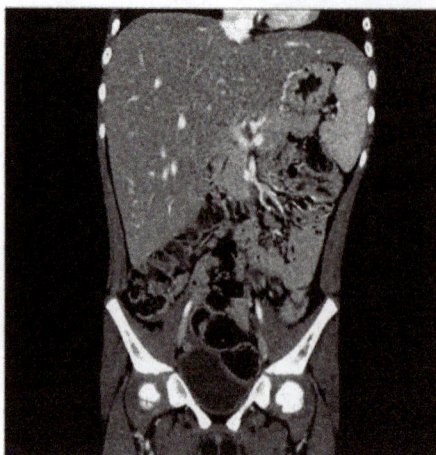

FIGURE 1: Computed tomography of abdomen and pelvis. The liver is enlarged, measuring up to 17 cm in width and craniocaudal dimension. The contour is smooth. The hepatic parenchyma is homogenous without a focal mass. There is no intrahepatic biliary dilatation. The portal and hepatic venous systems are patent and nondilated.

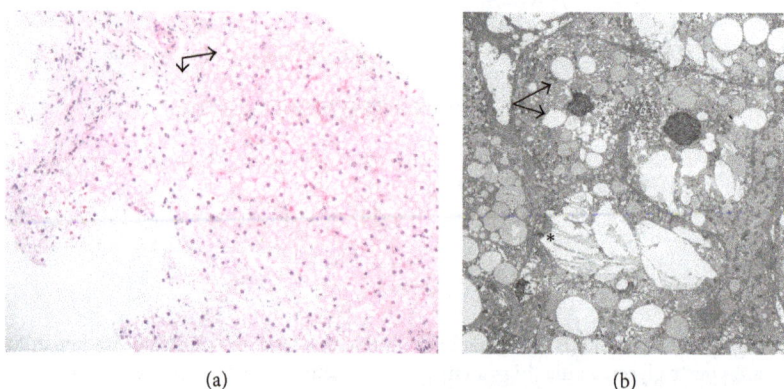

(a)   (b)

FIGURE 2: (a) Liver biopsy, periodic acid-Schiff stain with diastase (magnification, ×40). Lipid demonstrated within the hepatocellular cytoplasm (arrows). (b) Electron micrograph (direct magnification, ×2500). The hepatocellular cytoplasm in places has a moth-eaten appearance with lipid droplets (arrows). Additionally, some foci show cholesterol crystals (∗) free in the hepatocellular cytoplasm.

disease. A repeat ultrasound demonstrated persistent hepatomegaly. Her transaminases (AST 133 U/L, ALT 112 U/L) remained elevated. The infectious workup was negative for cytomegalovirus, hepatitis A, Lyme disease, and malaria. She did have a positive Epstein-Barr virus IgM. Repeat blood work was obtained at follow-up infectious disease clinic visit where she was again found to have hepatomegaly (7 cm below the costal margin) and mildly abnormal transaminases. A computed tomography of the abdomen and pelvis (Figure 1) was performed that demonstrated hepatomegaly but had otherwise normal findings. Her fever resolved within 2 weeks. She was otherwise well and was not on any medications. There was no family history of liver disease. Her immunizations were up to date. Because of persistent hepatomegaly, she was referred to the liver clinic.

In the liver clinic, she was noted to have an enlarged, firm liver, palpable 8 cm below the costal margin with no associated splenomegaly. Test results for autoimmune hepatitis, WD, and alpha-1-antitrypsin deficiency were negative. Nonfasting lipid levels were abnormal; repeat testing showed

a fasting total cholesterol of 305 mg/dL and a triglyceride level of 142 mg/dL.

On the basis of a clinical suspicion of a diagnosis of CESD, a liver biopsy was performed. It revealed diffuse, microvesicular steatosis in the hepatic parenchyma (Figure 2(a)). Portal tracts were expanded by foamy macrophages containing finely vacuolated material, which was periodic acid-Schiff positive and resistant to diastase digestion. Trichrome stain for collagen showed mild portal fibrosis with early delicate bridging fibrosis. Ultrastructurally, the cytoplasm had a moth-eaten appearance with the presence of lipid droplets and cholesterol crystals (Figure 2(b)). There was no evidence of hepatocellular necrosis, cholestasis, or bile duct proliferation.

Liver tissue was sent to Dr. D. Wenger's Lysosomal Diseases Testing Laboratory at Thomas Jefferson University. She was found to have a low acid lipase activity of 7.2 (no units provided by Dr. D. Wenger's laboratory) in the liver. Follow-up testing through a commercial laboratory demonstrated low level of lysosomal acid lipase activity (0.008 nmol/punch/h) in blood. Lysosomal acid lipase gene sequence analysis was performed, which demonstrated that she was heterozygous for the following two mutations: c.57_60delTGAG and c.894G>A. Both parents underwent mutation analysis. The mother was confirmed to have the c.894G>A mutation while the father carried the c.57_60delTGAG mutation. The c.57_60delTGAG is a new mutation not previously described in the literature in patients with CESD.

3. Discussion

Cholesterol ester storage disease is an autosomal recessive, chronic liver disease caused by LAL deficiency. Its cognate gene is located on chromosome 10q23.3-q23.3 [2]. Lysosomal acid lipase hydrolyzes cholesterol esters and triglycerides that are delivered to the lysosomes by receptor-mediated endocytosis, and deficiency states result in accumulation of both cholesterol esters and triglycerides in hepatocytes [2]. Mutations in this gene cause two distinct phenotypes: WD and CESD. Both are characterized by hypercholesterolemia, hypertriglyceridemia, HDL deficiency, and hepatomegaly secondary to hepatic steatosis [2]. Complete absence of LAL activity results in WD, whereas CESD is due to mutations that result in partial loss of enzyme activity. Children diagnosed with CESD generally have a better prognosis but may often still require liver transplantation during their lifetime. They are also at risk for developing complications from cardiac disease.

Our patient's symptoms and presentation are typical of CESD. The histologic and ultrastructural examination of the liver along with markedly low LAL activity confirmed this diagnosis. DNA sequencing confirmed the presence of a novel hepatic mutation. It is a four-nucleotide deletion, c.57_60delTGAG in exon 2 of the LIPA gene. This mutation is predicted to result in a premature translation stop downstream of the deletion (p.E20fs) and, therefore, is felt to be a disease-causing mutation [4]. The second mutation noted in our patient is a previously described disease-causing mutation, c.894G>A change in exon 8 of the LIPA gene, which results in altered mRNA splicing and exon 8 skipping [5].

Current management is limited to preventing adverse effects of dyslipidemia. The use of statins [6, 7] and other cholesterol lowering agents such as cholestyramine and ezetimibe [1, 8, 9] has been associated with decreasing total cholesterol and increasing HDL, which is cardioprotective. Due to the young age of our patient, neither statins nor ezetimibe were prescribed for her hypercholesterolemia. In addition, lipid accumulation in the liver is not reversed with these medications. Patients may go on to develop cirrhosis and liver failure. Liver transplantation as a therapeutic option has been successfully used [1, 10, 11]. Direct enzyme replacement therapy with sebelipase alfa has been recently developed by Synageva BioPharma (Lexington, MA, USA) and is currently undergoing human trials [3, 12]. It has been recently reported in a phase 3 double blind placebo controlled trial that sebelipase alfa replacement enzyme therapy resulted in an improvement in ALT and AST with a relative reduction in hepatic fat fraction [13]. Thus, enzyme replacement therapy is a promising therapy that may change the long term outcome for patients with WD and CESD.

Disclosure

Patrick Lin and Sheela Raikar are co-first authors.

Conflict of Interests

The authors declare that there is no conflict of interests regarding the publication of this paper.

References

[1] D. L. Bernstein, H. Hülkova, M. G. Bialer, and R. J. Desnick, "Cholesteryl ester storage disease: review of the findings in 135 reported patients with an underdiagnosed disease," *Journal of Hepatology*, vol. 58, no. 6, pp. 1230–1243, 2013.

[2] S. Muntoni, H. Wiebusch, M. Jansen-Rust et al., "Prevalence of cholesteryl ester storage disease," *Arteriosclerosis, Thrombosis, and Vascular Biology*, vol. 27, no. 8, pp. 1866–1868, 2007.

[3] T. Reynolds, "Cholesteryl ester storage disease: a rare and possibly treatable cause of premature vascular disease and cirrhosis," *Journal of Clinical Pathology*, vol. 66, no. 11, pp. 918–923, 2013.

[4] C. S. Richards, S. Bale, D. B. Bellissimo et al., "ACMG recommendations for standards for interpretation and reporting of sequence variations: revisions 2007," *Genetics in Medicine*, vol. 10, no. 4, pp. 294–300, 2008.

[5] H. Klima, K. Ullrich, C. Aslanidis, P. Fehringer, K. J. Lackner, and G. Schmitz, "A splice junction mutation causes deletion of a 72-base exon from the mRNA for lysosomal acid lipase in a patient with cholesteryl ester storage disease," *The Journal of Clinical Investigation*, vol. 92, no. 6, pp. 2713–2718, 1993.

[6] B. Dalgiç, S. Sari, M. Gündüz et al., "Cholesteryl ester storage disease in a young child presenting as isolated hepatomegaly treated with simvastatin," *The Turkish Journal of Pediatrics*, vol. 48, no. 2, pp. 148–151, 2006.

[7] S. A. Iverson, S. R. Cairns, C. P. Ward, and A. H. Fensom, "Asymptomatic cholesteryl ester storage disease in an adult controlled with simvastatin," *Annals of Clinical Biochemistry*, vol. 34, no. 4, pp. 433–436, 1997.

[8] L. Leone, P. F. Ippoliti, and R. Antonicelli, "Use of simvastatin plus cholestyramine in the treatment of lysosomal acid lipase deficiency," *The Journal of Pediatrics*, vol. 119, no. 6, pp. 1008–1009, 1991.

[9] V. T. Tadiboyina, D. M. Liu, B. A. Miskie, J. Wang, and R. A. Hegele, "Treatment of dyslipidemia with lovastatin and ezetimibe in an adolescent with cholesterol ester storage disease," *Lipids in Health and Disease*, vol. 4, article 26, 2005.

[10] J. N. Arterburn, W. M. Lee, R. P. Wood, B. W. Shaw, and R. S. Markin, "Orthotopic liver transplantation for cholesteryl ester storage disease," *Journal of Clinical Gastroenterology*, vol. 13, no. 4, pp. 482–484, 1991.

[11] G. D. Ferry, H. H. Whisennand, M. J. Finegold, E. Alpert, and A. Glombicki, "Liver transplantation for cholesteryl ester storage disease," *Journal of Pediatric Gastroenterology and Nutrition*, vol. 12, no. 3, pp. 376–378, 1991.

[12] H. Du, T. L. Cameron, S. J. Garger et al., "Wolman disease/cho-
     lesteryl ester storage disease: efficacy of plant-produced human
     lysosomal acid lipase in mice," *The Journal of Lipid Research*, vol.
     49, no. 8, pp. 1646–1657, 2008.

[13] M. Balwani, B. Burton, I. Baric et al., "Results of a global phase 3,
     randomized, double-blind, placebo-controlled trial evaluation
     the efficacy and therapy in children and adults with lysosomal
     acid lipase deficiency," *Hepatology*, vol. 60, no. 6, p. 127, 2014.

8

Exceptional Complex Chromosomal Rearrangements in Three Generations

Hannie Kartapradja,[1] **Nanis Sacharina Marzuki,**[1] **Mark D. Pertile,**[2]
David Francis,[2] **Lita Putri Suciati,**[1] **Helena Woro Anggaratri,**[1] **Debby Dwi Ambarwati,**[1]
Firman Prathama Idris,[1] **Harry Lesmana,**[1] **Hidayat Trimarsanto,**[1,3]
Chrysantine Paramayuda,[1] **and Alida Roswita Harahap**[1]

[1]*Eijkman Institute for Molecular Biology, Jl. Diponegoro 69, Jakarta 10430, Indonesia*
[2]*Victorian Clinical Genetics Services (VCGS), Royal Children's Hospital, Flemington Road, Melbourne, VIC 3052, Australia*
[3]*Agency for the Assessment and Application of Technology, Jl. MH Thamrin 8, Jakarta 10340, Indonesia*

Correspondence should be addressed to Hannie Kartapradja; hannie@eijkman.go.id

Academic Editor: Evica Rajcan-Separovic

We report an exceptional complex chromosomal rearrangement (CCR) found in three individuals in a family that involves 4 chromosomes with 5 breakpoints. The CCR was ascertained in a phenotypically abnormal newborn with additional chromosomal material on the short arm of chromosome 4. Maternal karyotyping indicated that the mother carried an apparently balanced CCR involving chromosomes 4, 6, 11, and 18. Maternal transmission of the derivative chromosome 4 resulted in partial trisomy for chromosomes 6q and 18q and a partial monosomy of chromosome 4p in the proband. Further family studies found that the maternal grandmother carried the same apparently balanced CCR as the proband's mother, which was confirmed using the whole chromosome painting (WCP) FISH. High resolution whole genome microarray analysis of DNA from the proband's mother found no evidence for copy number imbalance in the vicinity of the CCR translocation breakpoints, or elsewhere in the genome, providing evidence that the mother's and grandmother's CCRs were balanced at a molecular level. This structural rearrangement can be categorized as an exceptional CCR due to its complexity and is a rare example of an exceptional CCR being transmitted in balanced and/or unbalanced form across three generations.

1. Introduction

Constitutional complex chromosomal rearrangements (CCRs) usually involve at least two chromosomes and three breakpoints with varied outcomes (simple or 3-break insertions are excluded) [1–4]. These abnormalities may involve distal segments causing reciprocal translocation, or interstitial segments leading to insertion, inversion, deletion, or duplication, or they may involve a combination of both distal and interstitial segments [1, 3]. One chromosome may also have more than one aberration such as an inversion and a translocation that can coexist on the same chromosome [1].

The phenotype of the CCR carrier varies from normal to abnormal with congenital abnormalities and/or intellectual disability. The likelihood of an abnormal phenotype increases with the number of breakpoints associated with the de novo, apparently balanced CCR (BCCR) [5–7]. Approximately 255 cases of CCRs involving three or more chromosomes have been published. Cases involving 4 chromosomes with 5 breakpoints are classified as exceptional and can be highly complex in nature [4]. The risk of spontaneous abortion in a pregnancy from a CCR carrier can be as high as 50 to 100% [5], whereas 18% of all live births to CCR carriers result in phenotypically abnormal offspring [8]. According to Gardner and Sutherland [1], CCRs can be classified into three groups based on the number of breakpoints and type of arrangement. These are the following. (1) *Three-way exchange with three breaks from three chromosomes*: most three-way CCRs are

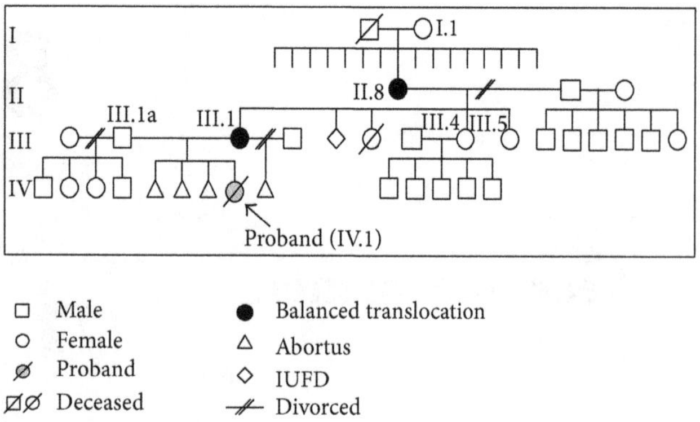

FIGURE 1: Pedigree of the family.

familial and are usually transmitted through the mother. They are the most common type of CCRs. (2) *Double two-way exchange with a coincidence of two separate simple reciprocal translocations*: the double two-way CCR is not a true CCR and might be described as a double or a multiple rearrangement. (3) *Exceptional CCRs with more complicated rearrangements*: most exceptional CCRs are de novo rearrangements and they are more commonly associated with abnormal phenotype.

Most familial transmissions of CCRs are through the mother [2, 6]. Phenotypically normal female BCCR carriers are usually ascertained following investigation for recurrent abortions or after the birth of an abnormal child. In contrast, phenotypically normal BCCR males are more frequently ascertained following investigation for infertility [6, 8–10]. Here we report a very rare familial exceptional CCR in 3 generations which includes two normal phenotype BCCR individuals.

2. Case Presentation

The proband was a one-day-old female referred to our clinic for chromosome analysis. She had multiple congenital anomalies with facial dysmorphism, cleft lip, micrognathia, and intrauterine growth retardation (IUGR). Her weight was 1630 grams and length 38 cm. The proband (individual IV.1) was delivered from an uneventful, full term pregnancy of a 30-year-old mother with an obstetrical status of $G_5P_1A_4$ from 2 marriages. The four previous pregnancies ended in abortions at around 20 weeks of gestation. The maternal grandmother of the proband (individual II.8) was the 8th of 16 normal phenotype siblings. Her 4th child, who died at 8 months old without any specific causes, was born prematurely with normal phenotype. The great grandmother from the mother's lineage (individual I.1) has 16 children with no miscarriage history. The proband's aunt (individual III.4) has 5 phenotypically normal sons and another aunt (individual III.5) was not involved in this study (Figure 1). Patient histories were negative for radiation exposure and drug consumption during pregnancy.

Cytogenetic investigations were carried out on 20 metaphase cells of phytohaemagglutinin- (PHA-) stimulated peripheral blood cultures using standard procedures,

and high resolution GTL banding was performed. Analysis undertaken on metaphase chromosomes from the proband at the 550-band level according to ISCN 2009 [11] showed the unbalanced karyotype: 46,XX,der(4)(18qter → q21.3::6q13q21::4p14 → qter)mat (Figure 2(a)). This result was determined after analysis of the mother's karyotype showed a BCCR with karyotype 46,XX,der(4)(18qter → q21.3::6q13q21::4p14 → qter),der(6)t(4;6)(p14;q21),der(11)t(6;11)(q21;q21),der(18)t(11; 18)(q21;q21.3) (Figure 2(b)). We extended our chromosome analysis to other family members and found the maternal grandmother (individual II.8) had the same BCCR as the proband's mother. The great grandmother (I.1) and another aunt of the proband (individual III.4) had normal karyotypes, which suggested that the BCCR arose as a de novo event in the proband's grandmother. This conclusion is based on the premise that the deceased great grandfather is very unlikely to have carried the BCCR, as he fathered 16 normal phenotype children in the absence of miscarriage.

To confirm the BCCR karyotyping result, we performed whole chromosome painting FISH (WCP FISH) (Cytocell Technologies Ltd., Cambridge, UK) using probes for chromosomes 4, 6, 11, and 18 on chromosome spreads from the mother and grandmother of the proband, using standard techniques. The hybridisation patterns were consistent with the karyotyping results (Figure 3). Figure 4 shows a cartoon summary of the BCCR based on the karyotype and whole chromosome painting FISH results.

To investigate whether the BCCR was balanced at a molecular level, we analysed DNA from the proband's mother using Affymetrix CytoScan HD microarray (Affymetrix, Santa Clara, CA, USA), with interpretation based on the NCBI36/hg18 (March 2006) human reference sequence. The microarray result showed no clinically significant genomic imbalance. In particular, there was no evidence for copy number imbalance on chromosomes 4, 6, 11, and 18 in the regions of the translocation breakpoints. Therefore, the CCR appeared to be balanced at the effective resolution of this array (approximately 25–50 kb).

3. Discussion

Complex chromosome rearrangements like the one segregating in this family are categorized as exceptional CCRs, which are the most complicated form of CCRs. This complexity results in a greater potential for producing unbalanced gametes during meiosis. A successful pregnancy is rare because the BCCR carrier has a risk for an abnormal conception due to either malsegregation of derivative chromosomes or generation of recombinant chromosomes [1]. According to Gorski et al. [8], there are 4 possible pregnancy outcomes for the BCCR carrier; these are abortion, a liveborn infant with unbalanced chromosomes, an infant carrying the BCCR, or a liveborn infant with normal chromosomes. In the familial exceptional CCR cases described here, we found one case of normal phenotype associated with de novo BCCR (maternal grandmother), one case of normal phenotype associated with maternal inheritance of the BCCR (mother), and one

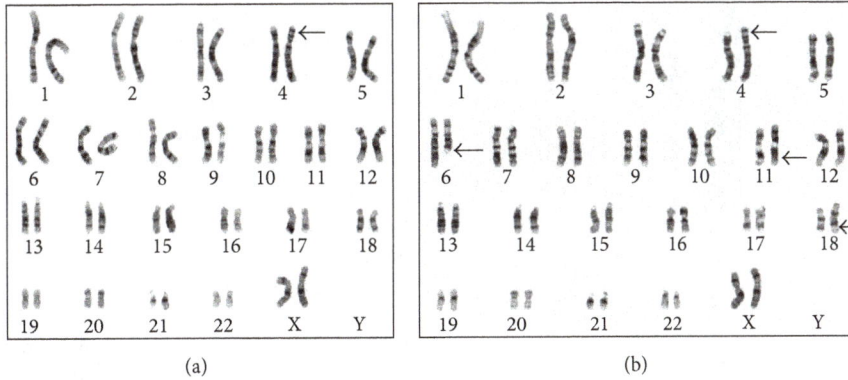

FIGURE 2: Karyotyping result: (a) proband and (b) mother and grandmother.

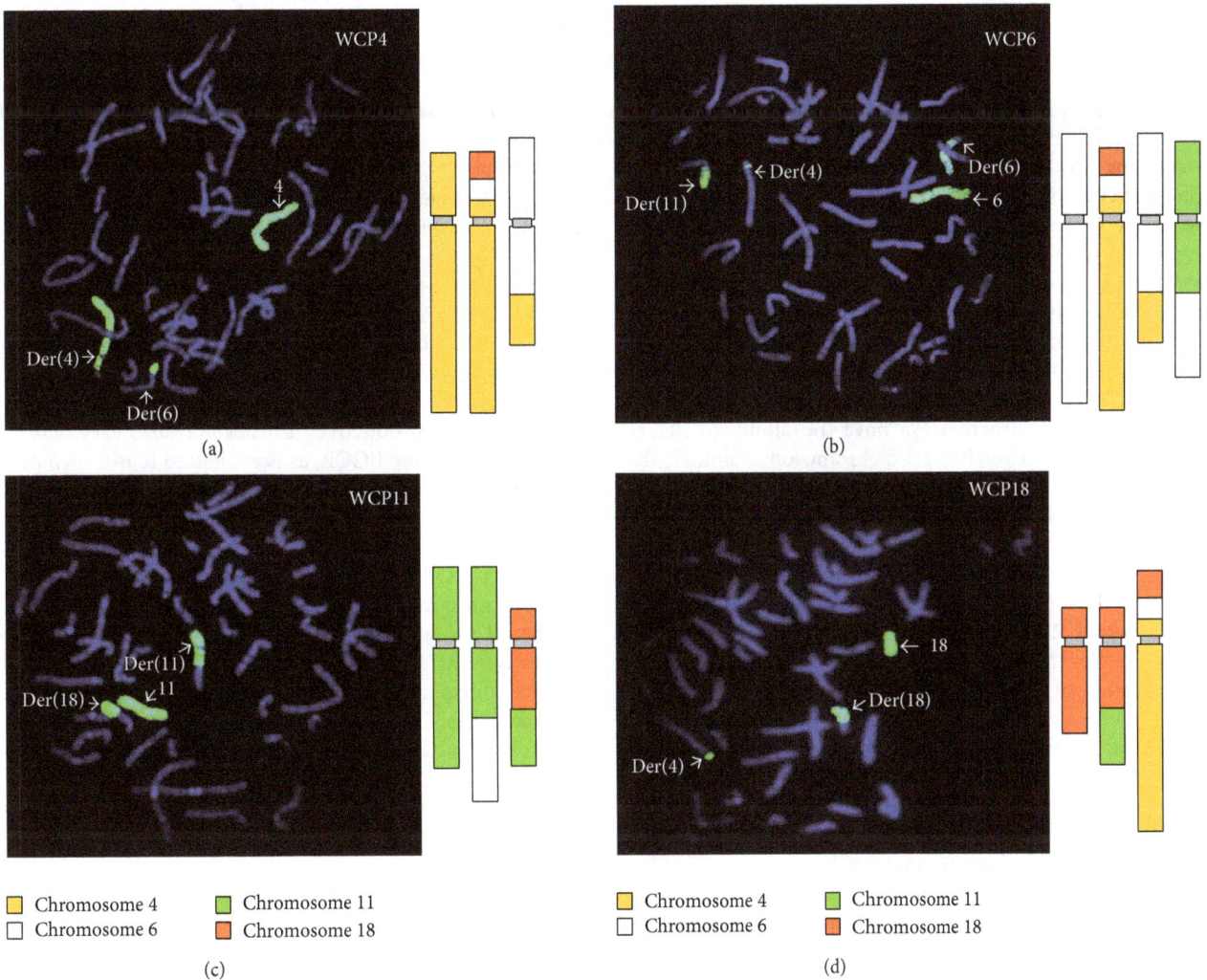

FIGURE 3: Whole chromosome painting FISH: (a) chromosome 4, (b) chromosome 6, (c) chromosome 11, and (d) chromosome 18.

case of abnormal phenotype due to maternal inheritance of an unbalanced form of the CCR (proband). Several familial CCRs reported previously described mostly unbalanced karyotypes [12–15]. In addition, the proband's aunty has inherited normal chromosomes from her BCCR carrier mother. Her normal karyotype result is consistent with her unremarkable reproductive history of 5 phenotypically normal sons and no miscarriages (Figure 1).

WCP FISH was performed to confirm the chromosome rearrangement identified by conventional karyotyping. WCP

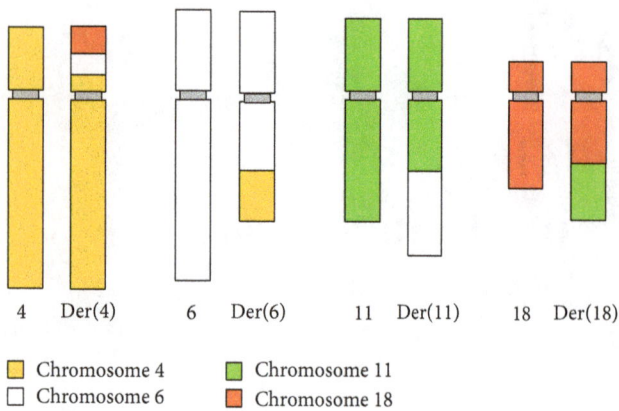

FIGURE 4: Cartoon summary of the BCCR carried by the proband's mother and grandmother.

FISH is a highly sensitive and specific technique that can be used to identify both numerical and structural chromosomal aberrations [16, 17], as well as cryptic genomic imbalances from individuals with apparently balanced chromosomal rearrangements [18, 19]. This technique is a very useful and necessary tool to help characterise the CCR [18–22]. As shown in Figure 3, the WCP FISH supported the karyotype findings and helped confirm the insertional rearrangement of a segment of chromosome 6q into the short arm of chromosome 4, lending support to this CCR being balanced at the cytogenetic level in the proband's mother and grandmother.

Whole genome microarrays have the ability to detect unbalanced de novo and inherited chromosomal abnormalities smaller than 3–5 Mb in size, which is below the resolution of conventional karyotyping [18, 19, 23, 24]. In this study, microarray analysis was used to confirm the apparently balanced nature of the CCR carried by the proband's mother. No evidence for copy number imbalance was observed around the CCR breakpoints, or elsewhere in the genome, which excludes the presence of smaller, cryptic imbalances at the resolution of this array. This analysis supports the CCR being balanced at a molecular level and is consistent with the normal phenotype of BCCR carriers in this pedigree. A repeat sample from the proband was not available for microarray analysis, which would have been helpful to more accurately characterise the CCR breakpoints in the derivative chromosome 4. Microarray analysis has become a valuable tool for investigating apparently balanced chromosomal rearrangements associated with abnormal phenotype, where cryptic deletions below the resolution of light microscopy are often detected around the translocation breakpoints [18, 19]. Unbalanced rearrangements can also be characterised more fully at the molecular level.

A minimum of 70 unbalanced gametes are theoretically possible due to 4:4, 5:3, 6:2, and 7:1 segregations from an octavalent in the case of a CCR involving five breakpoints in four chromosomes [1]. The proband's abnormal karyotype is the result of a 4:4 unbalanced segregation, which is responsible for her abnormal phenotype. The derivative chromosome 4 harbours two additional segments that involve an insertion from chromosome 6q and a translocation from chromosome 18q, which leads to partial trisomy for these chromosomes, in addition to a partial monosomy of 4p. This derivative chromosome is the result of meiotic events producing abnormal gametes [25]. The risk of abnormal offspring from BCCR carriers in this family is high due to the large number of chromosomes and breakpoints involved. Based on a calculation of 4:4 segregation, the possibility of inheriting the balanced form of this CCR is only 2.8% given random segregation of octavalent chromosomes. This is supported by several previous reports [8, 26]. Gorski et al. [8] reported that the higher the number of chromosomal breakpoints and the more complex the chromosomal rearrangement, the higher the ratio of gametes with abnormal chromosomes.

Familial transmission of the BCCR in our pedigree was through female carriers. This is supported by previous reports that record familial transmissions occurring mainly through female carriers [4, 6, 21]. Gardner and Sutherland [1] and Pellestor et al. [4] reported that BCCR in males can cause subfertility and sterility due to disturbances of gametogenesis, whereas in females gametogenesis can escape from this complexity. Thus, females with BCCR can be fertile, have pregnancies, and potentially deliver normal children. This is consistent with the evidence from our pedigree, which includes two healthy female carriers in whom the rearrangements are balanced and another who has inherited normal chromosomes from a BCCR carrier female.

Due to the complex nature of BCCRs, genetic counselling will always be difficult. The reproductive risk is very specific for each carrier, and the precise risk may be impossible to establish [9]. Reproductive histories may also vary between carriers of the same BCCR, as is evidenced in our own pedigree, where the proband's mother has a poorer reproductive history than the proband's grandmother.

In conclusion, the proband's abnormal clinical presentation was caused by inheriting a derivative chromosome 4, which is an unbalanced form of the BCCR carried by her mother. Although the possibility of having a normal child is greatly reduced, a daughter has inherited the CCR in its balanced form, and another daughter has inherited normal chromosomes. This case is instructive in demonstrating that an exceptional BCCR can be inherited in its full balanced form to the next generation.

Conflict of Interests

The authors declare that there is no conflict of interests regarding the publication of this paper.

Acknowledgments

The authors are extremely grateful to the family involved in this study. They thank Dr. Azen Salim, Sp.OG, and Dr. Idham Amir, Sp.A(K), who sent the proband's sample and inspired them to continue their study with this family. They also thank Dr. Iswari Setianingsih, Sp.A., Ph.D., for her encouragement and her critical reading of the paper and they thank the clinic staff, Klinik Genetik Yayasan Genneka, for their help and support.

References

[1] R. J. M. Gardner and G. R. Sutherland, *Chromosome Abnormalities and Genetic Counselling*, Oxford University Press, Oxford, UK, 2004.

[2] J. Lespinasse, M. O. North, C. Paravy, M. J. Brunel, P. Malzac, and J. L. Blouin, "A balanced complex chromosomal rearrangement (BCCR) in a family with reproductive failure," *Human Reproduction*, vol. 18, no. 10, pp. 2058–2066, 2003.

[3] P. C. Patsalis, "Complex chromosomal rearrangements," *Genetic Counseling*, vol. 18, no. 1, pp. 57–69, 2007.

[4] F. Pellestor, T. Anahory, G. Lefort et al., "Complex chromosomal rearrangements: origin and meiotic behavior," *Human Reproduction Update*, vol. 17, no. 4, pp. 476–494, 2011.

[5] D. A. S. Batista, G. S. Pai, and G. Stetten, "Molecular analysis of a complex chromosomal rearrangement and a review of familial cases," *American Journal of Medical Genetics*, vol. 53, no. 3, pp. 255–263, 1994.

[6] K. Madan, A. W. M. Nieuwint, and Y. van Bever, "Recombination in a balanced complex translocation of a mother leading to a balanced reciprocal translocation in the child. Review of 60 cases of balanced complex translocations," *Human Genetics*, vol. 99, no. 6, pp. 806–815, 1997.

[7] P. J. P. de Vree, M. E. H. Simon, M. F. van Dooren et al., "Application of molecular cytogenetic techniques to clarify apparently balanced complex chromosomal rearrangements in two patients with an abnormal phenotype: case report," *Molecular Cytogenetics*, vol. 2, article 15, 2009.

[8] J. L. Gorski, M. L. Kistenmacher, H. H. Punnett, E. H. Zackai, and B. S. Emanual, "Reproductive risks for carriers of complex chromosome rearrangements: analysis of 25 families," *The American Journal of Medical Genetics*, vol. 29, no. 2, pp. 247–261, 1988.

[9] I. Bartels, H. Starke, L. Argyriou, S. M. Sauter, B. Zoll, and T. Liehr, "An exceptional complex chromosomal rearrangement (CCR) with eight breakpoints involving four chromosomes (1;3;9;14) in an azoospermic male with normal phenotype," *European Journal of Medical Genetics*, vol. 50, no. 2, pp. 133–138, 2007.

[10] T. Cai, P. Yu, D. A. Tagle, D. Lu, Y. Chen, and J. Xia, "A de novo complex chromosomal rearrangement with a translocation 7;9 and 8q insertion in a male carrier with no infertility," *Human Reproduction*, vol. 16, no. 1, pp. 59–62, 2001.

[11] L. G. Shaffer, M. L. Slovak, and L. J. Campbell, *An International System for Human Cytogenetic Nomenclature*, S. Karger, Basel, Switzerland, 2009.

[12] H. Karmous-Benailly, F. Giuliano, C. Massol et al., "Unbalanced inherited complex chromosome rearrangement involving chromosome 8, 10, 11 and 16 in a patient with congenital malformations and delayed development," *European Journal of Medical Genetics*, vol. 49, no. 5, pp. 431–438, 2006.

[13] A. Kuechler, M. Ziegler, C. Blank et al., "A highly complex chromosomal rearrangement between five chromosomes in a healthy female diagnosed in preparation for intracytoplasmatic sperm injection," *Journal of Histochemistry & Cytochemistry*, vol. 53, no. 3, pp. 355–357, 2005.

[14] B. Meer, G. Wolff, and E. Back, "Segregation of a complex rearrangement of chromosomes 6, 7, 8, and 12 through three generations," *Human Genetics*, vol. 58, no. 2, pp. 221–225, 1981.

[15] R. Smigiel, I. Laczmanska, and M. Sasiadek, "Maternal complex chromosome rearrangements involving five chromosomes 1, 4, 10, 12 and 20 ascertained through a del(4)(p14p15) detected in a mother's first affected daughter," *Clinical Dysmorphology*, vol. 16, no. 1, pp. 63–64, 2007.

[16] W. P. Baker and C. B. Jones, "FISH-ing for genes: modeling fluorescence in situ hybridization," *The American Biology Teacher*, vol. 68, no. 4, pp. 227–231, 2006.

[17] T. Ried, E. Schröck, Y. Ning, and J. Wienberg, "Chromosome painting: a useful art," *Human Molecular Genetics*, vol. 7, no. 10, pp. 1619–1626, 1998.

[18] I. Feenstra, N. Hanemaaijer, B. Sikkema-Raddatz et al., "Balanced into array: genome-wide array analysis in 54 patients with an apparently balanced de novo chromosome rearrangement and a meta-analysis," *European Journal of Human Genetics*, vol. 19, no. 11, pp. 1152–1160, 2011.

[19] C. Schluth-Bolard, B. Delobel, D. Sanlaville et al., "Cryptic genomic imbalances in de novo and inherited apparently balanced chromosomal rearrangements: array CGH study of 47 unrelated cases," *European Journal of Medical Genetics*, vol. 52, no. 5, pp. 291–296, 2009.

[20] K. A. Kaiser-Rogers, K. W. Rao, R. C. Michaelis, C. M. Lese, and C. M. Powell, "Usefulness and limitations of FISH to characterize partially cryptic complex chromosome rearrangements," *The American Journal of Medical Genetics*, vol. 95, no. 1, pp. 28–35, 2000.

[21] P. C. Patsalis, P. Evangelidou, S. Charalambous, and C. Sismani, "Flourescence in situ hybridization characterization of apparently balanced translocation reveals cryptic complex chromosomal rearrangements with unexpected level of complexity," *European Journal of Human Genetics*, vol. 12, no. 8, pp. 647–653, 2004.

[22] M. Trimborn, T. Liehr, B. Belitz et al., "Prenatal diagnosis and molecular cytogenetic characterization of an unusual complex structural rearrangement in a pregnancy following intracytoplasmic sperm injection (ICSI)," *Journal of Histochemistry & Cytochemistry*, vol. 53, no. 3, pp. 351–354, 2005.

[23] X. Lu, C. A. Shaw, A. Patel et al., "Clinical implementation of chromosomal microarray analysis: summary of 2513 postnatal cases," *PLoS ONE*, vol. 2, no. 3, article e327, 2007.

[24] L. G. Shaffer, M. P. Dabell, A. J. Fisher et al., "Experience with microarray-based comparative genomic hybridization for prenatal diagnosis in over 5000 pregnancies," *Prenatal Diagnosis*, vol. 32, no. 10, pp. 976–985, 2012.

[25] P. A. Iyer, J. C. Vyas, P. Ranjan, and D. Saranath, "A de novo complex chromosomal rearrangement of 46,XX,t(7;15;13)(p15;q21;q31) in a female with an adverse obstetric history," *International Journal of Human Genetics*, vol. 9, no. 2, pp. 139–143, 2009.

[26] J. C. K. Barber, "Directly transmitted unbalanced chromosome abnormalities and euchromatic variants," *Journal of Medical Genetics*, vol. 42, no. 8, pp. 609–629, 2005.

9

Ellis-van Creveld Syndrome: Mutations Uncovered in Lebanese Families

Maria Valencia,[1] Lara Tabet,[2] Nadine Yazbeck,[3] Alia Araj,[3] Victor L. Ruiz-Perez,[1,4] Khalil Charaffedine,[2] Farah Fares,[3] Rebecca Badra,[2] and Chantal Farra[2,3]

[1]Instituto de Investigaciones Biomédicas, Consejo Superior de Científicas, Universidad Autónoma de Madrid, Madrid, Spain
[2]Department of Pathology and Laboratory Medicine, American University of Beirut Medical Center, P.O. Box 11-0236 Riad El Solh, Beirut 1107 2020, Lebanon
[3]Department of Pediatrics and Adolescent Medicine, American University of Beirut Medical Center, P.O. Box 11-0236 Riad El Solh, Beirut 1107 2020, Lebanon
[4]Centro de Investigación Biomédica en Red de Enfermedades Raras (CIBERER), Instituto de Salud Carlos III (ISCIII), Madrid, Spain

Correspondence should be addressed to Chantal Farra; cf07@aub.edu.lb

Academic Editor: Philip D. Cotter

Background. Ellis-van Creveld (EvC) syndrome is a rare, autosomal recessive disorder characterized by short stature, short limbs, growth retardation, polydactyly, and ectodermal defects with cardiac anomalies occurring in around 60% of cases. EVC syndrome has been linked to mutations in *EVC* and *EVC2* genes. *Case Presentation*. We report EvC syndrome in two unrelated Lebanese families both having homozygous mutations in the *EVC2* gene, c.2653C>T (p.(Arg885*)) and c.2012_2015del (p.(Leu671*)) in exons 15 and 13, respectively, with the latter being reported for the first time. *Conclusion*. Although EvC has been largely described in the medical literature, clinical features of this syndrome vary. While more research is required to explore other genes involved in EvC, early diagnosis and therapeutic care are important to achieve a better quality of life.

1. Introduction

Ellis-van Creveld (EvC) syndrome, also known as chondroectodermal and mesoectodermal dysplasia, was first described in 1940 by Elis and Creveld, as an autosomal recessive disorder characterized by short stature and ribs, polydactyly, and ectodermal defects [1–4]. More than half of EvC patients manifest congenital heart defects [5].

While relatively rare, with a prevalence of 0.7/100,000 live birth and only around 300 cases reported worldwide [1, 3, 6], it is mainly reported in highly consanguineous populations such as the Amish population [7]. The syndrome can be diagnosed either by ultrasonography starting from 18th week of gestation or through clinical examination right after birth [3]. Diagnosis after birth is based on clinical observation of features and symptoms described above. It is also supported by an X-ray of the skeleton, chest radiography, ECG, and echocardiography [1].

EvC is related to a group of diseases with alteration of cilia (ciliopathies). Such abnormalities are caused by mutations in the EvC genes (*EVC* and *EVC2*) found on chromosome 4p16 [5, 8] in around two-thirds of the cases.

In this paper, we report EvC syndrome in two unrelated Lebanese families both having homozygous mutations in the *EVC2* gene, NM_147127.4: c.2653C>T p.(Arg885*) and NM_147127.4: c.2012_2015del (p.(Leu671*)) TAAT (p.(Leu671*)) in exons 15 and 13, respectively. While the first one has been recently reported in a Chinese patient, the latter is a newly described mutation.

Informed consents were obtained from the patients' guardians. Genetic analysis was approved by the Institutional Review Board at the Instituto de Investigaciones Biomédicas. Patients were clinically assessed by an experienced clinical geneticist.

The pedigrees of families affected are shown in Figures 1 and 2.

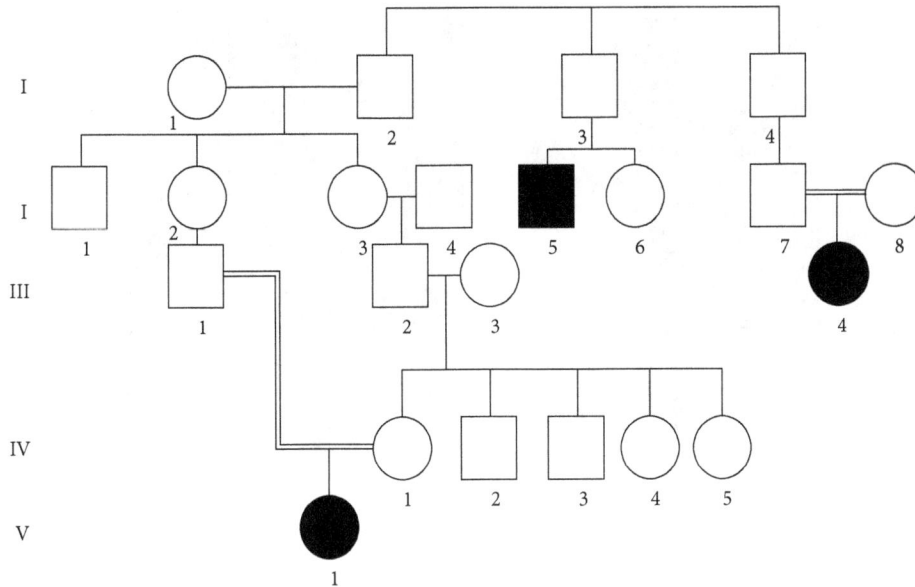

FIGURE 1: Pedigree of Family 1.

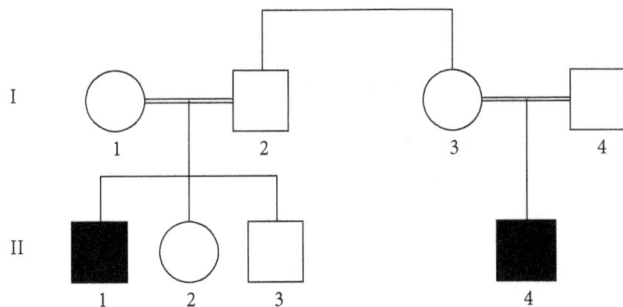

FIGURE 2: Pedigree of Family 2.

2. Case Presentations

2.1. Family 1. A two-year-old girl born to healthy, young consanguineous parents was referred to our genetics clinic at the American University of Beirut Medical Center (AUBMC) for short stature. The patient had a trial septal defect for which she underwent surgical repair. There was no family history of similar problems and the pregnancy and delivery were reportedly uneventful.

Upon physical examination, both height and weight were on the 10th percentiles according to CDC Growth Charts (Ht = 79 cm; <10th percentile; wt = 10 kg; <10th percentile). Upper and lower segment ratio was 34/17 (Figures 3(a) and 3(b)).

Radiology results showed shortening of the paired long bones and slight elongation of the thorax with relatively short ribs, early ossification of femoral heads, and irregular acetabular roofs. The patient had bone deformities and polydactyly with short fingers.

Laboratory work-up yielded a normal 46XX karyotype but a high thyroid hormone level (TSH = 18.27 μIU/mL) with free T4 within normal range. Gene sequencing showed

a NM_147127.4: c.2653C>T (p.(Arg885*)) stop codon mutation in exon 15 of *EVC2*.

2.2. Family 2. A one-year-old boy born to first degree cousins was referred to our genetics clinic for assessment because of short stature and polydactyly. He was the second child of first cousin Lebanese parents.

The patient was delivered at term via C-section to a 35-year-old mother (G5P4). His birth weight was 2260 grams (<5%), with a length of 42 cm (<5%) and a head circumference of 33.3 cm (<25). An echo done at the 7th month of gestation showed a bell-shaped chest. No otherwise prenatal complications were reported. An echocardiogram done at birth showed Patent Foramen Ovale (PFO).

Upon physical examination the patient's stature was below the 5th percentile (height: 69 cm <5th%; wt: 20 cm <25th%). Radiology results showed shortening of the limbs and ribs.

He had a brother who passed away at day 5 of age and who was born with cleft lip and palate and bilateral polydactyly. One of his paternal cousins, a 17-year-old male with normal karyotype (46, XY), was reported to have polydactyly, short stature, and dysplastic nails and teeth. He was labelled as having dwarfism without proper follow-up or accurate assessment. Upon examination, he had widely spaced conical shaped teeth and a height of 140 cm (Figure 1; Figures 4(a) and 4(b)).

DNA analyses for *EVC* and *EVC2* genes on both cousins revealed a NM_147127.4: c.2012_2015del TAAT in exon 13 of *EVC2*.

3. Discussion

EvC is a rare disorder involving several embryonic tissues and resulting in polymorphic symptoms. Although largely

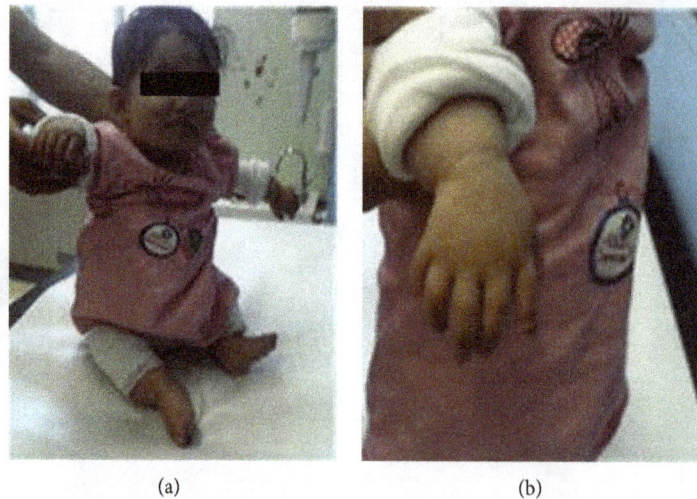

FIGURE 3: Clinical photos of patient from Family 1 depicting short upper and lower limbs and polydactyly.

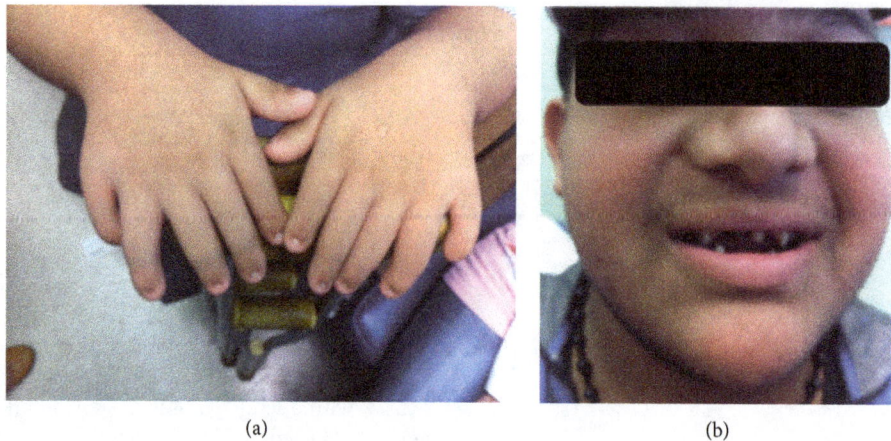

FIGURE 4: Clinical photos of patient from Family 2 showing conical shaped teeth and polydactyly.

described in the medical literature, the clinical features of this syndrome differ between patients [3, 7] with chondrodystrophia being the most commonly reported and the main reason behind short stature [1, 3, 5, 8].

Both families are consanguineous and presented with the classical findings of EvC syndrome. So far, around 93 mutations in either *EVC* or *EVC2* genes have been reported in the literature with the majority causing premature termination codons [5, 9, 10]. In both families, mutations were detected in *EVC2* gene. In the first family, a homozygous nonsense mutation c.2653C>T (p.(Arg885*)) was found. This mutation was previously reported in a 6-year-old Chinese female [10] who was a compound heterozygous for another mutation (IVS5-2A>G). Both our patient and the Chinese patient had similar clinical presentation [10]. In our second family, we detected a homozygous deletion of 4 nucleotides NM_147127.4: c.2012_2015del TAAT in exon 13 of *EVC2*. This deletion generates a frameshift that runs into a premature stop codon immediately. To our knowledge, this mutation is reported for the first time.

Amongst Arabs and Middle Eastern populations, mutation panels for recessive disorders in general differ from one country to another and in between religious denominations [11, 12] mainly because of the wide migratory movements that occurred over the centuries resulting in a great variability of ethnicity and origins that constitute these populations.

Lebanon is a small country with several ethnic and demographic groups originating in part, from European crusader Christians and Arabian Muslims, resulting in a heterogeneous background of our families [13]. Consanguineous marriages in Lebanon are relatively common (28.6%) leading to a high prevalence of autosomal recessive disorders [12, 14]. Despite this fact the need for genetic services in Lebanon is still not widely established. Indeed, lack of compliance for genetic referrals and testing is still witnessed mainly due to economic burdens since these tests do not benefit from third party coverage and also because of social taboos that are still associated with inherited diseases. For this reason, a substantial number of patients with genetic disorders may be misdiagnosed or not followed up properly. Reporting rare cases from our population will raise further awareness on the occurrence of these disorders and will increase the chance for a proper genetic assessment. This could also eventually contribute to unravel other genes that might be involved in EvC and to improve the quality of care for these patients.

Consent

The patients have given their consent for the case reports to be published.

Conflict of Interests

The authors declare that there is no conflict of interests regarding the publication of this paper.

References

[1] R. Kamal, P. Dahiya, S. Kaur, R. Bhardwaj, and K. Chaudhary, "Ellis-van Creveld syndrome: a rare clinical entity," *Journal of Oral and Maxillofacial Pathology*, vol. 17, no. 1, pp. 132–135, 2013.

[2] K. Hegde, R. M. Puthran, G. Nair, and P. P. Nair, "Ellis van Creveld syndrome—a report of two siblings," *The British Medical Journal Case Reports*, vol. 2011, 2011.

[3] G. Baujat and M. le Merrer, "Ellis-van creveld syndrome," *Orphanet Journal of Rare Diseases*, vol. 2, article 27, 2007.

[4] E. O. Da Silva, D. Janovitz, and S. Cavalcanti De Albuquerque, "Ellis-van Creveld syndrome: report of 15 cases in an inbred kindred," *Journal of Medical Genetics*, vol. 17, no. 5, pp. 349–356, 1980.

[5] V. L. Ruiz-Perez and J. A. Goodship, "Ellis-van Creveld syndrome and Weyers acrodental dysostosis are caused by cilia-mediated diminished response to Hedgehog ligands," *American Journal of Medical Genetics, Part C: Seminars in Medical Genetics*, vol. 151, no. 4, pp. 341–351, 2009.

[6] H. Saneifard and G. Amirhakimi, "Ellis van Creveld syndrome: report of a case and brief literature review," *Iranian Journal of Pediatrics*, vol. 18, no. 1, pp. 75–78, 2008.

[7] V. A. McKusick, "Ellis-van Creveld syndrome and the Amish," *Nature Genetics*, vol. 24, no. 3, pp. 203–204, 2000.

[8] L. Arya, V. Mendiratta, R. C. Sharma, and R. S. Solanki, "Ellis-van Creveld syndrome: a report of two cases," *Pediatric Dermatology*, vol. 18, no. 6, pp. 485–489, 2001.

[9] N. M. Suresh, K. T. S. Anand, P. Veena, K. K. Vinay, K. R. Asha, and M. Bhat, "Ellis-van Creveld Syndrome," *Anatomica Karnataka*, vol. 6, pp. 1–4, 2012.

[10] W. Shen, D. Han, J. Zhang, H. Zhao, and H. Feng, "Two novel heterozygous mutations of *EVC2* cause a mild phenotype of Ellis-van Creveld syndrome in a Chinese family," *American Journal of Medical Genetics Part A*, vol. 155, no. 9, pp. 2131–2136, 2011.

[11] C. Farra, R. Menassa, J. Awwad et al., "Mutational spectrum of cystic fibrosis in the Lebanese population," *Journal of Cystic Fibrosis*, vol. 9, no. 6, pp. 406–410, 2010.

[12] L. Al-Gazali, H. Hamamy, and S. Al-Arrayad, "Genetic disorders in the Arab world," *British Medical Journal*, vol. 333, no. 7573, pp. 831–834, 2006.

[13] S. Al-Nazhan, A. Al-Daafas, and N. Al-Maflehi, "Radiographic investigation of in vivo endodontically treated maxillary premolars in a Saudi Arabian sub-population," *Saudi Endodontic Journal*, vol. 2, no. 1, pp. 1–5, 2012.

[14] B. Barbour and P. Salameh, "Consanguinity in Lebanon: prevalence, distribution and determinants," *Journal of Biosocial Science*, vol. 41, no. 4, pp. 505–517, 2009.

10

Atypical Association of Angelman Syndrome and Klinefelter Syndrome in a Boy with 47,XXY Karyotype and Deletion 15q11.2-q13

Javier Sánchez,[1] **Ana Peciña,**[1,2] **Olga Alonso-Luengo,**[3] **Antonio González-Meneses,**[3] **Rocío Vázquez,**[4] **Guillermo Antiñolo,**[1,2] **and Salud Borrego**[1,2]

[1] *Department of Genetics, Reproduction and Fetal Medicine, Institute of Biomedicine of Seville (IBIS),*
 University Hospital Virgen del Rocío/CSIC/University of Seville, 41013 Seville, Spain
[2] *Centre of Biomedical Network Research on Rare Diseases (CIBERER), 41013 Seville, Spain*
[3] *Department of Pediatrics, University Hospital Virgen del Rocío, Avenida Manuel Siurot s/n, 41013 Seville, Spain*
[4] *Department of Neurophysiology, University Hospital Virgen del Rocío, Avenida Manuel Siurot s/n, 41013 Seville, Spain*

Correspondence should be addressed to Salud Borrego; salud.borrego.sspa@juntadeandalucia.es

Academic Editor: Jose Luis Royo

Angelman syndrome (AS, OMIM 105830) is a neurogenetic disorder with firm clinical diagnostic guidelines, characterized by severe developmental delay and speech impairment, balanced and behavioral disturbance as well as microcephaly, seizures, and a characteristic electroencephalogram (EEG). The majority of AS cases (70%) are caused by a 15q11.2-q13 deletion on the maternally derived chromosome. The frequency of AS has been estimated to be between 1/10000 and 1/20000. Klinefelter syndrome (KS) occurs due to the presence of an extra X chromosome (karyotype 47,XXY). The main features in KS are small testes, hypergonadotropic hypogonadism, gynecomastia, learning difficulties, and infertility. We present what is, to our knowledge, the first case of a patient with both KS and AS due to a 15q11.2-q13 deletion on the maternally derived chromosome and an extra X chromosome of paternal origin. He showed dysmorphic features, axial hypotonia, and delayed acquisition of motor skills. Early diagnosis is essential for optimal treatment of AS children; this is one of the earliest diagnosed cases of AS probably due to the presence of two syndromes. Clinical findings in this patient here described may be helpful to identify any other cases and to evaluate recurrence risks in these families.

1. Introduction

Angelman syndrome (AS, OMIM 105830) is a neurogenetic disorder with firm clinical diagnostic guidelines, characterized by severe developmental delay and speech impairment as well as balanced and behavioral disturbance. Other frequent clinical features include microcephaly, seizures, and a characteristic electroencephalogram (EEG) [1]. The majority of AS cases (70%) are caused by a 15q11.2-q13 deletion on the maternally derived chromosome. Other less frequent genetic mechanisms are paternal uniparental disomy of 15 chromosome (7%), imprinting defects (3%), or mutations in the maternal copy of the *UBE3A* gene (11%) [2]. The frequency of AS has been estimated to be between 1/10000

and 1/20000 [3]. Recurrence risk varies from <1% for deletion cases where no chromosome rearrangements or germinal mosaicism is present [4–6] to 50% for maternally inherited imprinting center deletions or UBE3A mutations [7].

Klinefelter syndrome (KS) also shows a clear clinical pattern, although no firm guidelines for diagnosis exist. The main features in KS are small testes, hypergonadotropic hypogonadism, gynecomastia, learning difficulties, and infertility [8]. KS occurs due to the presence of an extra X chromosome (karyotype 47,XXY) and the underlying putative genetic cause is that some genes escape inactivation of the extra X chromosome [9]. KS affects one in 150 per 100,000 male newborns and is the most common sex chromosome disorder in males. Since KS patients show great phenotypic variability, the majority of patients are diagnosed during the second decade of life and it is difficult to diagnose KS without cytogenetic analysis. In some instances chromosomal analysis is performed due to development delay, learning difficulties, or behavior problems [10].

Taking into account the incidence rates for both AS and KS, the anticipated incidence of both syndromes occurring together would be around 1 in 6–12 million by chance alone.

Here we present what is, to our knowledge, the first case of a patient with both KS and AS due to a 15q11.2-q13 deletion on the maternally derived chromosome. To date, few patients with KS and other microdeletion syndromes have been reported: six cases of KS and Prader-Willi syndrome (PWS) due to a 15q11.2-q13 deletion on the paternally derived chromosome have been published [11], a patient with KS and 22q11 microdeletion [12] and a combination of KS and 7q11.23 deletion (Williams syndrome) [13].

2. Patient Description

The propositus was the second child born to a healthy 33-year-old mother with a previous healthy son, now three years old. The parents were not consanguineous, and no remarkable family history was recorded. During pregnancy, she developed diabetes mellitus, which was well controlled by her diet. The mother reported the first fetal movements at 22-week gestation, with reduced fetal movements throughout the pregnancy. The propositus was delivered spontaneously at 37-week gestation. His birth weight was 3,190 g and head circumference was 34 cm. Apgar scores were 9 (1 min), 9 (5 min), and 10 (10 min). Severe hypotonia, feeding difficulties, and continuous crying were noted at birth.

At 8 months his head circumference was 46 cm (p75), weight 9,555 g (p90), and height 70 cm (p75–p90). He showed delayed acquisition of motor skills, he could not remain seated or handle objects, and axial hypotonia was observed. He showed dysmorphic features, occipital flattening, a thin upper lip, a wide mouth, tongue protrusion, a broad nasal root, and divergent strabismus (Figure 1). A brain MRI showed a structurally normal brain.

The EEG at 8 months showed diffuse high-amplitude 4–6 Hz activity and posterior intermittent rhythmic delta waves. No epileptiform discharges were observed. Three months later, the EEG showed no significant changes. Chromosome analysis and PWS/AS were performed due to dysmorphic features and hypotonia.

Informed consent was obtained from all participants for clinical and molecular genetic studies. The study conformed to the tenets of the declaration of Helsinki as well as the requirements established by our institutional review board.

Peripheral blood cytogenetic analysis revealed 47 chromosomes, with an extra X chromosome, karyotype 47,XXY (KS). FISH analysis with specific probes (D15Z1/SNRPN/PML) [Vysis, Downers Grove, IL] revealed a deletion of the SNRPN locus. Karyotype: 47,XXY.ish del (15)(q11.2q11.2)(SNRPN-)[20] (Figures 2 and 3).

No deletion or rearrangements were observed in the parents' karyotypes.

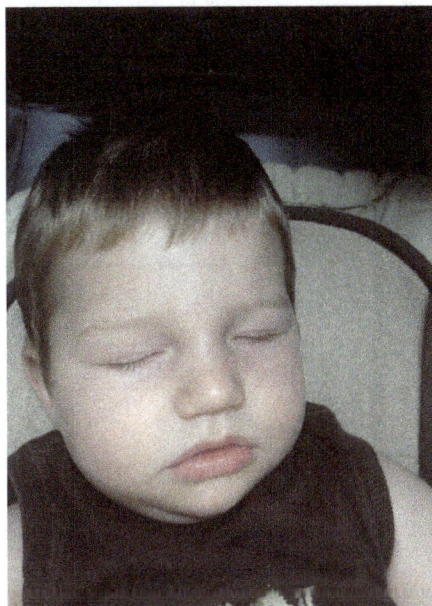

FIGURE 1: Facial appearance. Dysmorphic features, broad nasal root, and thin upper lip.

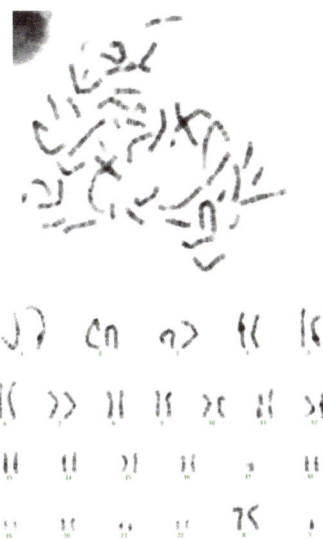

FIGURE 2: Karyotype showing the presence of an extra X chromosome.

Molecular analysis using Multiple Ligation Probe Amplification methodology (SALSA MLPA probemix kit P245-A2, MRC-Holland, Amsterdam, NL) confirmed the deletion of the PWS/AS critical region, while the dose of control probes located at 15q24.1 was normal. In order to determine the origin of the chromosome with the 15q11.2-q13 deletion, we analyzed five microsatellite markers: D15S541, D15S11, and GABR3, located within the critical region of PWS/AS, and D15S131 and D15S984 located outside of the critical region, which were used as controls. Analysis of D15S541, D15S11, and GABR3 markers confirmed the deletion of 15q11.2-q13 on

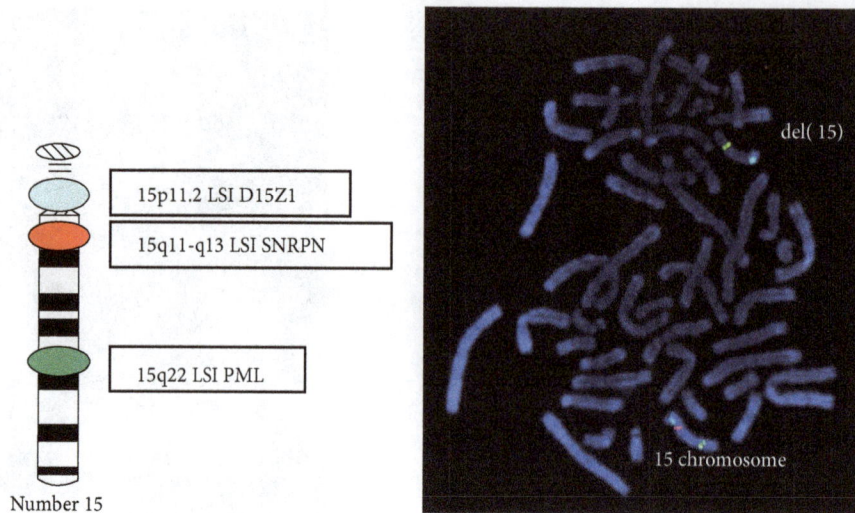

FIGURE 3: FISH analysis in metaphase with specific probes for 15 chromosome. Upper 15 chromosome with SNRPN deletion (del 15). D15Z1, SpectrumAqua; SNRPN, SpectrumOrange; PML, SpectrumGreen.

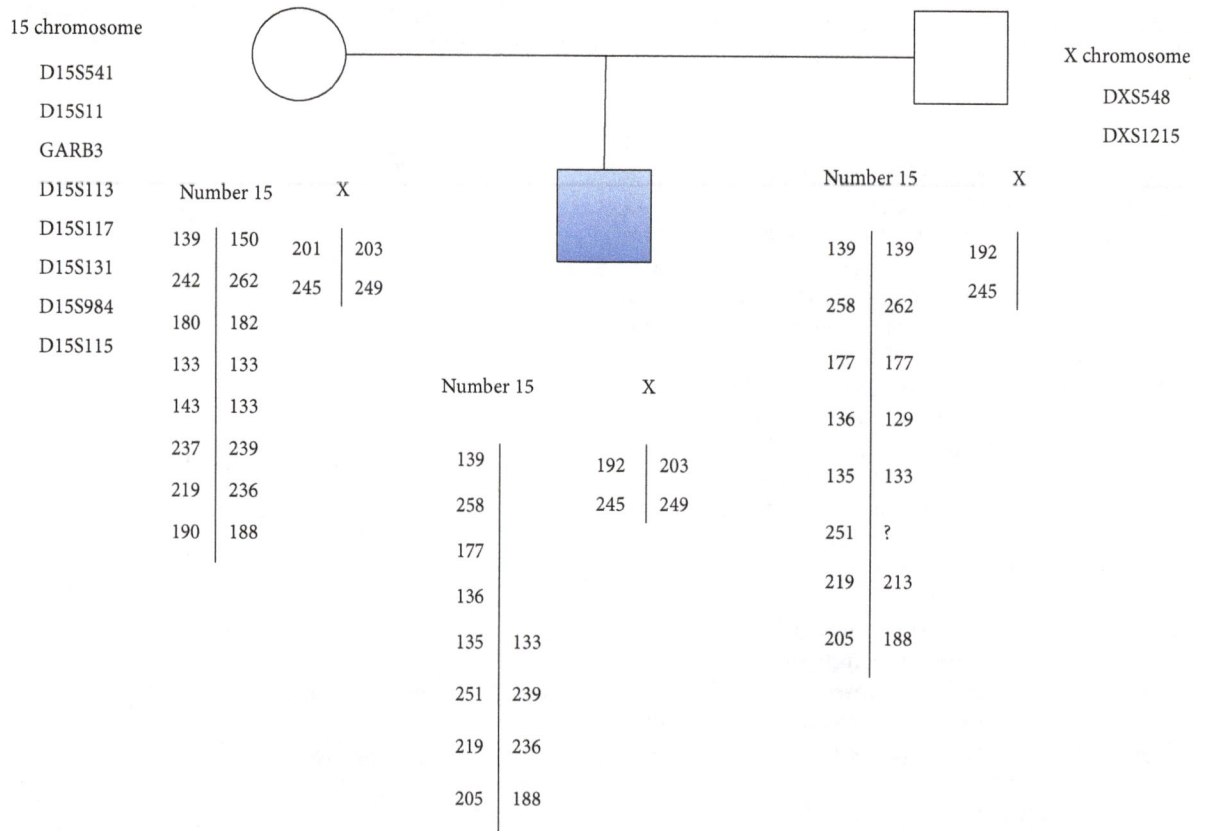

FIGURE 4: Microsatellite analysis and pedigree of the family. Microsatellite from X chromosome showed one of paternal origin and other of maternal origin. Microsatellite from 15 chromosome showed a deletion of D15S541, D15S11, GARB3, and D15S113 of maternal origin.

the maternal chromosome (AS) (Figure 4). Control markers showed paternal and maternal 15 chromosome.

The paternal origin of the extra X chromosome was determined by analysis of a set of microsatellites located on the X chromosome by multiplex PCR (Figure 3).

3. Discussion

To our knowledge, this is the first case of a patient with coexisting AS and KS. The combined effects of both syndromes are not clear, since the patient is currently only 11 months old.

The main phenotypic effects in KS are manifested in the mid-30s and in AS do not appear until 2-3 years after birth. This is one of the earliest diagnosed cases of AS, and it may be due to the presence of two syndromes. We can expect that the main phenotypic features that he will exhibit will be those of AS, since typical KS clinical features are much milder. We showed that the extra X chromosome was of paternal origin and the deletion in 15 chromosome was of maternal origin. Paternal and maternal sex chromosome nondisjunction contribute equally as causes of KS. Both parents were young and had normal karyotypes. Therefore, the abnormalities are most probably a coincidental event in our patient. In light of this, we estimate that the recurrence risk in the next pregnancy for both syndromes is low.

Early diagnosis is essential for optimal treatment of AS children. Abnormal EEG is used as diagnostic criteria since it is present in almost all AS patients [1, 14]. It has been suggested that EEG abnormalities are age-dependent: they usually appear early and decrease with age [15]. Seizures are a common feature observed in AS patients [1]. Seizures and EEG abnormalities were not detected in our patient, maybe because he is 11 months old and these do not usually occur until 22–24 months of age.

The most likely situation is that both conditions are coincidental. Therefore, to calculate risk, both conditions must be considered separately. Hence, KS patients with uncommon clinical features—such as the hypotonia, feeding difficulties, or frequent laughing observed in our patient— may be considered for assessment of another associated condition. Since there are no prenatal findings of AS and/or KS, for this couple we recommend offering cytogenetic prenatal diagnosis and FISH or array-CGH for AS.

Conflict of Interests

The authors declare no conflict of interests.

Acknowledgment

The authors would like to acknowledge the patient and his family for their kind cooperation and for providing the figure.

References

[1] C. A. Williams, A. L. Beaudet, J. Clayton-Smith et al., "Angelman syndrome 2005: updated consensus for diagnostic criteria," *American Journal of Medical Genetics*, vol. 140, no. 5, pp. 413–418, 2006.

[2] A. I. Dagli and C. A. Williams, "Angelman Syndrome," in *GeneReviews [Internet]*, R. A. Pagon, M. P. Adam, T. D. Bird et al., Eds., University of Washington, Seattle, Wash, USA, 2013, http://www.ncbi.nlm.nih.gov/books/NBK1144/.

[3] G. van Buggenhout and J.-P. Fryns, "Angelman syndrome (AS, MIM 105830)," *European Journal of Human Genetics*, vol. 17, no. 11, pp. 1367–1373, 2009.

[4] H. J. Stalker and C. A. Williams, "Genetic counseling in Angelman syndrome: the challenges of multiple causes," *American Journal of Medical Genetics*, vol. 77, no. 1, pp. 54–59, 1998.

[5] C. Camprubí, M. D. Coll, E. Gabau, and M. Guitart, "Prader-Willi and Angelman syndromes: genetic counseling," *European Journal of Human Genetics*, vol. 18, no. 2, pp. 154–155, 2010.

[6] J. Sánchez, R. Fernández, M. Madruga, J. Bernabeu-Wittel, G. Antiñolo, and S. Borrego, "Somatic and germ-line mosaicism of deletion 15q11.2-q13 in a mother of dyzigotic twins with Angelman syndrome," *American Journal of Medical Genetics Part A*, vol. 164, no. 2, pp. 370–376, 2014.

[7] C. A. Williams, D. J. Driscoll, and A. I. Dagli, "Clinical and genetic aspects of Angelman syndrome," *Genetics in Medicine*, vol. 12, no. 7, pp. 385–395, 2010.

[8] C. M. Smyth and W. J. Bremner, "Klinefelter syndrome," *Archives of Internal Medicine*, vol. 158, no. 12, pp. 1309–1314, 1998.

[9] K. A. Groth, A. Skakkebæk, C. Høst, C. H. Gravholt, and A. Bojesen, "Clinical review: Klinefelter syndrome—a clinical update," *Journal of Clinical Endocrinology and Metabolism*, vol. 98, no. 1, pp. 20–30, 2013.

[10] L. Aksglaede, K. Link, A. Giwercman, N. Jørgensen, N. E. Skakkebæk, and A. Juul, "47,XXY Klinefelter syndrome: Clinical characteristics and age-specific recommendations for medical management," *American Journal of Medical Genetics C: Seminars in Medical Genetics*, vol. 163, no. 1, pp. 55–63, 2013.

[11] P. C. Vasudevan and O. W. J. Quarrell, "Prader-willi and klinefelter syndrome: a coincidence or not?" *Clinical Dysmorphology*, vol. 16, no. 2, pp. 127–129, 2007.

[12] G. V. N. Velagaleti, A. Kumar, L. H. Lockhart, and R. Matalon, "Patent ductus arteriosus and microdeletion 22q11 in a patient with Klinefelter syndrome," *Annales de Génétique*, vol. 43, no. 2, pp. 105–107, 2000.

[13] Y. L. Le, C. Q. Swee, S. S. Chong, A. S. C. Tan, J. M. S. Lum, and D. L. M. Goh, "Clinical report: a case of Williams syndrome and Klinefelter syndrome," *Annals of the Academy of Medicine Singapore*, vol. 35, no. 12, pp. 901–904, 2006.

[14] R. L. Thibert, A. M. Larson, D. T. Hsieh, A. R. Raby, and E. A. Thiele, "Neurologic manifestations of Angelman syndrome," *Pediatric Neurology*, vol. 48, no. 4, pp. 271–279, 2013.

[15] N. Uemura, A. Matsumoto, M. Nakamura et al., "Evolution of seizures and electroencephalographical findings in 23 cases of deletion type Angelman syndrome," *Brain and Development*, vol. 27, no. 5, pp. 383–388, 2005.

11

Microduplication of 3p26.3 Implicated in Cognitive Development

Leah Te Weehi,[1] Raj Maikoo,[2] Adrian Mc Cormack,[1] Roberto Mazzaschi,[1] Fern Ashton,[1] Liangtao Zhang,[1] Alice M. George,[1] and Donald R. Love[1,3]

[1] Diagnostic Genetics, LabPLUS, Auckland City Hospital, P.O. Box 110031, Auckland 1148, New Zealand
[2] Pediatrics Department, Middlemore Hospital, Private Bag 93311, Auckland 1640, New Zealand
[3] School of Biological Sciences, University of Auckland, Private Bag 92019, Auckland 1142, New Zealand

Correspondence should be addressed to Donald R. Love; donaldl@adhb.govt.nz

Academic Editors: M. Chikri and L. Parnell

We report here a 34-month-old boy with global developmental delay referred for molecular karyotyping and fragile X studies. Molecular karyotype analysis revealed a microduplication in the 3p26.3 region involving part of the *CHL1* and *CNTN6* genes. Several deletions, one translocation, and one duplication have previously been described in this region of chromosome 3. The *CHL1* gene has been proposed as a dosage-sensitive gene with a central role in cognitive development, and so the microduplication reported here appears to be implicated in our patient's phenotype.

1. Introduction

Anomalies of the distal portion of the short arm of chromosome 3 are rare and not yet fully understood. The most well-characterised anomalies are deletions. For the most part, they occur *de novo*, although a few familial cases have been reported [1–8]. These deletions range from one to several megabases, but the extent of the deletion does not correlate with phenotypic severity. The clinical syndrome includes intellectual disability, low birth weight, micro- and trigonocephaly, and characteristic facial features such as ptosis, telecanthus, downslanting palpebral fissures, and micrognathia. Many genes have been implicated to play a role: *CRBN* and *CNTN4* have been suggested to cause typical 3p deletion syndrome [9, 10], and the *CHL1* gene has been proposed to play an additional role in cognitive impairment [8, 11–13]. The involvement of the *CHL1* gene has been reported in four previous case studies: three with deletions confined to 3p26.3 [6–8], including only the *CHL1* gene, a translocation [12], and one novel microduplication [13] (Figure 1). In these cases the growth abnormalities and typical facial features of 3p deletion syndrome were absent. Nonspecific intellectual disability was the main trait.

Interestingly, the previously reported 3p26.3 microduplication case manifested similar clinical features to those patients carrying a *CHL1* gene deletion, namely, nonspecific intellectual disability and epilepsy [13]. Epilepsy was also present in one child with a submicroscopic 3p26.3 noncontiguous terminal deletion containing only the *CHL1* gene [6].

We have identified a second case involving 3p26.3 microduplication that encompasses part of the *CHL1* gene as well as the *CNTN6* gene. Our case presents with motor and speech developmental delay and some autistic features.

2. Materials and Methods

Genomic deoxyribonucleic acid (DNA) was isolated from the peripheral blood using the Gentra Puregene Blood Kit (QIAGEN Genomics, Bothell, Washington, USA) according to the manufacturer's instructions. 0.1 micrograms of genomic DNA was labelled using the Affymetrix Cytogenetics Reagent Kit and labelled DNA was applied to an Affymetrix Whole-Genome 750K chip according to the manufacturer's instructions (Affymetrix Inc., CA, USA). The array was scanned and the data analysed using the Affymetrix Chromosome Analysis Suite (ChAS; version 1.0.1) and interpreted with the

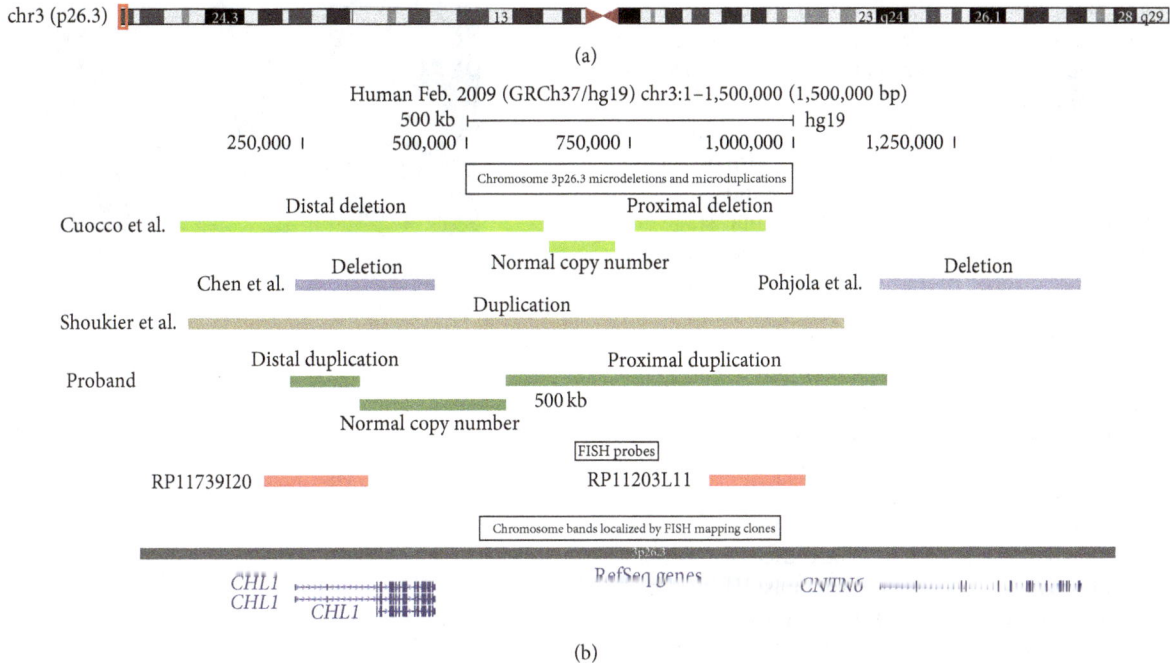

chr3 (p26.3)

(a)

Human Feb. 2009 (GRCh37/hg19) chr3:1–1,500,000 (1,500,000 bp)

(b)

FIGURE 1: Schematic of chromosome 3p26.3 showing microdeletions and microduplications. (a) Shows the ideogram of chromosome 3, together with the region encompassing microdeletions and microduplications (red box). (b) Shows the location and extent of the microdeletions and microduplications detected in the proband reported here and other cases reported in the literature [6–8, 13], BAC probes used in the FISH studies, and RefSeq genes that lie within this region of chromosome 3. These graphics were taken from the UCSC genome browser [14].

aid of the UCSC genome browser (http://genome.ucsc.edu/) [14]. All genomic coordinates were taken from the February 2009 (hg19) human reference sequence (NCBI Build 37), and gene and Online Mendelian Inheritance in Man (OMIM) references were from RefSeq and OMIM entries, respectively [14, 15].

A peripheral blood sample was collected in heparin from the proband and cultured according to standard cytogenetic protocols. Based on the duplicated region revealed by molecular karyotype analysis, two 3p26.3 locus-specific Bacterial Artificial Chromosome (BAC) probes, RP11-739I20 (SpG) (hg19 coordinates: chr3:190,761-349,109) and RP11-203L11 (SpO) (hg19 coordinates: chr3:871,241-1,019,847), were chosen from the Human BAC DNA library-32K set. They were labelled with green and orange fluorescent dyes, respectively. The Fluorescence *in situ* hybridisation (FISH) method followed the procedure of Pinkel et al. [16] with some modifications. Codenaturation was achieved by placing the slides into a thermal cycler (PTC-200) preheated to 87°C for 2 minutes. The slides were hybridized overnight in a humidified chamber at 37°C. The following day, the slides were subjected to a stringent wash in 0.4X SSC at 74°C for 2 minutes followed by 2X SSC at room temperature for 1 minute. After the slides were air-dried, 8 μL of mounting medium (Vectashield) was applied to each of the slides. FISH was performed on 10 metaphase cells. The images were captured using a MetaSystems ISIS imaging system on a Zeiss AXIO Imager, M1 fluorescence microscope with sequential DAPI, and spectral green and spectral orange filter settings.

3. Case Report

The patient is the second male child of healthy nonconsanguineous parents. There is no family history of syndromes or developmental delay. His four-year-old brother is normal. He was born at 38 weeks gestation via emergency caesarean section for breech position. He had a birth weight of 2930 g (2nd to 9th percentile) [17]. There were no antenatal problems or intrapartum complications. He was born with syndactyly of the right fourth and fifth metacarpals with shortened little finger and a hypoplastic right thumb. Careful examination revealed partial syndactyly of his second and third toes on both feet. He underwent surgical correction of his right hand syndactyly (division of synostosis and interlay of dermal fat graft) at almost 15 months and is awaiting surgery for his thumb.

The patient was referred to paediatric services at approximately 15 months of age for gross motor developmental concerns. These were first noticed at 5 months of age. He was able to sit with support at 10 months and independently at 13 months of age. By 15 months he was still not pulling himself to stand or crawling. Examination at 15 months showed a weight of 10.05 kg (10th to 25th percentile), length of 76.6 cm (25th percentile), and a head circumference of 47.5 cm (50th to 75th percentile). Prior to this, his growth parameters were reported to be tracking along the 10th to 25th percentiles. He had intact cranial nerves and normal neurology in his upper limbs. Lower limb examination revealed mild pes cavus and increased tone especially around the Achilles tendon. Both the cavus and tone were more significant on the left side. Knee and ankle jerks were hyperreflexic but plantars were both downgoing. The rest of the examination was unremarkable. The dominant finding was lower limb spasticity.

When seen again at 25 months of age, he was noted to be still delayed in the gross motor domain but also delayed in other domains. Fine motor skills and receptive and expressive language skills were at 18 months developmental stage and social and self-care skills at the 12 months stage. He was observed to have a large prominent forehead and button-shaped nose but no gross dysmorphic features. None of the characteristic facial features of the 3p deletions syndrome were observed. Features he demonstrated that were suggestive of autistic spectrum disorder were repetitive activities, preoccupation with spinning wheels, resistance to changes in routine, and heightened sensitivity to people touching his legs. Overall, however, he was not thought to have an autistic spectrum disorder.

He was referred to a speech language therapist, physiotherapist, and a neurodevelopmental therapist. Under these health professionals he made significant progress over several months. At 28 months of age, both receptive and expressive language domains were mildly delayed to the level of 22–24 months. His gross motor skills were similarly only mildly delayed. By 32 months he was able to mobilise 15 metres and transfer to standing through half-kneeling with one arm for support. The lower limb spasticity improved.

He underwent general investigations for developmental delay. The MRI scan of his brain was unremarkable and his creatinine kinase level was 35 U/L (normal age-specific range 30–150) [18]. Fragile X testing involved PCR amplification and then fluorescence-based capillary electrophoresis to determine the number of CGG repeats within the *FMR-1* gene [19]. He was found to have a normal CGG repeat length of 30.

Molecular karyotype analysis revealed a 913 kb region of allelic imbalance involving the 3p26.3 region (chr3:231,390-1,144,815; hg19 coordinates; data not shown). This allelic imbalance was complicated in that it comprised approximately 220 kb of neutral copy number flanked by regions with a copy number change consistent with duplication. These flanking regions, corresponding to chr3:231,390-336,272 and chr3:559,569-1,144,815, encompass the amino terminal regions of the *CHL1* and *CNTN6* genes, respectively (Figure 1).

FISH studies were undertaken of the proband's genome to determine if the copy number changes that were identified by molecular karyotyping were due to a tandem duplication event. Locus-specific probes showed target hybridisation to the short arm of both homologues of chromosome 3, with an enhanced signal for both probes on the same homologue (Figure 2). These results suggest the presence of two tandem duplications in close proximity to one another, supporting the molecular karyotyping findings.

4. Discussion

The *CHL1* gene encodes a protein that is part of the L1 gene family of neural adhesion molecules that regulate brain cell

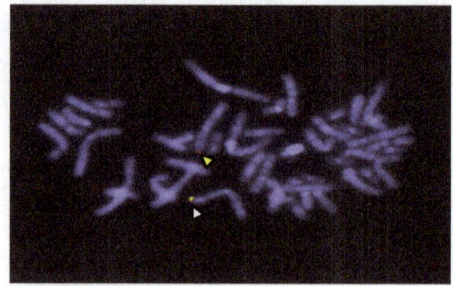

FIGURE 2: FISH analysis of metaphase cells using two BAC probes. The fluorescent signals identify the two homologues of chromosome 3 in cells of the proband. The orange and green signals (indicated by the yellow arrow head) show hybridisation of the BAC clones RP11-203L11 and RP11-739I20, respectively, to their normal sequences. The lower homolog shows a yellow signal, created from the combination of orange and green signals (indicated by a white arrow head), which is consistent with two tandem duplications on the same homologue.

migration and synaptogenesis [11]. It is highly expressed in the central and peripheral nervous systems. Our duplicated region includes three transcript variants; only the $5'$ untranslated regions of transcript variants 1 and 2 are included in the duplicated segment. The segment of the *CNTN6* gene that is duplicated also corresponds to an untranslated region. The *CNTN6* gene encodes a neural adhesion molecule that is part of the immunoglobulin superfamily [20, 21]. This gene plays important roles in the formation, maintenance, and plasticity of functional neuronal networks in the central nervous system.

The proposed pathogenic mechanism for the 3p deletion syndrome is haploinsufficiency of several crucial genes [12, 22]. The more proximal genes on 3p (*CRBN* and *CNTN4*) are thought to account for the dysmorphic features [9] and mental retardation [10], while the distal gene, *CHL1*, may also be involved in impaired cognitive functioning [12, 13].

In the limited number of case studies with anomalies restricted to the *CHL1* gene (Figure 1), the dysmorphic features have been varied but there is usually some degree of cognitive impairment. In one of the families reported by Pohjola et al. [7], both the proband and his mother carried the same 1.1 Mb deletion, containing only the *CHL1* gene. The proband's clinical presentation included slow physical development, microcephaly, reticular hyperpigmentation of the skin, temper tantrums, and severe learning disabilities. His facial dysmorphic features included hypotelorism, low forehead, and a long, thin, and pointed nose. His growth parameters, apart from head circumference, were within normal ranges. His mother shared similar facial features, except for hypotelorism and microcephaly. Her growth and development were completely normal. The authors suggested that the atypical presentation of the proband could possibly indicate two separate syndromes: the 3p deletion responsible for the mild mental retardation, and the other features, including skin hyperpigmentation, caused by a distinct but unknown aetiology [7].

In the case report by Cuoco et al. [6], the terminal deletion carrying only the *CHL1* gene was transmitted from a normal father to two affected sons. Both sons had mild mental retardation characterized by learning and language difficulties, but not the distinct features of the 3p deletion phenotype. The growth parameters for both brothers were within normal ranges. The first son also had tonic-clonic seizures, the first at 8 years of age, and required therapy with a single agent. The father, carrying the same 3p deletion, had completed studies as a dentist and never had any physical impairment [6].

A third case study identified a man with nonspecific mental retardation carrying a translocation 46, Y, t(X;3)(p22.1;p26.3) [12]. His clinical presentation included overall bradykinesia, low mental level, bradyphrenia, poor attention span, and mild echolalia. The Xp breakpoint did not affect a known or predicted breakpoint so the phenotype was presumably caused by disruption of one allele of the CHL1 gene alone. The second CHL1 allele was sequenced, and no intragenic mutation was identified. This case also supports the pathogenic mechanism of haploinsufficiency of CHL1 for nonspecific mental retardation. The authors went further to catalogue Chl1 expression levels in mice hipoccampi. Chl1 is the mouse ortholog of CHL1 (close homolog of L1). The authors found that found that Chl1 gene expression levels in the hippocampus of $Chl^{+/-}$ mice were half those found in wild type mice, but with normal through to abnormal behaviour.

In the first case study reporting microduplication in the CHL1 gene, the entire gene was duplicated [13]. The phenotype of the girl in this study included intellectual disability. Her gross development progressed normally and she reached her first motor milestones within the normal timeframes. She showed marked speech development delay after two years. She also displayed paroxysmal eyelid myoclonia from 3 months to 3 years and had generalised tonic-clonic seizures that commenced in her second year of life and required dual therapy. She was followed until 16 years of age and at this stage still showed significant intellectual disabilities. The authors did not postulate any models of pathogenesis for CHL1 gene duplication. They did suggest that the phenotypes for both microdeletion and microduplication were similar; however, they acknowledged that the number of reported patients was too low to claim this with confidence [13].

In addition, the correlation of genotype with phenotype is complicated by the observation that both deletion and duplication are associated with incomplete penetrance [13]. The two familial deletions of the CHL1 gene [6, 7] and the duplication [13] were all transmitted by healthy parents. In $Chl^{+/-}$ mice, there is a spectrum from normal to abnormal behaviour [12]. This spectrum may arise from different genetic backgrounds of the mice used in these studies; hence, genetic factors that lie outside the CNVs identified in human case reports may be playing a role in observed phenotypic variability.

Small scale duplications and their phenotypic spectrum are diverse, widespread, and incompletely understood [23]. They are thought to contribute significantly to genomic variation both in creating phenotypic diversity and in some cases causing disease [23]. With dosage-sensitive genes, under- and overexpression phenotypes can give rise to the same phenotype, or different phenotypes. In the case of the former, the gene balance hypothesis suggests that under- and overexpression of genes encoding for proteins that comprise a multimeric regulatory protein complex disturb the stoichiometry of protein subunits and can lead to the same clinical phenotype even though the underlying molecular mechanism differs [23]. This is contradicted by the insufficient amount hypothesis, which suggests that haploinsufficient genes are required at abnormally high levels, so they are more sensitive to reductions than increases in dosage. This hypothesis explains the different phenotypes seen in under- and overexpression of some genes.

Unfortunately, the case reported here has several major phenotypic and genotypic differences compared to the previous CHL1 duplication case so we are unable to confirm a clear phenotype that is distinct from patients carrying CHL1 gene deletions. In the case of phenotype, motor delay, a key feature in this case, is not apparent in the previous microduplication case. As mentioned above, the previous case reached her first motor milestones within the normal range, and no lower limb spasticity was reported. Additionally, her onset of speech delay was later than our case. The previous study had the advantage of following the subject until 16 years of age, when she continued to show significant intellectual disabilities [13]. Unfortunately, as our case is under 3 years of age, intellectual assessment is incomplete.

The distal duplicated region in our case (only 104 kb involving the 5' region of the CHL1 gene) is smaller than the previously reported microduplication of 1.07 Mb that encompasses the entire CHL1 gene [13]. The significance of duplicating the amino terminal regions of the CHL1 and CNTN6 genes is not known. It is possible that they affect the expression of their entire respective genes or even that of neighbouring genes. There are several proposed transcription factor binding sites upstream of the transcription start site of the CHL1 gene that are contained within the duplicated segment [14]. Therefore, the duplication breakpoints flanking the amino terminal region of the CHL1 gene may lead to gene disruption and hence reduced gene expression. In addition, there is a proposed 63 bp upstream open reading frame (uORF) that lies in the 5' untranslated region of transcripts 1 and 2 of the CHL1 gene [24]. uORFs have been suggested to regulate gene expression by largely reducing translational efficiency of the main ORF [25].

Another anomaly in our case is the area of copy-neutral allelic imbalance between the two duplicated regions. This region of approximately 220 kb contains the remainder of the CHL1 gene but no other genes. A proposed mechanism for a copy-neutral allelic imbalance region flanked by duplicated regions could involve two separate events. The first is a meiotic recombination event leading to a duplication of the 3pter region. Figure 3 shows a proposed mechanism of nonallelic homologous recombination involving repetitive elements flanking two genes. The maintenance of allelic imbalance in a copy-neutral region suggests two cell lines, both with the duplications present, but differing in the copy-neutral region. In one of the cell lines the region between the two duplications may have undergone interstitial segmental isodisomy due to an exchange between homologous

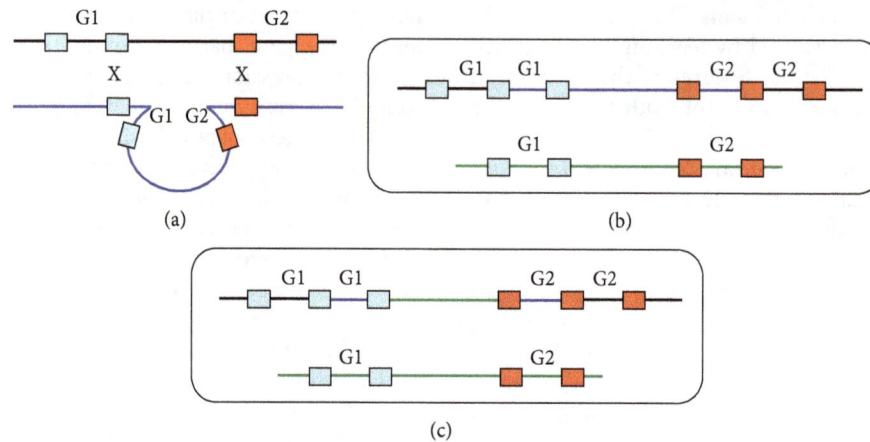

FIGURE 3: Schematic of hypothetical meiotic and mitotic recombination events leading to the observed allelic and copy number imbalances in the proband. (a) Shows a possible exchange between homologous chromosomes at meiosis that could lead to a copy number gain in two neighbouring genes (labelled G1 and G2); the coloured boxes represent flanking alleles of a repetitive sequence. (b) Shows the homologous chromosomes 3 of the proband at conception. (c) Shows a possible early mitotic event (between homologous copies of chromosome 3) during development of the proband that would give rise to interstitial segmental isodisomy in the region bounded by genes 1 and 2. The contribution of this cell line with that of the cell line represented in (b) would be consistent with the allelic imbalance and copy number data of the proband.

chromosomes and retention of only one of the recombinant outcomes [26]. It is possible that the flanking duplicated regions predispose the intervening region of chromosome 3 to this exchange event.

5. Conclusions

As previously recognised, the number of patients with duplications of the *CHL1* gene is too small to classify this anomaly as definitely disease causing [13]. This case adds to the limited literature and is complicated by a more complex chromosomal imbalance compared to other reports.

In support of other cases, the proband reported here demonstrates complex rearrangements within 3p26.3 and its correlation with neurodevelopment. Again, our analysis highlights the importance of understanding the pathogenic mechanism of dosage-sensitive genes in their under- and overexpressed states, and in particular the *CHL1* gene, given its vital function in cognitive development. In this respect, family studies are ongoing in the case reported here.

Conflict of Interests

The authors declare that there is no conflict of interests regarding the publication of this paper.

References

[1] M. Verjaal and M. B. De Nef, "A patient with a partial deletion of the short arm of chromosome 3," *American Journal of Diseases of Children*, vol. 132, no. 1, pp. 43–45, 1978.

[2] K. Narahara, K. Kikkawa, M. Murakami et al., "Loss of the 3p25.3 band is critical in the manifestation of del(3p) syndrome: karyotype-phenotype correlation in cases with deficiency of the distal portion of the short arm of chromosome 3," *American Journal of Medical Genetics*, vol. 35, no. 2, pp. 269–273, 1990.

[3] S. Kariya, K. Aoji, H. Akagi et al., "A terminal deletion of the short arm of chromosome 3: karyotype 46, XY, del (3) (p25-pter); a case report and literature review," *International Journal of Pediatric Otorhinolaryngology*, vol. 56, no. 1, pp. 71–78, 2000.

[4] C. B. Cargile, D. L.-M. Goh, B. K. Goodman et al., "Molecular cytogenetic characterization of a subtle interstitial del(3)(p25.3p26.2) in a patient with deletion 3p syndrome," *American Journal of Medical Genetics*, vol. 109, no. 2, pp. 133–138, 2002.

[5] C.-P. Chen, S.-P. Lin, C.-S. Ho et al., "Distal 3p monosomy associated with epilepsy in a boy," *Genetic Counseling*, vol. 16, no. 4, pp. 429–432, 2005.

[6] C. Cuoco, P. Ronchetto, S. Gimelli et al., "Microarray based analysis of an inherited terminal 3p26.3 deletion, containing only the CHL1 gene, from a normal father to his two affected children," *Orphanet Journal of Rare Diseases*, vol. 6, no. 1, article 12, 2011.

[7] P. Pohjola, N. de Leeuw, M. Penttinen, and H. Kääriäinen, "Terminal 3p deletions in two families—correlation between molecular karyotype and phenotype," *American Journal of Medical Genetics A*, vol. 152, no. 2, pp. 441–446, 2010.

[8] C.-P. Chen, Y.-N. Su, C.-Y. Hsu et al., "Mosaic deletion-duplication syndrome of chromosome 3: prenatal molecular cytogenetic diagnosis using cultured and uncultured amniocytes and association with fetoplacental discrepancy," *Taiwanese Journal of Obstetrics and Gynecology*, vol. 50, no. 4, pp. 485–491, 2011.

[9] T. Fernandez, T. Morgan, N. Davis et al., "Disruption of contactin 4 (CNTN4) results in developmental delay and other features of 3p deletion syndrome," *American Journal of Human Genetics*, vol. 74, no. 6, pp. 1286–1293, 2004.

[10] T. Dijkhuizen, T. van Essen, P. van der Vlies et al., "FISH and array-CGH analysis of a complex chromosome 3 aberration suggests that loss of CNTN4 and CRBN contributes to mental retardation in 3pter deletions," *American Journal of Medical Genetics A*, vol. 140, no. 22, pp. 2482–2487, 2006.

[11] M.-H. Wei, I. Karavanova, S. V. Ivanov et al., "In silico-initiated cloning and molecular characterization of a novel

human member of the L1 gene family of neural cell adhesion molecules," *Human Genetics*, vol. 103, no. 3, pp. 355–364, 1998.

[12] S. G. M. Frints, P. Marynen, D. Hartmann et al., "CALL interrupted in a patient with non-specific mental retardation: gene dosage-dependent alteration of murine brain development and behavior," *Human Molecular Genetics*, vol. 12, no. 13, pp. 1463–1474, 2003.

[13] M. Shoukier, S. Fuchs, E. Schawibold et al., "Microduplication of 3p26. 3 in nonsyndromic intellectual disability indicates an important role of CHL1 for normal cognitive function," *Neuropediatrics*, vol. 44, pp. 268–271, 2013.

[14] University of California Santa Cruz (UCSC) Genome Browser, http://genome.ucsc.edu/.

[15] Online Mendelian Inheritance in Man (OMIM) database, http://www.ncbi.nlm.nih.gov/omim.

[16] D. Pinkel, T. Straume, and J. W. Gray, "Cytogenetic analysis using quantitative, high-sensitivity, fluorescence hybridization," *Proceedings of the National Academy of Sciences of the United States of America*, vol. 83, no. 9, pp. 2934–2938, 1986.

[17] Ministry of Health Growth Charts, http://www.health.govt.nz/our-work/life-stages/child-health/well-child-tamariki-ora-services/growth-charts.

[18] S. Solidin, B. Brugnara, and E. Wong, *Pediatric Reference Ranges*, American Association for Clinical Chemistry, 4th edition, 2003.

[19] E. Doherty, R. O'Connor, A. Zhang et al., "Developmental delay referrals and the roles of Fragile X testing and molecular karyotyping: a New Zealand perspective," *Molecular Medicine Reports*, vol. 7, no. 5, pp. 1710–1714, 2013.

[20] Y. Takeda, K. Akasaka, S. Lee et al., "Impaired motor coordination in mice lacking neural recognition molecule NB-3 of the contactin/F3 subgroup," *Journal of Neurobiology*, vol. 56, no. 3, pp. 252–265, 2003.

[21] A. Zuko, K. T. Kleijer, A. Oguro-Ando et al., "Contactins in the neurobiology of autism," *European Journal of Pharmacology*, vol. 719, no. 1–3, pp. 63–74, 2013.

[22] T. Dijkhuizen, T. van Essen, P. van der Vlies et al., "FISH and array-CGH analysis of a complex chromosome 3 aberration suggests that loss of CNTN4 and CRBN contributes to mental retardation in 3pter deletions," *American Journal of Medical Genetics A*, vol. 140, no. 22, pp. 2482–2487, 2006.

[23] B. Conrad and S. E. Antonarakis, "Gene duplication: a drive for phenotypic diversity and cause of human disease," *Annual Review of Genomics and Human Genetics*, vol. 8, pp. 17–35, 2007.

[24] AceView, http://www.ncbi.nlm.nih.gov/IEB/Research/Acembly/av.cgi?db=human&c=Gene&l=CHL1.

[25] C. Barbosa, I. Peixeiro, and L. Romão, "Gene expression regulation by upstream open reading frames and human disease," *PLoS Genetics*, vol. 9, no. 8, Article ID e1003529, 2013.

[26] H. M. Kearney, J. B. Kearney, and L. K. Conlin, "Diagnostic implications of excessive homozygosity detected by SNP-Based microarrays: consanguinity, uniparental disomy, and recessive single-gene mutations," *Clinics in Laboratory Medicine*, vol. 31, no. 4, pp. 595–613, 2011.

12

Severe Psychomotor Delay in a Severe Presentation of Cat-Eye Syndrome

Guillaume Jedraszak,[1,2] Aline Receveur,[2] Joris Andrieux,[3] Michèle Mathieu-Dramard,[1] Henri Copin,[2] and Gilles Morin[1]

[1] *Unité de Génétique Médicale et Oncogénétique, Centre Hospitalier Universitaire Amiens-Picardie, 80054 Amiens Cedex, France*
[2] *Laboratoire de Cytogénétique et Biologie de la Reproduction, CECOS de Picardie, Centre Hospitalier Universitaire Amiens-Picardie, 80054 Amiens Cedex, France*
[3] *Laboratoire de Génétique Médicale, Hôpital Jeanne de Flandre, Centre Hospitalier Régional Universitaire de Lille, 59037 Lille Cedex, France*

Correspondence should be addressed to Guillaume Jedraszak; guillaumejedraszak@yahoo.fr

Academic Editor: Philip D. Cotter

Cat-eye syndrome is a rare genetic syndrome of chromosomal origin. Individuals with cat-eye syndrome are characterized by the presence of preauricular pits and/or tags, anal atresia, and iris coloboma. Many reported cases also presented with variable congenital anomalies and intellectual disability. Most patients diagnosed with CES carry a small supernumerary bisatellited marker chromosome, resulting in partial tetrasomy of 22p-22q11.21. There are two types of small supernumerary marker chromosome, depending on the breakpoint site. In a very small proportion of cases, other cytogenetic anomalies are reportedly associated with the cat-eye syndrome phenotype. Here, we report a patient with cat-eye syndrome caused by a type 1 small supernumerary marker chromosome. The phenotype was atypical and included a severe developmental delay. The use of array comparative genomic hybridization ruled out the involvement of another chromosomal imbalance in the neurological phenotype. In the literature, only a few patients with cat-eye syndrome present with a severe developmental delay, and all of the latter carried an atypical partial trisomy 22 or an uncharacterized small supernumerary marker chromosome. Hence, this is the first report of a severe neurological phenotype in cat-eye syndrome with a typical type 1 small supernumerary marker chromosome. Our observation clearly complicates prognostic assessment, particularly when cat-eye syndrome is diagnosed prenatally.

1. Introduction

Cat-eye syndrome (CES), also referred to as Schmid-Fraccaro syndrome (OMIM 115470), is a rare genetic disease with an estimated prevalence of between 1 in 50,000 and 1 in 150,000 individuals [1]. Individuals with CES are characterized by three main clinical features: preauricular pits and/or tags, anal atresia, and iris coloboma. However, many reported cases also feature congenital kidney abnormalities, congenital cardiac defects, intellectual disability, and growth delay. It has been observed that most patients diagnosed with CES carry a small supernumerary bisatellited marker chromosome (sSMC), which results in partial tetrasomy of 22p-22q11.21. There are two types of sSMC, depending on the breakpoint site: type 1,

the most frequent, involves the cat-eye syndrome critical region (CESCR) alone, whereas type 2, more rarely reported, involves both the CESCR and the DiGeorge syndrome critical region [2]. Other exceptional cytogenetic anomalies, such as partial trisomy of chromosome 22 [3] and intrachromosomal triplication of 22q11.21 region [4], are also reportedly associated with the CES phenotype.

Here, we report a patient who presented with typical features of CES: imperforate anus, severe preauricular and auricular anomalies, and cardiac malformation. Progression of the syndrome was marked by an uncommon, severe psychomotor delay. Cytogenetic analyses (including karyotyping, fluorescence *in situ* hybridization (FISH), and array comparative genomic hybridization (CGH)) revealed a typical

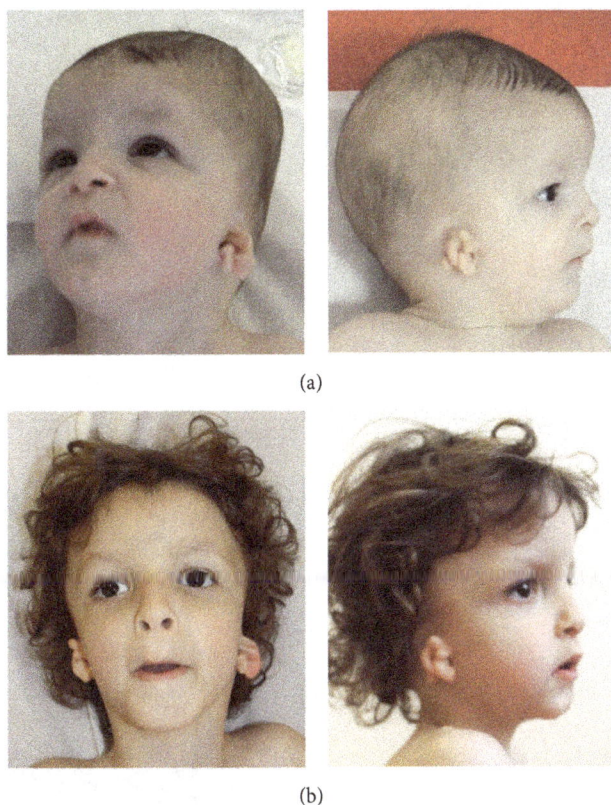

FIGURE 1: Craniofacial dysmorphism. Pictures of the patient at the age of 6 months (top panel) and 3 and a half (bottom panel). The facial dysmorphism consisted in hypertelorism, downslanting palpebral fissures, a thin upper lip, retrognathism, an irregularly shaped skull, and severe malformation of the external ears.

type 1 sSMC involving the 22p-22q11.21 region and ruled out other chromosomal imbalances.

2. Case Presentation

The patient was the second child born to healthy, unrelated parents with no family history of malformation or intellectual disability. The pregnancy featured an elevated risk score at the second-trimester trisomy 21 screening test (1 out of 198) and the development of intrauterine growth restriction during the third trimester. The parents did not wish amniocentesis to be performed. The patient was born after 38 weeks of gestation, with a birth weight of 2800 g (10th percentile) and a head circumference of 35 cm (50–75th percentile). A clinical examination revealed an imperforate anus, facial dysmorphism (Figure 1), general hypotonia, and bilateral malformation of the external ears (present as several tags, in combination with atresia of the external auditory canal) (Figure 1). Hearing tests evidenced a 70 dB bilateral conductive hearing loss. A CT scan showed bilateral hypoplasia of the tympanic cavity and right-side hypoplasia of the middle ear. Due to poor weight gain during the first weeks of life, the patient underwent gastrostomy. The subsequent course was marked by a severe global developmental delay: the child began sitting at the age of 2 years and 9 months and was unable to walk at

the age of 3 and a half. His language was also severely impaired, with the absence of distinctive words until the age of 3 years and a half. Brain MRI showed thickening of the upper two-thirds of the pituitary stalk but no other malformation, suggesting the presence of an ectopic posterior pituitary gland in addition to the normally situated posterior pituitary gland. The results of hormone assays (for IgF1, GH, ACTH, FSH, LH, TSH, FT3, FT4, and cortisol) were normal. Cryptorchidism and right-side Duane syndrome were also observed. At the age of 3 and a half, the patient weighed 10.4 kg (<3rd percentile), was 97 cm tall (25th–50th percentile), and had a head circumference of 49 cm (25th–50th percentile).

Karyotyping of a peripheral blood sample revealed an additional dicentric sSMC (Figures 2(a), 2(b), and 2(c)). The results of FISH analyses using probes RP11-112D4 (22q11.21—cat-eye syndrome critical region) and TBX1 (DiGeorge syndrome critical region) (Figure 2(d)) and oligonucleotide-based array-CGH using a 44K array (AgilentTM, Agilent Technologies, Santa Clara, CA, USA) showed a typical type 1 CES chromosome (Figure 2(e)), with the following results: 47,XY,+idic(22)(q11.21)[19].ish22q11.21(RP11-112D4)x4[15]. arr22q11.1q11.21(16,053,473-18,641,468)x4(hg19). The parents' karyotypes were normal, confirming the *de novo* occurrence of the sSMC.

(a)

(b)

(c)

(d)

(e)

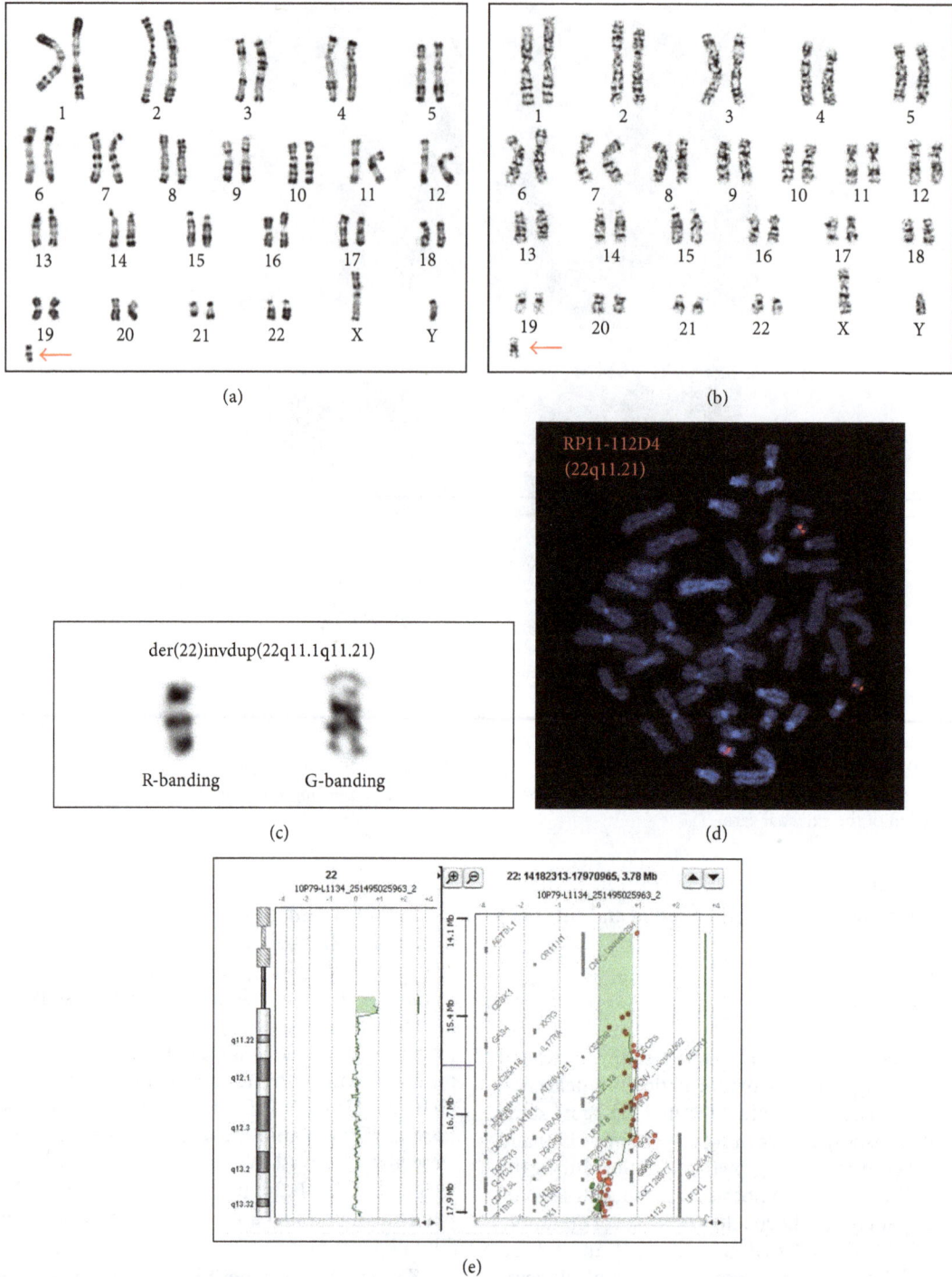

FIGURE 2: Cytogenetic testing. RHG-banding (a) and GTG-banding (b) karyotypes show the sSMC (red arrow). A zoomed image on the sSMC confirmed that the latter is dicentric and bisatellited (c). FISH analysis with an RP11-112D4 (22q11.21) probe shows two normal signals and one doubled signal, confirming the involvement of the CESCR (d).

3. Discussion

To the best of our knowledge, this is the first report of a very severe neurological phenotype in CES caused by an isolated type 1 sSMC (according to McTaggart et al.'s classification [2]).

The three main characteristic clinical symptoms identifying cat-eye syndrome are preauricular anomalies, anorectal malformations, and coloboma of the iris. Other recurrent observed features include variable congenital kidney abnormalities, congenital cardiac defects, and mild to severe growth delays. Symptoms and findings associated with CES are also extremely variable in range and severity among the affected patients.

This phenotypic variability in CES has been extensively studied [1, 5]. Our patient manifested only two of the three typical characteristics: an anal malformation and ear anomalies. Missing of one of the three main clinical sign is not so uncommon in CES patients: only 41% of them presented with the three main characteristic features. Iris coloboma is the most frequently missing typical feature, as 50% of patients with CES do not present with this eye anomaly [1]. Furthermore, the patient presented with other features commonly found in CES, such as cryptorchidism (24% of cases), impaired ocular motility (25 to 76% of cases), and facial dysmorphism.

Intellectual disability or psychomotor delay (ID/PD) can also be considered as a common feature in CES, since it is present in 32% of cases. However, the neurologic impairment is rarely prominent. Of the 50 patients carrying invdup(22) and with a detailed neurologic phenotype reviewed in [1], only 17 presented with mild-to-moderate ID/PD and none presented with severe ID/PD. Only a few patients diagnosed with CES have been reported as suffering from a severe developmental delay. These patients did not carry the common type 1 sSMC but carried other chromosomal anomalies rarely reported to be associated with the CES phenotype: partial trisomy 22q (more often associated with severe ID/DD [6, 7]) or a type 2 sSMC [8]. It is noteworthy that none of these patients have been assessed with array-CGH; hence, the presence of an additional, small, associated chromosomal imbalance (which may have been involved in the severe neurological phenotype) cannot be ruled out.

We reported the first case of severe developmental delay in a patient with CES caused by a typical type 1 sSMC. Absence of mosaicism for the sSMC could explain a part of the severity of the phenotype of our patient, even if previous reported studies did not show any impact of the mosaicism rate on the severity of the phenotype of CES patients [1]. Array-CGH ruled out the involvement of another chromosomal imbalance in the neurological phenotype. However, we cannot exclude the involvement of other genetics (point mutation in one of the genes comprised in the sSMC or in another gene responsible for developmental delay, uniparental disomy, etc.) or nongenetic factors in the severity of the phenotype of our patient.

In conclusion, this observation clearly complicates prognostic assessment when CES is diagnosed prenatally.

Conflict of Interests

The authors declare that they have no conflict of interests regarding the publication of this paper.

Acknowledgment

The authors wish to express their sincere gratitude to the patient and his family for their cooperation.

References

[1] M. J. W. Berends, G. Tan-Sindhunata, B. Leegte, and A. J. van Essen, "Phenotypic variability of cat-eye syndrome," *Genetic Counseling*, vol. 12, no. 1, pp. 23–34, 2001.

[2] K. E. McTaggart, M. L. Budarf, D. A. Driscoll, B. S. Emanuel, P. Ferreira, and H. E. McDermid, "Cat eye syndrome chromosome breakpoint clustering: identification of two intervals also associated with 22q11 deletion syndrome breakpoints," *Cytogenetics and Cell Genetics*, vol. 81, no. 3-4, pp. 222–228, 1998.

[3] M. Meins, P. Burfeind, S. Motsch et al., "Partial trisomy of chromosome 22 resulting from an interstitial duplication of 22q11.2 in a child with typical cat eye syndrome," *Journal of Medical Genetics*, vol. 40, no. 5, article e62, 2003.

[4] J. Knijnenburg, Y. van Bever, L. O. M. Hulsman et al., "A 600 kb triplication in the cat eye syndrome critical region causes anorectal, renal and preauricular anomalies in a three-generation family," *European Journal of Human Genetics*, vol. 20, no. 9, pp. 986–989, 2012.

[5] A. Schinzel, W. Schmid, M. Fraccaro et al., "The 'Cat Eye syndrome': dicentric small marker chromosome probably derived from a No. 22 (Tetrasomy 22pter → q11) associated with a characteristic phenotype—report of 11 patients and delineation of the clinical picture," *Human Genetics*, vol. 57, no. 2, pp. 148–158, 1981.

[6] A. Schinzel, W. Schmid, P. Auf der Maur et al., "Incomplete trisomy 22. I. Familial 11/22 translocation with 3:1 meiotic disjunction. Delineation of a common clinical picture and report of nine new cases from six families," *Human Genetics*, vol. 56, no. 3, pp. 249–262, 1981.

[7] E. S. Romagna, M. C. Appel da Silva, and P. A. Z. Ballardin, "Schmid-Fraccaro syndrome: severe neurologic features," *Pediatric Neurology*, vol. 42, no. 2, pp. 151–153, 2010.

[8] A. J. Mears, A. M. V. Duncan, M. L. Budarf et al., "Molecular characterization of the marker chromosome associated with cat eye syndrome," *The American Journal of Human Genetics*, vol. 55, no. 1, pp. 134–142, 1994.

13

Unexplained False Negative Results in Noninvasive Prenatal Testing: Two Cases Involving Trisomies 13 and 18

R. Hochstenbach,[1] G. C. M. L. Page-Christiaens,[2] A. C. C. van Oppen,[2] K. D. Lichtenbelt,[1] J. J. T. van Harssel,[1] T. Brouwer,[1] G. T. R. Manten,[2] P. van Zon,[1] M. Elferink,[1] K. Kusters,[1] O. Akkermans,[1] J. K. Ploos van Amstel,[1] and G. H. Schuring-Blom[1]

[1]Department of Medical Genetics, Division of Biomedical Genetics, University Medical Centre Utrecht, P.O. Box 85090, Mail Stop KC04.084.2, 3508 AB Utrecht, Netherlands
[2]Department of Obstetrics and Gynecology, University Medical Centre Utrecht, P.O. Box 85090, Mail Stop KE04.123.1, 3508 AB Utrecht, Netherlands

Correspondence should be addressed to R. Hochstenbach; p.f.r.hochstenbach@umcutrecht.nl

Academic Editor: Philip D. Cotter

Noninvasive prenatal testing (NIPT) validation studies show high sensitivity and specificity for detection of trisomies 13, 18, and 21. False negative cases have rarely been reported. We describe a false negative case of trisomy 13 and another of trisomy 18 in which NIPT was commercially marketed directly to the clinician. Both cases came to our attention because a fetal anatomy scan at 20 weeks of gestation revealed multiple anomalies. Karyotyping of cultured amniocytes showed nonmosaic trisomies 13 and 18, respectively. Cytogenetic investigation of cytotrophoblast cells from multiple placental biopsies showed a low proportion of nontrisomic cells in each case, but this was considered too small for explaining the false negative NIPT result. The discordant results also could not be explained by early gestational age, elevated maternal weight, a vanishing twin, or suboptimal storage or transport of samples. The root cause of the discrepancies could, therefore, not be identified. The couples involved experienced difficulties in accepting the unexpected and late-adverse outcome of their pregnancy. We recommend that all parties involved in caring for couples who choose NIPT should collaborate to clarify false negative results in order to unravel possible biological causes and to improve the process of patient care from initial counseling to communication of the result.

1. Introduction

Noninvasive prenatal testing (NIPT) based on massively parallel sequencing (MPS) of cell-free fetal DNA (cffDNA) fragments in the maternal circulation is rapidly becoming common clinical practice [1–5]. These DNA fragments are derived from apoptotic placental cytotrophoblast cells [4–6]. At approximately 10 weeks of gestation, the fraction of cffDNA fragments in the maternal circulation is about 10–20% of the total cell-free DNA while the remainder is of maternal origin [3–5].

NIPT enables testing for trisomies 13, 18, and 21 in pregnancies that are at elevated risk for aneuploidy, for example, because of maternal age, first trimester combined screening result, or ultrasound abnormalities [3–6]. Prospective studies show that trisomies 18 and 21 can also reliably be detected by NIPT in an unselected obstetric population [7–10]. In both groups the sensitivity and specificity of NIPT are 99-100% for trisomy 21. For trisomy 18, sensitivity is 90–100% and specificity is 99-100%; for trisomy 13, they are 93–100% and 99-100%, respectively [6–10]. Nevertheless, NIPT is not considered a diagnostic test and, in case of a positive NIPT result, follow-up invasive testing by chorionic villi sampling (CVS) or amniocentesis must be offered before a definitive diagnosis can be made [11, 12]. The major reason is that placental DNA is not representative of the fetus in all cases, a phenomenon that has been known for decades when performing cytogenetic analysis of chorionic villi [13–15].

Most laboratories adopt a minimum threshold of 4% cffDNA for yielding an accurate result by MPS [5]. Several factors influence the contribution of fetal cells to the total cell-free DNA. A low fetal DNA fraction has been attributed to early gestational age or high maternal weight [5, 16–18]. Also, prolonged (>24 hrs) storage of blood samples under suboptimal conditions prior to processing reduces the fetal DNA fraction because of an increase of maternal genomic DNA due to cell degradation [19, 20]. Furthermore, a reduction has been reported in the fetal DNA fraction in trisomy 13, trisomy 18, and monosomy X pregnancies as compared to euploid pregnancies [21, 22], but this has not been confirmed in all studies [23]. Finally, in cases of a mosaic placenta, the presence of euploid cells reduces the fetal DNA fraction contributed by the aneuploid cells. For example, if there is 50% mosaicism for a trisomy in the cytotrophoblast, a fetal DNA fraction of 10% is reduced to an effective fraction of 5% for detecting the trisomy [17]. There is little information on how frequently these parameters affect the clinical performance of NIPT. A review of 15 clinical validation studies, together incorporating more than 21,000 cases, shows that few of the trisomies are missed [6]. For trisomy 21, 3 out of 835 cases were false negative (0.36%), 6 out of 315 for trisomy 18 (1.90%) and 4 out of 60 for trisomy 13 (6.67%). In most of these studies, the fetal DNA fraction was not provided for the false negative cases, and follow-up by cytogenetic or molecular genetic investigation of the placenta and the newborn child was not included in the study design. Therefore, few data are available on the contribution of the diverse causes of false negative results. Problems with sample identity were reported in one study, leading to a false negative result in 2 out of 3,430 cases [24]. Published case reports of false negative NIPT results are summarized in Table 1, showing that, in cases with molecular or cytogenetic follow-up investigations, placental mosaicism was frequently involved and was the most likely cause of the false negative result. Here we report the cytogenetic follow-up of two novel false negative cases.

2. Case Reports

In neighboring countries of The Netherlands, commercial marketing of NIPT started in 2012, and several thousands of Dutch women, including women at low risk for fetal aneuploidy, have opted for "outsourced" NIPT testing via institutions abroad. The two cases described here came to our attention after a fetal anatomy scan at 20 weeks of gestation revealed anomalies indicative of trisomy 13 (Case 1) and trisomy 18 (Case 2). Case 1 has been referred to previously [35]. The relevant characteristics of these two cases are summarized in Table 2.

2.1. Case 1. In a 35-year-old, healthy woman (G1P0), first trimester combined testing for Down syndrome at 12 5/7 weeks of gestation showed a risk of 1/190 for trisomy 18; the nuchal translucency (NT) was 1.6 mm (1.18 MoM). She opted for NIPT to avoid potential complications of invasive testing. Blood was taken at 13 5/7 weeks of gestation and sent overseas via an intermediate party. Maternal weight and BMI (body

mass index) were 59 kg and 22.0, respectively. NIPT results were available at 15 weeks and indicated that she was at "low risk" for each of the three common trisomies (<1/10,000). The cffDNA fraction was reported to be 8.8%. Ultrasound examination at 19 5/7 weeks showed a small male fetus with a right-sided cleft of the lip and alveolar ridge and cerebellar vermis hypoplasia. There were no signs of a vanishing or demised fetus nor of an empty, second sac. Two days later, the couple was counseled by a clinical geneticist. Amniocentesis was performed at 20 5/7 weeks. The patient consented to have a blood sample taken for NIPT prior to amniocentesis. The blood sample was processed and analyzed in the laboratory of our department, at the time performing a NIPT validation study. The result of quantitative fluorescence polymerase chain reaction (QF-PCR) based on DNA extracted from uncultured amniocytes was indicative of nonmosaic trisomy 13, and the couple was informed at 21 weeks. Karyotyping of G-banded metaphases of cultured amniocytes (12 clones, *in situ* method) showed a 47,XY,+13 karyotype in all metaphases. NIPT in our department using the SOLiD Wildfire was performed as described [36]; the result was consistent with trisomy 13 (z-score 25.5). The couple was counseled by the clinical geneticist for a second time and was supported by a bereavement counselor for decision making. The pregnancy was terminated at 22 weeks. Postpartum karyotyping of 32 metaphases of cultured fetal fibroblasts showed a 47,XY,+13 karyotype in all cells. The placenta was sampled at 9 representative approximately equidistant positions, representing 9 equally large sections. For each biopsy, mesenchymal and cytotrophoblast cells were separated as published earlier [37, 38] and 100 interphase nuclei of each cell type were investigated by fluorescence *in situ* hybridization (FISH). This showed high percentages of cells with trisomy 13 throughout the placenta in both cytotrophoblast (average 96%; range 91–100%) and mesenchyme (average 96%; range 92–100%). A similar result was seen for the umbilical cord (97%).

2.2. Case 2. A 40-year-old, healthy woman (G2P1) had blood taken for NIPT at 11 0/7 weeks of gestation. The blood sample was sent overseas via an intermediate party. The cffDNA fraction was reported to be 10.7% and the test result indicated that there was a "low risk" for each of the three common trisomies (<1/10,000). Maternal weight and BMI were 70 kg and 22.4, respectively. At ultrasound examination at 19 5/7 weeks, multiple anomalies were noted in a female fetus, including a strawberry skull, bilateral plexus cysts, a complex cardiac anomaly (large ventricular septal defect, Ebstein anomaly of the tricuspid valve, and abnormal pulmonary venous connection), and bilateral clenched fists and rocker bottom feet. There were no indications for presence of a vanishing twin nor of an empty sac. The next day amniocentesis was performed and the patient agreed to have a blood sample taken, prior to amniocentesis, for NIPT. Results of QF-PCR based on DNA from uncultured amniocytes were available at 20 weeks and were indicative of nonmosaic trisomy 18. The couple was counseled by a clinical geneticist and assisted by a bereavement counselor. Karyotyping of metaphases of 30 clones of cultured amniocytes showed a 47,XX,+18 karyotype in all clones. In addition, FISH showed trisomy 18 in all

TABLE 1: Survey of published cases of false negative NIPT by massive parallel shotgun sequencing with (molecular) cytogenetic follow-up included[1].

Trisomy	Study [reference]	Indication for NIPT	Case, mat. age	Blood drawn at GA[2]	Fetal DNA fraction (effective fetal DNA fraction)	Result of NIPT	Karyotype	Explanation for false negative NIPT result
13	Canick et al. (2013) [17]	Ultrasound abnormalities	Case 1 34 yrs	14 w	6% (0.6%)	z-score 0.08 for chromosome 13	46,XX/47,XX,+13 in cultured amniocytes	Amniocentesis showed 10% mosaicism for a cell line with +13
18	Canick et al. (2013) [17]	Maternal age	Case 5 39 yrs	12 w	23% (10%)	z-score 0.22 for chromosome 18	47,XY,+21/48,XY,+18,+21 in CVS	CVS showed 45% mosaicism for a cell line with both +18 and +21
18	Gao et al. (2014) [25]	1/70 risk for tri-21 by combined 1st trim. test	43 yrs	13 w	7.4%	Low risk tri-13, tri-18, and tri-21, high risk XXX	48,XXX,+18 in cultured amniocytes	Estimated 20–30% of placental cells studied by FISH were +18, with QF-PCR showing variable levels of +18 cells across the placenta
18	Mao et al. (2014) [26]	1/313 risk for tri-18 by serum screening	22 yrs	17 w	11.6% (4.1%)	z-score 0.35 for tri-18; z-score 4.4 for tri-21	47,XX,+18 in cultured amniocytes	Placental biopsies showed on average 50% +21, 35% +18, and 15% normal cells, but at least one region had 61% +21 but only 22% +18
18	Pan et al. (2014) [27]	1/45 risk for tri-21 by combined test	24 yrs	18 w	Not provided	t-score −0.52 for tri-18; t-score −4.05 for X-chromosome	47,XX,+18 in cultured amniocytes, both by karyotyping and SNP-array	About 30% of placental cells studied by FISH were +18, and about 67% were 45, X; SNP-array was indicative of ~50% cells with +18
18	Zhang et al. (2015) [28]	1/360 risk for tri-21 by combined test	29 yrs	19 w	5.3% (1.1–2.2%)	Aneuploidy not detected	47,XY,+18 in products of conception	6 placental biopsies showed 20–40% cells with +18
18	Zhang et al. (2015) [28]	1/45 risk for tri-21 by combined test	24 yrs	20 w	9.5% (2.9%)	Indicative of 45,X	47,XX,+18 in cultured amniocytes	In placental tissue 30% of the cells showed +18 and 60% showed 45,X
21	Canick et al. (2013) [17]	Maternal age	Case 2 44 yrs	11 w	17% (1.7%)	z-score 2.03 for chromosome 21	46,XY[20]/47,XY,+21[2] in CVS	CVS showed 9% mosaicism for a cell line with +21
21	Canick et al. (2013) [17]	Maternal age	Case 3 41 yrs	12 w	9% (4.5%)	z-score −1.25 for chromosome 21	46,XY/47,XY,+21 in CVS	50% mosaicism by CVS; possibly this was lower in the placenta as a whole
21	Wang et al. (2013) [29]	1/370 risk for tri-21 by serum screening at 17 w	Case 1 32 yrs	18 w	15.6%	z-score 2.04[3] for chromosome 21	46,XX,der(21;21)(q10;q10),+21 in fetal blood (cordocentesis)	Placental biopsies had 17%, 21%, 23%, and 53% cells with +21
21	Wang et al. (2013) [29]	2 spontaneous abortions	Case 2 35 yrs	18 w	19.7%	z-score 1.33 for chromosome 21	47,XY,+21 in cultured amniocytes	Placental biopsies had 2%, 51%, and 76% cells with +21
21	Smith et al. (2014) [30]	CAVCD[4]	32 yrs	20 w	Not provided	"Negative" for trisomy 21	47,XX,+21 in postnatal blood	No study of placenta or umbilical cord; no explanation provided

Notes. [1] A false negative case of trisomy 21 was also mentioned by Wang et al. [31], 2 other false negative trisomy 21 cases were mentioned by Dar et al. [32], and another 6 false negative trisomy 21 cases were described by Zhang et al. [28]; a false negative case of trisomy 18 was mentioned by Beamon et al. [33], another one by Quezada et al. [34] and by Zhang et al. [28]; 3 false negative cases of tri-13 were reported by Quezada et al. [34]; all of these were without further investigation of the possible causes of the discrepant findings.
[2] GA: gestational age.
[3] In a repeat blood sample taken at 24 weeks the z-score for chromosome 21 was 4.0 and trisomy-21 was reported as a result.
[4] CAVCD: complete atrioventricular canal defect.

TABLE 2: Demographics and summary of laboratory testing in two cases with false negative NIPT.

Case; age (status)	BMI	Medication, alcohol, and drugs	1st trimester combined screening (NT)	Blood for NIPT drawn at GA[1]	Fetal fraction	Result of NIPT issued by a third party			Pregnancy outcome; cytogenetic follow-up
						Tri-13	Tri-18	Tri-21	
Case 1 35 yrs (G1P0)	22.0	Negative	1:190 risk for trisomy-18 (NT 1.6 mm)	13 5/7	8.8%	<1/10,000	<1/10,000	<1/10,000	Amniocentesis at 21 weeks showed a nonmosaic 47, XY, +13 karyotype; sampling of placenta (9 biopsies) gave no evidence for the presence of euploid cells
Case 2 40 yrs (G2P1)	22.4	Negative	Not performed	11 0/7	10.7%	<1/10,000	<1/10,000	<1/10,000	Amniocentesis at 20 weeks showed a nonmosaic 47, XX, +18 karyotype; sampling of placenta (10 biopsies) showed that a maximum of 20–30% euploid cells may have been present in the cytotrophoblast

Note. [1]GA: gestational age.

52 metaphases investigated after trypsinization of cells cultured *in situ*. NIPT performed in our department using the SOLiD Wildfire [36] was also consistent with trisomy 18 (z-score 25.4). The pregnancy was terminated at 23 2/7 weeks after repeated counseling sessions. In cultured lymphocytes from fetal blood, trisomy 18 was detected in all 89 metaphases investigated. Ten biopsies were taken from the placenta, representing 10 equally sized sections, and investigated as described above. Eight biopsies had ≥70% trisomy 18 cells in both cytotrophoblast (average 78%; range 70–90%) and mesenchyme (average 78%; range 73–83%). In two biopsies the cytotrophoblast showed 64% and 69% trisomy 18, respectively, whereas mesenchyme was 88% and 80%, respectively. In the umbilical cord biopsy, we found 80% trisomy 18. Presence of 20–30% euploid cells in the cytotrophoblast would reduce the 10.7% fetal fraction to an effective fetal fraction of 7.5–8.5%.

3. Discussion

We describe two cases in which "outsourced" NIPT gave a "low risk" result (<1/10,000) in women carrying a trisomic fetus. The patients received the NIPT result between 12 and 15 weeks of gestation. When, at 20 weeks of gestation, multiple fetal anomalies were detected by ultrasound examination, amniocentesis was performed. Analysis by QF-PCR and karyotyping revealed trisomy 13 in one case and trisomy 18 in the other. These unexpected, discrepant results caused disbelief and distress to the families, requiring multiple counseling sessions.

Several companies in the USA and Europe are marketing MPS-based NIPT directly to the clinician (e.g., Ariosa Diagnostics, Natera, Verinata Health, the Sequenom Center for Molecular Medicine, and LifeCodexx). Validation studies in high risk pregnancies (elevated maternal age, increased risk from first trimester combined testing) showed high sensitivity and specificity for the detection of each of the three common trisomies [3, 4, 6–10]. False negative results are inherent to this technique that is based on quantification of sequence reads of cffDNA fragments originating from the cytotrophoblast. This can be explained in several ways. NIPT depends on a statistical assessment of the sequence reads. Therefore, cutoff values must be defined for discrimination between normal and abnormal results, and, as a consequence, NIPT is still considered a screening test and not a diagnostic test [11]. In addition, false negative results can be caused by a low fetal fraction, for example, when NIPT is done too early in gestation (<10 weeks) [5, 14, 17], in obese women [5, 16–18], in cases of suboptimal, prolonged storage of blood samples prior to processing [19, 20], or if there is an euploid vanishing twin that contributed to the cffDNA. Finally, large-scale evaluation of CVS showed that in 0.8–1% of cases there is confined placental mosaicism, with a different karyotype in cytotrophoblast cells, the source of cffDNA, than that in the fetus proper [13, 14]. In a retrospective study based on 52,673 pregnancies, placental mosaicism was predicted to be the likely cause of a false negative NIPT result in 1/136 trisomy 13, 1/64 trisomy 18, and 1/135 trisomy 21 cases [39].

To systematically explore the possible causes of the false negative results in our two cases we first looked at factors known to cause a low fetal DNA fraction. An early gestational age (<10 weeks) or elevated maternal weight was not implied and we have no indications for suboptimal storage or transport conditions of the blood samples. Second trimester ultrasound examination did not indicate the presence of a vanishing twin or an empty, second sac, and we assume that this was also the case at the time of blood sampling for NIPT. To look for mosaicism as an explanation, we examined multiple placental biopsies and karyotyped fetal cells. The results are summarized in Table 2. In Case 1, the proportion of non-trisomic cells in the cytotrophoblast was 0% or close to 0%. In Case 2, on average not more than 20–30% nontrisomic cells were present in the cytotrophoblast. Given a cell-free fetal DNA fraction of 10.7%, this percentage of nontrisomic cells would not have been large enough to lower the fraction of aneuploid, fetal DNA below 4%. Case 2 differs in this respect from the cases described by Canick et al. [17], Wang et al. [29], Gao et al. [25], and Mao et al. [26] in which much larger fractions of nontrisomic cells were found in placental biopsies (Table 1). Thus, there is no evidence that the false negative NIPT results in Cases 1 and 2 are due to placental mosaicism. Because the NIPT tests were carried out by a third party we could not verify sample identity (as required according to ISO 15189 [40]). We conclude that in both cases the root cause of the discrepant NIPT results could not be identified.

So, how should the problem of unexpected false negative NIPT results be handled in clinical practice? During pretest counseling it must be clearly explained to the patient that NIPT is based on DNA fragments from the placenta, not from the fetus, and that a false positive or false negative result may occur. This will enable pregnant women and their partners to make informed choices between NIPT and alternative options and allows to reinforce the usefulness of a fetal anatomy scan at 20 weeks of gestation. Furthermore, the presence of a demised cotwin should always be excluded since this might cause false negative (or false positive) results. In addition, a systematic investigation into the cause of discrepancies as described in this paper will be helpful not only to understand the limitations of NIPT but also to improve its performance in daily clinical practice. This investigation should include verification of sample identity as required according to ISO 15189 [40]. Finally, an international registry for systematic recording of all discordant NIPT results and their causes, as was done when CVS was introduced in prenatal diagnosis more than 30 years ago [13, 14], will provide insight into the frequency and causes of false negative and false positive NIPT results [11, 41]. In clinical practice, reported frequencies of false negative results show a surprisingly large and unexplained variation, ranging from 1/16,000 [28] or 1/9,000 [32] to 1/200 [33] consecutive cases from a mixed low and high risk population. In case of a trisomy detected by NIPT, CVS or amniocentesis can be offered for confirmation, depending on the gestational age. In case CVS is opted, both cytotrophoblast and mesenchymal cells should be investigated, and, even so, one must be aware of the possibility that a trisomy can be confined to the placenta [15, 39], a problem that does not play a role when analyzing amniotic fluid cells.

Conflict of Interests

The authors declare that there is no conflict of interests regarding the publication of this paper.

Acknowledgments

The authors are indebted to their technicians for expert assistance in cytogenetic and molecular analysis. They also thank the two families involved for their cooperation.

References

[1] R. W. K. Chiu, K. C. A. Chan, Y. Gao et al., "Noninvasive prenatal diagnosis of fetal chromosomal aneuploidy by massively parallel genomic sequencing of DNA in maternal plasma," *Proceedings of the National Academy of Sciences of the United States of America*, vol. 105, no. 51, pp. 20458–20463, 2008.

[2] H. C. Fan, Y. J. Blumenfeld, U. Chitkara, L. Hudgins, and S. R. Quake, "Noninvasive diagnosis of fetal aneuploidy by shotgun sequencing DNA from maternal blood," *Proceedings of the National Academy of Sciences of the United States of America*, vol. 105, no. 42, pp. 16266–16271, 2008.

[3] P. Benn, H. Cuckle, and E. Pergament, "Non-invasive prenatal testing for aneuploidy: current status and future prospects," *Ultrasound in Obstetrics and Gynecology*, vol. 42, no. 1, pp. 15–33, 2013.

[4] E. R. Norwitz and B. Levy, "Noninvasive prenatal testing: the future is now," *Reviews in Obstetrics & Gynecology*, vol. 6, no. 2, pp. 48–62, 2013.

[5] D. W. Bianchi and L. Wilkins-Haug, "Integration of noninvasive DNA testing for aneuploidy into prenatal care: what has happened since the rubber met the road?" *Clinical Chemistry*, vol. 60, no. 1, pp. 78–87, 2014.

[6] G. J. W. Liao, A. M. Gronowski, and Z. Zhao, "Non-invasive prenatal testing using cell-free fetal DNA in maternal circulation," *Clinica Chimica Acta*, vol. 428, pp. 44–50, 2014.

[7] K. H. Nicolaides, A. Syngelaki, G. Ashoor, C. Birdir, and G. Touzet, "Noninvasive prenatal testing for fetal trisomies in a routinely screened first-trimester population," *American Journal of Obstetrics & Gynecology*, vol. 207, no. 5, pp. 374.e1–374.e6, 2012.

[8] S. Dan, W. Wang, J. Ren et al., "Clinical application of massively parallel sequencing-based prenatal noninvasive fetal trisomy test for trisomies 21 and 18 in 11 105 pregnancies with mixed risk factors," *Prenatal Diagnosis*, vol. 32, no. 13, pp. 1225–1232, 2012.

[9] D. W. Bianchi, R. Lamar Parker, J. Wentworth et al., "DNA sequencing versus standard prenatal aneuploidy screening," *The New England Journal of Medicine*, vol. 370, no. 9, pp. 799–808, 2014.

[10] M. E. Norton, B. Jacobsson, G. K. Swamy et al., "Cell-free DNA analysis for noninvasive examination of trisomy," *The New England Journal of Medicine*, vol. 372, no. 17, pp. 1589–1597, 2015.

[11] P. Benn, A. Borell, R. Chiu et al., "Position statement from the Aneuploidy Screening Committee on behalf of the Board of the International Society for Prenatal Diagnosis," *Prenatal Diagnosis*, vol. 33, no. 7, pp. 622–629, 2013.

[12] A. R. Gregg, S. J. Gross, R. G. Best et al., "ACMG statement on noninvasive prenatal screening for fetal aneuploidy," *Genetics in Medicine*, vol. 15, no. 5, pp. 395–398, 2013.

[13] D. H. Ledbetter, J. M. Zachary, J. L. Simpson et al., "Cytogenetic results from the U.S. collaborative study on CVS," *Prenatal Diagnosis*, vol. 12, no. 5, pp. 317–345, 1992.

[14] J. M. Hahnemann and L. O. Vejerslev, "Accuracy of cytogenetic findings on chorionic villus sampling (CVS)—diagnostic consequences of CVS mosaicism and non-mosaic discrepancy in centres contributing to eucromic 1986–1992," *Prenatal Diagnosis*, vol. 17, no. 9, pp. 801–820, 1997.

[15] P. Brady, N. Brison, K. Van Den Bogaert et al., "Clinical implementation of NIPT—technical and biological challenges," *Clinical Genetics*, 2015.

[16] G. Ashoor, A. Syngelaki, L. C. Y. Poon, J. C. Rezende, and K. H. Nicolaides, "Fetal fraction in maternal plasma cell-free DNA at 11-13 weeks' gestation: relation to maternal and fetal characteristics," *Ultrasound in Obstetrics and Gynecology*, vol. 41, no. 1, pp. 26–32, 2013.

[17] J. A. Canick, G. E. Palomaki, E. M. Kloza, G. M. Lambert-Messerlian, and J. E. Haddow, "The impact of maternal plasma DNA fetal fraction on next generation sequencing tests for common fetal aneuploidies," *Prenatal Diagnosis*, vol. 33, no. 7, pp. 667–674, 2013.

[18] E. Wang, A. Batey, C. Struble, T. Musci, K. Song, and A. Oliphant, "Gestational age and maternal weight effects on fetal cell-free DNA in maternal plasma," *Prenatal Diagnosis*, vol. 33, no. 7, pp. 662–666, 2013.

[19] M. R. Fernando, K. Chen, S. Norton et al., "A new methodology to preserve the original proportion and integrity of cell-free fetal DNA in maternal plasma during sample processing and storage," *Prenatal Diagnosis*, vol. 30, no. 5, pp. 418–424, 2010.

[20] A. N. Barrett, B. G. Zimmermann, D. Wang, A. Holloway, and L. S. Chitty, "Implementing prenatal diagnosis based on cell-free fetal DNA: accurate identification of factors affecting fetal DNA yield," *PLoS ONE*, vol. 6, no. 10, Article ID e25202, 2011.

[21] R. P. Rava, A. Srinivasan, A. J. Sehnert, and D. W. Bianchi, "Circulating fetal cell-free DNA fractions differ in autosomal aneuploidies and monosomy X," *Clinical Chemistry*, vol. 60, no. 1, pp. 243–250, 2014.

[22] E. Pergament, H. Cuckle, B. Zimmermann et al., "Single-nucleotide polymorphism-based noninvasive prenatal screening in a high-risk and low-risk cohort," *Obstetrics & Gynecology*, vol. 124, no. 2, part, pp. 210–218, 2014.

[23] A. Gerovassili, C. Garner, K. H. Nicolaides, S. L. Thein, and D. C. Rees, "Free fetal DNA in maternal circulation: a potential prognostic marker for chromosomal abnormalities?" *Prenatal Diagnosis*, vol. 27, no. 2, pp. 104–110, 2007.

[24] R. P. Porreco, T. J. Garite, K. Maurel et al., "Noninvasive prenatal screening for fetal trisomies 21, 18, 13 and the common sex chromosome aneuploidies from maternal blood using massively parallel genomic sequencing of DNA," *American Journal of Obstetrics and Gynecology*, vol. 211, pp. 365.e1–365.e12, 2014.

[25] Y. Gao, D. Stejskal, F. Jiang, and W. Wang, "False-negative trisomy 18 non-invasive prenatal test result due to 48,XXX,+18 placental mosaicism," *Ultrasound in Obstetrics and Gynecology*, vol. 43, no. 4, pp. 477–478, 2014.

[26] J. Mao, T. Wang, B.-J. Wang et al., "Confined placental origin of the circulating cell free fetal DNA revealed by a discordant non-invasive prenatal test result in a trisomy 18 pregnancy," *Clinica Chimica Acta*, vol. 433, pp. 190–193, 2014.

[27] Q. Pan, B. Sun, X. Huang et al., "A prenatal case with discrepant findings between non-invasive prenatal testing and fetal genetic testings," *Molecular Cytogenetics*, vol. 7, article 48, 2014.

[28] H. Zhang, Y. Gao, F. Jiang et al., "Non-invasive prenatal testing for trisomies 21, 18 and 13: clinical experience from 146, 958 pregnancies," *Ultrasound in Obstetrics & Gynecology*, vol. 45, no. 5, pp. 530–538, 2015.

[29] Y. Wang, J. Zhu, Y. Chen et al., "Two cases of placental T21 mosaicism: challenging the detection limits of non-invasive prenatal testing," *Prenatal Diagnosis*, vol. 33, no. 12, pp. 1207–1210, 2013.

[30] M. Smith, K. M. Lewis, A. Holmes, and J. Visootsak, "A case of false negative NIPT for Down syndrome-lessons learned," *Case Reports in Genetics*, vol. 2014, Article ID 823504, 3 pages, 2014.

[31] J.-C. Wang, T. Sahoo, S. Schonberg et al., "Discordant noninvasive prenatal testing and cytogenetic results: a study of 109 consecutive cases," *Genetics in Medicine*, vol. 17, no. 3, pp. 234–236, 2015.

[32] P. Dar, K. J. Curnow, S. J. Gross et al., "Clinical experience and follow-up with large scale single-nucleotide polymorphism-based noninvasive prenatal aneuploidy testing," *American Journal of Obstetrics & Gynecology*, vol. 211, no. 5, pp. 527.e1–527.e17, 2014.

[33] C. J. Beamon, E. E. Hardisty, S. C. Harris, and N. L. Vora, "A single center's experience with noninvasive prenatal testing," *Genetics in Medicine*, vol. 16, no. 9, pp. 681–687, 2014.

[34] M. S. Quezada, M. M. Gil, C. Francisco, G. Oròsz, and K. H. Nicolaides, "Screening for trisomies 21, 18 and 13 by cell-free DNA analysis of maternal blood at 10-11 weeks' gestation and the combined test at 11-13 weeks," *Ultrasound in Obstetrics & Gynecology*, vol. 45, no. 1, pp. 36–41, 2015.

[35] P. J. Willems, H. Dierickx, E. Vandenakker et al., "The first 3,000 non-invasive prenatal tests (NIPT) with the harmony test in Belgium and the Netherlands," *Facts, Views & Vision in ObGyn*, vol. 6, no. 1, pp. 7–12, 2014.

[36] R. Hochstenbach, P. G. Nikkels, M. G. Elferink et al., "Cell-free fetal DNA in the maternal circulation originates from the cytotrophoblast: proof from an unique case," *Clinical Case Reports*, 2015.

[37] G. H. Shuring-Blom, M. Keijzer, M. E. Jakobs et al., "Molecular cytogenetic analysis of term placentae suspected of mosaicism using fluorescence in situ hybridization," *Prenatal Diagnosis*, vol. 13, no. 8, pp. 671–679, 1993.

[38] G. H. Schuring-Blom, K. Boer, and N. J. Leschot, "A placental diploid cell line is not essential for ongoing trisomy 13 or 18 pregnancies," *European Journal of Human Genetics*, vol. 9, no. 4, pp. 286–290, 2001.

[39] F. R. Grati, F. Malvestiti, J. C. Ferreira et al., "Fetoplacental mosaicism: potential implications for false-positive and false-negative noninvasive prenatal screening results," *Genetics in Medicine*, vol. 16, no. 8, pp. 620–624, 2014.

[40] International Organization for Standardization, "Medical laboratories—requirements for quality and competence," ISO 15189:2012, International Organization for Standardization, Geneva, Switzerland, 2012.

[41] M. T. Mennuti, A. M. Cherry, J. J. D. Morrissette, and L. Dugoff, "Is it time to sound an alarm about false-positive cell-free DNA testing for fetal aneuploidy?" *American Journal of Obstetrics and Gynecology*, vol. 209, no. 5, pp. 415–419, 2013.

14

A Case of Acute Myeloid Leukemia with a Previously Unreported Translocation (14; 15) (q32; q13)

Mohamad Khawandanah,[1,2] Bradley Gehrs,[3] Shibo Li,[4] Jennifer Holter Chakrabarty,[1] and Mohamad Cherry[1]

[1] *Hematology-Oncology Section, Department of Medicine, The University of Oklahoma Health Sciences Center, Oklahoma City, OK 73104, USA*
[2] *University of Oklahoma Health Sciences Center, Stephenson Cancer Center, 800 NE 10th Street, Oklahoma City, OK 73102, USA*
[3] *Department of Pathology, The University of Oklahoma Health Sciences Center, Oklahoma City, OK 73104, USA*
[4] *Department of Pediatrics, The University of Oklahoma Health Sciences Center, Oklahoma City, OK 73104, USA*

Correspondence should be addressed to Mohamad Khawandanah; mohamad-khawandanah@ouhsc.edu

Academic Editor: Philip D. Cotter

Background. We hereby describe what we believe to be the first reported case of t (14; 15) (q32; q13) associated with acute myeloid leukemia (AML). *Methods.* PubMed, Embase, and OVID search engines were used to review the related literature and similar published cases. *Case.* A 47-year-old female presented in December 2011 with AML (acute myelomonocytic leukemia) with normal cytogenetics; molecular testing revealed FLT-3 internal tandem duplication (ITD) mutation, while no mutations involving FLT3 D385/I836, NPM1 exon 12, or KIT exons 8 and 17 were detected. She was induced with 7 + 3 (cytarabine + idarubicin) and achieved complete remission after a second induction with high-dose cytarabine (HiDAC) followed by uneventful consolidation. She presented 19 months after diagnosis with relapsed disease. Of note, at relapse cytogenetic analysis revealed t (14; 15) (q32; q13), while FLT-3 analysis showed a codon D835 mutation (no ITD mutation was detected). She proved refractory to the initial clofarabine-based regimen, so FLAG-idarubicin then was used. She continued to have persistent disease, and she was discharged on best supportive care. *Conclusion.* Based on this single case of AML with t (14; 15) (q32; q13), this newly reported translocation may be associated with refractory disease.

1. Introduction

Genetic evaluation plays an integral role in the classification of AML [1–3]. Approximately 50% of patients with de novo AML have cytogenetics abnormalities. As reflected in the latest WHO classification scheme for AML, certain cytogenetic abnormalities are used to diagnose patients with AML regardless of the blast count. Cytogenetic analysis also identifies abnormalities with prognostic and therapeutic implications, it can aid in monitoring the therapeutic response, and in the future it likely will have a greater role in abnormality-tailored approaches.

Similarly, mutational analysis plays an important and expanding role in the diagnosis and management of AML. FLT3 is a member of the class III receptor tyrosine kinase family important for the normal development of hematopoietic stem cells and the immune system. FLT3 is the most commonly mutated gene in AML, with mutations occurring in about 30% of cases overall. There are several known activating mutations of FLT3 in AML, including internal tandem duplications (ITD) and mutations in the activation loop of the second tyrosine kinase domain (TKD) such as *FLT-3 D835/I836*. FLT3-ITD mutations are an adverse prognostic factor. However, the significance of FLT3-TKD mutations is unclear; they are overrepresented in the PML-RARA and inv(16) AML subtypes and more generally in the intermediate-risk cytogenetic subgroup [2].

We hereby describe what we believe to be the first reported case of t (14; 15) (q32; q13) associated with AML. Relapse in this case also is notable for alterations in the FLT3

(a)

(b)

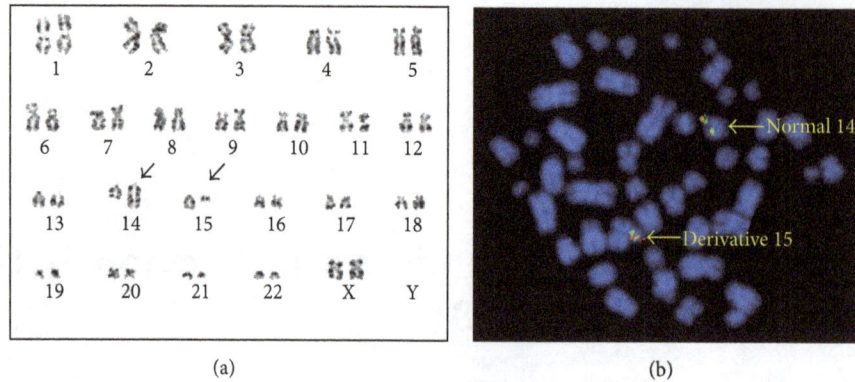

FIGURE 1: (a) G-banded chromosome analysis showed an apparently balanced translocation between chromosomes 14 and 15 at breakpoints of 14q32 and 15q13, respectively. (b) FISH analysis using IGHG1 break-apart probe revealed intact signals on a normal chromosome 14 and a derivative chromosome 15.

status (isolated FLT3-ITD mutation at diagnosis; isolated FLT3 D835 mutation at relapse) in addition to the appearance of this newly described translocation.

2. Case Presentation

The patient was a 47-year-old white female who initially presented with abdominal pain. She was noted to have leukocytosis with numerous blasts in her peripheral blood; her CBC included a WBC count of 16,900/mm^3 (with a differential of 56% blasts, 1% promyelocytes, 1% myelocytes, 1% metamyelocytes, 1% bands, 2% neutrophils, 30% lymphocytes, and 8% monocytes), a hemoglobin of 7.5 g/dL, and a platelet count of 43,000/mm^3. She did not have a significant medical or surgical history, although she had a 27-pack-year smoking history. Her father died from pancreatic cancer. On exam her vital signs were within normal limits. No splenomegaly or lymphadenopathy was noted.

Bone marrow specimens were obtained for morphologic, immunophenotypic, and genetic analyses. Based on morphology and flow cytometric analysis, the patient was diagnosed with AML (acute myelomonocytic leukemia). Flow cytometry showed 25% blasts expressing CD45 (moderate intensity), CD34, CD13, CD117 (partial), CD33 (partial), HLA-DR (partial), CD4 (partial), and CD15 (partial); the blasts had no significant expression of CD14, CD64, CD10, CD19, CD20, surface immunoglobulin light chains, CD2, CD3, CD5, CD7, CD8, or CD56. It also noted 31% monocytes expressing CD45 (bright), CD13, CD33, CD4, CD64, HLA-DR, CD14 (partial), and CD15 (partial) with possible slight expression of CD34 and CD2; the monocytes exhibited no expression of CD117 or the other analyzed lymphoid antigens.

Routine cytogenetic analysis revealed a normal female karyotype (46, XX [21]). A multiplex, nested reverse transcription PCR assay for 16 of the more common recurrent chromosomal rearrangements associated with acute leukemia did not detect any abnormalities. Molecular assays for detection of mutations involving FLT3 ITD, FLT3 D835/I836, NPM1 exon 12, and KIT exons 8 and 17 were performed; only a FLT3 ITD mutation was detected.

The patient was started on induction chemotherapy with 7 + 3 (cytarabine 100 mg/m^2/day continuous IV infusion on days 1–7 and idarubicin 12 mg/m^2/d IV on days 1–3). The day 18 bone marrow evaluation was suspicious for residual AML, so a second induction was completed with HiDAC (cytarabine 3 g/m^2 IV q12 hour × 6 doses on days 1, 3, and 5). A bone marrow evaluation after the second induction revealed no evidence of residual AML. She was consolidated with 4 additional cycles of HiDAC. She achieved complete remission with a normal CBC and transfusion independence. She was not a candidate for allogeneic stem cell transplantation due to the lack of an appropriate donor and concerning psychosocial assessment.

Fourteen months later, she presented with relapsed AML. Her CBC showed a WBC count of 4,000/mm^3 (53% blasts, 1% bands, 4% neutrophils, 41% lymphocytes, and 1% monocytes), a hemoglobin of 11.0 g/dL, and a platelet count of 83,000/mm^3.

A restaging bone marrow confirmed relapsed AML. Flow cytometry showed somewhat similar results to those at diagnosis. There were 36% blasts expressing CD45 (dim), CD13, CD117 (partial), CD33, CD4 (partial), and CD15 (partial); the blasts exhibited minimal expression of CD34 and HLA-DR and no significant expression of CD14, CD64, CD10, CD19, CD20, surface immunoglobulin light chains, CD2, CD3, CD5, CD7, CD8, or CD56. There also were 25% monocytes expressing CD45 (bright), CD13 (partial), CD33, CD4, CD64, HLA-DR (partial), CD14 (partial), and CD15; the monocytes exhibited no expression of CD34, CD117, or the analyzed lymphoid antigens.

Repeated routine cytogenetic analysis revealed an abnormal karyotype with t (14; 15) (q32; q13) in 16 of 20 analyzed cells (Figure 1). Molecular studies no longer showed a FLT-3 ITD mutation, but a FLT-3 D835 mutation was detected (Table 1).

Her relapse initially was treated with a clofarabine-based regimen (clofarabine 30 mg/m^2/day IV on days 1–5, cytarabine 20 mg/m^2/day SC on days 1–14, and sorafenib 400 mg PO BID on days 1–14). Unfortunately the postinduction day 22 bone marrow showed persistent AML, including the presence

TABLE 1: Molecular and cytogenetic test results at initial diagnosis and at time of relapse.

Test	Result at diagnosis	Repeated result at time of relapse
FLT-3 ITD	Detected	Not detected
FLT-3 D835	Not detected	Detected
FLT-3 I836	Not detected	Not detected
NPM1 exon 12	Not detected	Not performed
Cytogenetics	46, XX [21]	46, XX, t (14; 15) (q32; q13) [16]/46, XX [4]

of t (14; 15) (q32; q13). A second induction was performed with FLAG-idarubicin (fludarabine $30 \, mg/m^2$/day IV on days 1–5, cytarabine $3000 \, mg/m^2$/day IV on days 1–5, and idarubicin $10 \, mg/m^2$/day IV on days 1–3); this treatment was complicated with prolonged neutropenia and a disseminated Fusarium infection involving sinus and cutaneous tissues. The day 40 bone marrow biopsy was consistent with persistent AML; it was hypocellular with left-shifted granulocytic maturation, decreased erythropoiesis, and dysmegakaryopoiesis. As a result, the patient was discharged on hospice care.

3. Discussion

To the best of our knowledge, this is the first described case of AML with t (14; 15) (q32; q13). The genes activated or inactivated as a result of this translocation as well as the overall significance of this translocation in the disease process are unclear. Chromosome 14q32 encodes the IgH gene, which produces heavy chain immunoglobulin. Translocations involving the IgH gene/14q32 are well established in multiple hematologic malignancies including diffuse large B-cell lymphoma [3], mantle cell lymphoma [4], precursor T cell acute lymphoblastic leukemia/lymphoma [5], chronic lymphocytic leukemia [6], and multiple myeloma [7]. Another gene located at chromosome 14q32 is BCL11B (B-cell lymphoma/leukemia 11B), which plays a critical role in T-cell differentiation and proliferation and typically is associated with T-lymphoid malignancies. BCL11B encodes a C2H2-type zinc finger protein and is closely related to BCL11A, a gene whose translocation may be associated with B-cell malignancies [8]. BCL11B was first associated with hematological malignancies due to its recurrent involvement along with the homeobox transcription factor TLX3 (previously HOX11L2) in a significant percentage of pediatric T-cell acute lymphoblastic leukemia (T-ALL) cases carrying the cryptic t (5; 14) (q35; q32) [9]. Interestingly, in 2004 Bezrookove et al. [10] described an unusual case of AML with t (6; 14) (q25–q27; q32) affecting the BCL11B gene. In 2011 Oliveira et al. described a case of a child with bilineal T/myeloid acute leukemia associated with del (9q) (q13q22) and TLX3/BCL11B fusion due to the cryptic t (5; 14) (q35; 32) [11]. More recently Ahmad et al. [12] suggested that BCL11B could be a potential oncogene involved in AML with 14q32 aberrations; the identified 4 cases of AML with BCL11B rearrangements (each with a different partner chromosome) expressed both myeloid and T-cell markers and carried AML-associated FLT3 internal tandem duplications (one case also

had a FLT-3 D835 mutation). Given the absence of pan-T-cell markers in our case, potential involvement by BCL11B certainly is only conjecture.

Additional sporadic cases of AML with translocations involving 14q32 have been reported. For example, Tecimer et al. [13] reported a case of AML (AML-M0) with t (1; 14) (p13; q32). Ahmad et al. [12] reported a case of AML (AML-M0/M1) with t (14; 17) (q32; q11.2).

In our case the relapsed leukemia demonstrated refractoriness to multiagent chemotherapy regimens. This may represent either clonal evolution or an entirely new clone which can reflect a therapy related resistant disease after exposure to leukemia treatment on initial presentation. The lack of the FLT-3 ITD mutation, the presence of a FLT-3 D835 codon mutation, and the new onset of t (14; 15) (q32; q13) could support the second interpretation. In the setting of AML, this translocation is of unknown potential but may be linked to refractoriness to chemotherapy. However, potential unidentified mutation involving partner genes can lead also refractory disease. Collecting and reporting data of rare chromosomal abnormalities will potentially add more information concerning the pathogenesis and prognosis of AML. Additionally, it may translate to improved patient outcome and management in the future if identified earlier in the clinical course which may aid in selecting patients to undergo more aggressive chemotherapy regimens and allogeneic stem cell transplant.

Conflict of Interests

The authors declare that there is no conflict of interests regarding the publication of this paper.

References

[1] D. Gary Gilliland and J. D. Griffin, "The roles of FLT3 in hematopoiesis and leukemia," *Blood*, vol. 100, no. 5, pp. 1532–1542, 2002.

[2] C. H. Kok, A. L. Brown, M. Perugini, D. G. Iarossi, I. D. Lewis, and R. J. D'Andrea, "The preferential occurrence of FLT3-TKD mutations in inv(16) AML and impact on survival outcome: a combined analysis of 1053 core-binding factor AML patients," *British Journal of Haematology*, vol. 160, no. 4, pp. 557–559, 2013.

[3] J. C. Cigudosa, N. Z. Parsa, D. C. Louie et al., "Cytogenetic analysis of 363 consecutively ascertained diffuse large B-cell lymphomas," *Genes Chromosomes Cancer*, vol. 25, pp. 123–133, 1999.

[4] N. L. Harris, E. S. Jaffe, H. Stein et al., "A revised European-American classification of lymphoid neoplasms: a proposal

from the International Lymphoma Study Group," *Blood*, vol. 84, no. 5, pp. 1361–1392, 1994.

[5] N. A. Heerema, H. N. Sather, M. G. Sensel et al., "Frequency and clinical significance of cytogenetic abnormalities in pediatric T-lineage acute lymphoblastic leukemia: a report from the Children's Cancer Group," *Journal of Clinical Oncology*, vol. 16, no. 4, pp. 1270–1278, 1998.

[6] M. Hanada, D. Delia, A. Aiello, E. Stadtmauer, and J. C. Reed, "bcl-2 Gene hypomethylation and high-level expression in B-cell chronic lymphocytic leukemia," *Blood*, vol. 82, no. 6, pp. 1820–1828, 1993.

[7] H. Avet-Loiseau, T. Facon, B. Grosbois et al., "Oncogenesis of multiple myeloma: 14q32 and 13q chromosomal abnormalities are not randomly distributed, but correlate with natural history, immunological features, and clinical presentation," *Blood*, vol. 99, no. 6, pp. 2185–2191, 2002.

[8] Y. Gao, H. Wu, D. He et al., "Downregulation of BCL11A by siRNA induces apoptosis in B lymphoma cell lines," *Biomedical Reports*, vol. 1, pp. 47–52, 2013.

[9] O. A. Bernard, M. Busson-LeConiat, P. Ballerini et al., "A new recurrent and specific cryptic translocation, t(5;14)(q35;q32), is associated with expression of the Hox11L2 gene in T acute lymphoblastic leukemia," *Leukemia*, vol. 15, no. 10, pp. 1495–1504, 2001.

[10] V. Bezrookove, S. L. van Zelderen-Bhola, A. Brink et al., "A novel t(6;14)(q25~q27;q32) in acute myelocytic leukemia involves the BCL11B gene," *Cancer Genetics and Cytogenetics*, vol. 149, no. 1, pp. 72–76, 2004.

[11] J. L. Oliveira, R. Kumar, S. P. Khan et al., "Successful treatment of a child with T/myeloid acute bilineal leukemia associated with *TLX3/BCL11B* fusion and 9q deletion," *Pediatric Blood & Cancer*, vol. 56, no. 3, pp. 467–469, 2011.

[12] F. Ahmad, R. Dalvi, S. Mandava, and B. R. Das, "Acute Myelogeneous Leukemia (M0/M1) with novel chromosomal abnormality of t(14;17) (q32; q11.2)," *The American Journal of Hematology*, vol. 82, no. 7, pp. 676–678, 2007.

[13] C. Tecimer, B. A. Loy, and A. W. Martin, "Acute myeloblastic leukemia (M0) with an unusual chromosomal abnormality: Translocation (1;14)(p13;q32)," *Cancer Genetics and Cytogenetics*, vol. 111, no. 2, pp. 175–177, 1999.

15

Mitchell-Riley Syndrome: A Novel Mutation in RFX6 Gene

Marta Zegre Amorim,[1] **Jayne A. L. Houghton,**[2] **Sara Carmo,**[3] **Inês Salva,**[4]
Ana Pita,[4] **and Luis Pereira-da-Silva**[4]

[1]*Genetics Department, Hospital Dona Estefânia, Centro Hospitalar de Lisboa Central, 1169-045 Lisbon, Portugal*
[2]*Royal Devon and Exeter Hospital, Exeter, Devon EX2 5DW, UK*
[3]*Pediatric Surgery Department, Hospital Dona Estefânia, Centro Hospitalar de Lisboa Central, 1169-045 Lisbon, Portugal*
[4]*NICU, Hospital Dona Estefânia, Centro Hospitalar de Lisboa Central, 1169-045 Lisbon, Portugal*

Correspondence should be addressed to Luis Pereira-da-Silva; l.pereira.silva@chlc.min-saude.pt

Academic Editor: Philip D. Cotter

A novel RFX6 homozygous missense mutation was identified in an infant with Mitchell-Riley syndrome. The most common features of Mitchell-Riley syndrome were present, including severe neonatal diabetes associated with annular pancreas, intestinal malrotation, gallbladder agenesis, cholestatic disease, chronic diarrhea, and severe intrauterine growth restriction. Perijejunal tissue similar to pancreatic tissue was found in the submucosa, a finding that has not been previously reported in this syndrome. This case associating RFX6 mutation with structural and functional pancreatic abnormalities reinforces the RFX6 gene role in pancreas development and β-cell function, adding information to the existent mutation databases.

1. Introduction

In the rare Mitchell-Riley syndrome (OMIM #601346) recently described, severe neonatal diabetes associated with hypoplastic or annular pancreas, duodenal or jejunal atresia, intestinal malrotation, gallbladder hypoplasia or agenesis, and cholestatic disease are the most common features described [1, 2].

Homozygosity mapping has identified chromosomal regions linked to Mitchell-Riley syndrome, in which the regulatory factor X 6 (RFX6) gene was identified [3]. The RFX family has 7 members of transcription factors with a highly conserved DNA-binding domain. The RFX3 and RFX6 members are important for β-cell formation and function [4]. Mutations in RFX6 are assumed to be the cause of neonatal diabetes in this syndrome, through the production of a defective RFX6 protein [2–5]. Recently, Concepcion et al. [2] reviewed the RFX6 mutations found in the eight patients (seven probands) reported to date with neonatal diabetes and multiple congenital digestive tract anomalies.

Herein, a novel RFX6 mutation is reported in an infant with Mitchell-Riley syndrome.

2. Case Report

We report a girl, the second child of first-cousin Gipsy parents. Before the proband, the 28-year-old mother had 3 spontaneous abortions in the first trimester and a child with isolated congenital anorectal malformation.

The ultrasound scanning at 33 weeks of gestation revealed intrauterine growth restriction without umbilical artery flow changes, and a "double bubble" suggestive of duodenal atresia. A normal 46, XX karyotype was observed in fetal cells and the fetal echocardiogram was normal. She was born at 35 weeks of gestation by spontaneous vaginal delivery. At birth she appeared malnourished with weight, length, and head circumference below the 3rd centile, respectively, 1370 g, 44 cm, and 29.5 cm. No dysmorphic features were noted, except for anteriorly placed anus. The first hours after birth were complicated with anemia (hemoglobin 9.8 g/dL), oliguria, and metabolic acidosis, improving with volume expansion and red blood cell transfusion. On day 2 hyperglycemia (415 mg/dL) occurred, requiring continuous insulin infusion along with parenteral nutrition with glucose rates around 5-6 mg/Kg/min. On day 3 the blood insulin level was 0.12 μUI/mL and C peptide was <0.1 ng/mL during an episode of hyperglycemia (312 mg/dL). Glutamic acid decarboxylase (GADA), islet cell (ICA), and islet antigen 2 (IA-2) autoantibodies were negative.

On day 4 laparotomy confirmed duodenal atresia (type II) that was associated with annular pancreas, malrotation, and gallbladder agenesis. Perijejunal tissue in the submucosa was found with macroscopic appearance of ectopic pancreatic tissue; instability of the patient during surgery precluded the biopsy of the tissue for histological confirmation. Duodenoduodenostomy and Ladd's procedures were performed. Preoperative analyses showed bilirubin and liver enzymes within normal values. From D6 cholestasis appeared and progressively worsened reaching levels of conjugated bilirubin of 3.07 mg/dL, gamma-glutamyl transpeptidase of 458 IU/L, with relatively normal alkaline phosphatase 94–149 IU/L and transaminases. Subsequently, cholestasis progressively improved and normalization occurred by two months of age without any specific treatment. On day 7 the abdominal ultrasound showed biliary duct dilation with 3 mm greater axis, slightly tortuous, with diminished caliber of intrahepatic right and left biliary ducts; the cephalic region of pancreas was disproportionately larger than the body with unidentifiable tail.

Enteral nutrition was initiated on day 9; however diarrhea developed when enteral volume of breast milk and/or extensively hydrolyzed formula was increased. Exocrine pancreatic supplementation has been unsuccessful and even with free amino acids formula she maintained diarrhea, limiting enteral feeding progression.

Currently she is seven months old and still has malabsorption with failure to thrive (weight 4865 g). Insulin was administered by continuous infusion up to age of five months and subsequently by insulin pump. Complementary feeding was initiated at the age of six months, but she is still dependent on free amino acids formula and parenteral nutrition which provides approximately 60% of daily energy.

The proband and her parents underwent genetic analysis of RFX6 gene. Genomic DNA was extracted from peripheral leukocytes using standard procedures and the coding region and intron/exon boundaries of the RFX6 gene were amplified by PCR (primers available on request). Amplicons were sequenced using the Big Dye Terminator Cycler Sequencing Kit v3.1 (Applied Biosystems, Warrington, UK) according to manufacturer's instructions and reactions were analysed on an ABI 3730 Capillary sequencer (Applied Biosystems, Warrington, UK). Sequences were compared with the reference sequences (NM_173560.3) using Mutation Surveyor v3.24 software (SoftGenetics, State College, PA). A homozygous missense mutation was identified on exon 4, c.541C>T, p.R181W in the proband. Both parents are heterozygous.

3. Discussion

In permanent neonatal diabetes mellitus a genetic cause can be identified in around half the cases and the altered gene expression usually affects pancreas development, β-cell mass, or β-cell function [4]. The most frequent gene with identified mutations is KCNJ11 and to a lesser extent GCK, ABCC8,

and HNF1β. Most patients with neonatal diabetes do not have other congenital abnormalities [6]. The association of the particular phenotype of Martinez-Frias syndrome with a mutation on the RFX6 gene and neonatal diabetes has been called Mitchell-Riley syndrome, and it was suggested that both syndromes represent a symptom continuum or an RFX6 malformation complex [7].

The most common features described in Mitchell-Riley syndrome were present in the reported case, including severe neonatal diabetes associated with annular pancreas, intestinal malrotation, gallbladder agenesis, abnormal biliary tract, cholestatic disease, chronic diarrhea, intrauterine growth restriction, and consanguinity [1, 2, 4]. Some less common features have also been reported [1, 2]. Similarly to our case, anemia at birth requiring prompt red blood cell transfusion has been previously described [1, 5, 8]. Precocious anemia may have been due to fetomaternal transfusion, but this was not investigated. A novel feature found in our case was the perijejunal tissue similar to pancreatic tissue in the submucosa. Unfortunately, instability of the patient during surgery precluded the biopsy for histological confirmation. Two theories have been suggested for heterotopic pancreatic tissue: during embryological development buds of embryonic tissue penetrate into the wall of the growing gut separating from the main pancreas; alternatively, inappropriate expression of pluripotent embryonic mesenchymal tissue of the gastrointestinal tract may lead to pancreatic metaplasia [9–11].

All the seven probands previously reported with Mitchell-Riley syndrome presented RFX6 mutations [2]. To the best of our knowledge this is the eighth proband with Mitchell-Riley syndrome and RFX6 mutation, in whom the novel p.R181W mutation was found. The arginine residue at codon 181, located in the DNA binding domain, is highly conserved across species and this change affects protein function. This mutation was not listed before and is likely pathogenic.

A different mutation at the same residue has already been reported in patients with Mitchell-Riley syndrome (p.R181Q) [4].

In Mitchell-Riley syndrome accurate genetic counselling is inseparable from molecular diagnosis, offering better reproductive options and prenatal diagnosis to the couple and genetic counselling to family members at risk.

The present report reinforces that severe neonatal diabetes associated with RFX6 gene mutation constitutes a distinct phenotype presently described as Mitchell-Riley syndrome. This strongly suggests that RFX6 has a specific role in pancreas development and β-cell function. The novel mutation herein described may contribute to clarifying the reported genetic heterogeneity and adds valuable information to the existent mutation databases.

Conflict of Interests

The authors have no conflict of interests to declare.

Acknowledgment

Genetic testing for neonatal diabetes was performed at the University of Exeter Medical School (UK) with funding from the Wellcome Trust to Professors Andrew Hattersley and Sian Ellard.

References

[1] J. Mitchell, Z. Punthakee, B. Lo et al., "Neonatal diabetes, with hypoplastic pancreas, intestinal atresia and gall bladder hypoplasia: search for the aetiology of a new autosomal recessive syndrome," *Diabetologia*, vol. 47, no. 12, pp. 2160–2167, 2004.

[2] J. P. Concepcion, C. S. Reh, M. Daniels et al., "Neonatal diabetes, gallbladder agenesis, duodenal atresia, and intestinal malrotation caused by a novel homozygous mutation in RFX6," *Pediatric Diabetes*, vol. 15, no. 1, pp. 67–72, 2014.

[3] S. B. Smith, H.-Q. Qu, N. Taleb et al., "Rfx6 directs islet formation and insulin production in mice and humans," *Nature*, vol. 463, no. 7282, pp. 775–780, 2010.

[4] E. J. Pearl, Z. Jarikji, and M. E. Horb, "Functional analysis of Rfx6 and mutant variants associated with neonatal diabetes," *Developmental Biology*, vol. 351, no. 1, pp. 135–145, 2011.

[5] R. Spiegel, A. Dobbie, C. Hartman, L. de Vries, S. Ellard, and S. A. Shalev, "Clinical characterization of a newly described neonatal diabetes syndrome caused by RFX6 mutations," *American Journal of Medical Genetics Part A*, vol. 155, no. 11, pp. 2821–2825, 2011.

[6] L. Chappell, S. Gorman, F. Campbell et al., "A further example of a distinctive autosomal recessive syndrome comprising neonatal diabetes mellitus, intestinal atresias and gall bladder agenesis," *American Journal of Medical Genetics Part A*, vol. 146, no. 13, pp. 1713–1717, 2008.

[7] L. Cruz, R. E. Schnur, E. M. Post et al., "Clinical and genetic complexity of Mitchell-Riley/Martinez-Frias syndrome," *Journal of Perinatology*, vol. 34, no. 12, pp. 948–950, 2014.

[8] D. Martinovici, V. Ransy, S. Vanden Eijnden et al., "Neonatal hemochromatosis and Martinez-Frias syndrome of intestinal atresia and diabetes mellitus in a consanguineous newborn," *European Journal of Medical Genetics*, vol. 53, no. 1, pp. 25–28, 2010.

[9] E. C. S. Lai and R. K. Tompkins, "Heterotopic pancreas. Review of a 26 year experience," *The American Journal of Surgery*, vol. 151, no. 6, pp. 697–700, 1986.

[10] H. R. Makhlouf, J. L. Almeida, and L. H. Sobin, "Carcinoma in jejunal pancreatic heterotopia," *Archives of Pathology and Laboratory Medicine*, vol. 123, no. 8, pp. 707–711, 1999.

[11] I. Jovanovic, S. Knezevic, M. Micev, and M. Krstic, "EUS mini probes in diagnosis of cystic dystrophy of duodenal wall in heterotopic pancreas: a case report," *World Journal of Gastroenterology*, vol. 10, no. 17, pp. 2609–2612, 2004.

16

The Use of High-Density SNP Array to Map Homozygosity in Consanguineous Families to Efficiently Identify Candidate Genes: Application to Woodhouse-Sakati Syndrome

Molly B. Sheridan,[1] **Elizabeth Wohler,**[2] **Denise A. S. Batista,**[1,2,3]
Carolyn Applegate,[1] **and Julie Hoover-Fong**[1]

[1]*McKusick-Nathans Institute of Genetic Medicine, Johns Hopkins University School of Medicine, Baltimore, MD 21287, USA*
[2]*Cytogenomics Laboratory, Johns Hopkins Hospital, Baltimore, MD 21287, USA*
[3]*Department of Pathology, Johns Hopkins University School of Medicine, Baltimore, MD 21287, USA*

Correspondence should be addressed to Molly B. Sheridan; msherid3@jhmi.edu

Academic Editor: Mohnish Suri

Two consanguineous Qatari siblings presented for evaluation: a 17-4/12-year-old male with hypogonadotropic hypogonadism, alopecia, intellectual disability, and microcephaly and his 19-year-old sister with primary amenorrhea, alopecia, and normal cognition. Both required hormone treatment to produce secondary sex characteristics and pubertal development beyond Tanner 1. SNP array analysis of both probands was performed to detect shared regions of homozygosity which may harbor homozygous mutations in a gene causing their common features of abnormal pubertal development, alopecia, and variable cognitive delay. Our patients shared multiple homozygous genomic regions; ten shared regions were >1 Mb in length and constituted 0.99% of the genome. *DCAF17*, encoding a transmembrane nuclear protein of uncertain function, was the only gene identified in a homozygous region known to cause hypogonadotropic hypogonadism. *DCAF17* mutations are associated with Woodhouse-Sakati syndrome, a rare disorder characterized by alopecia, hypogonadotropic hypogonadism, sensorineural hearing loss, diabetes mellitus, and extrapyramidal movements. Sequencing of the coding exons and flanking intronic regions of *DCAF17* in the proband revealed homozygosity for a previously described founder mutation (c.436delC). Targeted *DCAF17* sequencing of his affected sibling revealed the same homozygous mutation. This family illustrates the utility of SNP array testing in consanguineous families to efficiently and inexpensively identify regions of genomic homozygosity in which genetic candidates for recessive conditions can be identified.

1. Introduction

Woodhouse-Sakati syndrome (WSS, MIM 241080) is a rare, multisystem autosomal recessive disorder that was first described in two consanguineous families from Saudi Arabia in 1983 [1]. To date, approximately 84 WSS patients in 29 families have been reported in the literature [2–16]. While WSS has been identified predominantly in patients of Middle Eastern origin, it has been described in four European families (Italy, France, and Eastern Europe) and two patients from South Asia (South India and Pakistan) [2, 3, 5–10].

The WSS phenotype is variable within and among families but is characterized overall by alopecia, hypogonadotropic hypogonadism (HH), sensorineural hearing loss, diabetes mellitus, and extrapyramidal movements. The alopecia is often present in early childhood in affected individuals, potentially involving scalp hair, eyebrows, eyelashes, and pubic and axillary hair [15]. HH becomes apparent when pubertal development is delayed or fails to occur, thus a later sign of WSS [16]. Exogenous hormone therapy can promote secondary sex characteristic development, as in our male patient presented here. Streak, hypoplastic, and absent gonads and uterine structures have also been described in WSS [5, 7, 10, 11, 15, 16]. Hearing loss may be mild to profound though not present in all affected individuals. The diabetes which develops in the majority of WSS patients may require insulin for adequate glucose control though insulin resistance is not common. The extrapyramidal features of WSS are varied, ranging from focal dystonia and chorea which evolves to be generalized. Several published reports of the movement disorder associated with WSS indicate that it begins in the 2nd decade or beyond but is not identified in all patients with WSS [4, 9, 16]. A wide range of cognitive abilities has also been reported in WSS patients, with most exhibiting mild to moderate intellectual disability. Rare instances of WSS patients with normal cognition have been reported [4, 7]. Additional, less consistent features of WSS include anodontia, dysrhythmia, keratoconus, and syndactyly. Some who have undergone brain imaging have revealed white matter changes [4, 8–10, 14].

Interestingly, WSS has been described almost exclusively in consanguineous families ($n = 27/29$, 93.1%). Two nonconsanguineous families were described prior to the discovery of the gene associated with WSS; thus, molecular confirmation of this diagnosis has not been published [4]. WSS is caused by mutations in the gene encoding DCAF17 (DDB1 and CUL4 associated factor 17, C2ORF37), a transmembrane nuclear protein of uncertain function. Nine putative loss of function mutations in *DCAF17* have been reported in association with WSS [6, 9–13, 15]: three nonsense mutations [c.341C>A (p.S114X), c.387G>A (p.W129X), and c.906G>A (p.W302X)], four intronic mutations that are predicted to result in *DCAF17* missplicing (c.127+3delTAGinsAA, c.321+1G>A, c.1091+6T>G, and c.1422+5G>T), and two single nucleotide deletions (c.50delC and c.436delC). With the exception of c.436delC, a founder mutation identified in multiple families from the Arabian Peninsula [6], each of these is a private mutation found in a single consanguineous family. To our knowledge, no WSS patients with compound heterozygote *DCAF17* mutations have been reported. In this paper, we describe an additional consanguineous family with features of WSS. Homozygosity mapping using SNP array was used to identify *DCAF17* as a candidate gene.

2. Materials and Methods

Peripheral blood samples were obtained from Patients 1 and 2 with informed consent following the guidelines of the Institutional Review Board at the Johns Hopkins School of Medicine. Genomic DNA was extracted using the QIAamp DNA Blood Midi kit (Qiagen, Valencia, CA, USA) and SNP array was performed using the Illumina HumanOmni1-Quad (1 million markers; Illumina, San Diego, CA, USA). Bead-Chips were imaged using the Illumina Bead Array reader and allele ratios/signal intensities were analyzed with the CNV Partition 2.4.4.0 algorithm in KaryoStudio (v.1.4.3.0) and GenomeStudio (v.2010.3) (Illumina). The coding exons and flanking intronic regions of *DCAF17* were sequenced at Centogene (Rostock, Germany). All genomic coordinates are based on February 2009 Human Genome Build (hg19).

3. Case Presentations

3.1. Patient 1. Patient 1 (pedigree position V-3) presented with his family from Qatar on referral from a local pediatric endocrine colleague to our clinic at the age of 17-4/12 years for evaluation of a potential unifying diagnosis for his constellation of features including HH, cognitive delay, pectus carinatum, and microcephaly. History included an uncomplicated pregnancy and delivery. He had early delays, walking at 16–18 months and using his first words at 18 months. Formal developmental assessment at 6 years of age revealed no specific delays; yet his parents reported consistent global inability to keep up with peers. Though attending 11th grade at the time of clinical presentation, his parents estimate he is at least 4 grade levels behind age-matched peers. In terms of his physical features, patient 1 had thick, dark hair of normal texture until 6 years of age when it began to thin. Initially there was diffuse hair loss over the scalp, then localized to the bitemporofrontal region, as in male-pattern progressive alopecia. At 15 years of age, he was evaluated for lack of all sexual development. Laboratory evaluations at that time revealed low LH (0.51 μIU/mL; normal 1.1–7.0), FSH (0.38 μIU/mL; normal 1.7–12.0), and testosterone (0.27 ng/mL; normal 3.0–10.6), making the diagnosis of HH. After treatment with testosterone, the patient's voice deepened, he developed mild axillary and facial and pubic hair (Tanner IV), and there was mild genital development. He had delayed primary and secondary tooth eruption and now has multiple caries throughout. He has poor oral hygiene, reported to be similar to that of his brother, yet the latter does not have caries and neither has tooth breakage. On review, he has grossly normal hearing, no additional chronic medical conditions, and no motor movement abnormalities and he is able to smell. He wears glasses for mixed hyperopia and myopia with astigmatism. His growth has always been at low average for height and weight. On exam, weight is just above the 3rd percentile, height is 10th percentile, and his OFC is <−2 SD below the mean (50% for 7-year-old male). He appears to be microcephalic with a horizontal ridge on the superior forehead and bitemporal narrowing. The auricles (>2 SD) and nose are large. Chest circumference is 75th percentile with low, widely spaced nipples, and he has an asymmetric pectus carinatum with a bell-shaped inferior rib margin. He appears to be dolichostenomelic though arm span : height ratio is upper-normal at 1.05. Upper segment lower segment ratio is 1.05 (normal) and limb segments are proportionate with full range of motion of small, medium, and large joints throughout. Several keloid-type scars are present on the posterior right shoulder, back, and foot from a prior accident.

3.2. Patient 2. Patient 2 (V-2) presented at 19-0/12 years of age with her brother on referral from a local adult endocrinologist for evaluation of a potential genetic cause for her primary amenorrhea and gonadal dysgenesis. Her parents were first concerned about her lack of pubertal development at 15 years of age. Laboratory evaluations at that time revealed elevated FSH, LH and low estradiol (exact values unavailable), and a normal karyotype (46,XX). She was treated with hormone therapy (i.e., oral estrogens and progesterone; dose

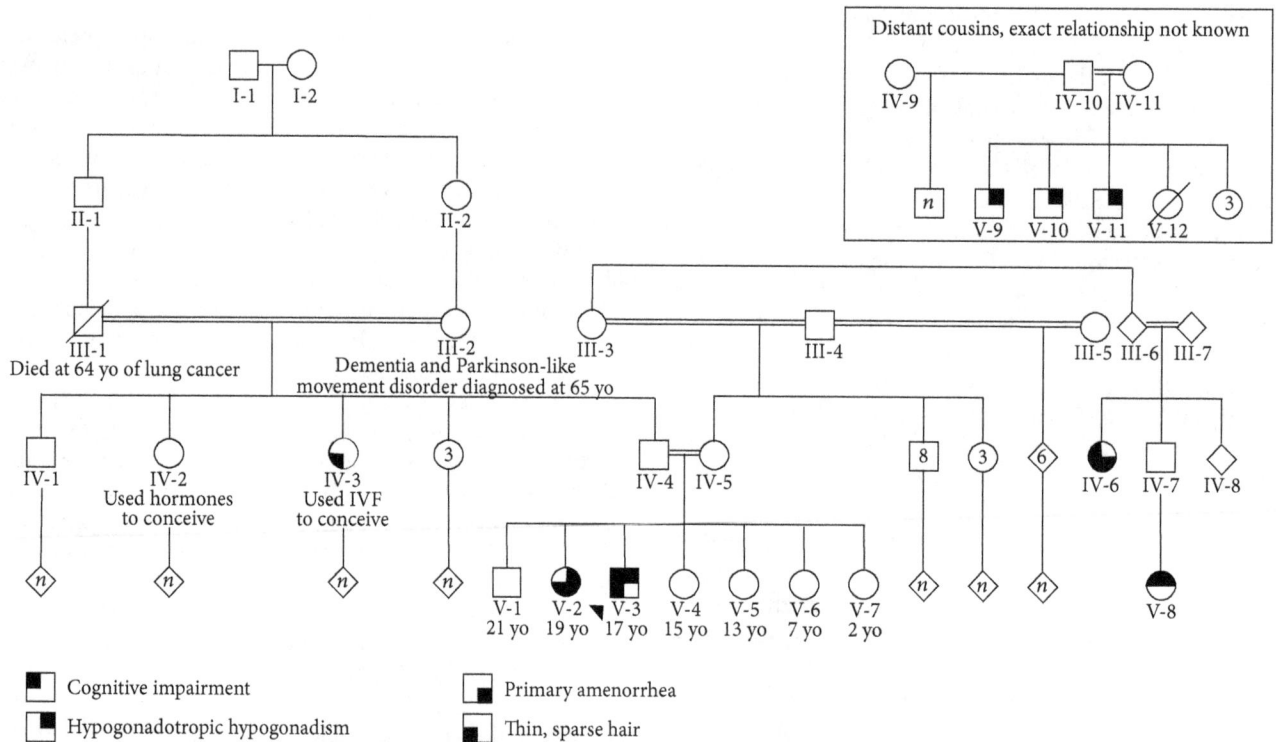

FIGURE 1: Pedigree illustrating multiple instances of consanguinity. Patient 1 (V-3), the proband, is indicated with an arrow. The proband's parents (IV-4 and IV-5) shared a common grandfather approximately 5 generations ago. Individual's clinical phenotypes are specified according to the key. The individuals in the inset are related to both the maternal and paternal lineages, but exact relationships are not known.

unknown) to induce secondary sexual characteristics and menses, now monthly. There was one low platelet value prior to presentation at our institution (111K). The patient denied bleeding problems, palpable bruising, or petechiae and none of these features were appreciated on exam. Pelvic ultrasound imaging showed hypoplastic ovaries and uterus. Her scalp hair began to thin at 11 years of age and she was recently treated with minoxidil, a topical vasodilator, to promote scalp hair growth. On review, her family reports her speech has become less clear over the last few months. She is otherwise healthy without other chronic medical conditions and she has always had normal, age-matched global development. On exam, her weight is 25–50th percentile and height is 50th percentile and she is normocephalic with sparse hair around the temporal region. She has no pectus and breast development is Tanner 3 with pubic hair at Tanner 3. Limb segments and limbs to trunk are proportionate with full range of motion of all joints and no camptodactyly.

Family history for both patients is significant for multiple instances of consanguinity throughout the pedigree and several family members were significant for infertility (Figure 1). Patients 1 and 2 have a 21-year-old brother (V-1) and 4 sisters ranging in age from 2 to 15 years of age who are all healthy with normal pubertal development, hair, and cognition (V-4 to V-7). The parents of our patients entered puberty at 16

years of age and they are at average height (180 cm and 158 cm) with normal hair, cognitive development, and fertility. There are 2 paternal aunts (IV-2 and IV-3) who underwent infertility treatment (i.e., IVF, hormone treatment) to conceive additional pregnancies after initial successful spontaneous gestations; one paternal aunt (IV-3) also has a history of hair loss. The paternal grandmother (III-2) carries a diagnosis of dementia since 65 years of age, complicated by a Parkinson-like movement disorder; she conceived all her pregnancies naturally per available history. The paternal grandfather (III-1) died at 64 years of age from lung cancer though he was not a smoker. The mother of our patients (IV-5) is alive and well with 8 full brothers, 3 full sisters, and 6 paternal half-siblings. There is a maternal cousin once-removed from our patients (IV-6) who never entered puberty and has hair loss and cognitive delay and another maternal second cousin (V-8) without pubertal development and difficulty in school. There are several distant cousins (multiple siblings sharing the same mother and father, V-9 to V-11) related through both the maternal and paternal sides of our patients who are described to have a similar body shape as patient 1, did not develop secondary sexual characteristics, and were infertile. The father of one of these affected family branches (IV-10) remarried and had several subsequent children with normal pubertal development.

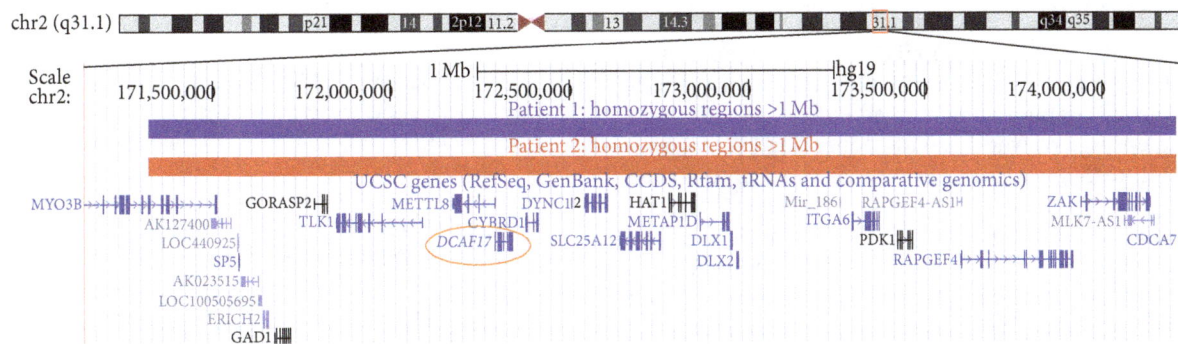

FIGURE 2: Illumina HumanOmni1-Quad SNP array indicates a shared region of homozygosity on chromosome 2q31.1. This region is approximately 2.9 Mb and contains *DCAF17*, the gene associated with WSS. This graphic was constructed using the UCSC Genome Browser (GRCh37/hg19).

4. Results

Based on the highly suggestive autosomal recessive pedigree, we performed a SNP array on patients 1 and 2 to examine shared areas of homozygosity for genes associated with HH. The SNP arrays revealed a male genotype and female genotype with no significant copy number alterations for patients 1 and 2, respectively. However, as expected due to the consanguineous family history, in each individual there were multiple, large homozygous regions (>1 Mb in length) with normal copy number. These homozygous regions ranged in size from 1 Mb to 12.5 Mb and represented approximately 2.8% of the genome in each patient. Overall, the two siblings shared 10 homozygous regions totaling to 30.5 Mb (0.99% of genome). The Genomic Oligoarray and SNP array evaluation tool v3.0 (http://firefly.ccs.miami.edu/cgi-bin/ROH/ROH_analysis_tool.cgi) was used to search for genes associated with HH in the shared regions of homozygosity [17]. A search of OMIM Clinical Synopsis fields using the term "hypogonadism" identified *DCAF17* as the only candidate gene in the shared regions of homozygosity (Figure 2). Sequencing of the coding exons and flanking intronic regions of *DCAF17* in patient 1 revealed homozygosity for the previously described founder mutation (c.436delC; p.Ala147Hisfs*9) [6]. Targeted *DCAF17* sequencing in patient 2 identified the same homozygous mutation. Monetary resources were not available to confirm the heterozygous carrier status of the parents. However, as noted, this family's *DCAF17* mutation was previously described, there was no evidence of a large *DCAF17* deletion, and our patients' phenotype was consistent with WSS.

5. Discussion

In this report, we have presented the clinical and molecular findings for two new WSS patients. Similar to most patients described in the literature, these patients are from a consanguineous family from the Middle East. Despite the identification of a Middle Eastern *DCAF17* founder mutation associated with WSS, we suggest that the presence of HH manifesting as delayed pubertal development in any consanguineous family should prompt consideration of

this syndrome. There is a general paucity of WSS patients reported in the literature, therefore, the validity of this apparent geographic distribution cannot be determined. It is possible that the diagnosis of WSS is not considered in other populations because individuals do not have all the cardinal features of the condition (i.e., HH, diabetes mellitus, alopecia, and sensorineural hearing loss). Even in the family presented here, the phenotype is more variable among the affected individuals than presented in earlier articles. Overall, it is likely that there are more individuals with WSS in whom the diagnosis has not been considered and testing has not been pursued.

Although we have only been able to confirm the WSS diagnosis in patients 1 and 2 from this Qatari family, we suspect, based on the family history, that there are additional family members who are affected (Pedigree positions: IV-2, IV-3, IV-6, V-8, V-9, V-10, and V-11). Of those, 2 paternal aunts (IV-2 and IV-3) to patients 1 and 2 demonstrated infertility which was reportedly treated successfully with hormone supplementation and IVF, resulting in pregnancy. Unfortunately additional details of their clinical course are not available from these individuals and molecular testing has not been possible to validate that pregnancy is possible in WSS patients with HH. A survey of the literature revealed one female who potentially had WSS that may have been able to bear children [8]. Although molecular testing of this mother was not possible, she was thought to have WSS and was able to conceive and deliver four live-born offspring. It is unknown if assisted reproductive technologies were utilized to achieve these pregnancies (personal communication). This is an intriguing point for patients and families with WSS and the associated HH in that fertility may be possible for affected individuals. It should be noted that there is a wide range of cognitive abilities in affected individuals. Individuals with WSS with normal cognition would be able to raise children and therefore could benefit from a variety of reproductive technologies including sperm or egg retrieval, ICSI, IVF, and/or surrogacy if uterine or gonadal development was insufficient. Clinicians are encouraged to report such events in patients confirmed to have WSS to allow other patients and their healthcare providers to benefit from this experience.

This study further illustrates the utility of SNP array in consanguineous families to efficiently and inexpensively direct further study of shared genomic regions for disease-causing gene variants among affected individuals [18]. Even with the upsurge of whole exome sequencing (WES), SNP array still remains a cost effective method of mapping homozygous regions in consanguineous families, particularly those with distinct phenotypes [19]. Despite the falling price of WES, it is still costly to perform WES for multiple individuals in a single family. High resolution SNP array can be used to determine regions containing potential candidate genes in consanguineous families and can be followed by WES in a single individual or Sanger sequencing of candidate genes in multiple affected individuals. In addition, homozygosity mapping using high resolution SNP array can assess regions of the genome that are not represented in WES data including noncoding regions or those not covered due to technical limitations including low read depth or overlap with paralogous sequences [18]. In this study, cost and the high likelihood of finding a small number of candidate genes that could be followed up with Sanger sequencing were both considerations when choosing the SNP array-first testing strategy. Homozygosity mapping using SNP array is not without limitations, however. The resolution of homozygous regions that can be detected by SNP array is directly proportional to the number of SNPs on the array. Thus, use of a high resolution array is particularly important in consanguineous families manifesting phenotypes with high locus heterogeneity to limit the number of candidate genes that require follow-up testing.

In summary, this family illustrates the variable phenotype associated with WSS and suggests that this diagnosis should be considered in any consanguineous family presenting with HH manifesting as delayed pubertal development, alopecia, intellectual compromise, and/or extrapyramidal movements.

Abbreviations

HH: Hypogonadotropic hypogonadism
WES: Whole exome sequencing
WSS: Woodhouse-Sakati syndrome.

Conflict of Interests

The authors have no conflict of interests to declare related to this paper.

Acknowledgments

The authors would also like to acknowledge Dr. Fowzan S. Alkuraya, Dr. Susanne Schneider, and Dr. Kailash Bhatia for their personal communication regarding their previously reported patients. In addition, they thank the members of the Kennedy Krieger Institute Cytogenetics and Microarray laboratory for technical assistance. DCAF17 sequencing was performed by Centogene (Rostock, Germany). Most of all, they would like to thank the patients and their family for their willingness to participate in this study.

References

[1] N. J. Y. Woodhouse and N. A. Sakati, "A syndrome of hypogonadism, alopecia, diabetes mellitus, mental retardation, deafness, and ECG abnormalities," *Journal of Medical Genetics*, vol. 20, no. 3, pp. 216–219, 1983.

[2] D. Gul, M. Ozata, H. Mergen, Z. Odabasi, and M. Mergen, "Woodhouse and Sakati syndrome (MIM 241080): report of a new patient," *Clinical Dysmorphology*, vol. 9, no. 2, pp. 123–125, 2000.

[3] S. A. Al-Swailem, A. A. Al-Assiri, and A. A. Al-Torbak, "Woodhouse Sakati syndrome associated with bilateral keratoconus," *British Journal of Ophthalmology*, vol. 90, no. 1, pp. 116–117, 2006.

[4] A. Al-Semari and S. Bohlega, "Autosomal-recessive syndrome with alopecia, hypogonadism, progressive extra-pyramidal disorder, white matter disease, sensory neural deafness, diabetes mellitus, and low IGF1," *American Journal of Medical Genetics A*, vol. 143, no. 2, pp. 149–160, 2007.

[5] I. Medica, J. Sepčić, and B. Peterlin, "Woodhouse-Sakati syndrome: case report and symptoms review," *Genetic Counseling*, vol. 18, no. 2, pp. 227–231, 2007.

[6] A. M. Alazami, A. Al-Saif, A. Al-Semari et al., "Mutations in C2orf37, encoding a nucleolar protein, cause hypogonadism, alopecia, diabetes mellitus, mental retardation, and extrapyramidal syndrome," *The American Journal of Human Genetics*, vol. 83, no. 6, pp. 684–691, 2008.

[7] G. Koshy, S. Danda, N. Thomas, V. Mathews, and V. Viswanathan, "Three siblings with Woodhouse-Sakati syndrome in an Indian family," *Clinical Dysmorphology*, vol. 17, no. 1, pp. 57–60, 2008.

[8] S. A. Schneider and K. P. Bhatia, "Dystonia in the woodhouse sakati syndrome: a new family and literature review," *Movement Disorders*, vol. 23, no. 4, pp. 592–596, 2008.

[9] A. M. Alazami, S. A. Schneider, D. Bonneau et al., "C2orf37 mutational spectrum in Woodhouse-Sakati syndrome patients," *Clinical Genetics*, vol. 78, no. 6, pp. 585–590, 2010.

[10] K. L. Steindl, A. M. Alazami, K. P. Bhatia et al., "A novel C2orf37 mutation causes the first Italian cases of woodhouse Sakati syndrome," *Clinical Genetics*, vol. 78, no. 6, pp. 594–597, 2010.

[11] T. Ben-Omran, R. Ali, M. Almureikhi et al., "Phenotypic heterogeneity in woodhouse-sakati syndrome: two new families with a mutation in the C2orf37 gene," *American Journal of Medical Genetics Part A*, vol. 155, no. 11, pp. 2647–2653, 2011.

[12] R. Habib, S. Basit, S. Khan, M. N. Khan, and W. Ahmad, "A novel splice site mutation in gene C2orf37 underlying Woodhouse-Sakati syndrome (WSS) in a consanguineous family of Pakistani origin," *Gene*, vol. 490, no. 1-2, pp. 26–31, 2011.

[13] M. Rachmiel, T. Bistritzer, E. Hershkoviz, A. Khahil, O. Epstein, and R. Parvari, "Woodhouse-sakati syndrome in an israeli-arab family presenting with youth-onset diabetes mellitus and delayed puberty," *Hormone Research in Paediatrics*, vol. 75, no. 5, pp. 362–366, 2011.

[14] M. Kojovic, I. Pareés, T. Lampreia et al., "The syndrome of deafness-dystonia: clinical and genetic heterogeneity," *Movement Disorders*, vol. 28, no. 6, pp. 795–803, 2013.

[15] A. Nanda, S. M. Pasternack, N. Mahmoudi, R. Ishorst, R. Grimalt, and R. C. Betz, "Alopecia and hypotrichosis as characteristic findings in woodhouse-sakati syndrome: report of a family with mutation in the C2orf37 gene," *Pediatric Dermatology*, vol. 31, no. 1, pp. 83–87, 2014.

[16] M. Agopiantz, P. Corbonnois, A. Sorlin et al., "Endocrine disorders in Woodhouse-Sakati syndrome: a systematic review of the literature," *Journal of Endocrinological Investigation*, vol. 37, no. 1, pp. 1–7, 2014.

[17] K. J. Wierenga, Z. Jiang, A. C. Yang, J. J. Mulvihill, and N. F. Tsinoremas, "A clinical evaluation tool for SNP arrays, especially for autosomal recessive conditions in offspring of consanguineous parents," *Genetics in Medicine*, vol. 15, no. 5, pp. 354–360, 2013.

[18] F. S. Alkuraya, "Homozygosity mapping: one more tool in the clinical geneticist's toolbox," *Genetics in Medicine*, vol. 12, no. 4, pp. 236–239, 2010.

[19] F. S. Alkuraya, "The application of next-generation sequencing in the autozygosity mapping of human recessive diseases," *Human Genetics*, vol. 132, no. 11, pp. 1197–1211, 2013.

17

Identification of Novel Mutations in *Spatacsin* and *Apolipoprotein B* Genes in a Patient with Spastic Paraplegia and Hypobetalipoproteinemia

Leema Reddy Peddareddygari[1] and Raji P. Grewal[2]

[1]The Neuro-Genetics Institute, 501 Elmwood Avenue, Sharon Hill, PA 19079, USA
[2]Neuroscience Institute, Saint Francis Medical Center, 601 Hamilton Avenue, Trenton, NJ 08629, USA

Correspondence should be addressed to Raji P. Grewal; rgrewal@stfrancismedical.org

Academic Editor: Mogens Fenger

Complicated hereditary spastic paraplegia (HSP) presents with complex neurological and nonneurological manifestations. We report a patient with autosomal recessive (AR) HSP in whom laboratory investigations revealed hypobetalipoproteinemia raising the possibility of a shared pathophysiology of these clinical features. A lipid profile of his parents disclosed a normal maternal lipid profile. However, the paternal lipid profile was similar to that of the patient suggesting autosomal dominant transmission of this trait. Whole exome sequence analysis was performed and novel mutations were detected in both the *SPG11* and the *APOB* genes. Genetic testing of the parents showed that both *APOB* variants were inherited from the father while the *SPG11* variants were inherited one from each parent. Our results indicate that, in this patient, the hypobetalipoproteinemia and spastic paraplegia are unrelated resulting from mutations in two independent genes. This clinical study provides support for the use of whole exome sequencing as a diagnostic tool for identification of mutations in conditions with complex presentations.

1. Introduction

Hereditary spastic paraplegias (HSPs) are a genetically heterogeneous group of neurodegenerative disorders with autosomal dominant, recessive, or an X-linked pattern of inheritance. Clinically they can be classified as pure (or uncomplicated) form or the complicated form of HSP where spasticity may be associated with a combination of neurological or nonneurological manifestations. These can include cerebellar ataxia, dysarthria, mental retardation, optic atrophy, retinitis pigmentosa, hearing loss, a thin corpus callosum, or peripheral neuropathy. HSP can also be genetically classified depending on their specific locus which at present ranges from SPG1 to SPG72 (http://neuromuscular.wustl.edu/spinal/fsp.html).

Familial hypobetalipoproteinemia (FHBL) is an autosomal dominant condition characterized by low plasma concentrations of total cholesterol, low-density lipoprotein cholesterol, and apolipoprotein B (apoB). Mutations in several different genes can cause hypobetalipoproteinemia, the most common of which are a result of truncating mutations in the *APOB* gene [1].

Several different mechanisms have been proposed regarding the pathogenesis of HSP including defective subcellular transportation, mitochondrial malfunction, and increased oxidative stress. Most recently the identification of 1088C > T (S363F) mutation in exon 5 of *cytochrome P450-7B1* in SPG5 disease locus provides a link between cholesterol metabolism and neuronal degeneration in HSPs [2]. The association of HSP with familial hypobetalipoproteinemia is rare and has been reported only once previously [3]. Although a disease causing mutation in this family was identified in the *APOB* gene, they were not able to identify the genetic cause of HSP.

We report a patient with HSP and associated hypobetalipoproteinemia in whom whole exome sequencing was performed to identify the disease causative mutation(s) after initial diagnostic testing for HSP was negative.

TABLE 1: Lipid profile values of the patient and his parents.

Lipid profile	Patient	Mother	Father	Normal range
Total cholesterol	82 mg/dL	214 mg/dL	117 mg/dL	<200 mg/dL
Triglycerides	104 mg/dL	163 mg/dL	120 mg/dL	<150 mg/dL
HDL	39 mg/dL	51 mg/dL	50 mg/dL	≤40 mg/dL
VLDL	17 mg/dL	28 mg/dL	17 mg/dL	<30 mg/dL
LDL	25 mg/dL	135 mg/dL	50 mg/dL	<130 mg/dL
apoB-100-calc	41 mg/dL	109 mg/dL	53 mg/dL	<109 mg/dL

2. Case Presentation

This is a 30-year-old man who was well until the age of 13 years when he started tripping and falling. He was observed to be dragging his feet and developed a clumsy gait. These symptoms progressed and he started to use a cane at the age of 16, a walker at the age of 18, and, ultimately, a wheelchair at the age of 24 years. During this time period he had numerous neurological evaluations and was diagnosed with spastic paraparesis. He has had no associated complaints of pain, numbness, bowel or bladder symptoms, seizures, visual abnormalities, or vertigo. In the last few years, he has developed symptoms of dysarthric speech and clumsiness of his upper extremities. He was diagnosed with attention deficit disorder and further evaluations showed IQ scores (Wechsler Intelligence Scale for Children) of 107 (verbal), 100 (performance), with an overall score of 103. He went on to complete high school and postsecondary education.

He is the product of a normal full term pregnancy and although both parents are of Italian origin, there is no consanguinity. There is no family history of any neurological disorder on either the paternal or maternal branches of the family. The patient has no siblings.

General physical examination revealed no abnormalities. Neurological examination performed showed a minimental status score of 30/30. His speech was dysarthric but otherwise the cranial nerve and sensory examinations were normal. The stretch reflexes were diffusely pathologically brisk and he had sustained clonus at the ankles with bilateral extensor responses. Motor examination revealed a marked hypertonia across all joints bilaterally. Both lower extremities were extended at the knee joint and very spastic. Power was full in the upper extremities (MRC Grade 5/5) and reduced in the lower extremities (MRC Grade 3/5 distally). He could not stand unassisted. A neurological examination was performed on both parents and revealed no abnormalities.

During the course of his medical care many investigations were performed and the following tests were either normal or negative: routine serum chemistries, cell count and differential, creatine phosphokinase, renal and thyroid function studies, and serology for HTLV1.

In addition, magnetic resonance imaging studies of his spinal cord and brain were normal. An electromyography indicated no evidence of neuropathy or myopathy.

A lipid profile of the patient had been performed as part of routine screening and was abnormal. Subsequently, lipid profiles of both parents were performed (Table 1).

3. Genetic Testing

All of the genetic investigations performed on this patient and his family members were done after informed consent was obtained following local IRB policies and procedures. Prior genetic testing performed at a number of commercial laboratories was negative for specific genes tested, including DYT1, SPG3A, SPG4, and NIPA1. However, the spastic paraplegia 11 (SPG11) gene had not been tested. We elected to perform whole exome sequencing through a commercial lab using Illumina HiSeq 2000 platform; sequence capture was done using Agilent SureSelect. The paired-end raw reads were aligned to the hg19 (USCS version) human genome reference and variant list compiled. The raw variant list was analyzed for variants in the known SPG genes and since the patient's lipid profile was consistent with hypobetalipoproteinemia, the variants in APOB gene were also analyzed.

The nucleotide level variant analysis of SPG genes revealed two novel variants on chromosome 15 located in SPG11 gene. Both of the single nucleotide polymorphisms (SNPs) were reconfirmed in the patient by Sanger sequencing (Figure 1). One variant at genomic position, 44905652, resulted in a heterozygous c.1322G > A change in exon 6 (ENSE00001183238, NM_025137). This change results in premature truncation of the spatacsin protein p.W441X (Figure 1(a)). The second variant at genomic position 44943823 results in a c.3121C > T change in the exon 17 (ENSE00001287244, NM_025137) of the SPG11 gene also resulting in premature truncation of the spatacsin protein p.R1041X (Figure 1(b)).

The nucleotide level variant analysis of APOB gene on chromosome 2 revealed two SNPs that were reconfirmed by Sanger sequencing (Figure 2). A previously described change at genomic position 21238413 that causes c.3337G > C change in exon 22 (ENSE00000542198, NM_000384), resulting in a missense mutation from substitution of amino acid, p.D1113H (Figure 2(a)). A novel SNP was also identified, a G to T change at genomic position 21228407. This heterozygous c.11333C > A variant in the exon 26 (ENSE00001183453, NM_000384) results in a stop codon leading to premature truncation of the protein p.S3778X (Figure 2(b)).

The patient is a compound heterozygous for two truncating mutations in the SPG11 gene. Sanger sequencing of the exons containing these individual SNPs on DNA obtained from his parents indicates that the patient has inherited the p.W441X mutation from the mother and p.R1041X mutation from the father (Figure 3). The parents were also tested for

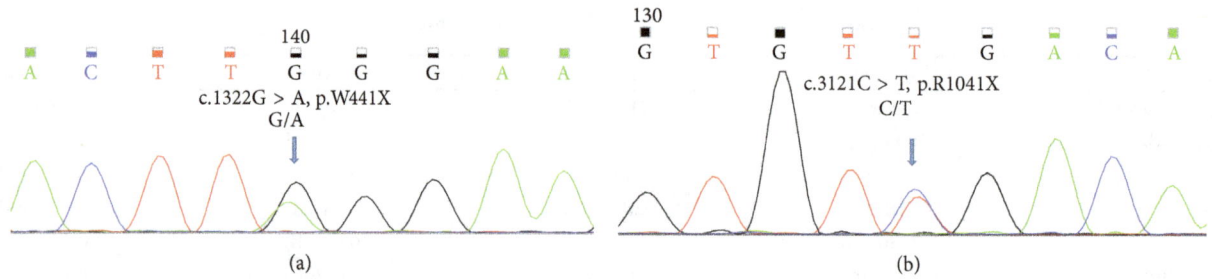

FIGURE 1: Sangers sequencing results of the *SPG11* (NM_025137.3) variants identified by whole exome sequencing of the patient. (a) Showing the c.1322G > A mutation in exon 6 and (b) showing the c.3121C > T mutation in exon 17 of the *SPG11* gene.

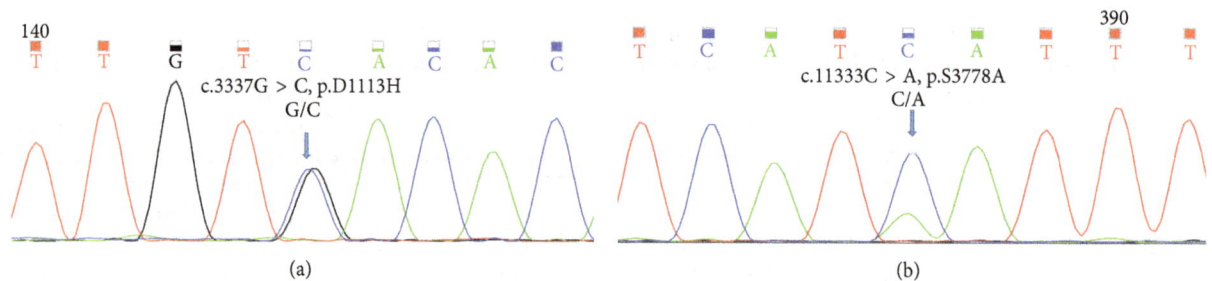

FIGURE 2: Sangers sequencing results of the *APOB* (NM_000384.2) variants identified by whole exome sequencing of the patient. (a) Showing the variant c.3337G > C in exon 22 and (b) showing the variant c.11333C > A in exon 26 of the *APOB* gene.

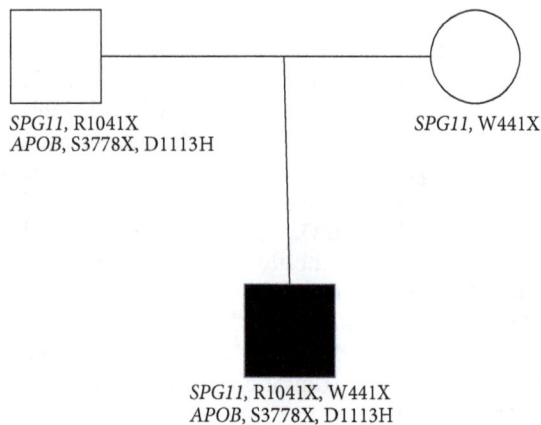

FIGURE 3: Pedigree of the family showing the parents and the affected individual with mutations in the *SPG11* and *APOB* gene. The son is compound heterozygous for *SPG11* mutations, inheriting one variant from each of the parents. Both *APOB* variants were inherited from the father.

the *APOB* mutations and no mutations were detected in the mother. However, analysis of the paternal DNA shows the presence of both *APOB* variants (Figure 3).

4. Discussion

Spastic paraplegia 11 (SPG11) is an autosomal recessive disorder caused by loss of function mutations in the *spatacsin* (*SPG11*) gene on chromosome 15q21.1. This patient's phenotype is consistent with that described in previously reported

patients with genetically confirmed SPG11 (http://neuromuscular.wustl.edu/spinal/fsp.html#spgmu). There are 98 pathogenic/likely pathogenic SNPs that have been reported (http://www.ncbi.nlm.nih.gov/clinvar/). Our patient inherited two losses of function mutations, one from each parent. Both of these mutations are novel and result in premature truncation of the protein strongly suggesting that they are disease producing mutations causing HSP.

The *APOB* gene is translated into both apoB-100 and apoB-48 proteins. The shorter apoB-48 protein is produced after RNA editing of the apoB-100 transcript at residue 2180 (CAA → UAA), resulting in a stop codon producing early termination. The majority of reported *APOB* mutations result in premature truncation of the protein. In heterozygous *APOB* mutation, the normal apoB-100 product is produced at a lower rate while truncated apoB is cleared too rapidly resulting in the low apoB-100 levels [4]. Nonsynonymous, nontruncating *APOB* mutations have also been reported [5, 6]. It was reported that a nontruncated mutant protein can result in impaired secretion compared with the normal secretion of the mutant truncated proteins [7]. All of the previously reported nontruncating mutations are observed in residues 292–593.

Heterozygotes for FHBL have less than half-normal LDL-cholesterol and apoB concentrations, whereas homozygotes have extremely low or undetectable LDL-cholesterol and apoB levels. Both the father and the son have variants in exons 22 and 26. The exon 22 variant causes a substitution of aspartic acid at position 1113 with histidine and affects both apoB-100 and apoB-48. This SNP has been reported in the 1000-genome project with a minor allele frequency of G = 0.003/7 and this change is predicted to be damaging to the protein by both Sift (score 0.02) and PolyPhen (score 0.999) analysis (http://www.ensembl.org/index.html, rs12713844). This variant does not involve the N-terminal $\beta\alpha1$ domain (residues 1–930) of the protein which is important for effective secretion and in subpopulation of Utah residents (CEPH) with Northern and Western European ancestry the frequency of allele G is reported to be as high as 2%. Therefore APOB p.D1113H may not be a disease producing variant. The exon 26 (ENSE00001183453, NM_000384) encodes amino acids 1406 to 3931. The exon 26 variant, 3778 (TCA → TAA), inherited by the patient from his father results in a stop codon leading to premature truncation of the protein p.S3778X. Therefore, it is more likely that the disease causing mutation in the father and son is this exon 26 variant which does not affect apoB-48 but does cause premature truncation of the apoB-100 at residue 3778. In previous reports of heterozygotes for point mutations located in the exon 26 of the *APOB* gene it was found that the clinical manifestations of FHBL are dependent on the size of the resultant truncated apoB [7]. This variant likely accounts for the low LDL-cholesterol, total cholesterol, and apoB-100 observed in the father and son.

When the patient was first encountered, similar to the previously reported family [3], it was hypothesized that there may be connection between the abnormal cholesterol profile and spasticity. However, the genetic analysis performed indicates that these are disparate clinical features.

This case provides support for the value of whole exome sequencing as a diagnostic tool for identification of mutations in conditions where the commercial testings were negative. We were able to identify the genetic cause for hereditary spastic paraplegia and hypobetalipoproteinemia in this patient presenting with a rare combination of autosomal recessive progressive spastic paraparesis and autosomal dominant hypobetalipoproteinemia with normal triglycerides.

Conflict of Interests

The authors declare that there is no conflict of interests regarding the publication of this paper.

Acknowledgments

The authors thank all members of this family for their cooperation and are grateful for the support from the Neuro-Genetics Institute, Sharon Hill, PA, and the Neurogenetics Foundation, NJ.

References

[1] P. Tarugi and M. Averna, "Hypobetalipoproteinemia: genetics, biochemistry, and clinical spectrum," *Advances in Clinical Chemistry*, vol. 54, pp. 81–107, 2011.

[2] M. K. Tsaousidou, K. Ouahchi, T. T. Warner et al., "Sequence alterations within CYP7B1 implicate defective cholesterol homeostasis in motor-neuron degeneration," *The American Journal of Human Genetics*, vol. 82, no. 2, pp. 510–515, 2008.

[3] A. J. Hooper, B. Akinci, A. Comlekci, and J. R. Burnett, "Familial hypobetalipoproteinemia in a Turkish family with hereditary spastic paraplegia," *Clinica Chimica Acta*, vol. 390, no. 1-2, pp. 152–155, 2008.

[4] G. Schonfeld, X. Lin, and P. Yue, "Familial hypobetalipoproteinemia: genetics and metabolism," *Cellular and Molecular Life Sciences*, vol. 62, no. 12, pp. 1372–1378, 2005.

[5] J. R. Burnett, J. Shan, B. A. Miskie et al., "A novel nontruncating *APOB* gene mutation, R463W, causes familial hypobetalipoproteinemia," *The Journal of Biological Chemistry*, vol. 278, no. 15, pp. 13442–13452, 2003.

[6] J. R. Burnett, S. Zhong, Z. G. Jiang et al., "Missense mutations in *APOB* within the $\beta\alpha1$ domain of human APOB-100 result in impaired secretion of ApoB and ApoB-containing lipoproteins in familial hypobetalipoproteinemia," *The Journal of Biological Chemistry*, vol. 282, no. 33, pp. 24270–24283, 2007.

[7] R. Martín-Morales, J. D. García-Díaz, P. Tarugi et al., "Familial hypobetalipoproteinemia: analysis of three Spanish cases with two new mutations in the *APOB* gene," *Gene*, vol. 531, no. 1, pp. 92–96, 2013.

18

Concomitant Alpha- and Gamma-Sarcoglycan Deficiencies in a Turkish Boy with a Novel Deletion in the Alpha-Sarcoglycan Gene

Gulden Diniz,[1] Hulya Tosun Yildirim,[2] Sarenur Gokben,[3] Gul Serdaroglu,[3] Filiz Hazan,[4] Kanay Yararbas,[5,6] and Ajlan Tukun[5,6,7]

[1] Neuromuscular Diseases Centre, Tepecik Research Hospital, Kibris Sehitleri Caddesi 51/11, Alsancak, 35220 Izmir, Turkey
[2] Pathology Department, Dr. Behcet Uz Children's Research Hospital, 35210 İzmir, Turkey
[3] Pediatric Neurology Department, Faculty of Medicine, Ege University, 35100 İzmir, Turkey
[4] Medical Genetics Department, Dr. Behcet Uz Children's Research Hospital, 35210 Izmir, Turkey
[5] Medical Genetics Department, Duzen Laboratories, Istanbul, Turkey
[6] Medical Genetics Department, Duzen Laboratories, Ankara, Turkey
[7] Medical Genetics Department, Faculty of Medicine, Ankara University, 06100 Ankara, Turkey

Correspondence should be addressed to Gulden Diniz; agdiniz@gmail.com

Academic Editor: Patrick Morrison

Limb-girdle muscular dystrophy type 2D (LGMD-2D) is caused by autosomal recessive defects in the alpha-sarcoglycan gene located on chromosome 17q21. In this study, we present a child with alpha-sarcoglycanopathy and describe a novel deletion in the alpha-sarcoglycan gene. A 5-year-old boy had a very high serum creatinine phosphokinase level, which was determined incidentally, and a negative molecular test for the dystrophin gene. Muscle biopsy showed dystrophic features. Immunohistochemistry showed that there was diminished expression of alpha- and gamma-sarcoglycans. DNA analysis revealed a novel 7 bp homozygous deletion in exon 3 of the alpha-sarcoglycan gene. His parents were consanguineous heterozygous carriers of the same deletion. We believe this is the first confirmed case of primary alpha-sarcoglycanopathy with a novel deletion in Turkey. In addition, this study demonstrated that both muscle biopsy and DNA analysis remain important methods for the differential diagnosis of muscular dystrophies because dystrophinopathies and sarcoglycanopathies are so similar.

1. Introduction

Limb girdle muscular dystrophy type 2D (LGMD-2D) is an autosomal recessive muscular disease caused by genetic defects in sarcolemmal alpha sarcoglycan (α-SGC) glycoprotein. Alpha-SGC or adhalin, one of the four sarcoglycans (SGCs), is essential for membrane integrity during muscle contraction and provides a scaffold for important signaling molecules [1–3]. Alpha-SGC is encoded by the sarcoglycan alpha gene (SGCA) located on chromosome 17q21 [1, 4]. LGMD-2D predominantly affects proximal muscles around the scapular and the pelvic girdles. LGMD-2D has a very heterogeneous phenotype. The age of onset, rate of progression, and the severity of disease can vary between and also within affected families. The most clinically severe course is generally observed when the sarcolemmal α-SGC is totally absent whereas milder phenotypes are observed when residual proteins are present [1–4]. Interestingly, a mutation in any SGC gene can lead to a reduction or absence of the other SGCs [4–7]. It was previously reported that the SGCA gene must be evaluated first if there is a concomitant absence of α-SGC and gamma- (γ-) SGC [4].

The differential diagnosis for LGMD-2D includes Duchenne and Becker muscular dystrophies (DMD/BMD) and it is impossible to reach a diagnosis on clinical grounds alone. Therefore, immunohistochemical staining of a muscle biopsy and molecular genetic analysis are mandatory for the correct diagnosis [3, 5, 8, 9]. In this report, the patient's

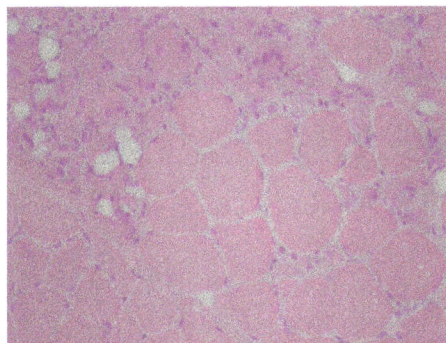

FIGURE 1: Differences in the size and shape of myofibers as well as regeneration (HEx 200).

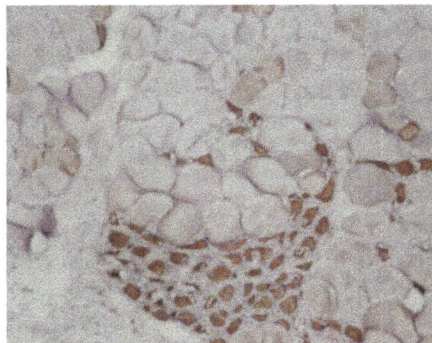

FIGURE 2: Immature pathological fibers visualized with anti-neonatal myosin antibody staining (DABx 100).

genotype was a previously unknown 7 bp deletion in exon 3. This finding adds to the growing spectrum of mutations in the alpha-sarcoglycan gene. Finally, we also discuss important considerations in the differential diagnosis of the muscular dystrophies.

2. Case Report

A 5-year-old boy had second degree consanguineous parents from Turkey without an ancestral history of neuromuscular disorders. There were no complications during pregnancy, and antenatal signs of muscular disorders such as polyhydramnios and reduced fetal movements were not noted. Cognitive and motor development was normal. At the time of presentation, his previously undetected mild muscle weakness was predominantly proximal. Deep tendon reflexes were present and he had no contractures. He was walking normally but he had mild difficulty when climbing stairs and running. Pulmonary function tests were normal. His creatinine phosphokinase (CPK) levels were between 9000 and 15000 units per liter (normal < 250 U/L), and there were myopathic changes on electromyography. Because of the very high CPK level, muscular dystrophy was suspected and, after informed consent, samples were obtained for histopathology, immunohistochemistry, and molecular genetics testing.

A muscle biopsy specimen from the left gastrocnemius muscle of the patient was frozen in isopentane that was precooled to −160°C in liquid nitrogen. Cryosections were immunostained for dystrophin using a polyclonal antibody (Neomarkers), with a monoclonal spectrin antibody (Novocastra) as a control. A neonatal myosin heavy chain (Neonatal myosin, Novocastra) antibody was used for the identification of pathological immature myofibers. SGCs were detected with anti-α-, -β-, -δ-, and -γ-SGC antibodies (Novocastra).

Peripheral blood specimens were collected from the proband and parents. Genomic DNA was extracted from whole blood using a commercial DNA extraction kit (Qia-Gen, USA) following the standard manufacturer's protocol. The concentration of sample DNA was determined by a NanoDrop spectrophotometer (NanoDrop Technologies, Wilmington, DE). The exon regions and flanking short intronic sequences of the SGCA gene were amplified using polymerase chain reaction (PCR), followed by direct sequencing of the PCR products (ABI, US) (NCBI Reference Sequence: NG_0088891). Hitherto reported genetic abnormalities in LGMD-2D are listed in Table 1.

3. Results

The muscle biopsy showed dystrophic changes like contraction, regeneration (Figure 1), degeneration, necrosis, nuclear internalization, and fibrosis. In addition, many pathological immature myofibers were visualized using the neonatal myosin staining (Figure 2). Based on immunostaining, dystrophin and spectrin expressions were normal. Except for isolated deficient fibers, beta (β) sarcoglycan and delta (δ) sarcoglycan were present at normal levels, whereas α-SGC and γ-SGC were diffusely absent (Figure 3).

Based on analysis of the proband, we have identified a previously undetermined homozygous 7 bp deletion in exon 3 (Figure 4). A similar heterozygous deletion was found in both parents (Figures 5 and 6). Location of this deletion was also indicated in Table 1. In addition, there were no abnormalities in the dystrophin gene and the other sarcoglycan genes (SGCB, SGCD, and SGCG) in the patient and his parents.

4. Discussion

Human SGCA cDNA from a human skeletal muscle library was isolated and sequenced in 1993. This gene consisted of 10 exons. The protein product of SGCA gene consisted of 387 amino acids with an extracellular N-terminus, a transmembrane domain, and an intracellular C-terminus. Northern blot analysis showed that human adhalin mRNA was expressed at the highest levels in skeletal muscle. It was also expressed in cardiac muscle and in the lung, but at much lower levels. On the contrary, adhalin mRNA was not detected in the brain. It was also reported that the adhalin mRNA from cardiac muscle was shorter relative to skeletal muscle and that the base sequence encoding the transmembrane domain was absent. It is known that LGMD-2D primarily affects skeletal muscles while brain and peripheral nerve functions are largely preserved. Briefly, the less severe cardiac dysfunction and lack of mental retardation

TABLE 1: Nucleotide and amino acid sequences of α-SGC gene.

Pos	1	2	3	4	5	6	7	8	9	10	11	12	13	14	15
1	ATG	GCT	GAG	ACA	CTC	TTC	TGG	ACT	CCT	CTC	CTC	GTG	GTT	CTC	CTG
1	Met	Ala	Glu	Thr	Leu	Phe	Trp	Thr	Pro	Leu	Leu	Val	Val	Leu	Leu
46	GCA	GGG	CTG	GGG	GAC	ACC	GAG	GCC	CAG	CAG	ACC	ACG	CTA	CAC	CCA
16	Ala	Gly	Leu	Gly	Asp	Thr	Glu	Ala	Gln	Gln	Thr	Thr	Leu	His	Pro#
91	CTT#	GTG	GGC	CGT#	GTC	TTT	GTG	CAC	ACC	TTG	GAC	CAT	GAG	ACG	TTT
31	Leu#	Val	Gly	Arg#	Val	Phe	Val	His	Thr	Leu	Asp	His	Glu	Thr	Phe
136	CTG	AGC	CTT	CCT	GAG	CAT	GTC	GCT#	GTC	CCA	CCC	GCT	GTC	CAC	ATC
46	Leu	Ser	Leu	Pro	Glu	His	Val	Ala#	Val	Pro	Pro	Ala	Val	His	Ile
181	ACC	TAC#	CAC	GCC	CAC	CTC	CAG	GGA#	CAC	CCA	GAC	CTG	CCC	CGG#	TGG
61	Thr	Tyr#	His	Ala	His	Leu	Gln	Gly#	His	Pro	Asp	Leu	Pro	Arg#	Trp
226	CTC	CGC#	TAC##	ACC##	CAG##	CGC#	AGC	CCC	CAC	CAC	CCT	GGC	TTC	CTC#	TAC#
76	Leu	Arg#	Tyr##	Thr##	Gln##	Arg#	Ser	Pro	His	His	Pro	Gly	Phe	Leu#	Tyr#
271	GGC#	TCT	GCC#	ACC	CCA	GAA	GAT#	CGT#	GGG	CTC	CAG	GTC	ATT#	GAG	GTC
91	Gly#	Ser	Ala#	Thr	Pro	Glu	Asp#	Arg#	Gly	Leu	Gln	Val	Ile#	Glu	Val
316	ACA	GCC	TAC	AAT	CGG#	GAC	AGC	TTT	GAA	ACC	ACT	CGG	CAG	AGG	CTG
106	Thr	Ala	Tyr	Asn	Arg#	Asp	Ser	Phe	Glu	Thr	Thr	Arg	Gln	Arg	Leu
361	GTG	CTG	CTG	ATT#	GGG	GAC	CCA	GAA	GGC	CCC	CTG	CTG	CCA	TAC	CAA
121	Val	Leu	Leu	Ile#	Gly	Asp	Pro	Glu	Gly	Pro	Leu	Leu	Pro	Tyr	Gln
406	GCC	GAG#	TTC	CTG#	GTG	CGC#	AGC	CAC	GAT	GCG	GAG	GAG	GTG	CTG	CCC
136	Ala	Glu#	Phe	Leu#	Val	Arg#	Ser	His	Asp	Ala	Glu	Glu	Val	Leu	Pro
451	TCA	ACA	CCT	GCC	AGC	CGC	TTC	CTC#	TCA	GCC	TTG	GCC	GGA	CTC	TGG
151	Ser	Thr	Pro	Ala	Ser	Arg	Phe	Leu#	Ser	Ala	Leu	Ala	Gly	Leu	Trp
496	GAG	CCC	GGA	GAG	CTT	CAG	CTG	AAC	AAC	GTC#	ACC	TCT	GGG	TTG	GAC
166	Glu	Pro	Gly	Glu	Leu	Gln	Leu	Asn	Asn	Val#	Thr	Ser	Gly	Leu	Asp
541	CGT#	GGG	GGC	CGT	GTC	CCC	CTT	CCC	ATT	GAG	GGC	CGA	AAA	GAA	GAC
181	Arg#	Gly	Gly	Arg	Val	Pro	Leu	Pro	Ile	Glu	Gly	Arg	Lys	Glu	Asp
586	GTA#	TAC	ATT	AAG	GTG	GGT	TCT	GCC	TCA	CCT#	TTT	TCT	ACT#	TGC	GGG#
196	Val#	Tyr	Ile	Lys	Val	Gly	Ser	Ala	Ser	Pro#	Phe	Ser	Thr#	Cys	Gly#
631	AAG	ATG	GTG	GCA	TCC#	CGC#	GAT	AGC	CAC	GCC	CGC#	TGT	GCC	CAG#	CTG
211	Lys	Met	Val	Ala	Ser#	Arg#	Asp	Ser	His	Ala	Arg#	Cys	Ala	Gln#	Leu
676	CAG	CCT#	CCA#	CTT	CTG	TTC	TGC#	TAC	GAC	ACC	TTG	GCA	CCC#	CAC	TTC
226	Gln	Pro#	Pro#	Leu	Leu	Phe	Cys#	Tyr	Asp	Thr	Leu	Ala	Pro#	His	Phe
721	CGC	GTT#	GAC	TGG	TGC	AAT	GTG#	ACC	CTG	GTG	GAT	CCC	TCA	GTG	CCG
241	Arg	Val#	Asp	Trp	Cys	Asn	Val#	Thr	Leu	Val	Asp	Pro	Ser	Val	Pro
766	GAG	CCT	GCA	GAT	GAG	GTG	CCC#	ACC	CCA	CCA	GAT	CCA	ATC	CTG	GAG
256	Glu	Pro	Ala	Asp	Glu	Val	Pro#	Thr	Pro	Pro	Asp	Pro	Ile	Leu	Glu
811	CAT	GAC#	CCG	TTC	TTC	TGC	CCA	CCC	ACT	GAG	GCC	CCA	GCC	CGT#	GAC
271	His	Asp#	Pro	Phe	Phe	Cys	Pro	Pro	Thr	Glu	Ala	Pro	Ala	Arg#	Asp
856	TTC	TTG	GTG	GCT	CTC	CTG	GTC	CTG	CTC	GTG	CTG	CCC	GTC	CTG	GTG
286	Phe	Leu	Val	Ala	Leu	Leu	Val	Leu	Leu	Val	Leu	Pro	Val	Leu	Val
901	GCC	CTG	CTT	CTC	TAT	TTG	CTG	GCC	GCC	TTG	GTC	ATG#	TGC	TGC	CGG
301	Ala	Leu	Leu	Leu	Tyr	Leu	Leu	Ala	Ala	Leu	Val	Met#	Cys	Cys	Arg
946	CGG	GAG	GGA	AGG	CTG	AAG	AGA	GAC	CTG	GCT	ACC	TCC	GAC	ATC	CAG
316	Arg	Glu	Gly	Arg	Leu	Lys	Arg	Asp	Leu	Ala	Thr	Ser	Asp	Ile	Gln

TABLE 1: Continued.

991	ATG	GTC	CAC	CAC	TGC	ACC	ATC	CAC	GGG	AAC	ACA	GAG	GAG	CTG	CGG
331	Met	Val	His	His	Cys	Thr	Ile	His	Gly	Asn	Thr	Glu	Glu	Leu	Arg
1036	CAG	ATG	GCG	GCC	AGC	CGC	GAG	GTG	CCC	CGG	CCA	CTC	TCC	ACC	CTG
346	Gln	Met	Ala	Ala	Ser	Arg	Glu	Val	Pro	Arg	Pro	Leu	Ser	Thr	Leu
1081	CCC	ATG	TTC	AAT	GTG	CAC	ACA	GGT	GAG	CGG	CTG	CCT	CCC	CGC	GTG
361	Pro	Met	Phe	Asn	Val	His	Thr	Gly	Glu	Arg	Leu	Pro	Pro	Arg	Val
1126	GAC	AGC	GCC	CAG	GTG	CCC	CTC	ATT	CTG	CAC	CAG	CAC	TGA		
376	Asp	Ser	Ala	Gln	Val	Pro	Leu	Ile	Leu	Asp	Gln	His	Ter		

* Note the previously determined missense mutations marked with #. The present deletion was marked with ## and bold letters.

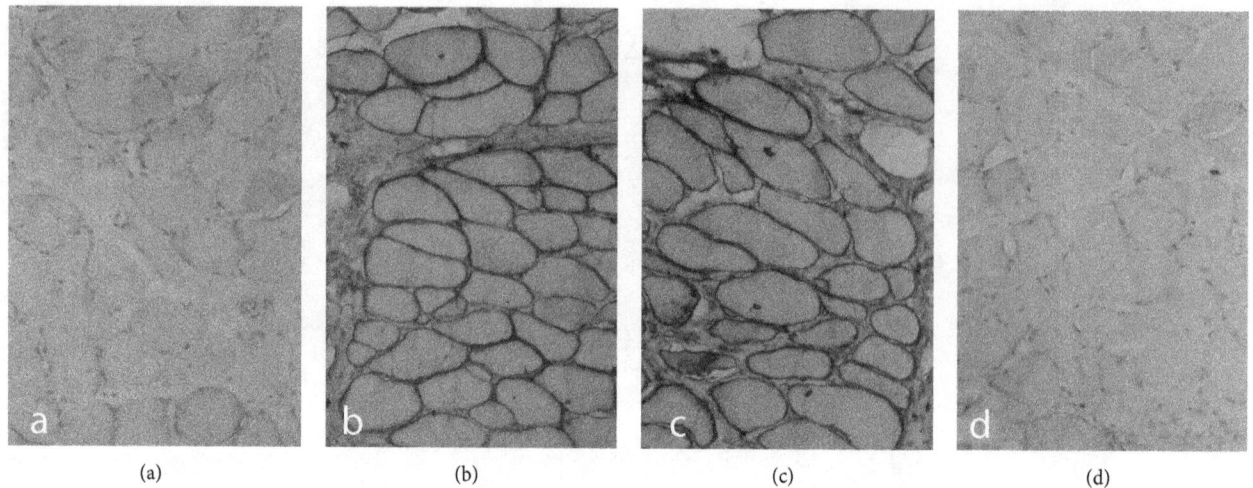

FIGURE 3: Diffuse absence of sarcolemmal α-SGC (a) and γ-SGC (d) expression and normal β-SGC (b) and δ-SGC (c) expression (DABx 200).

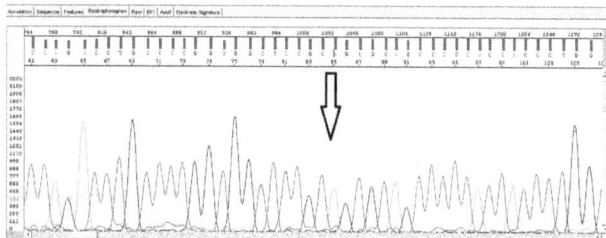

FIGURE 4: Proband exon 3 homozygous del TACACCC site.

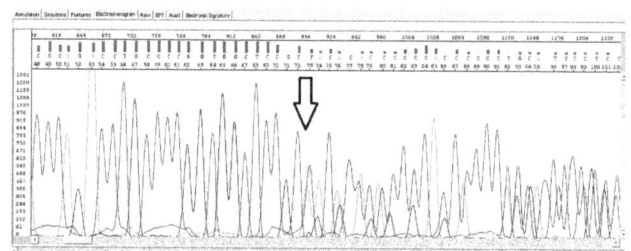

FIGURE 6: Paternal heterozygous del TACACCC site.

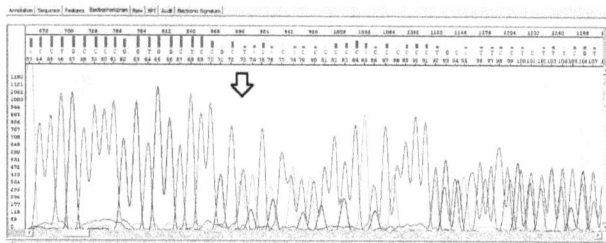

FIGURE 5: Maternal heterozygous del TACACCC site.

in patients with LGMD-2D may be explained by the lower expression of α-SGC in cardiac muscle and the absence of adhalin expression in the brain [1, 3, 10]. In the patient described in this report, we did not find clinical evidence of cardiac involvement, decreased intellectual capacity, or denervation (as demonstrated by electromyography). The course of the disease in this case suggests that this novel deletion may cause a milder phenotype of LGMD-2D despite the diffuse absence of α-SGC and γ-SGC.

Immunohistochemical analysis of sarcolemmal proteins in muscle biopsies like dystrophin, SGCs, merosin, and dysferlin is an important part of the diagnostic evaluation of patients with muscular dystrophy. Reduced or absent sarcolemmal expression of one of the 4 SGCs can be found in patients with any type of LGMDs and also in patients with dystrophinopathies. It has previously been suggested that different patterns of SGC expression could predict the primary genetic defect and that genetic analysis could be directed by these patterns [5–8]. However, Klinge et al. [9] reported that residual SGC expression could be highly variable and an accurate prediction of the genotype could not be achieved. Babameto-Laku et al. [4] also determined that the concomitant absence of α-SGC and γ-SGC expression was caused by defects in the SGCA gene. Therefore, they recommended using antibodies against all four SGCs for immunoanalysis of skeletal muscle sections. Similarly, a concomitant reduction in dystrophin and any of the SGCs may illustrate the importance of considering coexisting dystrophinopathies in patients with sarcoglycan-deficient LGMD [9–13]. For this reason, it is not easy to decide whether the disease is a dystrophinopathy with defective expressions of SGCs or a LGMD with defective expression of dystrophin. However, in the patient described in this report, dystrophinopathies, such as DMD and BMD, were ruled out because the expression of sarcolemmal dystrophin was diffusely present and molecular tests for dystrophin gene were normal.

At present, more than 70 mutations have been reported in the SGCA gene that cause changes in the α-SGC glycoprotein. Approximately a two-thirds of mutations are missense mutations that generate a complete protein with a single residue substitution, whereas other mutations like nucleotide replacements, duplications, deletions, or insertions produce truncated, incomplete, or anomalous proteins. Almost all missense mutations map to the extracellular domain which is a critical region for the organization of SGCs and their association with dystroglycan. Only a single missense mutation maps to the intracellular domain and causes LGMD-2D in homozygous cases. Similarly, two mutations caused by deletions generate a normal extracellular portion of α-SGC and truncated intracellular tails. At present, there is no data about the intracellular tail of the α-SGC protein and its function [1, 10–14]. In the family described in this report, we discovered a novel deletion in the TACACCC site of exon 3 that would cause a frame-shift mutation. The past literature highlights that the prediction of pathological consequences associated with different mutations of SGCA gene is very complex. It is not clear whether this novel deletion generates a severe disease phenotype or whether it also has additional, undetermined consequences.

Patients with any of the LGMDs may be clinically indistinguishable from those with the primary dystrophinopathies. It is likely that the prevalence of LGMD is underestimated and a number of male patients are incorrectly diagnosed with DMD or BMD [13]. A definitive diagnosis rests on performing the appropriate immunohistochemical examination as well as doing a molecular analysis. A normal dystrophin staining pattern should be seen as well as an autosomal recessive mode of inheritance. In contrast, the patients with dystrophinopathies may show variable findings from a normal to a regional absence or a mosaic pattern of sarcolemmal staining with anti-SGCs antibodies which correspond to an abnormal organization of the cell-membrane-associated dystrophin glycoprotein complex. Therefore, it is necessary to perform a careful examination of the immunohistochemical staining as well as a genetic study in order to make the correct diagnosis.

In summary, this report describes a novel deletion that adds to the growing list of defects associated with LGMD-2D and further emphasizes the importance of systematic analysis of all related genes, instead of limiting the analysis to the one SGC gene that is hypothesized to be the cause of the abnormalities. In this study, we also highlight the complexity of staining patterns associated with sarcolemmal proteins and the importance of careful analysis of this staining pattern in order to narrow the differential diagnosis of muscular dystrophies.

Conflict of Interests

The authors declare that there is no conflict of interests.

References

[1] D. Sandonà and R. Betto, "Sarcoglycanopathies: molecular pathogenesis and therapeutic prospects," *Expert Reviews in Molecular Medicine*, vol. 11, p. e28, 2009.

[2] A. Carrié, F. Piccolo, F. Leturcq et al., "Mutational diversity and hot spots in the α-sarcoglycan gene in autosomal recessive muscular dystrophy (LGMD2D)," *Journal of Medical Genetics*, vol. 34, no. 6, pp. 470–475, 1997.

[3] B. Eymard, N. B. Romero, F. Leturcq et al., "Primary adhalinopathy (α-sarcoglycanopathy): clinical, pathologic, and genetic correlation in 20 patients with autosomal recessive muscular dystrophy," *Neurology*, vol. 48, no. 5, pp. 1227–1234, 1997.

[4] A. Babameto-Laku, M. Tabaku, V. Tashko, M. Cikuli, and V. Mokini, "The first case of primary alpha-sarcoglycanopathy identified in Albania, in two siblings with homozygous alpha-sarcoglycan mutation," *Genetic Counseling*, vol. 22, no. 4, pp. 377–383, 2011.

[5] V. Dubowitz, C. A. Sewry, and A. Oldfors, *Muscle Biopsy: A Practical Approach*, Saunders, Philadelphia, Pa, USA, 2013.

[6] I. Higuchi, H. Kawai, Y. Umaki et al., "Different manners of sarcoglycan expression in genetically proven α-sarcoglycan deficiency and γ-sarcoglycan deficiency," *Acta Neuropathologica*, vol. 96, no. 2, pp. 202–206, 1998.

[7] E. S. Moreira, M. Vainzof, O. T. Suzuki, R. C. Pavanello, M. Zatz, and M. R. Passos-Bueno, "Genotype-phenotype correlations in 35 Brazilian families with sarcoglycanopathies including the description of three novel mutations," *Journal of Medical Genetics*, vol. 40, no. 2, p. E12, 2003.

[8] R. Pogue, L. V. B. Anderson, A. Pyle et al., "Strategy for mutation analysis in the autosomal recessive limb-girdle muscular dystrophies," *Neuromuscular Disorders*, vol. 11, no. 1, pp. 80–87, 2001.

[9] L. Klinge, G. Dekomien, A. Aboumousa et al., "Sarcoglycanopathies: can muscle immunoanalysis predict the genotype?" *Neuromuscular Disorders*, vol. 18, no. 12, pp. 934–941, 2008.

[10] M. Trabelsi, N. Kavian, F. Daoud et al., "Revised spectrum of mutations in sarcoglycanopathies," *European Journal of Human Genetics*, vol. 16, no. 7, pp. 793–803, 2008.

[11] R. M. Quinlivan, S. A. Robb, C. Sewry, V. Dubowitz, F. Piccolo, and J. C. Kaplan, "Absence of alpha-sarcoglycan and novel missense mutations in the alpha-sarcoglycan gene in a young British girl with muscular dystrophy," *Developmental Medicine and Child Neurology*, vol. 39, no. 11, pp. 770–774, 1997.

[12] S. Ávila De Salman, A. L. Taratuto, G. Dekomien, and R. Carrero-Valenzuela, "Alpha vs. gamma sarcoglycanopathy: DNA tests solve a case from Argentina," *Acta Myologica*, vol. 26, no. 2, pp. 115–118, 2007.

[13] U. Schara, M. Gencik, J. Mortier et al., "Alpha-sarcoglycanopathy previously misdiagnosed as Duchenne muscular dystrophy: implications for current diagnostics and patient care," *European Journal of Pediatrics*, vol. 160, no. 7, pp. 452–453, 2001.

[14] G. Diniz, H. Tosun Yildirim, G. Akinci et al., "Sarcolemmal alpha and gamma sarcoglycan protein deficiencies in Turkish siblings with a novel missense mutation in the alpha sarcoglycangene," *Pediatric Neurology*, vol. 50, no. 6, pp. 640–647, 2014.

19

Warfarin Dosing in a Patient with *CYP2C9** 3* 3 and *VKORC1-1639 AA* Genotypes

Mark Johnson,[1] **Craig Richard,**[1] **Renee Bogdan,**[2] **and Robert Kidd**[1]

[1] *Bernard J. Dunn School of Pharmacy, Shenandoah University, Winchester, VA 22601, USA*
[2] *PinnacleHealth, Harrisburg, PA 17109, USA*

Correspondence should be addressed to Robert Kidd; rkidd@su.edu

Academic Editors: F.-C. Hsu, B. Melegh, L. Parnell, and P. Saccucci

Genetic factors most correlated with warfarin dose requirements are variations in the genes encoding the enzymes cytochrome P450 2C9 (CYP2C9) and vitamin K epoxide reductase (VKOR). Patients receiving warfarin who possess one or more genetic variations in *CYP2C9* and *VKORC1* are at increased risk of adverse drug events and require significant dose reductions to achieve a therapeutic international normalized ratio (INR). A 74-year-old white female with atrial fibrillation was initiated on a warfarin dose of 2 mg PO daily, which resulted in multiple elevated INR measurements and three clinically significant hemorrhagic events and four vitamin K antidote treatments over a period of less than two weeks. Genetic analysis later revealed that she had the homozygous variant genotypes of *CYP2C9** 3* 3 and *VKORC1-1639 AA*. Warfarin dosing was subsequently restarted and stabilized at 0.5 mg PO daily with therapeutic INRs. This is the first case report of a white female with these genotypes stabilized on warfarin, and it highlights the value of pharmacogenetic testing prior to the initiation of warfarin therapy to maximize efficacy and minimize the risk of adverse drug events.

1. Introduction

Warfarin is the most widely used anticoagulant in the world and has been consistently shown to be effective at preventing emboli in patients with prosthetic heart valves or atrial fibrillation [1]. Achieving a safe and effective warfarin maintenance dose can take weeks or months after the initiation of therapy due to its narrow therapeutic range and wide interindividual dose variation [2]. Unexpected sensitivity to warfarin commonly results in prolonged bleeding caused by excessive anticoagulation and warfarin is the number one cause of hospitalization due to an adverse drug event in the USA [3].

Clinical factors including age, height, weight, gender, race, diet, smoking, comorbidities, prosthetic heart valve, and other medications contribute to the dose variability of warfarin, but genetic factors have been shown to be the largest contributor to the dose variability of warfarin [2, 3]. The two genetic factors that are most correlated with warfarin dose requirements are variations in the genes encoding the enzymes cytochrome P450 2C9 (CYP2C9) and vitamin K epoxide reductase (VKOR) [1].

CYP2C9 is the primary enzyme responsible for inactivating warfarin. The *CYP2C9** 3 variant allele has been shown to cause an 80% decrease in enzymatic activity of CYP2C9 and therefore contributes to the dose variance of warfarin [4]. The pharmacological target for warfarin is inhibition of the VKOR enyzme, a product of the *VKORC1* gene [5]. The VKOR enzyme reduces vitamin K 2,3-epoxide to the active vitamin K hydroquinone which is a required cofactor in the production of several procoagulation factors [6]. The *VKORC1-1639 G > A* gene variant results in a 50% decreased transcription of the *VKOR* gene and increases a patient's sensitivity to warfarin [7]. Therefore, the *VKORC1-1639 A* variant contributes significantly to the variability of warfarin dosing [2]. Patients who are homozygous variant for *CYP2C9** 3 and homozygous variant for *VKORC1-1639 A* are expected to be extremely sensitive to warfarin. Therefore, these patients will require very low doses of warfarin to achieve appropriate therapeutic effect and minimize risk of adverse drug events.

The first detailed clinical report of an individual patient with a genotype of *CYP2C9*3*3* and *VKORC1-1639 AA* was a Japanese female stabilized on a maintenance dose of warfarin that was about 90% less than the average starting dose for warfarin [8]. Herein, we provide the first case report of a white female with a genotype of *CYP2C9*3*3* and *VKORC1-1639 AA* stabilized on the same maintenance dose of warfarin. This report details the clinical course of the patient, summarizes findings from related case reports, and highlights the value of pharmacogenetic testing for warfarin patients.

2. Case Report

2.1. Clinical Course. The patient was a 74-year-old (height 157.5 cm and weight 54 kg) white female of Ashkenazi Jewish descent. Her past medical history was significant for atrial fibrillation, hypertension, diabetes mellitus, coronary artery disease, cardiomyopathy, hypothyroidism, myelodysplastic syndrome with chronic anemia, cerebrovascular accident, chronic kidney disease, peptic ulcer disease, peripheral vascular disease, and pulmonary hypertension. The patient reported a previous "hypersensitivity" to warfarin six years earlier at a different institution. Medications included aspirin 81 mg PO daily, isosorbide mononitrate 40 mg PO daily, furosemide 10 mg alternating with 20 mg PO daily, ramipril 10 mg PO daily, amiodarone 200 mg PO daily, atorvastatin 80 mg PO daily, metoprolol 25 mg PO daily, multiple vitamin PO daily, insulin glargine 14 units subcutaneously daily, epoetin alfa 40,000 units subcutaneously weekly, levothyroxine 100 mcg PO daily, calcitriol 0.25 mcg alternating with 0.5 mcg PO daily, and polysaccharide iron complex 150 mg PO twice daily. Due to a recurrence of atrial fibrillation, the patient was initiated on warfarin (Jantoven) at 2 mg PO daily with an international normalized ratio (INR) goal of 2.0–3.0 which would indicate the appropriate level of anticoagulation for this patient.

The timeline of the subsequent clinical course is outlined in Figure 1. Three days after initiation of warfarin, the patient's INR was 1.4 and the dose remained unchanged. Six days later the patient's INR was 9.1, so warfarin was held and phytonadione (vitamin K) 2.5 mg PO was administered as an antidote to counteract the excessive anticoagulation. One day later the INR had fallen to 4.6, and no additional vitamin K was administered. However, three days later the INR had risen to 7.9, and the patient reported bleeding from her left hand for one hour after accidentally hitting it. As a result, vitamin K was administered a second time at a dose of 5 mg PO. Two days later the INR had decreased to 1.8, yet the patient reported her lip bleeding for approximately 30 minutes after accidentally biting it. Two days later the INR had risen to 3.8, and the patient reported her elbow bleeding for an undetermined period of time after injuring it. Vitamin K was then administered a third time at a dose of 2.5 mg PO. Three days later, the INR had risen to 4.0 and vitamin K was administered a fourth time at a dose of 5 mg PO. Upon subsequent follow-up the INR had decreased to 1.3 after two

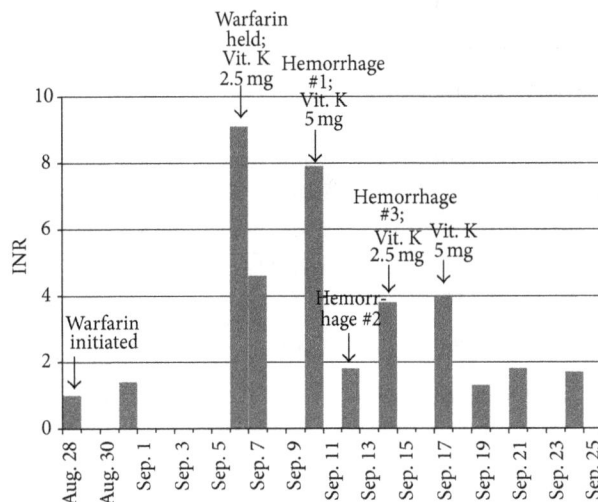

FIGURE 1: Timeline of INR and significant events after patient was initiated on warfarin 2 mg per day.

more days and increased to 1.8 over the next two days, but it then decreased three days later to 1.7. At this time, the decision was made to not restart warfarin due to the supratherapeutic response and to increase the aspirin dose to 325 mg PO daily.

Due to this hypersensitivity to warfarin, the patient consented to genetic testing which revealed *CYP2C9*3*3* and *VKORC1-1639 AA* genotypes. The patient received a second opinion, and it was decided to restart warfarin to decrease risks of a thromboembolic event. Seven months after the previous discontinuation of warfarin, a baseline INR of 1.0 confirmed that the patient's untreated INR was not elevated. Warfarin was then reinitiated at 0.5 mg PO two times weekly and slowly titrated up to 0.5 mg PO daily over the next three months to achieve therapeutic INRs. No hemorrhages were reported during this time.

2.2. Genetic Analyses. This study was approved by the Shenandoah University Institutional Review Board. The patient signed an informed consent and provided a cheek swab sample for DNA collection at the time of a scheduled appointment. Genomic DNA was isolated from the cheek swab sample using a Qiagen QiaCube automated DNA isolation instrument (Qiagen Inc, Chatsworth, CA) following the manufacturer's protocol and then frozen at −20°C until the time of genotyping. The DNA sample was genotyped for *CYP2C9*2* (rs1799853), *3* (rs1057910), *5* (rs28371686), *6* (rs9332131), *7* (rs67807361), *8* (rs7900194), *9* (rs2256871), *11* (rs28371685), *12* (rs9332239), *13* (rs72558187), and *VKORC1-1639 G > A* (rs9923231). All genotyping was performed by allelic discrimination using real-time PCR 5' nuclease assays (Life Technologies, Grand Island, NY) on an Applied Biosystems 7300 real-time PCR (Life Technologies).

3. Discussion

This report summarizes the clinical course of a supratherapeutic response to warfarin in a 74-year-old white female due

TABLE 1: Case reports of warfarin-dosing in patients with CYP2C9*3*3 and VKORC1-1639 AA genotypes.

Age (yrs)	Weight (kg)	Gender	Ethnicity	Indication	Target INR	Drug Interaction(s)	Therapeutic warfarin dose (mg/d)	Reference
69	79.8	Female	Japanese	AFib	1.5–20	NR	0.5	[8]
71	82	Male	White	AFib	2.0–3.0	Amiodarone	0.9	[11]
58	70	Male	Japanese	AFib	NR	Propafenone	0.25–0.75	[12]
68	70	Female	Chinese	AFib	2.0–3.0	NR	0.63	[13]
50	88	Male	Chinese	AFib	2.0–3.0	NR	1.25	[13]
74	54	Female	White	AFib	2.0–3.0	Amiodarone/ Atorvastatin	0.5	Present case

AFib: atrial fibrillation; NR: none reported.

to impaired warfarin metabolism as a result of a CYP2C9*3*3 genotype as well as increased pharmacodynamic sensitivity due to the presence of two variant alleles of VKORC1. Patients who possess one or more genetic variations in CYP2C9 and VKORC1 are at an increased risk of adverse drug events with warfarin and require significant dose reductions to achieve therapeutic INRs [1]. Patients with the CYP2C9*3*3 and VKORC1-1639 AA genotypes are expected to be extremely warfarin sensitive and to require very small doses to achieve the desired therapeutic effect. Additionally, the time required to achieve a maximum, stable INR from a warfarin dosage regimen is delayed due to the impaired metabolic clearance and longer elimination half-life. It has been estimated that, with CYP2C9*3*3 genotype, patients will require at least two to four weeks to reach a maximum, stable INR from a given dose of warfarin [9]. Therefore, dosage adjustments should be made much less frequently than normal.

In this case report, the patient initially received only two mg per day for one week; yet this very conservative dose still resulted in three clinically significant hemorrhagic events and required four vitamin K antidote treatments over a period of less than two weeks after the warfarin was held. This prolonged effect was a direct result of her deficient capacity to metabolize warfarin as a consequence of possessing two CYP2C9 variant alleles resulting in a much longer elimination half-life of warfarin. The patient also possessed two variant alleles of VKORC1 which resulted in an increased pharmacodynamic sensitivity to the vitamin K antagonistic effects of warfarin. The combination of these two factors could have resulted in more severe outcomes. Fortunately, this patient received immediate medical care for her hemorrhagic events and appropriate vitamin K antidote treatments.

Patients with this combination of genotypes are rare, and therefore only a limited number of patients with the CYP2C9*3*3 and VKORC1-1639 AA genotypes receiving warfarin have been reported in the literature. The VKORC1-1639 AA and the CYP2C9*3*3 genotypes have been reported to occur at frequencies of 32.5% and 0.4% in a mixed ethnic population, respectively [10]. A literature search yielded four case reports (one in the form of a letter to the editor) with detailed clinical courses of five patients

including demographic information, comorbidities, and concomitant medications. A summary of these case reports and the current one is presented in Table 1.

The Coumadin package insert provides ranges of expected maintenance doses based on genotypes [9]. The expected maintenance dose range in the package insert for a patient with CYP2C9*3 and VKORC1-1639 AA genotypes is 0.5–2.0 mg per day. This expected dose range in the package insert may be higher than the observed dose range of 0.25–1.25 mg per day in the case report patients in Table 1 because it does not incorporate additional factors (e.g., age, body size, gender, diet, ethnicity, comorbidities, and concomitant drug therapy) that are known to influence warfarin dosing. Several pharmacogenetic-based warfarin dosing nomograms which incorporate additional clinical factors are now available, and the two most commonly cited ones can be accessed at http://www.warfarindosing.org/ [10, 14]. For the present patient case, these nomograms yielded estimated therapeutic warfarin doses of 0.9 and 0.2 mg per day. Interestingly, the average of these estimated doses would be approximately 0.5 mg per day, and this was the dose the patient was stabilized on after pharmacogenetic testing.

If this patient had been genotyped for CYP2C9 and VKORC1 variant alleles prior to the selection of her warfarin dose, one can only speculate what actual warfarin dose would have been chosen. However, given the dosing guidelines described above, the patient would have likely received a significantly lower dose than two mg per day and may have avoided the hemorrhagic events. Due to the complications with her initial warfarin dose, she was also not optimally anticoagulated for an extended period of time which put her at increased risk of a thromboembolic event. Klein et al. reported that approximately 66% of patients of mixed ethnicities had at least one VKORC1 variant and 24% had at least one CYP2C9 variant [10]. Therefore, the majority of patients could benefit from pharmacogenetic testing prior to the initiation of warfarin therapy. Our case report details the potential challenges and risks for patients and clinicians alike in the absence of CYP2C9 and VKORC1 pharmacogenetic testing.

Conflict of Interests

The authors declare that there is no conflict of interests regarding the publication of this paper.

References

[1] N. Eriksson and M. Wadelius, "Prediction of warfarin dose: why, when and how?" *Pharmacogenomics*, vol. 13, no. 4, pp. 429–440, 2012.

[2] J. F. Carlquist and J. L. Anderson, "Using pharmacogenetics in real time to guide warfarin initiation: a clinician update," *Circulation*, vol. 124, no. 23, pp. 2554–2559, 2011.

[3] D. S. Budnitz, M. C. Lovegrove, N. Shehab, and C. L. Richards, "Emergency hospitalizations for adverse drug events in older Americans," *The New England Journal of Medicine*, vol. 365, no. 21, pp. 2002–2012, 2011.

[4] K. Takanashi, H. Tainaka, K. Kobayashi, T. Yasumori, M. Hosakawa, and K. Chiba, "CYP2C9 Ile359 and Leu359 variants: enzyme kinetic study with seven substrates," *Pharmacogenetics*, vol. 10, no. 2, pp. 95–104, 2000.

[5] T. Li, C.-Y. Chang, D.-Y. Jin, P.-J. Lin, A. Khvorova, and D. W. Stafford, "Identification of the gene for vitamin K epoxide reductase," *Nature*, vol. 427, no. 6974, pp. 541–544, 2004.

[6] M. J. Rieder, A. P. Reiner, B. F. Gage et al., "Effect of VKORC1 haplotypes on transcriptional regulation and warfarin dose," *The New England Journal of Medicine*, vol. 352, no. 22, pp. 2285–2293, 2005.

[7] H.-Y. Yuan, J.-J. Chen, M. T. M. Lee et al., "A novel functional VKORC1 promoter polymorphism is associated with inter-individual and inter-ethnic differences in warfarin sensitivity," *Human Molecular Genetics*, vol. 14, no. 13, pp. 1745–1751, 2005.

[8] T. Fukuda, T. Tanabe, M. Ohno et al., "Warfarin dose requirement for patients with both VKORC1 3673A/A and CYP2C9*3/*3 genotypes," *Clinical Pharmacology and Therapeutics*, vol. 80, no. 5, pp. 553–554, 2006.

[9] Coumadin, *Package Insert*, Bristol-Myers Squibb, Princeton, NJ, USA, 2011.

[10] T. E. Klein, R. B. Altman, N. Eriksson et al., "Estimation of the warfarin dose with clinical and pharmacogenetic data," *The New England Journal of Medicine*, vol. 360, no. 8, pp. 753–764, 2009.

[11] G. R. Grice, P. E. Milligan, C. Eby, and B. F. Gage, "Pharmacogenetic dose refinement prevents warfarin overdose in a patient who is highly warfarin-sensitive," *Journal of Thrombosis and Haemostasis*, vol. 6, no. 1, pp. 207–209, 2008.

[12] T. Goto, M. Miura, A. Murata et al., "Standard warfarin dose in a patient with the CYP2C9*3/*3 genotype leads to hematuria," *Clinica Chimica Acta*, vol. 411, no. 17-18, pp. 1375–1377, 2010.

[13] L. Gao, L. He, J. Luo et al., "Extremely low warfarin dose in patients with genotypes of CYP2C9*3/*3 and VKORC1-1639A/A," *Chinese Medical Journal*, vol. 124, no. 17, pp. 2767–2770, 2011.

[14] B. F. Gage, C. Eby, J. A. Johnson et al., "Use of pharmacogenetic and clinical factors to predict the therapeutic dose of warfarin," *Clinical Pharmacology and Therapeutics*, vol. 84, no. 3, pp. 326–331, 2008.

20

Mild Phenotype in a Patient with a *De Novo* 6.3 Mb Distal Deletion at 10q26.2q26.3

George A. Tanteles,[1] **Elpiniki Nikolaou,**[1] **Yiolanda Christou,**[2]
Angelos Alexandrou,[3] **Paola Evangelidou,**[3] **Violetta Christophidou-Anastasiadou,**[1]
Carolina Sismani,[3] **and Savvas S. Papacostas**[2]

[1]*Clinical Genetics Department, The Cyprus Institute of Neurology and Genetics and Archbishop Makarios III Medical Centre,*
 2370 Nicosia, Cyprus
[2]*Clinical Sciences Neurology Clinic B, The Cyprus Institute of Neurology and Genetics, 2370 Nicosia, Cyprus*
[3]*Cytogenetics and Genomics Department, The Cyprus Institute of Neurology and Genetics, 2370 Nicosia, Cyprus*

Correspondence should be addressed to George A. Tanteles; gtanteles@cing.ac.cy

Academic Editor: Mohnish Suri

We report on a 29-year-old Greek-Cypriot female with a *de novo* 6.3 Mb distal 10q26.2q26.3 deletion. She had a very mild neurocognitive phenotype with near normal development and intellect. In addition, she had certain distinctive features and postural orthostatic tachycardia. We review the relevant literature and postulate that certain of her features can be diagnostically relevant. This report illustrates the powerful diagnostic ability of array-CGH in the elucidation of relatively mild phenotypes.

1. Introduction

Distal deletions of the long arm of chromosome 10 are uncommon. Since the first published report of an individual with a distal 10q deletion in 1978 [1], there have been over 30 cases with deletions involving either the 10q26.2 or the 10q26.3 breakpoint reported in the literature. The exact locations and sizes of distal 10q deletions vary and involve either the terminal or subterminal region of chromosome 10q [2].

Deletions or duplications of the telomeric region of chromosome 10q have not previously been associated with a clearly recognizable phenotype. However, patients with a 10q monosomy present with certain clinical characteristics which include facial dysmorphism, congenital heart defects, and varying degrees of developmental delay and intellectual disability [2–5]. Other common findings include strabismus, neurobehavioral manifestations, and urogenital anomalies [2, 5, 6].

We report on a 29-year-old lady with a 6.3 Mb *de novo* distal 10q26.2q26.3 deletion associated with a mild phenotype which includes distinctive facial features, strabismus, tachyarrhythmia, and relatively mild cognitive issues.

2. Patient and Methods

2.1. Clinical Description. Review of the family history revealed that the proband was the third child born to non-consanguineous parents, a 32-year-old father and a 27-year-old mother. Her father had a history of type II diabetes while her mother underwent ablation for ventricular ectopics. Her younger brother also had a history of tachyarrhythmias and her eldest sister was affected with Turner syndrome. She was born following a normal vaginal delivery at 37-week gestation with a birth weight of 2.6 kg. Soon after birth, she developed jaundice and severe hyperbilirubinemia for which she required exchange transfusion thrice. In addition, she had unspecified breathing difficulties requiring NICU admission for approximately three weeks. She had congenital strabismus for which she underwent corrective surgeries at the ages of 2.5 years and 15 years. There were no other major issues reported during childhood. Developmentally, there were no concerns and she completed a senior high school without requiring support. She described herself as an average pupil and there was no clear evidence of significant learning issues. Her motor and intellectual developments were reported as normal.

She presented at the age of 21 years with recurrent episodes of brief sudden loss of consciousness. During such episodes, she would lose muscle tone and fall without injuring herself. In their maximum frequency, these episodes occurred 2-3 times daily but subsequently became less frequent occurring at least once or twice per week. The patient did not report any associated bladder or bowel control loss or postepisode confusion. Most of the times, these episodes followed stressful events or could occur when she became tired. On a few occasions, blurring of vision could precede the episode. In addition to these paroxysmal episodes, she had a history of iron deficiency anaemia.

On examination, at the age of 29 years, her height was 155 cm (9th centile), her weight was 57 kg (25th–50th centile), and her occipitofrontal circumference (OFC) was 54 cm (25th–50th centile). She had distinctive facial features with upslanting palpebral fissures, a long tubular nose with a prominent nasal bridge and tip, an overhanging columella, and a short philtrum. She had right-sided strabismus and asymmetry of the angles of the mouth with retrognathia. She had a left-sided posteriorly rotated ear with an overfolded helix. She had a small hypomelanotic macule over the left shoulder and 2-3 small hypomelanotic macules over the right shoulder. She had transverse creases in the mid phalanges of the index fingers bilaterally. She had curled 2nd, 3rd, and 4th toes on the right (Figures 1 and 2). Her patellae were present. Cardiovascular and neurological examinations were otherwise unremarkable.

During follow-ups, the patient reported occasional episodes of palpitations for which she remained under the care of a cardiologist, while her episodes of loss of consciousness subsequently resolved. The patient seemed to have very few problems with regard to her independence and could manage her finances and personal hygiene without any difficulties. She obtained a college degree as a nursery teacher, could hold a job, and drive a car.

Previous normal or negative investigations included a full blood count, biochemistry, liver and thyroid function tests, plasma lactate, CK, a basic metabolic screen, vitamin B12, folate, molecular test for fragile X syndrome, an abdominal ultrasound scan, and an ophthalmology evaluation including visual evoked potentials. A brain MRI scan revealed small white matter lesions at the trigons of the lateral ventricles. Several EEGs did not reveal any evidence of epileptiform activity. Echocardiography, cardiac electrophysiological studies, and abdominal ultrasound scans were unremarkable. Tilt table test was positive for postural orthostatic tachycardic syndrome with normal cardiac anatomy.

On the basis of her clinical presentation and facial features, array-CGH analysis was requested. Informed consent was obtained by the patient.

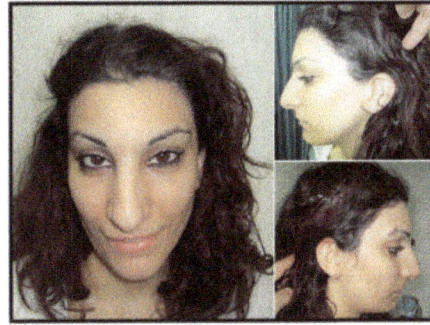

FIGURE 1: Frontal and profile views of our patient.

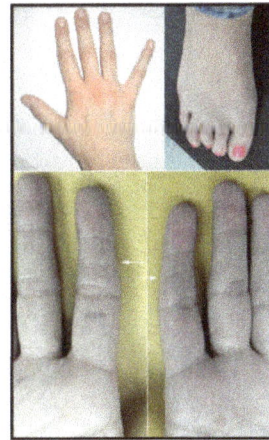

FIGURE 2: Hand and foot views. Note the curled toes and in particular the distinctive bilateral transverse creases involving the middle phalanx of the index finger (white arrows).

2.2. Cytogenetic and Molecular Analyses. DNA of the index patient and her parents was isolated from peripheral blood using the QIAamp DNA Midi Kit (Qiagen, Hidden, Germany) according to the supplier's protocol. Array-CGH (comparative-genomic-hybridization) was carried out using the Cytochip ISCA array (BlueGnome, version 1.0) with 180,000 oligos in a 4 × 180 k format according to the recommendations of the manufacturer. Briefly, 500 ng of patient and pooled reference gDNA were differentially labeled using the Bioprime DNA Labeling System (Invitrogen, Carlsbad, CA) and the Cy3 and Cy5 fluorescent dyes (GE Healthcare, UK, Ltd.), respectively. Hybridization was carried out using an automated slide processor HS 400 PRO Hybridization Station (Tecan Inc., Männedorf, Switzerland). The array was scanned at 3 um resolution using the Agilent DNA microarray scanner (Agilent Technologies Inc., Santa Clara, CA, USA) and fluorescent ratios were calculated using the BlueFuse Multi software V4.2 (BlueGnome Ltd., Cambridge, UK). Fluorescence *in situ* hybridization (FISH) analysis was carried out on metaphase preparations using subtelomeric specific probes for the short (p-arm) and long arms (q-arm) of chromosome 10 (Cytocell, Cambridge, UK) according to the recommendations of the manufacturer.

(a)

(b)

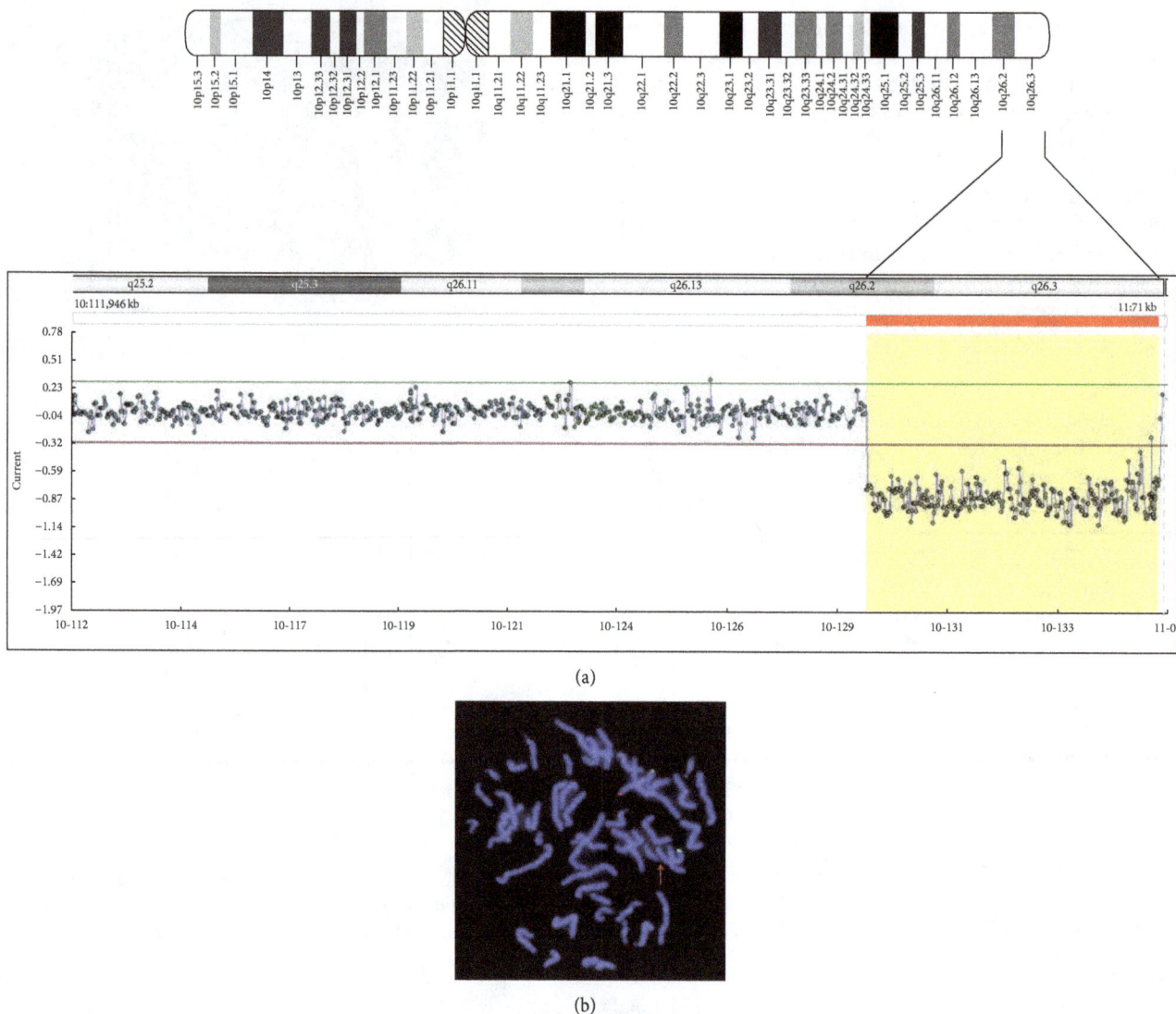

FIGURE 3: (a) Array-CGH analysis result demonstrating the 6.3 Mb distal deletion of chromosome 10 (q-arm) at chromosomal band 10q26.2 extending to band 10q26.3. (b) FISH analysis of the index patient's metaphases showing two signals of the 10p region and only one signal of the 10q region.

3. Results

Array-CGH analysis revealed a distal deletion of approximately 6.3 Mb in size on the long arm of chromosome 10 (q-arm) at chromosomal band 10q26.2 extending to band 10q26.3 (location 129,142,062–135,434,149 using build GRCh37 (hg19)). The region spans approximately 6.3 Mb and encompasses several known genes (DECIPHER: https://decipher.sanger.ac.uk/) including *CALY* and partially deleted *DOCK1*. In order to confirm the deletion, FISH analysis showed positive 10ptel (green) and 10qtel signals (red) on the normal chromosome 10 but only a positive 10ptel (green) signal on the del(10) (Figure 3), therefore confirming the distal deletion on the long arm of chromosome 10 detected by array-CGH analysis. Furthermore, FISH analyses were performed for both parents to determine whether the deletion originated from any chromosomal rearrangement is present in one of the parents. Parental FISH analyses

showed normal hybridization pattern on both chromosomes 10, indicating that the deletion originated in the patient as a *de novo* event.

4. Discussion

Constitutional subterminal 10q deletions are rare and attempts to correlate deletion size to phenotype have been reported. These deletions have been associated with a wide range of clinical findings including facial dysmorphism, learning difficulties, varying degrees of developmental delay, and intellectual disability as well as cardiovascular abnormalities [5, 7]. Other common findings include strabismus, urogenital anomalies, cryptorchidism in males, and behavioral problems [3, 5–7]. In this report, we describe a female patient with a *de novo* distal 10q26.2q26.3 deletion of approximately 6.3 Mb who presented with distinctive

TABLE 1: OMIM genes located in the deleted 10q26.2q26.3 region.

Gene symbol	Gene title	Function	OMIM
DOCK1	Dedicator of cytokinesis 1	Cell migration, phagocytosis [7]	601403
PPP2R2D	Protein phosphatase 2, regulatory subunit B, and delta	Cause of developmental delay or intellectual disability [4]	613992
BNIP3	BCL2/adenovirus E1B 19 kDa interacting protein 3	Cause of developmental delay or intellectual disability [4]	603293
DPYSL4	Dihydropyrimidinase-like 4	Neuronal differentiation [3, 5]	608407
INPP5A	Inositol polysphosphate-5-phosphatase	Central nervous system development [2]	600106
GPR123	G protein-coupled receptor 123	Central nervous system development [2]	612302
ADAM8	ADAM metallopeptidase domain 8	Neurogenesis, muscle development [7]	602267
CALY	Calcyon neuron-specific vesicular protein	Vesicle trafficking-related functions [2]	604647

OMIM: Online Mendelian Inheritance in Man.

facial features, strabismus, postural orthostatic tachycardic syndrome, and relatively mild cognitive deficits. Despite the fact that no formal neurocognitive evaluation was performed (including IQ measurement), her social and practical skills, including communication, social interaction, taking care of her personal hygiene, managing her finances, effective use of independent transportation, level of independence, fine and gross motor skills, are evidence of normal or near normal development and intellect.

The wide variability in phenotypic expression of 10q deletions has been suggested to correlate to deletion size [3, 4]. However, there does not seem to be clear evidence to support this observation [2]. The variable degree of intellectual disability also seems to exhibit great interfamilial variability and this has been shown in familial cases that share the same deletion [3, 5].

Interrogation of the Database of Genomic Variants revealed that the deleted region encompasses 35 genes, 23 of which are listed in OMIM. There were very few candidates for specific correlations with the patient's phenotype. Eight genes namely, DOCK1, PPP2R2D, BNIP3, DPYSL4, INPP5A, GPR123, ADAM8, and CALY, are notable as they have been associated with certain clinical manifestations (Table 1). The CALY gene encodes a single transmembrane protein expressed in the brain which is involved in vesicle trafficking-related functions, important for efficient synaptic transmission in the central nervous system [2]. Deletion of CALY has been reported in patients with behavioral problems and it has been suggested that haploinsufficiency of this gene could partially contribute to the development of behavioral disturbances [2]. In addition, deletions of the INPP5A and GPR123 genes, which encode proteins involved in central nervous system development, could lead to neurobehavioral abnormalities [2]. Furthermore, it has been suggested that DPYSL4 gene deletion could be associated with behavioral problems and/or intellectual disability because its function is involved in neuronal differentiation [2, 3, 5]. The ADAM8 gene encodes a protein that is implicated in neurogenesis and muscle development and has been associated with susceptibility to autism [8]. According to Iourov et al., haploinsufficiency of PPP2R2D and BNIP3 is likely to cause

a phenotypic effect such as developmental delay or intellectual disability [4]. Our patient had near normal intelligence and did not exhibit significant neurobehavioral issues. Although our patient's phenotype could not be supported by the published literature as described above, her presentation could reflect variability in phenotypic expression as it has been suggested that alterations in genes involved in signaling and regulation pathways could be responsible for the wide degree of phenotypic variability observed in patients with 10q deletions [7]. Finally, the phenotypic heterogeneity could result from incomplete penetrance or due to other genetic, epistatic, epigenetic, or environmental factors.

The DOCK1 gene (partially deleted in our patient) is known to be involved in several biological processes including cell migration and phagocytosis [7]. DOCK1 haploinsufficiency can result in craniofacial dysmorphism and cardiac and urinary anomalies [8]. There is a hypothesis which suggests that a critical region containing the DOCK1 gene could cause the characteristic clinical phenotype seen in 10q deletions [2]. It remains plausible that haploinsufficiency of DOCK1 could be associated with our patient's distinctive facial features. In addition to the facial features, of note are the distinctive bilateral transverse creases involving the middle phalanx of the index finger which we postulate that it could represent a diagnostic clue. She also had a history of postural orthostatic tachycardic syndrome, the significance of which remains unclear. The positive family history of arrhythmias could however point towards an independent to the 10q26.2q26.3 deletion, factor as potentially causal.

In conclusion, a female with a de novo 6.3 Mb distal deletion of chromosome 10q at chromosomal band 10q26.2 extending to 10q26.3 displaying a very mild phenotype compared to previous reports of similar deletions is reported. She had near normal development and intellect, postural orthostatic tachycardic syndrome and certain distinctive features. This report illustrates the powerful diagnostic ability of array-CGH in the elucidation of relatively mild phenotypes. Further molecular studies should be performed to further establish the genotype-phenotype correlations of these deletions with a view to clarify the role and influence of the genes involved in this region.

Conflict of Interests

The authors declare that there is no conflict of interests regarding the publication of this paper.

Acknowledgment

The authors would like to thank the patient for consenting to this publication.

References

[1] R. C. Lewandowski Jr., M. K. Kukolich, J. W. Sears, and C. B. Mankinen, "Partial deletion 10q," *Human Genetics*, vol. 42, no. 3, pp. 339–343, 1978.

[2] J. Plaisancié, L. Bouneau, C. Cances et al., "Distal 10q monosomy: new evidence for a neurobehavioral condition?" *European Journal of Medical Genetics*, vol. 57, no. 1, pp. 47–53, 2014.

[3] W. Courtens, W. Wuyts, L. Rooms, S. B. Pera, and J. Wauters, "A subterminal deletion of the long arm of chromosome 10: a clinical report and review," *American Journal of Medical Genetics*, vol. 140, no. 4, pp. 402–409, 2006.

[4] I. Y. Iourov, S. G. Vorsanova, O. S. Kurinnaia et al., "An interstitial deletion at 10q26.2q26.3," *Case Reports in Genetics*, vol. 2014, Article ID 505832, 3 pages, 2014.

[5] M. Irving, H. Hanson, P. Turnpenny et al., "Deletion of the distal long arm of chromosome 10; is there a characteristic phenotype? A report of 15 de novo and familial cases," *American Journal of Medical Genetics*, vol. 123, no. 2, pp. 153–163, 2003.

[6] A. Vera-Carbonell, V. López-González, J. A. Bafalliu et al., "Clinical comparison of 10q26 overlapping deletions: delineating the critical region for urogenital anomalies," *American Journal of Medical Genetics A*, vol. 167, pp. 786–790, 2015.

[7] Y.-T. Chang, I.-C. Chou, C.-H. Wang et al., "Chromosome 10q deletion del (10)(q26.1q26.3) is associated with cataract," *Pediatrics and Neonatology*, vol. 54, no. 2, pp. 132–136, 2013.

[8] S. A. Yatsenko, M. C. Kruer, P. I. Bader et al., "Identification of critical regions for clinical features of distal 10q deletion syndrome," *Clinical Genetics*, vol. 76, no. 1, pp. 54–62, 2009.

21

Novel *SMAD3* Mutation in a Patient with Hypoplastic Left Heart Syndrome with Significant Aortic Aneurysm

Kristi K. Fitzgerald,[1] Abdul Majeed Bhat,[1] Katrina Conard,[2,3] James Hyland,[4] and Christian Pizarro[1]

[1] Nemours Cardiac Center, Nemours/Alfred I. duPont Hospital for Children, 1600 Rockland Road, Wilmington, DE 19803, USA
[2] Department of Pathology, Nemours/Alfred I. duPont Hospital for Children, Wilmington, DE 19803, USA
[3] Anatomy and Cell Biology, Thomas Jefferson University Hospital, Philadelphia, PA 19107, USA
[4] Connective Tissue Gene Tests, Allentown, PA 18106, USA

Correspondence should be addressed to Kristi K. Fitzgerald; kristi.fitzgerald@nemours.org

Academic Editors: C.-W. Cheng, M. Fenger, C.-S. Huang, P. Morrison, and G. Vogt

Aneurysms-osteoarthritis syndrome (AOS) caused by haploinsufficiency of *SMAD3* is a recently described cause of syndromic familial thoracic aortic aneurysm and dissection (TAAD). We identified a novel *SMAD3* mutation in a patient with hypoplastic left heart syndrome (HLHS) who developed progressive aortic aneurysm requiring surgical replacement of the neoaortic root, ascending aorta, and proximal aortic arch. Family screening for the mutation revealed that his father, who has vascular and skeletal features of AOS, and his brother, who is asymptomatic, also have the pathogenic mutation. This is the first case report of a *SMAD3* mutation in a patient with hypoplastic left heart syndrome. This case highlights the importance of genetic testing for known causes of aneurysm in patients with congenital heart disease who develop aneurysmal disease as it may significantly impact the management of those patients and their family members.

1. Introduction

Familial thoracic aortic aneurysm can be divided into syndromic and nonsyndromic forms. While abdominal aortic aneurysm generally occurs sporadically, thoracic aortic aneurysm and dissection (TAAD) is inherited in an autosomal dominant manner with decreased penetrance and variable expression [1]. The genes causing syndromic and nonsyndromic forms of TAAD encode proteins that compose the structural components associated with connective tissue, key members of the TGF-β signaling pathway, or components of the contractile unit of smooth muscle cells. The genetic etiology of nonsyndromic causes of familial TAAD is largely unknown; however, several genes including, *MYH11*, *ACTA2*, and *MYLK* have been implicated [2–4]. The genetic cause of syndromic forms of TAAD include *FBN1*, the cause of Marfan syndrome, *SLC2A10*, the cause of arterial tortuosity

syndrome, and *TGFβR1*, *TGFβR2*, and the recent identification of *TGFβ2*, all of which cause Loeys-Dietz syndrome [5–9].

In 2011 *SMAD3*, was shown to cause a new syndromic form of thoracic aortic aneurysm and dissection. The features of this condition included early onset osteoarthritis in the majority of patients and the authors proposed the name aneurysms-osteoarthritis syndrome (AOS) [10]. In addition to aneurysm and dissection, early osteoarthritis, and other systemic findings, congenital heart disease including persistent ductus arteriosus, atrial septal defect, pulmonary valve stenosis, atrial fibrillation, and bicuspid aortic valve have also been observed in patients with defects in *SMAD3* [11]. *SMAD3* encodes an intracellular member of the TGF-β signaling pathway that activates or represses gene transcription. Heterozygous mutations in *SMAD3* lead to increased expression of several components of the TGF-β pathway

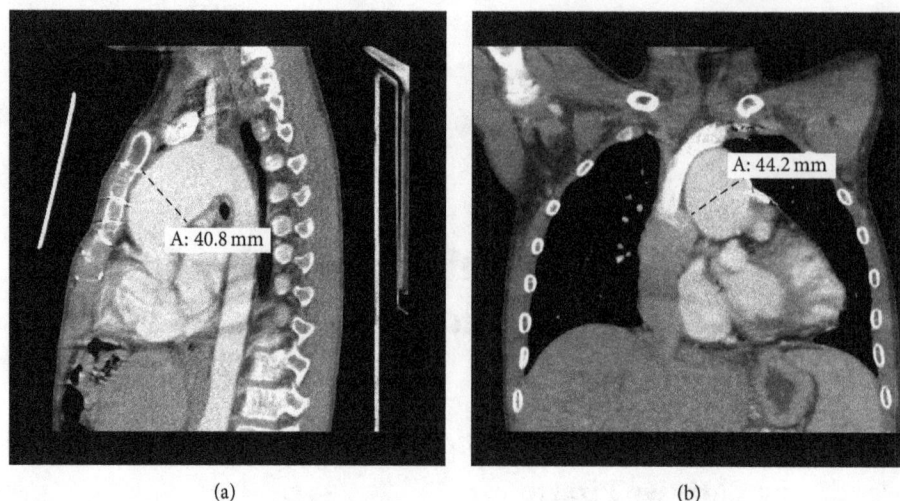

(a)

(b)

FIGURE 1: Optiray contrast-enhanced computed tomography images of the chest with sagittal (a) and coronal (b) reconstructions in the 14-year-old proband revealing aneurysmal dilation of the ascending aorta.

including phosphorylated SMAD2, total *SMAD3*, *TGFβ1*, and connective tissue growth factor [10].

We present a 14-year-old boy born with hypoplastic left heart syndrome (HLHS) who developed significant aneurysm of the neoaorta and proximal arch after completed, staged palliation and who was found to have a novel, pathogenic *SMAD3* mutation. Further testing in the family revealed additional at risk family members and who were offered appropriate cardiovascular and orthopedic screening.

2. Case Presentation

The proband, a 14-year-old male, was conceived via in vitro fertilization secondary to infertility and was diagnosed prenatally with hypoplastic left heart syndrome with mitral valve hypoplasia and aortic valve stenosis. He underwent palliative staged reconstruction including modified Fontan procedure. He developed significant aneurysmal dilatation of his reconstructed ascending aorta and neoaortic root and regurgitation of his native pulmonic valve. He underwent partial replacement of his neoaortic root with a 24 mm Hemashield graft at an outside institution. Due to significant residual neoaortic regurgitation, he underwent neoaortic valve replacement with a 25 mm On-X prosthetic. Subsequently, over a few years, he exhibited progressive dilatation of the remaining neoaorta reaching a maximal dimension of 5.2 cm. He presented to the emergency room with history of severe chest pain radiating to the neck following exercise. Computed tomography scan ruled out the presence of an aneurysmal rupture or dissection but revealed a fusiform aneurysmal dilatation of the ascending aorta with greatest dimensions of the ascending aorta of 4.1 cm (AP) × 4.4 cm (RL) (Figures 1(a) and 1(b)). He underwent aortic root, ascending aorta, and partial transverse aortic arch replacement with a 26 mm woven Dacron (Hemashield) graft, reimplantation of the mechanical prosthesis into the graft as well as reimplantation of the proximal native ascending

aorta on the side of the graft. Microscopic examination of the resected ascending aorta and native pulmonary artery showed elastic artery with mucopolysaccharide rich areas and fibrosis with fragmentation and disorganization of the elastic fibers. Additionally, the aorta showed dystrophic calcification (Figures 2(a) and 2(b)).

The proband underwent sequencing of genes known to cause thoracic aortic aneurysm and dissection. Next generation sequencing followed by Sanger sequencing revealed that the proband has a novel, pathogenic *SMAD3* mutation, c.3G>A (p. Met1Ile) (Figure 3). First degree relatives were screened for the *SMAD3* mutation. The proband's 46-year-old father and 9-year-old brother were also found to have the *SMAD3* c.3G>A mutation. The affected family members underwent transthoracic echocardiography and magnetic resonance angiography (MRA) of the brain, neck, chest, abdomen, and pelvis; the proband's MRA was normal. The father, now 46 years, has intervertebral disc degeneration of his cervical spine and osteoarthritis of his knee. Echocardiogram revealed aortic root dilation with a diameter of 4.0 cm and mitral valve prolapse with mild to moderate mitral regurgitation. MRAs of the neck, chest, abdomen, and pelvis were normal. The proband's brother had a normal echocardiogram and total body MRA. His past medical history is significant for left sided inguinal hernia requiring surgical repair. Of note, the proband has no evidence of osteoarthritis. Additional screening for the *SMAD3* mutation in extended relatives was recommended.

3. Discussion

In this report, we describe a proband with HLHS who developed significant aortic aneurysm in whom clinical sequencing for genetic causes of TAAD revealed a pathogenic mutation in *SMAD3*. Testing of the proband's family members lead to identification of a serious health risk for thus far two additional family members. Identification of the *SMAD3*

(a)

(b)

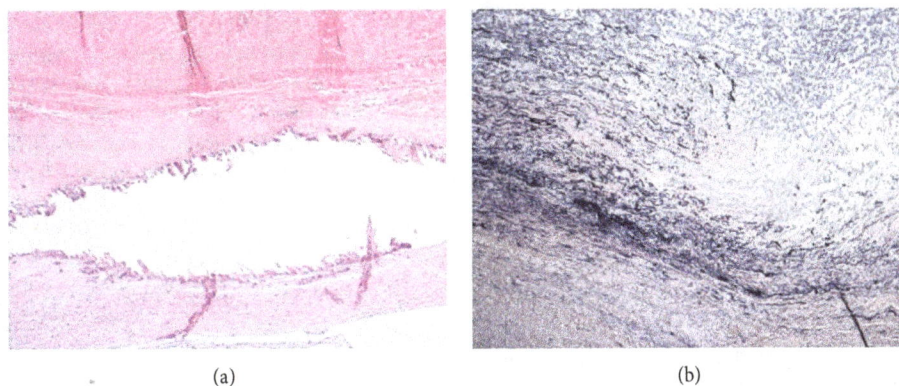

FIGURE 2: (a) Ascending aorta: medial fibrosis and dystrophic calcification (Hematoxylin and Eosin) and (b) fragmentation and disorganization of the elastic fibers (Verhoeff Van Gieson's elastic stain).

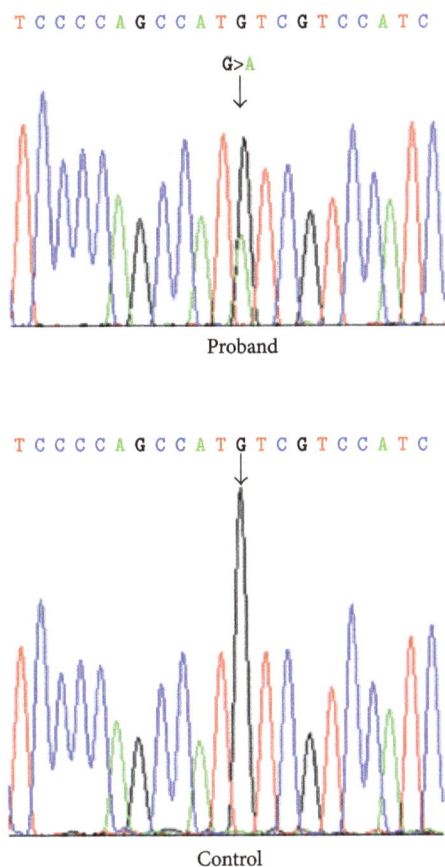

FIGURE 3: Sanger sequencing chromatogram revealing the pathogenic *SMAD3* mutation, c.3G>A (p. MetIIle) in the proband versus the normal sequence in a control.

mutation in the proband's father also explains his orthopedic complications. While other congenital heart defects such as persistent ductus arteriosus, atrial septal defect, and pulmonary valve stenosis have been observed in patients with *SMAD3* mutations, to our knowledge, this is the first case reported with HLHS.

The findings in this family are consistent with the phenotype previously described in patients with AOS. The majority of previously described mutations in *SMAD3* were observed in families with TAAD, implying a bias towards an aortic aneurysm and dissection phenotype [10, 11]. The patients in this family were ascertained only after screening in the proband, who developed significant neoaortic aneurysm following extensive cardiac surgical history for his congenital heart defect.

The phenotype of AOS in this family is age dependent with the 46-year-old father exhibiting both vascular and skeletal features while the 9-year-old brother has neither. This is consistent with many previous reports; however, a recent study by Wischmeijer et al. reported pathologic aortic dilation in a patient as young as 12 months [12]. The report by Hilhorst-Hofstee et al. of an unanticipated copy number variant of chromosome 15 disrupting *SMAD3* revealed a three generation family at risk for aortic dissection. This included the 12-year-old proband initially investigated for mild mental retardation and a 4-year-old asymptomatic cousin. The two children in this family had the abnormal feature of ascending aorta wider than the sinotubular junction; the authors queried if this may be the first sign of future dilation [13]. In our case, the proband's 9-year-old brother (whose transthoracic echocardiogram and MRA were normal) also had an ascending aorta wider than the sinotubular junction (ascending aorta = 2.4 cm, sinotubular junction = 2.2 cm).

Aortic dilations in congenital aortic diseases such as bicuspid aortic valve and coarctation of the aorta are well described, and of the cyanotic congenital heart diseases, Tetralogy of Fallot has been the most widely studied with dilation at the annulus and sinus occurring in 88% and 87% of patients respectively [14]. Neoaortic root dilation has also been observed in other CHD's including transposition of the great arteries following aortic switch operation, [15, 16] following Ross procedure for congenital aortic valve disease, [17] and truncus arteriosus [18]. Specific to our case, neoaortic root dilation and valve regurgitation were reported in a group of patients with HLHS following staged palliation by Cohen et al. [19] in their cohort of 53 patients; aortic root dilation and aortic valve regurgitation were observed in 98%

and 61%, respectively. Transection of the main pulmonary artery followed by reconstruction, exposing the neoaortic root (native pulmonary root) at systemic pressure, is the common denominator for all surgical interventions where the pulmonary valve becomes the neoaortic valve. It has been suggested that under these circumstances, aortic dilatation could be a result of blood flow to the vessel wall being compromised [19].

While neoaortic root dilation and aortic valve regurgitation are commonly observed in HLHS patients following staged palliation, the degree of aneurysm observed in our patient is not commonly observed in this patient cohort. Additionally, significant aneurysm formation leading to dissection is not typical based on the literature. Aortic dissection was reported in one 26-year-old male with HLHS where the aortic root measured 7.8 cm by transthoracic echocardiogram [20]. Additional information regarding the phenotype of this patient or his family history was not reported.

The phenotype of the proband and his father is consistent with what has been described thus far for the aneurysms-osteoarthritis syndrome, which leads us to conclude that the c.3G>A mutation in *SMAD3* found in this family is pathogenic and is an explanation for their clinical findings. Identification of AOS in this family allowed for the screening of at risk family members, identification of early vascular disease, and it offers an explanation for the aneurysmal history in the proband and degenerative disk disease and arthritic history in his father. This case highlights the importance of screening patients with congenital heart defects for genetic causes of known aneurysmal disease.

Conflict of Interests

The authors declare that there is no conflict of interests regarding the publication of this paper.

References

[1] D. M. Milewicz, H. Chen, E.-S. Park et al., "Reduced penetrance and variable expressivity of familial thoracic aortic aneurysms/dissections," *American Journal of Cardiology*, vol. 82, no. 4, pp. 474–479, 1998.

[2] L. Zhu, R. Vranckx, P. K. Van Kien et al., "Mutations in myosin heavy chain 11 cause a syndrome associating thoracic aortic aneurysm/aortic dissection and patent ductus arteriosus," *Nature Genetics*, vol. 38, no. 3, pp. 343–349, 2006.

[3] D.-C. Guo, H. Pannu, V. Tran-Fadulu et al., "Mutations in smooth muscle α-actin (ACTA2) lead to thoracic aortic aneurysms and dissections," *Nature Genetics*, vol. 39, no. 12, pp. 1488–1493, 2007.

[4] L. Wang, D.-C. Guo, J. Cao et al., "Mutations in myosin light chain kinase cause familial aortic dissections," *American Journal of Human Genetics*, vol. 87, no. 5, pp. 701–707, 2010.

[5] H. C. Dietz, G. R. Cutting, R. E. Pyeritz et al., "Marfan syndrome caused by a recurrent de novo missense mutation in the fibrillin gene," *Nature*, vol. 352, no. 6333, pp. 337–339, 1991.

[6] P. J. Coucke, A. Willaert, M. W. Wessels et al., "Mutations in the facilitative glucose transporter GLUT10 alter angiogenesis and cause arterial tortuosity syndrome," *Nature Genetics*, vol. 38, no. 4, pp. 452–457, 2006.

[7] B. L. Loeys, J. Chen, E. R. Neptune et al., "A syndrome of altered cardiovascular, craniofacial, neurocognitive and skeletal development caused by mutations in TGFBR1 or TGFBR2," *Nature Genetics*, vol. 37, no. 3, pp. 275–281, 2005.

[8] C. Boileau, D. C. Guo, N. Hanna et al., "TGFB2 mutations cause familial thoracic aortic aneurysms and dissections associated with mild systemic features of Marfan syndrome," *Nature Genetics*, vol. 44, no. 8, pp. 916–921, 2012.

[9] M. E. Lindsay, D. Schepers, N. A. Bolar et al., "Loss-of-function mutations in TGFB2 cause a syndromic presentation of thoracic aortic aneurysm," *Nature Genetics*, vol. 44, no. 8, pp. 922–927, 2012.

[10] I. M. B. H. van de Laar, R. A. Oldenburg, G. Pals et al., "Mutations in SMAD3 cause a syndromic form of aortic aneurysms and dissections with early-onset osteoarthritis," *Nature Genetics*, vol. 43, no. 2, pp. 121–126, 2011.

[11] I. M. B. H. van de Laar, D. van der Linde, E. H. G. Oei et al., "Phenotypic spectrum of the SMAD3-related aneurysms-osteoarthritis syndrome," *Journal of Medical Genetics*, vol. 49, no. 1, pp. 47–57, 2012.

[12] A. Wischmeijer, L. Van Lear, G. Tortora et al., "Thoracic aortic aneurysm in infancy in aneurysms-osteoarthritis syndrome due to a novel SMAD3 mutation: further delineation of the phenotype," *American Journal of Medical Genetics Part A*, vol. 161, no. 5, pp. 1028–1035, 2013.

[13] Y. Hilhorst-Hofstee, A. J. Scholte, M. E. Rijlaarsdam et al., "An unanticipated copy number variant of chromosome 15 disrupting SMAD3 reveals a three-generation family at serious risk for aortic dissection," *Clinical Genetics*, vol. 83, no. 4, pp. 337–344, 2013.

[14] W.-Y. Chong, W. H. S. Wong, C. S. W. Chiu, and Y.-F. Cheung, "Aortic root dilation and aortic elastic properties in children after repair of tetralogy of Fallot," *American Journal of Cardiology*, vol. 97, no. 6, pp. 905–909, 2006.

[15] M. Hourihan, S. D. Colan, G. Wernovsky, U. Maheswari, J. E. Mayer Jr., and S. P. Sanders, "Growth of the aortic anastomosis, annulus, and root after the arterial switch procedure performed in infancy," *Circulation*, vol. 88, no. 2, pp. 615–620, 1993.

[16] B. S. Marino, G. Wernovsky, D. B. McElhinney et al., "Neo-aortic valvar function after the arterial switch," *Cardiology in the Young*, vol. 16, no. 5, pp. 481–489, 2006.

[17] R. C. Elkins, D. M. Thompson, M. M. Lane, C. C. Elkins, and M. D. Peyton, "Ross operation: 16-year experience," *Journal of Thoracic and Cardiovascular Surgery*, vol. 136, no. 3, pp. 623–630, 2008.

[18] W. F. Carlo, E. D. Mckenzie, and T. C. Slesnick, "Root dilation in patients with truncus arteriosus," *Congenital Heart Disease*, vol. 6, no. 3, pp. 228–233, 2011.

[19] M. S. Cohen, B. S. Marino, D. B. McElhinney et al., "Neo-aortic root dilation and valve regurgitation up to 21 years after staged reconstruction for hypoplastic left heart syndrome," *Journal of the American College of Cardiology*, vol. 42, no. 3, pp. 533–540, 2003.

[20] M. Egan, A. Phillips, and S. C. Cook, "Aortic dissection in the adult fontan with aortic root enlargement," *Pediatric Cardiology*, vol. 30, no. 4, pp. 562–563, 2009.

22

A Rare, Recurrent, *De Novo* 14q32.2q32.31 Microdeletion of 1.1 Mb in a 20-Year-Old Female Patient with a Maternal UPD(14)-Like Phenotype and Intellectual Disability

Almira Zada,[1,2] **Farmaditya E. P. Mundhofir,**[2] **Rolph Pfundt,**[1] **Nico Leijsten,**[1] **Willy Nillesen,**[1] **Sultana M. H. Faradz,**[2] **and Nicole de Leeuw**[1]

[1] *Department of Human Genetics, Radboud University Medical Center, The Netherlands Division of Human Genetics, P.O. Box 9101, 6500 HB Nijmegen, The Netherlands*
[2] *Center for Biomedical Research (CEBIOR), Faculty of Medicine, Diponegoro University, GSG 2nd Floor, Jl. Dr. Sutomo 14, Semarang 50244, Indonesia*

Correspondence should be addressed to Almira Zada; almira.zd@gmail.com

Academic Editors: C. López Ginés and G. Perez de Nanclares

We present a 20-year-old female patient from Indonesia with intellectual disability (ID), proportionate short stature, motor delay, feeding problems, microcephaly, facial dysmorphism, and precocious puberty who was previously screened normal for conventional karyotyping, fragile X testing, and subtelomeric MLPA analysis. Subsequent genome wide array analysis was performed on DNA from blood and revealed a 1.1 Mb deletion in 14q32.2q32.31 (chr14:100,388,343-101,506,214; hg19). Subsequent carrier testing in the parents by array showed that the deletion had occurred *de novo* in the patient and that her paternal 14q32 allele was deleted. The deleted region encompasses the *DLK1/GTL2* imprinted gene cluster which is consistent with the maternal UPD(14)-like phenotype of the patient. This rare, recurrent microdeletion was recently shown not to be mediated by low copy repeats, but by expanded TGG repeats, flanking the 14q32.2q32.21 deletion boundaries, a novel mechanism of recurrent genomic rearrangement. This is another example how the application of high resolution genome wide testing provides an accurate genetic diagnosis, thereby improving the care for patients and optimizing the counselling for family.

1. Introduction

The application of high resolution genome wide array analysis provides an accurate genetic diagnosis in many patients with ID and/or congenital anomalies caused by genomic imbalances. The use of this technology has led to the discovery of several novel microdeletion and microduplication syndromes. Although several patients have been reported with a terminal 14q32 deletion, patients with an in terstitial microdeletion in the 14q32 region seem to be rare. To our knowledge, only two patients with an interstitial 1.1 Mb deletion in q32.2q32.31 have previously been reported [1, 2].

Human chromosome 14q32.2 is the critical region for uniparental disomy of chromosome 14 (UPD(14)) phenotypes because it carries a cluster of imprinted genes, including the paternally expressed genes (PEGs) such as *DLK1&RTL1* and the maternally expressed genes (MEGs) such as *GTL2* (also known as *MEG3*), *RTL1as* (RTL1 antisense), and *MEG8*. Deletion of the paternal allele in this region causes a UPD(14)mat-like phenotype [3]. Uniparental disomy (UPD) occurs when the two copies of a chromosome pair are inherited from only one parent [4]. Maternal UPD of chromosome 14 (UPD(14)mat) is characterized by pre- and postnatal growth retardation, hypotonia, feeding problems, motor delay, short stature, early onset of puberty, and minor dysmorphic features of the face, hands, and feet [5]. Seven out of eleven UPD(14)mat-like cases without UPD have been reported to carry a deletion in the 14q32.2 region [2, 3, 6–9].

Here we report an additional female patient with a 1.1 Mb deletion of chromosome 14 in the q32.2q32.31 region identified by high resolution genome wide SNP array analysis.

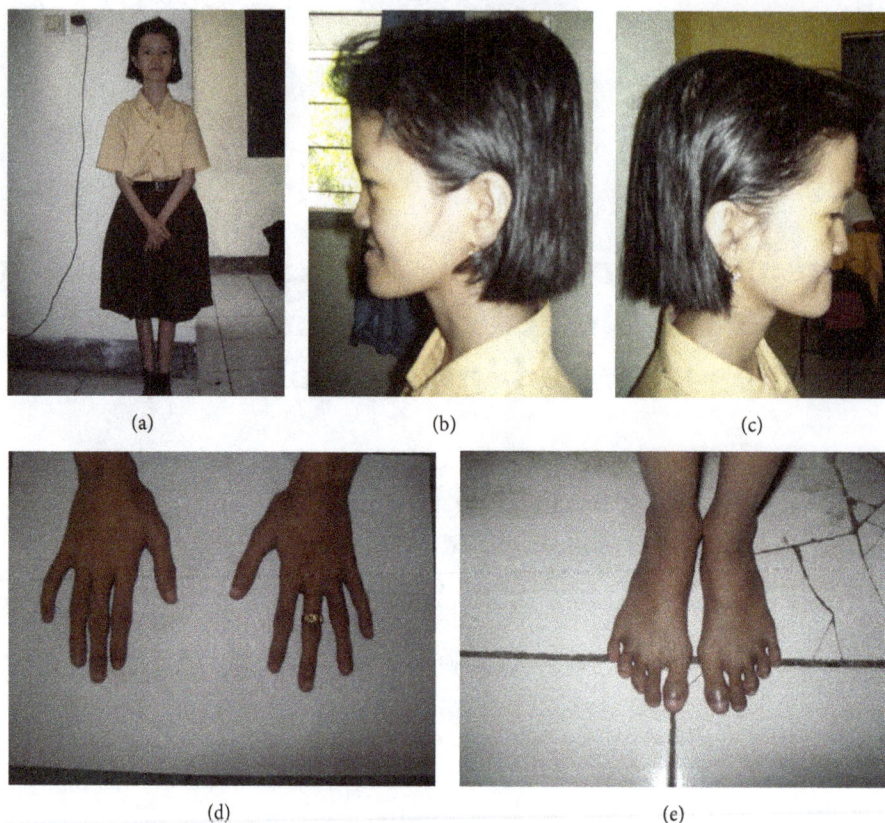

FIGURE 1: Photograph of Indonesian patient with a 14q32.2 microdeletion. Our 20-year-old patient showed extremely short and thin stature, flat face, flat philtrum, thin lips, tapering fingers, clinodactyly of the fifth finger on the right hand, and clubbing feet toes.

2. Case Report

A 20-year-old female Indonesian Javanese patient presented with extremely thin and short stature, microcephaly, motor delay, hypotonia, mild intellectual disability, flat face, flat philtrum, thin lips, tapering fingers, clinodactyly of her fifth finger on the right hand, clubbing feet toes, feeding problems, and precocious puberty (Figure 1). She was born at 32 weeks of pregnancy with a low birth weight of 1,800 g (p5–10) as the second child of healthy, unrelated parents. At the time of her birth, her mother was 24 years of age, and her father was 33 years of age. There was no family history of intellectual disability. Postnatally, she was found to have feeding problem, motor delay, hypotonia, and precocious puberty. She was able to walk at three years of age and able to speak at two years of age. When she was examined at 20 years of age, her body height was 130 cm ($P < 3$), her weight was 18 kg ($P < 3$), and her arm span was 125 cm. Her ratio height to arm span was 0.96 cm, thus showing proportionate short stature. She has microcephaly with an occipital frontal circumference (OFC) of 50 cm ($P < 3$). Previously, genetic tests were done, including conventional karyotyping, subtelomeric MLPA, and fragile X testing, all of which showed normal results [10]. Informed consent for publishing results and photos has been obtained from the patient's parents.

We performed genome wide array analysis on DNA from blood using the Affymetrix CytoScan HD Array platform (Affymetrix, Inc., Santa Clara, CA, USA) following the manufacturer's protocols, which showed a 1.1 Mb deletion in 14q32.2q32.31 (chr14:100,388,343-101,506,214; hg19) as depicted in Figure 2(a). Subsequent carrier testing with the same array platform in the parents revealed that the deletion had occurred *de novo* in the patient (Figure 2(b)) and that her paternal 14q32 allele was deleted. The possible presence of either a balanced chromosomal rearrangement and/or mosaic imbalance in the father was subsequently studied by fluorescence in situ hybridization (FISH) analysis using a FISH probe (RP11-123M6; BlueGnome Ltd., Cambridge, UK) specific for the 14q32.2q32.31 region. These FISH results showed that the father did not carry a balanced rearrangement and/or mosaic imbalance (Figure 3).

3. Discussion

Here we report an additional patient with a rare, recurrent, *de novo* 14q32.2q32.31 microdeletion of 1.1 Mb. Two other (female) patients have been reported in the literature with a similar 1.1 Mb microdeletion in 14q32.2q32.31 [1, 2]. Comparable to our patient, it concerned a *de novo* loss of paternal

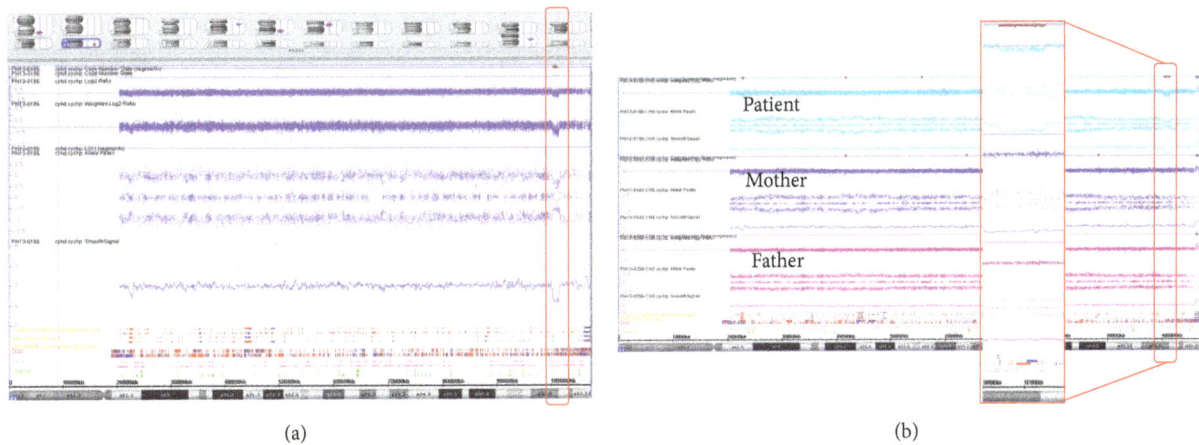

FIGURE 2: (a) Array plots of chromosome 14, visualized using the Affymetrix Chromosome Analysis Suite (ChAS) Software. A 1.1 Mb loss in 14q32.2q32.31 was detected in Patient 1 (arr[hg19] 14q32.2q32.31(100,388,343-101,506,214)x1 dn) as indicated by the red rectangle. (b) Trio analysis confirms that the deletion has occurred *de novo* in the patient.

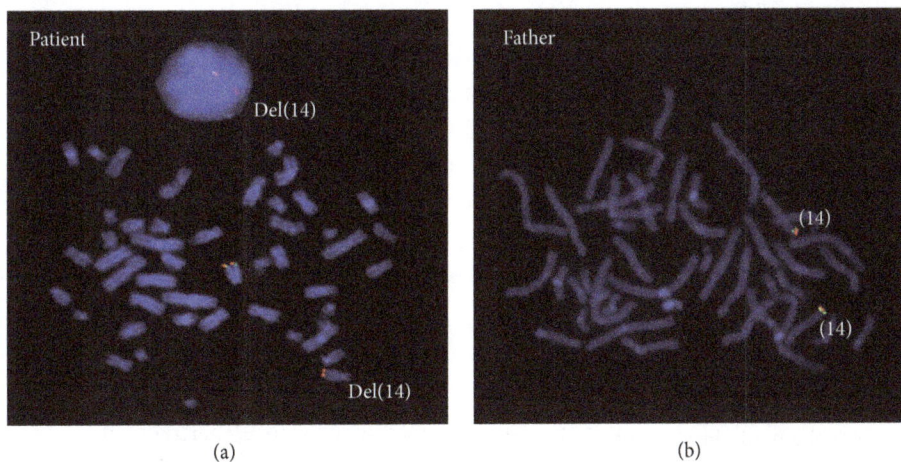

FIGURE 3: FISH study in the patient and her father. In each of them, 30 metaphases from cultured peripheral blood lymphocytes were analysed. (a) Patient metaphase showing one normal chromosome 14 [RP11-123M6 (green)/14 qter 9 (red)] and the del(14)(q32.2q32.31) with only 14 qter signal (red). (b) Metaphase from the father with a normal FISH pattern, indicating two normal chromosomes 14.

14q32 allele in both patients, who exhibited clinical features compatible with UPD-(14)-mat (genomic coordinates and clinical features in hg 19 are shown in Table 1).

This deleted region comprises a snoRNA, part of a microRNA cluster, and 15 protein-coding genes, containing a cluster of imprinted genes including paternally expressed genes *DLK1&RTL1* and maternally expressed genes *GTL2* (also known as *MEG3*), *RTL1as,* and *MEG8.* The deleted paternal 14q32 allele causes a maternal UPD(14)-like phenotype [3]. The other 10 genes are not imprinted (*EVL, DEGS2, YY1, SLC25A29, c14orf68, WARS, WDR25, BEGAIN, c14orf70,* and the 3'end of *EML1*).

Other than pre- and postnatal growth retardation, precocious puberty, and feeding problems, which are compatible with UPD(14)mat phenotypes, the patient reported here also manifested intellectual disability (ID) which is not or rarely observed in patients with UPD(14)mat. Considering that the 1.1 Mb 14q32 deletion also encompasses many nonimprinted

genes, it is likely that the ID in this patient is caused by haploinsufficiency of one or more dosage-sensitive genes. For example, the *BEGAIN* (brain-enriched guanylate kinase-associated protein) gene represents a good candidate based on its localization in the neuronal synapse [11]. The recently reported *YY1* gene is considered to be an ID disease gene based on the exome sequencing in a patient with unexplained ID in whom a missense mutation c.1138G>T with protein level change p.Asp380Tyr was found [12]. This gene implicates chromatin remodelling as its main function by encoding the ubiquitously expressed transcription factor yin-yang 1 and directing histone acetylases and histone acetyltransferases. Experiments with Yy1 knockdown mice resulted in growth retardation, neurulation defects, and brain abnormalities [13].

Most recurrent genomic rearrangements are due to non-allelic homologous recombination (NAHR) between misaligned low copy repeats resulting in a microdeletion or

TABLE 1: Genomic coordinates and clinical features of all cases.

	Buiting et al., 2008 [2]	Béna et al., 2010 [1]	Present case
Deletion positions (Mb) in chromosome 14 (hg 19)	100.396–101.502	100.400–101.500	100.388–101.506
Sex	Female	Female	Female
Age (years)	$14\frac{1}{4}$	4	20
Pre- and postnatal growth retardation	+	+	+
Hypotonia	+	+	+
Feeding problems	+	+	+
Precocious puberty	+	?	+
Intellectual disability	+	+	+
Dysmorphism	–	High forehead, small chin, posteriorly rotated ears, and flat feet	Flat face, flat philtrum, thin lips, tapering fingers, clinodactyly of the fifth finger on the right hand, and clubbing feet toes
Others	–	Hypermetropia	–

+: present; –: not present; ?: undetermined yet.

a microduplication [14]. However, a recent paper by Béna et al. [1] reported the observations regarding the mechanism underlying the recurrent 14q32.2 deletion described here. They found that large (TGG)n tandem repeat tracts of about 500 bp are at both boundaries of the deletion (chr14:100,394,091-100,394,594 and chr14:101,504,592-101,505,016; hg19). The TGG repeats are the longest type of triplets motif and highly capable of forming G4 DNA. Some theories might explain how these triplet repeats can cause genomic rearrangement. First, expanded triplet repeats would provide an aggravated substrate for genomic rearrangement through the NAHR mechanism [15, 16]. Second, expanded triplet repeats have the tendency to form intramolecular secondary structures termed guanine quadruplexes or G4 DNA which could promote double strand chromosome breaks [17]. Therefore, it is suggested that this recurrent 14q32.2 microdeletion is mediated by expanded TGG repeats, a novel mechanism of recurrent genomic rearrangement that is shown not to be mediated by low copy repeats.

In conclusion, we were able to detect a rarely identified 14q32.2 microdeletion by using high resolution genome wide array analysis in a patient whose genotype and phenotype are in agreement with those of two previously reported patients in the literature. This case report demonstrates the value of applying high resolution genome wide testing for accurate genetic diagnosis that can help to improve the care for patients and to optimize the counselling for family.

Conflict of Interests

The authors declare that there is no conflict of interests regarding the publication of this paper.

Acknowledgments

This research study was partly funded by the Excellent Scholarship Program of the Bureau of Planning and International Cooperation, Ministry of National Education, Government of Indonesia, in collaboration with the Radboud University Medical Centre (Radboud UMC) in Nijmegen, The Netherlands. The authors thank the family for their cooperation and permission to publish this paper. They also thank the laboratory staff of Department of Human Genetics, Radboud UMC, Nijmegen, The Netherlands, and CEBIOR, Faculty of Medicine, Diponegoro University, Semarang, Indonesia.

References

[1] F. Béna, S. Gimelli, E. Migliavacca et al., "A recurrent 14q32.2 microdeletion mediated by expanded TGG repeats," *Human Molecular Genetics*, vol. 19, no. 10, pp. 1967–1973, 2010.

[2] K. Buiting, D. Kanber, J. I. Martín-Subero et al., "Clinical features of maternal uniparental disomy 14 in patients with an epimutation and a deletion of the imprinted DLK1/GTL2 gene cluster," *Human Mutation*, vol. 29, no. 9, pp. 1141–1146, 2008.

[3] M. Kagami, Y. Sekita, G. Nishimura et al., "Deletions and epimutations affecting the human 14q32.2 imprinted region in individuals with paternal and maternal upd(14)-like phenotypes," *Nature Genetics*, vol. 40, no. 2, pp. 237–242, 2008.

[4] E. Engel, "A new genetic concept: uniparental disomy and its potential effect, isodisomy," *American Journal of Medical Genetics*, vol. 6, no. 2, pp. 137–143, 1980.

[5] V. R. Sutton and L. G. Shaffer, "Search for imprinted regions on Chromosome 14: comparison of maternal and paternal UPD cases with cases of chromosome 14 deletions," *American Journal of Medical Genetics*, vol. 93, pp. 381–387, 2000.

[6] D. Mitter, K. Buiting, F. Von Eggeling et al., "Is there a higher incidence of maternal uniparental disomy 14 [upd(14)mat]? Detection of 10 new patients by methylation-specific PCR,"

American Journal of Medical Genetics A, vol. 140, no. 19, pp. 2039–2049, 2006.

[7] K. Hosoki, T. Ogata, M. Kagami, T. Tanaka, and S. Saitoh, "Epimutation (hypomethylation) affecting the chromosome 14q32.2 imprinted region in a girl with upd(14)mat-like phenotype," *European Journal of Human Genetics*, vol. 16, no. 8, pp. 1019–1023, 2008.

[8] A. Schneider, B. Benzacken, A. Guichet et al., "Molecular cytogenetic characterization of terminal 14q32 deletions in two children with an abnormal phenotype and corpus callosum hypoplasia," *European Journal of Human Genetics*, vol. 16, no. 6, pp. 680–687, 2008.

[9] U. Zechner, N. Kohlschmidt, G. Rittner et al., "Epimutation at human chromosome 14q32.2 in a boy with a upd(14)mat-like clinical phenotype," *Clinical Genetics*, vol. 75, no. 3, pp. 251–258, 2009.

[10] F. E. Mundhofir, T. I. Winarni, B. W. van Bon et al., "A cytogenetic study in a large population of intellectually disabled Indonesians," *Genetic Test Molecular Biomarkers*, vol. 16, pp. 412–417, 2012.

[11] I. Yao, J. Iida, W. Nishimura, and Y. Hata, "Synaptic and nuclear localization of brain-enriched guanylate kinase-associated protein," *Journal of Neuroscience*, vol. 22, no. 13, pp. 5354–5364, 2002.

[12] L. E. L. M. Vissers, J. De Ligt, C. Gilissen et al., "A de novo paradigm for mental retardation," *Nature Genetics*, vol. 42, no. 12, pp. 1109–1112, 2010.

[13] Y. He and P. Casaccia-Bonnefil, "The Yin and Yang of YY1 in the nervous system," *Journal of Neurochemistry*, vol. 106, no. 4, pp. 1493–1502, 2008.

[14] P. J. Hastings, J. R. Lupski, S. M. Rosenberg, and G. Ira, "Mechanisms of change in gene copy number," *Nature Reviews Genetics*, vol. 10, no. 8, pp. 551–564, 2009.

[15] J. Rubnitz and S. Subramani, "The minimum amount of homology required for homologous recombination in mammalian cells," *Molecular and Cellular Biology*, vol. 4, no. 11, pp. 2253–2258, 1984.

[16] A. S. Waldman and R. M. Liskay, "Dependence of intrachromosomal recombination in mammalian cells on uninterrupted homology," *Molecular and Cellular Biology*, vol. 8, no. 12, pp. 5350–5357, 1988.

[17] K. Usdin, "NGG-triplet repeats form similar intrastrand structures: implications for the triplet expansion diseases," *Nucleic Acids Research*, vol. 26, no. 17, pp. 4078–4085, 1998.

23

Whole Exome Sequencing Reveals Compound Heterozygosity for Ethnically Distinct PEX7 Mutations Responsible for Rhizomelic Chondrodysplasia Punctata, Type 1

Jessie C. Jacobsen,[1] Emma Glamuzina,[2] Juliet Taylor,[3] Brendan Swan,[1] Shona Handisides,[4] Callum Wilson,[2] Michael Fietz,[5,6] Tessa van Dijk,[7] Bart Appelhof,[7] Rosamund Hill,[8] Rosemary Marks,[9] Donald R. Love,[10] Stephen P. Robertson,[11] Russell G. Snell,[1] and Klaus Lehnert[1]

[1] Centre for Brain Research and School of Biological Sciences, The University of Auckland, Auckland 1010, New Zealand
[2] Adult and Paediatric National Metabolic Service, Auckland City Hospital, Auckland 1142, New Zealand
[3] Genetic Health Service New Zealand, Auckland City Hospital, Auckland 1142, New Zealand
[4] Department of Radiology, Auckland City Hospital, Auckland 1142, New Zealand
[5] Department of Biochemical Genetics, SA Pathology, North Adelaide, SA 5006, Australia
[6] Department of Diagnostic Genomics, PathWest, Nedlands, WA 6009, Australia
[7] Department of Genome Analysis, Academic Medical Centre, 1105 Amsterdam, Netherlands
[8] Department of Neurology, Auckland City Hospital, Auckland 1142, New Zealand
[9] Developmental Paediatric Service, Starship Children's Health, Auckland 1142, New Zealand
[10] Diagnostic Genetics, LabPLUS, Auckland City Hospital, Auckland 1142, New Zealand
[11] Dunedin School of Medicine, University of Otago, Dunedin 9016, New Zealand

Correspondence should be addressed to Russell G. Snell; r.snell@auckland.ac.nz

Academic Editor: Mohnish Suri

We describe two brothers who presented at birth with bone growth abnormalities, followed by development of increasingly severe intellectual and physical disability, growth restriction, epilepsy, and cerebellar and brain stem atrophy, but normal ocular phenotypes. Case 1 died at 19 years of age due to chronic respiratory illnesses without a unifying diagnosis. The brother remains alive but severely disabled at 19 years of age. Whole exome sequencing identified compound heterozygous stop mutations in the *peroxisome biogenesis factor 7* gene in both individuals. Mutations in this gene cause rhizomelic chondrodysplasia punctata, type 1 (RCDP1). One mutation, p.Arg232*, has only been documented once before in a Japanese family, which is of interest given these two boys are of European descent. The other mutation, p.Leu292*, is found in approximately 50% of RCDP1 patients. These are the first cases of RCDP1 that describe the coinheritance of the p.Arg232* and p.Leu292* mutations and demonstrate the utility of WES in cases with unclear diagnoses.

1. Introduction

Rhizomelic chondrodysplasia punctata, type 1 (RCDP; OMIM 215100), resulting from mutations in *peroxisome biogenesis factor 7* (*PEX7*; OMIM 601757) is typically characterised by severe, prenatal defects in bone growth resulting in short stature, neurological impairment, and cataracts. Milder phenotypes with a growing genotypic and biochemical spectrum have been reported [1–3]. RCDP is estimated to affect approximately 1 per 100,000 children [1, 4], with type 1 accounting for greater than 90% of cases [3]. The *PEX7* gene encodes the receptor required for the targeting of peroxisomal proteins containing the peroxisome targeting signal 2, including the enzymes phytanoyl-CoA hydroxylase and alkyl-dihydroxyacetone phosphate synthase. These enzymes are involved in peroxisomal α-oxidation of phytanic acid and the synthesis of plasmalogen ether lipids, respectively. Interruption of these processes results in the key biochemical hallmarks of RCDP1, elevated plasma phytanic acid and low erythrocyte plasmalogen levels, which occur in the presence of normal plasma very long chain fatty acid (VLCFA) levels (reviewed by Wanders [5]). We describe a sib-pair with variable phytanic acid levels coupled with normal levels of VLCFA who presented with global developmental delay, mild epiphyseal dysplasia, epilepsy, poor growth, subtle dysmorphism, and cerebellar and brain stem atrophy. The two affected individuals are the only live-born children (seven miscarriages) to unrelated parents of European descent. Using whole exome sequencing we identified two stop mutations in the *PEX7* gene, and a subsequent diagnosis of RCDP1 was made.

2. Case 1

Case 1 was born at term after a pregnancy complicated by deficiency in amniotic fluid. He had low muscle tone and required oxygen and bag-mask resuscitation immediately after birth. He breathed normally at 3 minutes (Apgar [6] scores of 3 and 9 at one and five minutes after birth, resp.). Birth weight (3210 g) and head circumference (34 cm) were on the 25th percentile. He was noted initially to have micrognathia and contractures of the hands and feet but fed well and was discharged at day 3. By 6 months, developmental delay across all milestones was apparent and growth was well below the 3rd percentile (6 kg at 7 months). At 3 years of age, growth defects at the ends of his long bones (epiphyseal dysplasia with flared metaphyses and small epiphyseal ossification centres) were reported. Radiographs at 12 years of age showed punctate patellar ossification centres and marked metaphyseal splaying (Supplementary Figure 1 in Supplementary Material available online at http://dx.doi.org/10.1155/2015/454526). Development remained markedly delayed with treatment-refractory epilepsy resulting in regression. Growth remained poor with a weight of 10 kg at 6 years of age ($\ll$ 3rd percentile) despite supplemental feeding, and vision assessments were normal (last performed at 10 years). A peroxisomal disorder was initially considered, and elevated phytanic acid level with normal VLCFAs was reported at 6 years of age. However, repeat phytanic acid level was normal, and thus a peroxisomal disorder was thought to have been excluded (Supplementary Table 1). Brain magnetic resonance imaging (MRI) at 10 years of age revealed delayed myelination and atrophy of the brain stem and cerebellum (Supplementary Figure 2). He developed progressive scoliosis and recurrent chest infections and died at 19 years of age with no unifying diagnosis. Postmortem examination confirmed an abnormal hindbrain and brainstem.

3. Case 2

Case 2 was born at 35 weeks' gestation by elective caesarean section due to poor fetal growth and decreasing liquor from

32 weeks. Apgar scores were within normal range (8^1 and 9^5). He had flexion contractures of the knees and required respiratory support for 24 hours. Punctate calcifications of his patellae, proximal femurs, and humerus (head and medial epicondyles) were evident, but there were no reports of shortened limbs. He later developed evidence of epiphyseal dysplasia with metaphyseal flaring (Supplementary Figure 1). He had slightly more prominent facial dysmorphism and was less alert and interactive but otherwise followed a similar developmental and growth trajectory to his brother. At 17 years of age he weighed 19.6 kg. He had severe intellectual and physical impairment with increasing encephalopathy and treatment-refractory epilepsy which started at 6 years of age. He was dependant for all activities of daily living and was largely noncommunicative. There was no clear evidence of multisystem disease and no cataracts. Brain MRI at 6 years of age was similar to his brother and a repeat scan at 17 years of age revealed moderate atrophy of the cerebellum (Supplementary Figure 2). A neurometabolic workup was completed. The only abnormalities were elevated neopterin and low biogenic monoamine metabolites, which were thought to be secondary to brain disease. Phytanic acid was elevated and VLCFAs were reported as normal (Supplementary Table 1).

4. Exome Sequencing

To identify the causal mutations underlying this sib-pair, we performed whole exome sequencing of both brothers. The study was approved by the New Zealand Northern B Health and Disability Ethics Committee (12/NTB/59), and parents provided written informed consent. We obtained average coverage of 71 and 74, respectively, across the targeted regions and discovered 46,794 high-quality variants with concordant genotypes in the sib-pair. The 19,439 homozygous variants were filtered to remove genotypes observed more than once in 123 control New Zealand exomes and variants with alleles frequently observed in Europeans (Supplementary Table 2). Only one of the remaining 114 homozygous variants was potentially functional (*RTKN2*) but was not located in a gene related to cerebellar ataxia or atrophy.

Of the 27,355 heterozygous variants identified in both siblings, 1,447 were rare or absent in the surveyed European population or control exomes; of these, 238 variants were potentially functional. Five genes carried more than one rare and functional variant and met our minimum criteria for potentially compound recessive inheritance (Supplementary Table 2). Nonsynonymous mutations in *CHTF18*, *FSIP2*, and *MYOM2* were excluded from further consideration based on the genes' known biological functions or disease associations. Two nonsynonymous mutations were identified in *CACNA1H* (RefSeq accession NG_012647.1; OMIM 607904), which is a susceptibility gene for childhood absence epilepsy (OMIM 611942). Two stop-gain variants, c.694C>T, p.Arg232* (rs121909153) and c.875T > A, p.Leu292* (rs1805137), in the *PEX7* gene (RefSeq accession NG_008462.1) were the most functionally significant mutations and were validated by PCR and Sanger sequencing in the affected children and their unaffected parents, confirming

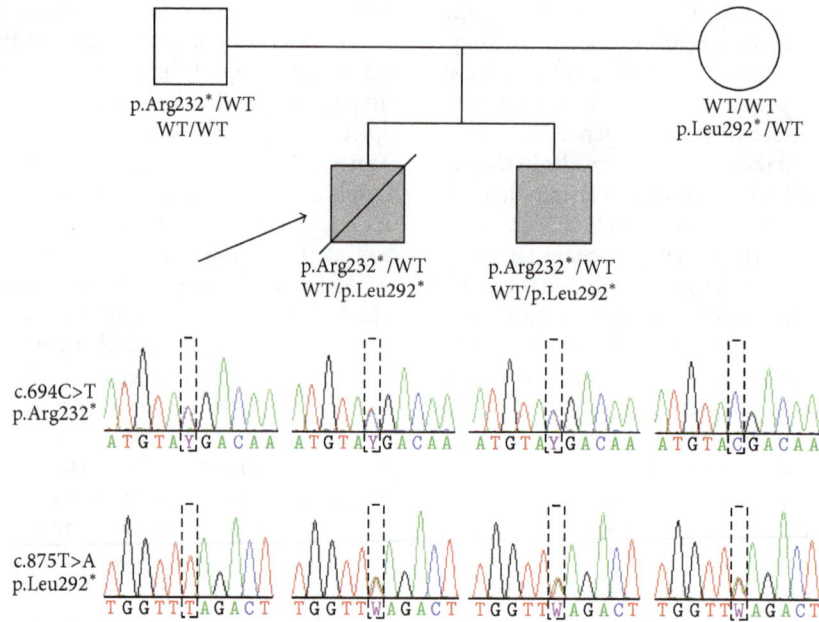

FIGURE 1: Family pedigree and transmission of the c.694C>T and c.875T>A mutations in the *PEX7* gene. The arrow identifies case 1. Protein genotypes are indicated immediately below each family member's pedigree symbol, and Sanger sequencing electropherograms for both loci are shown below the corresponding family member in the lower part of the figure. The couple's seven miscarriages are not depicted. WT, wild-type allele.

compound heterozygous inheritance (Figure 1). Both mutations are extremely rare and have been previously identified as pathogenic, causing RCDP1. The p.Leu292* mutation is estimated to account for >50% of RCDP1 cases [1, 2, 7]. The p.Arg232* mutation has only been published in a single consanguineous Japanese parent-child trio [8, 9] and reported in a heterozygous carrier from South Asia [10]. This is the first time, to our knowledge, it has been identified in individuals of European ancestry. Following genetic diagnosis (at 18 years of age) erythrocyte phospholipids (plasmalogens) were also found to be markedly reduced, which is consistent with a diagnosis of RCDP1 (Supplementary Table 1).

5. Discussion

Whole exome sequencing identified two compound heterozygous stop-gain mutations in the *PEX7* gene in two New Zealand children of European descent who primarily presented with global developmental delay, mild bone growth defects, epilepsy, poor growth, subtle facial dysmorphism, and cerebellar and brain stem atrophy. Cerebellar atrophy is a well-documented phenomenon in RCDP1 and brainstem pathology has been previously reported in peroxisomal disorders [11–13]. Ichthyotic skin, cleft palate, and congenital heart disease were not observed in either case. Proximal limb shortening and cataracts were not noted in the children, and their neurological deterioration and poor growth were severe but attenuated compared to classical RCDP1. Interestingly, bilateral cataracts were also not observed in the only other case reported with an Arg232* mutation [9], broadening the phenotypic spectrum of RCDP1 and emphasising the importance of diagnosis by next generation sequencing. The *PEX7*

mutations described here have been previously reported, but not in this combination. One of the mutations, p.Leu292*, accounts for ~50% of RCDP1 cases and is due to a founder effect in Northern European Caucasian populations [1]. The second mutation, p.Arg232*, has only been published in a single family of Japanese descent, and a single heterozygous individual from South Asia has been reported in the ExAc database [10] (global allele frequency = 8.23×10^{-6}). The presented sib-pair shows that the mutation is not confined to Asian populations and suggests it should be screened in European cases.

In neonates suspected of RCDP1, biochemical diagnosis of the disorder is traditionally performed by the detection of reduced erythrocyte plasmalogen levels; elevated phytanic acid levels are usually only observed after 6–12 months of age, due to phytanic acid being derived from the diet. However, in older patients (greater than 12 months of age), plasma phytanic acid analysis is often used as a primary biochemical tool for the diagnosis of RCDP1. In this study, analysis of the older sibling at 6 years of age yielded an elevated and then normal phytanic acid level. Fluctuating phytanic acid levels were also obtained in case 2. These results, coupled with normal levels of VLCFA, and more subtle clinical features than expected resulted in the erroneous exclusion of a peroxisomal disorder despite reviews from multiple specialists. Although earlier studies have shown the presence of normal phytanic acid levels in children with milder presentations of RCDP1 [11, 14], the relatively severe clinical presentation of both siblings, together with the presence of two previously described nonsense variants in the *PEX7* gene, makes the observed oscillating phytanic acid levels quite unexpected.

This result emphasises the biochemical spectrum of RCDP1 and indicates that, in cases suspected of RCDP1, erythrocyte plasmalogen analysis should always be performed in parallel with phytanic acid testing.

Interestingly, the children also harbour two previously identified variants (rs57552791 and rs58173258) in the *CACNA1H* gene (inherited in a recessive compound heterozygous fashion), which is a susceptibility gene for childhood absence epilepsy. The rs58173258 variant (p.A876T) has been found to segregate with disease status in one family with epilepsy studied by Heron et al. [15]; however, the phenotypes within the family were diverse. When studied *in vitro*, the variant was found to alter channel activity resulting in an increase in channel function [15]. Therefore, it is possible that these two single nucleotide variants contribute to the epilepsy phenotype observed in these two children, although their seizures do not appear to be more pronounced than those observed in other RCDP1 patients and their MRI findings were typical of those with severe RCDP1 [11]. Given that the majority of RCDP1 patients develop seizures, further research would need to be conducted to deduce the underlying role of these *CACNA1H* variants.

The rapid developments and decreasing cost of exome and whole genome sequencing are making diagnosis of phenotypically diverse conditions such as RCDP1 easier. This is exemplified by the sib-pair presented here where diagnosis through whole exome sequencing provided the scaffold for interpretation of their clinical histories and biochemical results, which did not entirely fit the classical description of RCDP1. This methodology allowed the unifying diagnosis to be made 26 years after birth of case 1, vouching for the use of next generation sequencing for the diagnosis of severe neurodevelopmental disabilities.

Conflict of Interests

The authors declare that there is no conflict of interests regarding the publication of this paper.

Acknowledgments

The authors would like to thank the Centre for Genomics, Proteomics and Metabolomics at The University of Auckland for Sanger sequencing services and the New Zealand eScience Infrastructure for high-performance computing support. Jessie C. Jacobsen is supported by a Rutherford Discovery Fellowship from government funding, administered by the Royal Society of New Zealand, Stephen P. Robertson is supported by Cure Kids NZ, and Klaus Lehnert is supported by the Minds for Minds Charitable Trust. The research was funded by the Neurological Foundation of New Zealand and the Oakley Mental Health Research Foundation. They would like to thank the family for consenting to participate in this study.

References

[1] N. E. Braverman, A. B. Moser, and S. J. Steinberg, "Rhizomelic chondrodysplasia punctata type 1," in *GeneReviews*, R. A. Pagon, M. P. Adam, H. H. Ardinger et al., Eds., University of Washington, Seattle, Wash, USA, 2001.

[2] A. M. Motley, P. Brites, L. Gerez et al., "Mutational spectrum in the PEX7 gene and functional analysis of mutant alleles in 78 patients with rhizomelic chondrodysplasia punctata type 1," *The American Journal of Human Genetics*, vol. 70, no. 3, pp. 612–624, 2002.

[3] M. Noguchi, M. Honsho, Y. Abe et al., "Mild reduction of plasmalogens causes rhizomelic chondrodysplasia punctata: functional characterization of a novel mutation," *Journal of Human Genetics*, vol. 59, no. 7, pp. 387–392, 2014.

[4] C. Stoll, B. Dott, M.-P. Roth, and Y. Alembik, "Birth prevalence rates of skeletal dysplasias," *Clinical Genetics*, vol. 35, no. 2, pp. 88–92, 1989.

[5] R. J. Wanders, "Metabolic and molecular basis of peroxisomal disorders: a review," *American Journal of Medical Genetics Part A*, vol. 126, no. 4, pp. 355–375, 2004.

[6] V. Apgar, "A proposal for a new method of evaluation of the newborn infant," *Current Researches in Anesthesia & Analgesia*, vol. 32, no. 4, pp. 260–267, 1953.

[7] P. Brites, A. Motley, E. Hogenhout et al., "Molecular basis of rhizomelic chondrodysplasia punctata type I: high frequency of the Leu-292 Stop mutation in 38 patients," *Journal of Inherited Metabolic Disease*, vol. 21, no. 3, pp. 306–308, 1998.

[8] N. Shimozawa, Y. Suzuki, Z. Zhang et al., "A novel nonsense mutation of the PEX7 gene in a patient with rhizomelic chondrodysplasia punctata," *Journal of Human Genetics*, vol. 44, no. 2, pp. 123–125, 1999.

[9] Y. Suzuki, N. Shimozawa, K. Izai et al., "Peroxisomal 3-ketoacyl-CoA thiolase is partially processed in fibroblasts from patients with rhizomelic chondrodysplasia punctata," *Journal of Inherited Metabolic Disease*, vol. 16, no. 5, pp. 868–871, 1993.

[10] Exome Aggregation Consortium (ExAC), Cambridge, Mass, USA, May 2015, http://exac.broadinstitute.org.

[11] A. M. Bams-Mengerink, J. H. T. M. Koelman, H. Waterham, P. G. Barth, and B. T. Poll-The, "The neurology of rhizomelic chondrodysplasia punctata," *Orphanet Journal of Rare Diseases*, vol. 8, no. 1, article 174, 2013.

[12] N. Braverman, C. Argyriou, and A. Moser, "Human disorders of peroxisome biogenesis: zellweger spectrum and rhizomelic chondrodysplasia punctata," in *Molecular Machines Involved in Peroxisome Biogenesis and Maintenance*, C. Brocard and A. Hartig, Eds., pp. 63–90, Springer, Vienna, Austria, 2014.

[13] S. Ferdinandusse, S. Barker, K. Lachlan et al., "Adult peroxisomal acyl-coenzyme A oxidase deficiency with cerebellar and brainstem atrophy," *Journal of Neurology, Neurosurgery and Psychiatry*, vol. 81, no. 3, pp. 310–312, 2010.

[14] P. G. Barth, R. J. A. Wanders, R. B. H. Schutgens, and C. R. Staalman, "Variant rhizomelic chondrodysplasia punctata (RCDP) with normal plasma phytanic acid: clinico-biochemical delineation of a subtype and complementation studies," *American Journal of Medical Genetics*, vol. 62, no. 2, pp. 164–168, 1996.

[15] S. E. Heron, H. Khosravani, D. Varela et al., "Extended spectrum of idiopathic generalized epilepsies associated with CACNA1H functional variants," *Annals of Neurology*, vol. 62, no. 6, pp. 560–568, 2007.

24

Neurofibromatosis Type 1: A Novel NF1 Mutation Associated with Mitochondrial Complex I Deficiency

Sara Domingues,[1] **Lara Isidoro,**[2] **Dalila Rocha,**[2] **and Jorge Sales Marques**[2]

[1] *Pediatrics Department, Centro Hospitalar do Tâmega e Sousa, EPE, Unidade Padre Américo 4564-007 Penafiel, Portugal*
[2] *Pediatrics Department, Centro Hospitalar de Vila Nova de Gaia/Espinho, EPE, Unidade II, 4400-129 Vila Nova de Gaia, Portugal*

Correspondence should be addressed to Sara Domingues; saradomingues@hotmail.com

Academic Editors: P. D. Cotter and P. Morrison

Background. Neurofibromatosis type 1 is a multisystemic, progressive disease, with an estimated incidence of 1/3500-2500. Mitochondrial diseases are generally multisystemic and may be present at any age, and the global prevalence is 1/8500. The diagnosis of these disorders is complex because of its clinical and genetic heterogeneity. *Case Report.* We present a rare case of the association of these two different genetic diseases, in which a heterozygous missense mutation in the NF1 gene was identified which had not yet been described (p.M1149 V). Additionally, the patient is suspected of carrying an unspecified mutation causing respiratory chain complex I deficiency. Clinical presentation included hypotonia, global development delay, reduced growth rate, progressive microcephaly, and numerous *café-au-lait* spots. *Discussion.* To the best of our knowledge this is the first report of complex I deficiency in a patient with neurofibromatosis type 1. It is very important to maintain a high index of suspicion for the diagnosis of mitochondrial disorders. In this patient, both the laboratory screening and muscle histology were normal and only the biochemical study of muscle allowed us to confirm the diagnosis.

1. Introduction

Neurofibromatosis type 1 (NF1), first described in 1882 by von Recklinghausen [1, 2], is a multisystemic [1, 3], progressive disease [2], with an estimated incidence of 1/3500-2500 [1–4]. In about half of the cases, it is an autosomal dominant inherited disorder, and in the remaining cases, it results from *de novo* mutations [1, 3]. It has high penetrance and variable phenotypic expression between and within families [1]. It results from mutations in the NF1 tumor suppressor gene located on chromosome 17 [2], responsible for encoding neurofibromin [1]. The three main characteristics of this disease are *café-au-lait* spots, multiple neurofibromas, and Lisch nodules (pigmented *hamartomas* of the Iris) [5].

Mitochondrial disorders are a heterogeneous group of diseases characterized by defects of mitochondrial structure and oxidative phosphorylation [6–8]. These disorders are generally multisystemic [6, 8] and may be present at any age [7], and the global prevalence, probably underestimated,

is 1/8500 [7]. The organs with highest energy demand, such as, heart, brain, skeletal muscle tissue, and liver, are preferentially involved [6, 8–11]. Treatment is supportive [7, 12] and does not influence the natural course of the disease [8, 13], and the prognosis is often poor [11, 14]. Mitochondrial complex I deficiency is the most common defect of the oxidative phosphorylation system [10]. The diagnosis of mitochondrial disease is complex because of its clinical and genetic heterogeneity [7, 12, 14]. We present a case report on a child with NF1 and deficiency of the mitochondrial complex I, an association not described before.

2. Case Report

The patient, a boy, was born after a normal pregnancy of 39 weeks, through an instrumented vaginal delivery. His birth weight was 2970 g. At birth, he had a low Apgar score (3/6/8 at the first, fifth, and tenth minute of life, resp.), hypotonia, grunt, and respiratory depression, requiring noninvasive ventilation. During neonatal intensive care stay, he maintained hypotonia and feeding difficulties. Inborn errors of metabolism (including twenty four diseases of three main groups: aminoacidopathies, organic acidemias, and mitochondrial fatty-acid oxidation disorders) and congenital hypothyroidism were not detected in the analysis of the Guthrie card. The metabolic study (plasma lactate, pyruvate, ammonia, amino acids, carbohydrate deficient transferrin, acylcarnitines, and urinary organic acids profile plus amino acids) and brain magnetic resonance (MRI) were normal. He was discharged from hospital at 28 days of life to continue followup as an outpatient and was referred to a developmental early intervention program.

Family history was notable for the mother, uncles, and grandmother having various *café-au-lait* spots, negative for Leigh syndrome or mitochondrial dysfunction.

Regarding the milestones, he just reached the sitting position after twelve months. Gait and first words were present at twenty-four months. At three years of age, he maintained low weight and short stature for his age, hypotonia, and global development delay. Physical examination revealed progressive microcephaly, more than six *café-au-lait* spots, greater than 0.5 cm in diameter, (these appeared in the first year of life and increased progressively in number and size) and a systolic murmur.

Molecular study confirmed an heterozygous mutation in the NF1 gene (mutation c.3445A>G(p.Met1149Val)-exon 26). Liver, renal, and hemopoietic function were normal along with plasma lactate, pyruvate, amino acids, and urinary organic acids profile. Magnetic resonance spectroscopy and deltoid muscle histology were normal. The analysis of enzymatic activity of mitochondrial respiratory chain complexes I–V in muscle (spectrophotometric assay) revealed partial (29%) deficit of complex I activity relative to citrate synthase (5.7, normal: 8.8–30.8). In the molecular research, we used the technique of *polymerase chain reaction* followed by direct sequencing of genes encoding subunits of complex I. The most common mutations and mitochondrial DNA deletions of large size (3243A>G, 3271T>C, 8344A>G, 8356T>C, and 8993T>C/G) (5, 10, and 11) were sent to research. Then we studied the seven mitochondrial genes (MTND1-MTND6, and MTND4L) and subsequently sequenced the eleven nuclear genes in which mutations have been so far described—NDUF1, NDUFS2, NDUFS3, NDUFS4, NDUFS6, NDUFS7, NDUFS8, NDUFV1, NDUFV2, and NDUFA1 NDUFA8. All the molecular study was negative. Cardiac evaluation detected a low grade pulmonary stenosis; cardiomyopathy and arrhythmia were not observed. Subclinical hypothyroidism (thyroid-stimulating hormone 7.45 μUI/mL, normal: 0.27–4.2; free thyroxine 1.18 ng/dL, normal: 0.93–1.7; antithyroid peroxidase and thyroglobulin antibodies: negative) was also detected. The remaining studies (karyotype including fluorescence in situ hybridization, screening for celiac disease, and abdominal and pelvic ultrasound) were normal. Ophthalmologic and audiologic evaluations were normal.

He started treatment with coenzyme Q_{10} plus levothyroxine and maintained dietary supplementation as well as occupational and speech therapies.

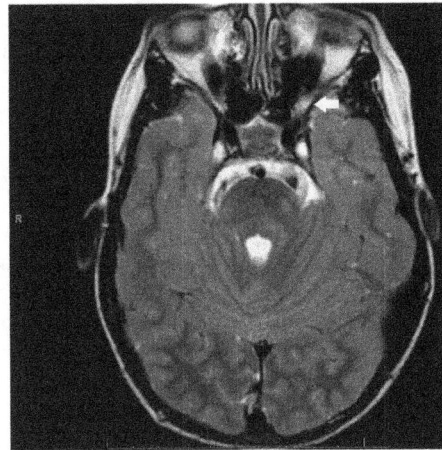

FIGURE 1: Brain MRI: axial section (T2) showing optic nerve glioma.

At the age of six, the brain MRI revealed subthalamus lesions of probable hamartomatous nature. At this age, evaluation with the Ruth Griffiths scale revealed global developmental delay involving uniformly motor, verbal, and cognition skills (general developmental quotient: 73%). According to the classification of the Diagnostic and Statistical Manual of Mental Disorders Fifth Edition (DSM-V) and the Conner's Ratting Scales, the patient did not meet criteria for attention-deficit/hyperactivity disorder (ADHD).

Currently, he is eight years old and is clinically well and asymptomatic. Nevertheless, cranial magnetic resonance imaging revealed a left optic nerve glioma in its prechiasmatic segment (Figure 1). After evaluation by a multidisciplinary team, it was decided to pursue a conservative approach with regular clinical and neuroimagiological followups (at 3 to 12 months intervals). There is no tumor progression until now in our patient.

3. Discussion

The authors present a child with NF1 in which a heterozygous missense mutation in the NF1 gene was identified that had not yet been described. Since NF1 is a very common disease [2], its association with other diseases is likely to occur coincidentally. Nevertheless, to the best of our knowledge, this is the first report of complex I deficiency in a patient with NF1.

These two diseases share important characteristics: they are both multisystemic and progressive [2, 7]. It is thus important for the physician to be alert to the characteristic signs and symptoms. Patients with NF1 are not expected to present microcephaly [2], and if it occurs, they should be appropriately investigated. It is among these atypical cases that mitochondrial disease is more common [7, 13]. It would thus be prudent to evaluate such patients with unexplained combination of multisystem symptoms and progressive clinical course for possible mitochondrial disease [15]. Consequently, we suggest that screening for mitochondrial disorders is included in the investigation of microcephaly in patients with NF1.

These diseases are frequently associated with neurocognitive deficits, including ADHD, autism spectrum disorders, behavioral abnormalities, and psychosocial issues [4, 14]. We highlight the importance of early (prescholar) and complete evaluation in these patients, to prepare the child, family, and technical education in the prevention of learning difficulties, promoting self-esteem, and social integration [2].

Optic nerve glioma developed in approximately 15% of patients with NF1 [1–3, 16]. It is the more feared complication, and also the one that leads to more doubts regarding treatment and followup [2]. It generally occurs before eight years of life and may present with visual impairment, facial asymmetry, proptosis, strabismus, and endocrine signs or symptoms (elevated growth velocity, precocious puberty) [2, 16]. In patients with NF1, optic pathway gliomas are typically low-grade pilocytic astrocytomas [3, 4] and grow more insidiously [16], leading to a better prognosis than in other patients [1, 3]. In our patient, the tumor was not progressive or clinically significant. Thus, as recommended by different authors [1, 16], a conservative approach, with regular followup was elected. If the disease becomes progressive, the patient should start treatment with chemotherapy [1, 4]. Radiotherapy is contraindicated [1, 4] and surgical treatment is not recommended unless the lesion exhibits rapid growth or the patient's clinical state deteriorates [4].

It is very important to maintain a high index of suspicion for the diagnosis of mitochondrial disease, because most patients do not present easily recognizable disorders [15]. Except for some specific mitochondrial encephalomyopathic syndromes, the clinical features are rarely pathognomonic for the diagnosis of mitochondrial disorders and symptoms can be difficult to assimilate into a unifying diagnosis particularly in the case of pediatric patients [15]. Pediatric mitochondrial disorders can be accompanied by normal muscle morphology, normal plasma lactate, normal mitochondrial enzymes on skeletal muscle, normal mitochondrial DNA mutation screening, and a nonclassical clinical presentation because none of these criteria has absolute sensitivity to detect mitochondrial disease [11]. In the present patient, both the laboratory screening and muscle histology were normal and only the biochemical study of muscle allowed us to confirm the diagnosis. It is well known that mitochondrial respiratory chain enzymatic defects are not specific, because they are also found in other disorders [14]. Therefore it is difficult to ascertain in this case if the enzymatic defect results from a primary or secondary cause [14].

Mitochondrial complex I deficiency is the most common defect of the oxidative phosphorylation system [10]. Most cases result from autosomal recessive inheritance; less frequently the disorder is maternally inherited or sporadic and the genetic defect is in the mtDNA [9]. At present, the diagnosis is often only based on biochemical measurements of the single enzyme activities of the oxidative phosphorylation system as the genetic cause is still unknown in many patients [8, 10]. The investigation of the deficits of complex I is highly complex due to the large number of subunits that comprise it, thus hindering the molecular characterization of these patients [8]. In our center it is intended to extend the molecular study to known genes encoding processing factors

(NDUFAF1 and B17.2L) as well as those that encode subunits of complex I, in which no mutations have been described to date, hoping that further investigation will allow us to increase the number of patients with definite diagnosis [8]. Enhanced methods are important to identify new mutations causing complex I deficiency; they may be useful tools in the near future, improving genetic counseling and prenatal diagnosis in at-risk families [8, 10].

Arun et al. [17] demonstrated a novel interaction between neurofibromin and leucine-rich pentatricopeptide repeat motif-containing protein, which subsequently links NF1 and Leigh syndrome French Canadian variant, at the molecular level. They further show that this interaction occurs as part of a ribonucleoprotein complex consistent with RNA granules, which are important epigenetic regulators. Further studies into the etiopathogenesis of NF1 and Leigh syndrome and mitochondrial dysfunction may contribute to our understanding of the molecular mechanisms that contribute to the complex developmental phenotypes associated with these syndromes.

Conflict of Interests

The authors declare that they have no conflict of interests regarding the publication of this paper.

References

[1] C. Couto, T. Monteiro, L. Araújo, and T. Temudo, "Neurofibromatosis type 1: diagnosis and follow-up in paediatrics," *Acta Pediátrica Portuguesa*, vol. 43, no. 2, pp. 75–83, 2012.

[2] C. L. Martins, J. P. Monteiro, A. Farias, R. Fernandes, and M. J. Fonseca, "Managing children with neurofibromatosis type 1: what should we look for?" *Acta Médica Portuguesa*, vol. 20, no. 5, pp. 393–400, 2007.

[3] I. Pascual-Castroviejo, S. I. Pascual-Pascual, R. Velazquez-Fragua, and J. Viaño, "Corpus callosum tumor as the presenting symptom of neurofibromatosis type 1 in a patient and literature review," *Revista de Neurologia*, vol. 55, no. 9, pp. 528–532, 2012.

[4] V. C. Williams, J. Lucas, M. A. Babcock, D. H. Gutmann, B. Bruce, and B. L. Maria, "Neurofibromatosis type 1 revisited," *Pediatrics*, vol. 123, no. 1, pp. 124–133, 2009.

[5] P. F. Chinnery, "Mitochondrial disorders overview," in *GeneReviews*, R. A. Pagon, Ed., University of Washington, Seattle, Wash, USA, 1993.

[6] C. C. Ferreiro-Barros, C. H. Tengan, M. H. Barros et al., "Neonatal mitochondrial encephaloneuromyopathy due to a defect of mitochondrial protein synthesis," *Journal of the Neurological Sciences*, vol. 275, no. 1-2, pp. 128–132, 2008.

[7] S. Challa, M. A. Kanikannan, M. M. K. Jagarlapudi, V. R. Bhoompally, and M. Surath, "Diagnosis of mitochondrial diseases: clinical and histological study of sixty patients with ragged red fibers," *Neurology India*, vol. 52, no. 3, pp. 353–358, 2004.

[8] M. Ferreira, T. Aguiar, and L. Vilarinho, "Cadeia respiratória mitocondrial aspectos clínicos, bioquímicos, enzimáticos e moleculares associados ao défice do complexo I," *Arquivos de Medicina*, vol. 22, no. 2-3, pp. 49–56, 2008.

[9] The United Mitochondrial Disease Foundation, "Mito profile complex I information," 2013, http://www.umdf.org/atf/cf/%7B8d4a231c12fb4a219a8593c7bd0c5a5a%7D/COMPLEX_1_DEFICIENCY.PDF.

[10] S. J. G. Hoefs, F. J. van Spronsen, E. W. H. Lenssen et al., "*NDUFA10* mutations cause complex I deficiency in a patient with Leigh disease," *European Journal of Human Genetics*, vol. 19, no. 3, pp. 270–274, 2011.

[11] F. Scaglia, J. A. Towbin, W. J. Craigen et al., "Clinical spectrum, morbidity, and mortality in 113 pediatric patients with mitochondrial disease," *Pediatrics*, vol. 114, no. 4, pp. 925–931, 2004.

[12] A. Mattman, M. O'Riley, P. J. Waters et al., "Diagnosis and management of patients with mitochondrial disease," *BC Medical Journal*, vol. 53, no. 4, pp. 177–182, 2011.

[13] R. K. Naviaux, "Overview the spectrum of mitochondrial disease," in *Mitochondrial and Metabolic Disorders: A Primary Care Physician's Guide*, Exceptional Parent Magazine Reprint, pp. 3–10, 1997.

[14] L. Diogo, M. Grazina, P. Garcia et al., "Pediatric mitochondrial respiratory chain disorders in the centro region of Portugal," *Pediatric Neurology*, vol. 40, no. 5, pp. 351–356, 2009.

[15] R. L. Costa, A. S. Martha, N. Steffen, and V. F. Martha, "Neurofibromatose tipo 1 em criança com manifestação parafaríngea," *X Salão de Iniciação científica—PUCRS*, pp. 797–803, 2009.

[16] M. J. Binning, J. K. Liu, J. R. W. Kestle, D. L. Brockmeyer, and M. L. Walker, "Optic pathway gliomas: a review," *Neurosurgical Focus*, vol. 23, no. 5, article E2, 2007.

[17] V. Arun, J. C. Wiley, H. Kaur, D. R. Kaplan, and A. Guha, "A novel neurofibromin (NF1) interaction with the leucine-rich pentatricopeptide repeat motif-containing protein links neurofibromatosis type 1 and the French Canadian variant of Leigh's syndrome in a common molecular complex," *Journal of Neuroscience Research*, vol. 91, no. 4, pp. 494–505, 2013.

25

A Case of 17q21.31 Microduplication and 7q31.33 Microdeletion, Associated with Developmental Delay, Microcephaly, and Mild Dysmorphic Features

**Adrian Mc Cormack,[1] Juliet Taylor,[2] Leah Te Weehi,[1]
Donald R. Love,[1,3] and Alice M. George[1]**

[1] Diagnostic Genetics, LabPlus, Auckland City Hospital, P.O. Box 110031, Auckland 1148, New Zealand
[2] Genetic Health Service New Zealand-Northern Hub, Auckland City Hospital, Private Bag 92024, Auckland 1142, New Zealand
[3] School of Biological Sciences, University of Auckland, Private Bag 92019, Auckland 1142, New Zealand

Correspondence should be addressed to Alice M. George; aliceg@adhb.govt.nz

Academic Editors: D. J. Bunyan, P. D. Cotter, A. DeWan, and S. Ennis

Concurrent cryptic microdeletion and microduplication syndromes have recently started to reveal themselves with the advent of microarray technology. Analysis has shown that low-copy repeats (LCRs) have allowed chromosome regions throughout the genome to become hotspots for nonallelic homologous recombination to take place. Here, we report a case of a 7.5-year-old girl who manifests microcephaly, developmental delay, and mild dysmorphic features. Microarray analysis identified a microduplication in chromosome 17q21.31, which encompasses the CRHR1, MAPT, and KANSL1 genes, as well as a microdeletion in chromosome 7q31.33 that is localised within the GRM8 gene. To our knowledge this is one of only a few cases of 17q21.31 microduplication. The clinical phenotype of patients with this microduplication is milder than of those carrying the reciprocal microdeletions, and suggests that the lower incidence of the former compared to the latter may be due to underascertainment.

1. Introduction

Since the advent of microarray technology considerable progress has been made in identifying small scale chromosome imbalances. The existence of colocalized microdeletion and microduplication syndrome sites has come to the fore in the recent years and a significant number of new microduplication syndromes have emerged such as 17p11.2 [1] and 22q11.21 [2]. These syndromes, like the corresponding microdeletion syndromes at these locations, appear to be driven by nonallelic homologous recombination (NAHR) involving low-copy repeats (LCRs or segmental duplications) [3–8]. LCRs are DNA fragments greater than 1 Kb in size, have 90% DNA sequence homology, and are thought to account for approximately 3–10% of the total genome.

The MAPT gene located on chromosome 17q21.31 is flanked by LCRs and two extended haplotypes, designated H1

and H2, have been identified [9, 10]. The H2 haplotype is a 900 kb inversion polymorphism that has been reported as the likely ancestral state and which has a tendency to undergo recombination [11] leading to the 17q21.31 microdeletion syndrome. This syndrome has been well characterised and appears to be caused by haploinsufficiency of at least one gene, KANSL, within the deleted region [12, 13]. The more common H1 haplotype appears to be overrepresented in patients manifesting progressive supranuclear palsy [14].

Here, we report a 7.5-year-old girl with a 647 kb duplication involving interstitial chromosome region 17q21.31 as well as a 232 kb heterozygous interstitial deletion involving chromosome region 7q31.33. We review this case in conjunction with other 17q21.31 microduplication cases described by Kirchhoff et al. [15], Kitsiou-Tzeli et al. [16], and Grisart et al. [17]. Our case shares some common phenotypic features with previously reported patients, including developmental delay, microcephaly, and mild dysmorphisms, which are milder than those identified in patients with the 17q21.31 microdeletion syndrome.

2. Clinical Report

The proband was the first born girl to nonconsanguineous Iraqi and Afghani parents. Family history on the mother's side was unremarkable. The father reportedly struggled at school and it has been suggested that he may have been microcephalic. The child was delivered at 38-week gestation via induction as there were concerns about IUGR. She was born in good condition and did not require resuscitation. Birth weight was 2490 g (3rd to 10th centile) and there were no other antenatal complications. Milestones were appropriate for age, walking at 15 months but always on her toes. She was initially referred to a child development service as she was falling a lot when walking and was prescribed orthoses. At the age of 2 years and 7 months she was further referred to a pediatric clinic because of her gait pattern. It was noted that she still had difficulty with toe walking, lack balance, and control when walking along slopes and stairs and was still learning how to do other developmental skills such as climbing, jumping, and pushing a bike. There were no obvious dysmorphic features. Her weight was 15.55 kg (90th centile), height was 92 cm (25th–50th centile), and head circumference was 46 cm (25th centile). A follow-up visit at 3 years of age showed that the idiopathic toe walking had resolved and that gross motor skills were continuing to develop. At the age of 5.5 years, she was found to be functioning at a level well below chronological age and was noted to be microcephalic (head circumference of 47 cm; 2nd centile) as well as developmentally delayed. Dysmorphic features were not observed at this visit, but some mild autistic traits were seen.

Developmental delay was further confirmed 2 years later, functioning at 4-5-years old level both academically and for fine motor skills. She required significant assistance with activities of daily life. It was also noticed at this visit that she had some dysmorphic features with possible almond shaped eyes and small hands.

3. Cytogenetic and Molecular Studies

Genome-wide copy number analysis of the proband was undertaken using an Affymetrix CytoScan 750 K Array, according to the manufacturer's instructions. Regions of copy number change were determined using the Affymetrix Chromosome Analysis Suite software (ChAS) v.1.2.2 and interpreted with the aid of the UCSC genome browser (http://genome.ucsc.edu/; Human Feb. 2009 GRCh37/hg19 assembly). The array showed a female molecular karyotype with a 232 kb heterozygous interstitial deletion involving chromosome region 7q31.33 [hg19 coordinates chr7:126,531,039-126,763,294] and a 647 kb duplication involving interstitial chromosome region 17q21.31 [hg 19 coordinates chr17:43,645,879-44,292,742]. The 7q31.33 microdeletion contains part of one gene, GRM8 (OMIM

601116), while the 17q21.31 microduplication contains a number of genes including *CRHR1* (OMIM 122561), *IMP5* (*SPPL2C*; OMIM 608284), *MAPT* (OMIM 157140), and *STH* (OMIM 607067) and a partial duplication of the *KANSL1* gene (also known as *KIAA1267*, OMIM 612452); see Figure 1.

In order to determine the genotype encompassing the *MAPT* gene, we focused on amplifying the region of intron 9 of the *MAPT* gene that carries a polymorphic 238 bp deletion, which is a characteristic marker of the H1/H2 genotypes. Fifty nanograms of genomic DNA was subjected to PCR amplification using Roche FastStart buffer (without Mg), 1.5 mM $MgCl_2$, 0.4 mM dNTPs, 1 unit Roche Faststart Taq DNA polymerase, and 0.8 μM of each forward and reverse primer [14]. PCR cycle conditions comprised 95°C for 5 minutes and then 35 cycles of 94°C for 30 seconds, 55°C for 30 seconds, and 72°C for 30 seconds, with a final extension at 72°C for 10 minutes. Amplified DNAs were electrophoretically separated in a 2% E-gel (Life Technologies) and the amplicons visualised under UV light. Only the 246 bp fragment was detected, suggesting the H2 genotype, hence an H2/H2/H2 haplotype.

4. Discussion

From the literature review, six cases of 17q21.31 microduplication syndrome have been previously reported [15–17]. Our patient together with two others also had an additional CNV. Kitsiou-Tzeli et al. [16] reported an additional 413 kb 15q11.2 deletion, and these authors have stated that this deletion may have contributed to some of the phenotypic symptoms of their patient. Patient 3 reported by Grisart et al. [17] had the common 17p11.2 deletion but was asymptomatic for NHPP (OMIM 162500) associated with this anomaly.

Molecular characterisation of our patient showed two abnormalities. In the case of the 7q31.33 microdeletion, the pathological significance of a partial deletion of the *GRM8* gene in this region has not been determined. The *GRM8* gene encodes a neurotransmitter receptor that responds to glutamate stimulation [18]. A partial duplication of the *GRM8* gene has been discovered in an individual with autistic spectrum disorder [19]. Further studies have indicated that deletions in this gene may be over-represented in some patients with ADHD [20]. While our patient does show some traits of autism, she has excellent social skills so she has not been further investigated for this condition. Therefore, we are uncertain if this partial deletion of the *GRM8* gene has a significant effect on the phenotype of our patient.

The duplicated region of 17q21.31 contains a small number of genes (Figure 1). Some are linked to a specific phenotype such as the *MAPT* gene (microtubule associated protein *TAU*). This gene encodes proteins that stabilise microtubules, which are mostly found in neurons. Loss of function abnormalities of this gene is associated with neurodegenerative disorders such as frontotemporal dementia with Parkinson's disease, progressive supranuclear palsy, and Alzheimer's disease [21, 22]. Interestingly, these disorders have also been reported to be associated with over-expression of other genes such as α synuclein gene in some cases of Parkinson's disease

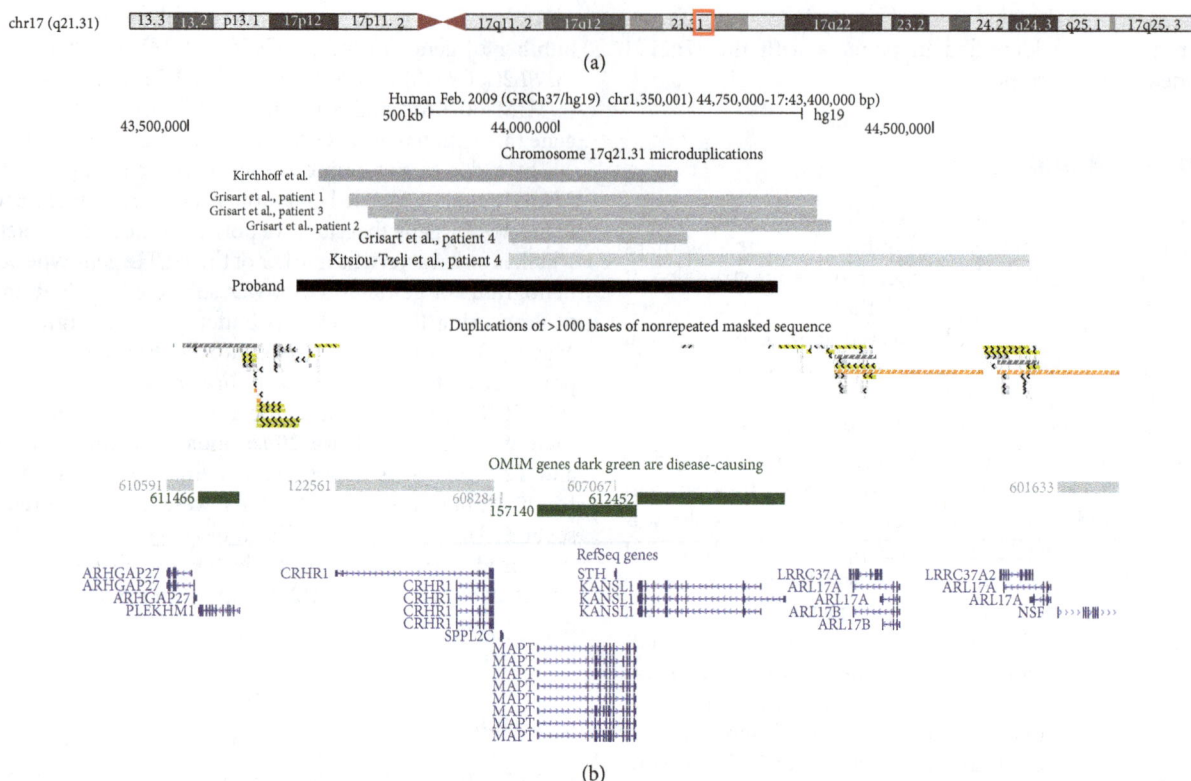

FIGURE 1: Schematic of the chromosome 17 region containing the microduplication. Panel A shows an ideogram of chromosome 17, together with the region encompassing the microduplications. Panel B shows the location and extent of the duplications detected in the proband reported here, other cases reported in the literature, LCRs (segmental duplications), and OMIM and Refseq genes that lie within the microduplicated region. These graphics were taken from the UCSC genome browser (http://genome.ucsc.edu/).

and amyloid precursor protein (APP gene) in Alzheimer's disease [23, 24].

Mouse models have shown that over-expression of the murine homologue of the TAU gene models the impact of human H1/H1 MAPT haplotype, increasing the expression of the tau protein and thereby the risk of the development of associated tauopathies [25]. However, larger screening of the MAPT gene has shown that copy number gains have not so far been implicated in neurodegenerative diseases [26].

The CRHR1 gene encodes a corticotrophin releasing hormone receptor type 1 and is involved in coordinating the endocrine, autonomic, behavioural, and immune responses to stress through actions in the brain and the periphery [27]. Polymorphisms in this gene have commonly been associated with depression and panic disorder [28, 29]. The IMP5 gene encodes intramembrane protease 5, which is a part of a class of enzymes which cleave integral membrane proteins [30]. The KANSL1 gene encodes a nuclear protein which plays a role in chromatin modification. It encodes two subunits which play a role in a histone acetyltransferase complex [31]. Finally, the STH gene is a polymorphic gene nested within an intron of the MAPT gene and encodes the protein Saitohin [32], the function of which is not yet known.

Table 1 summarises the clinical phenotypes of the limited number of 17q21.31 microduplication cases reported thus far.

In most cases pregnancies tend to be very uneventful (5/7) and early milestones normal (7/7). One of the first main signs has been hypotonia (3/7 cases), with tiptoe walking (3/7 cases) and microcephaly (3/7). Verbal skills vary widely from normal to very poor, while motor skills also appear to vary in the number of cases (3/7). Dysmorphic features have in general not been noticed until later in life and are often quite subtle, while some dysmorphic features like clinodactyly, syndactyly (2/7), and hypogonadism (1/7) have been reported infrequently. Both our patient and patient 3 reported by Grisart et al. [17] do not appear to suffer any increased phenotypic severity despite the presence of an additional CNV.

In contrast to the above, the corresponding 17q21.31 microduplication syndrome is characterised by developmental delay, hypotonia, facial dysmorphisms, and a friendly, amiable behaviour [33–35]. A number of recent reports have shown that loss of function of the KANSL1 gene within this region is sufficient to cause the syndrome [12, 13]. The 17q21.31 microduplication phenotype appears milder, while some of the more severe congenital malformations seen in the microdeletion syndrome such as urological anomalies, ventriculomegaly, musculoskeletal problems, dental abnormalities, and epilepsy have not been reported in patients with the corresponding microduplication [33–35]. Also of

TABLE 1: Comparison of main clinical indications reported on seven patients with 17q21.31 microduplications.

Reference	Present case	Kirchhoff et al. [15]	Kitsiou-Tzeli et al. [16] Patient 4	Grisart et al. [17] Patient 1	Grisart et al. [17] Patient 2	Grisart et al. [17] Patient 3	Grisart et al. [17] Patient 4
hg19 coordinates	43,645,879–44,292,742	43,675,408–44,159,862	43,993,055–44,628,150	43,717,703–44,345,038	43,773,601–44,344,056	~43,744,217–~44,344,223	43,932,635–44,172,437
Pregnancy	38 weeks, suspected IUGR	Uneventful 42 weeks	40 weeks	Placental detachment at term	Normal at term	Normal at term	Normal at term
Birth (gms)	2.490	3.070	2500	3.570 (P50)	3.500 (P50)	2.890 (−2SD)	5.100 (+3SD)
Walk (months)	15	60	13	12	24	14–16	27
Tiptoe walking	+	ND	ND	+	–	+	–
Psychomotor Development							
Hypotonia	ND	+	–	–	–	–	+
Hyperactivity	ND	+	ND	+	–	ND	+
Passivity	ND	ND	ND	ND	–	ND	ND
Obsessive behaviour	ND	ND	ND	ND	–	ND	–
Social interaction	ND	ND	Outburst of temper	Poor	Poor	Poor, anxious	Poor
Intelligence							
Psychomotor retardation	ND	Severe	ND	Mild	Mild	Mild	Mild
Verbal skills	Normal	Very poor	ND	Limited	Normal	Poor	Normal
Motor skills	Poor	ND	ND	Poor	Poor	ND	Normal
Dysmorphism							
Microcephaly	+	+	ND	Mild	–	–	–
Synophrys	ND	ND	ND	+	Bushy eyebrows	–	–
Epicanthic folds	ND	ND	ND	–	–	–	–
Dysplastic ears	ND	+	ND	+	–	–	+
Nose	ND	Short	Short nose, prominent nasal tip, and columella	Upturned	Short, upturned	–	–
Philtrum	ND	Smooth	Smooth	Short	Short	–	–
Midface	ND	ND	Small mouth	–	Flat	–	Flat
Palate	ND	High arched	ND	–	High arched	–	–
Prominent incisor	ND	+	ND	+	+	–	–
Micrognathia	ND	+	Mild	ND	–	ND	–
Finger	ND	Broad	ND	Clinodactyly of 5th	Tapering	ND	Clinodactyly of 5th
Palmar crease	ND	ND	ND	Single on right hand	–	ND	ND
Feet	ND	Broad	ND	Partial syndactyly	–	ND	2-3 Syndactyly
Others	Almond shaped eyes, small hands	Hirsutism on back	Global hirsutism, ataxic gait, VSD	Hirsutism on back	Low posthairline		Hypogonadism

ND: not determined, +/−: trait present/not present in patient.

interest is a recent report of a *de novo* triplication of the *MAPT* and *KANSL1* genes which extends into the polymorphic region of 17q21.31 [36]. The phenotype of this patient included behavioural and social problems, muscular hypotonia, hypoplastic genitalia, cryptorchidism, clinodactyly, and mild facial dysmorphisms, which is largely similar to the microduplication cases with minor facial features, behavioural problems, and moderate mental impairment.

The extent of the 17q21.32 microduplication among the patients shown in Table 1 varies from approximately 239 kb to 736 kb. An assessment of published cases and information from the DECIPHER database (http://decipher.sanger.ac.uk/) suggests that none of the cases contained full duplications of all of the main genes contained within the *MAPT* haplotype. Our patient contained a full copy of *MAPT* and *CRHR1* and a partial copy of *KANSL1* genes. Two patients reported by Kitsiou-Tzeli et al. [16] and Grisart et al. [17] (patients 4, Figure 1) appear to be the only cases reported thus far that do not contain a full or partial duplication of *CRHR1* gene. Our patient has a similar duplication to that of patient 1 reported by Grisart et al. [17] who has a 646 kb deletion, but with slightly varying breakpoints and with only a partial duplication of *CRHR1*. Both phenotypes were similar with common features including tiptoe walking, microcephaly, and poor motor skills. The main difference between these two cases appeared to be hypotonia and more severe dysmorphic features. Patient 4 reported by Grisart et al. [17] carries the smallest microduplication reported so far of 0.24 Mb. It contains a full duplication of the *MAPT* gene and a very small partial duplication of the *KANSL1* gene. This patient's phenotype appears to be the mildest of the cases reported with normal verbal and motor skills, psychomotor development and retardation similar to other cases, and mild dysmorphic features. Interestingly, the patient reported by Kirchhoff et al. [15] appears to lack a duplication of the *KANSL1* gene but has a full duplication of the *MAPT* and *CRHR1* genes and manifests similar psychomotor development, more severe psychomotor retardation, poorer verbal skills, and microcephaly in comparison to this case. A degree of variable penetrance may exist within the phenotype of the cases reported so far. Therefore while we cannot rule out the contribution of any gene or part of gene in the haplotype to the overall phenotype, patient 4 reported by Grisart et al. [17] may represent the minimum duplication of the 17q21.31 region that characterises this microduplication syndrome. It is possible that a minimum critical region encompassing the *MAPT* gene may emerge when further cases become apparent.

The *MAPT* gene is flanked by LCRs (Figure 1). NAHR involving LCRs can lead to deletion and duplication events, and the complex structure of LCRs that comprise both direct and indirect repeat elements can lead to inversions [5–8, 37]. While still to be determined for humans, *in vivo* experiments using mouse cells have shown that a minimum efficient processing segment (MEP) between 134 and 232 bp of perfect shared sequence identity is required for homologous recombination [3]. Koolen et al. [33] have identified an approximate 500 bp within an L2 LINE repetitive element motif at 17q21.31, representing a possible proximal hotspot

for NAHR within this haplotype. The distal breakpoint in the 17q21.31 microdeletion syndrome cases has been determined to be more variable due to it being located in a polymorphic region adjacent to the critical deletion region [33].

Compared to the corresponding microdeletion syndrome, 17q21.31 microduplications have been seen less frequently. A recent study [15] reported the frequency among live births of 1/55,000 and 1/327,000 for microdeletions and microduplications, respectively, which suggests a ratio of 6 : 1, which is lower than expected of NAHR [6]. Importantly, these ratios should be viewed against the molecular background in which they occur and the genomic region being investigated in that the H2 inversion haplotype is expected to favour microdeletions as opposed to microduplications [11]. The case reported here carries the H2 haplotype but is associated with a copy number gain rather than loss. Finally, it is possible that cases of 17q21.31 microduplication syndrome have been underascertained due to the milder phenotype and later onset.

Conflict of Interests

The authors declare that there is no conflict of interests regarding the publication of this paper.

References

[1] L. Potocki, K.-S. Chen, S.-S. Park et al., "Molecular mechanism for duplication 17p11.2—the homologous recombination reciprocal of the Smith-Magenis microdeletion," *Nature Genetics*, vol. 24, no. 1, pp. 84–87, 2000.

[2] T. M. Yobb, M. J. Somerville, L. Willatt et al., "Microduplication and triplication of 22q11.2: a highly variable syndrome," *The American Journal of Human Genetics*, vol. 76, no. 5, pp. 865–876, 2005.

[3] A. S. Waldman and R. M. Liskay, "Dependence of intrachromosomal recombination in mammalian cells on uninterrupted homology," *Molecular and Cellular Biology*, vol. 8, no. 12, pp. 5350–5357, 1988.

[4] J. A. Bailey, A. M. Yavor, H. F. Massa, B. J. Trask, and E. E. Eichler, "Segmental duplications: organization and impact within the current human genome project assembly," *Genome Research*, vol. 11, no. 6, pp. 1005–1017, 2001.

[5] J. R. Lupski, "Hotspots of homologous recombination in the human genome: not all homologous sequences are equal," *Genome Biology*, vol. 5, no. 10, article 242, 2004.

[6] J. R. Lupski and P. Stankiewicz, "Genomic disorders: molecular mechanisms for rearrangements and conveyed phenotypes," *PLoS Genetics*, vol. 1, no. 6, article e49, 2005.

[7] D. J. Turner, M. Miretti, D. Rajan et al., "Germline rates of de novo meiotic deletions and duplications causing several genomic disorders," *Nature Genetics*, vol. 40, no. 1, pp. 90–95, 2008.

[8] P. Stankiewicz and J. R. Lupski, "Structural variation in the human genome and its role in disease," *Annual Review of Medicine*, vol. 61, pp. 437–455, 2010.

[9] H. Stefansson, A. Helgason, G. Thorleifsson et al., "A common inversion under selection in Europeans," *Nature Genetics*, vol. 37, no. 2, pp. 129–137, 2005.

[10] P. N. Rao, W. Li, L. E. L. M. Vissers, J. A. Veltman, and R. A. Ophoff, "Recurrent inversion events at 17q21.31 microdeletion locus are linked to the MAPT H2 haplotype," *Cytogenetic and Genome Research*, vol. 129, no. 4, pp. 275–279, 2010.

[11] M. C. Zody, Z. Jiang, H.-C. Fung et al., "Evolutionary toggling of the MAPT 17q21.31 inversion region," *Nature Genetics*, vol. 40, no. 9, pp. 1076–1083, 2008.

[12] D. A. Koolen, J. M. Kramer, K. Neveling et al., "Mutations in the chromatin modifier gene *KANSL1* cause the 17q21.31 microdeletion syndrome," *Nature Genetics*, vol. 44, no. 6, pp. 639–641, 2012.

[13] M. Zollino, D. Orteschi, M. Murdolo et al., "Mutations in *KANSL1* cause the 17q21.31 microdeletion syndrome phenotype," *Nature Genetics*, vol. 44, no. 6, pp. 636–638, 2012.

[14] M. Baker, I. Litvan, H. Houlden et al., "Association of an extended haplotype in the tau gene with progressive supranuclear palsy," *Human Molecular Genetics*, vol. 8, no. 4, pp. 711–715, 1999.

[15] M. Kirchhoff, A.-M. Bisgaard, M. Duno, F. J. Hansen, and M. Schwartz, "A 17q21.31 microduplication, reciprocal to the newly described 17q21.31 microdeletion, in a girl with severe psychomotor developmental delay and dysmorphic craniofacial features," *European Journal of Medical Genetics*, vol. 50, no. 4, pp. 256–263, 2007.

[16] S. Kitsiou-Tzeli, H. Frysira, K. Giannikou et al., "Microdeletion and microduplication 17q21.31 plus an additional CNV, in patients with intellectual disability, identified by array-CGH," *Gene*, vol. 492, no. 1, pp. 319–324, 2012.

[17] B. Grisart, L. Willatt, A. Destrée et al., "17q21.31 microduplication patients are characterised by behavioural problems and poor social interaction," *Journal of Medical Genetics*, vol. 46, no. 8, pp. 524–530, 2009.

[18] S. W. Scherer, S. Soder, R. M. Duvoisin, J. J. Huizenga, and L.-C. Tsui, "The human metabotropic glutamate receptor 8 (GRM8) gene: a disproportionately large gene located at 7q31.3-q32.1," *Genomics*, vol. 44, no. 2, pp. 232–236, 1997.

[19] F. J. Serajee, H. Zhong, R. Nabi, and A. H. M. M. Huq, "The metabotropic glutamate receptor 8 gene at 7q31: partial duplication and possible association with autism," *Journal of Medical Genetics*, vol. 40, no. 4, p. e42, 2003.

[20] J. Elia, J. T. Glessner, K. Wang et al., "Genome-wide copy number variation study associates metabotropic glutamate receptor gene networks with attention deficit hyperactivity disorder," *Nature Genetics*, vol. 44, no. 1, pp. 78–84, 2011.

[21] A. Delacourte and L. Buee, "Tau pathology: a marker of neurodegenerative disorders," *Current Opinion in Neurology*, vol. 13, no. 4, pp. 371–376, 2000.

[22] A. M. Pittman, A. J. Myers, P. Abou-Sleiman et al., "Linkage disequilibrium fine mapping and haplotype association analysis of the tau gene in progressive supranuclear palsy and corticobasal degeneration," *Journal of Medical Genetics*, vol. 42, no. 11, pp. 837–846, 2005.

[23] A. B. Singleton, M. Farrer, J. Johnson et al., "α-Synuclein locus triplication causes Parkinson's disease," *Science*, vol. 302, no. 5646, p. 841, 2003.

[24] A. Rovelet-Lecrux, D. Hannequin, G. Raux et al., "APP locus duplication causes autosomal dominant early-onset Alzheimer disease with cerebral amyloid angiopathy," *Nature Genetics*, vol. 38, no. 1, pp. 24–26, 2006.

[25] S. J. Adams, R. J. P. Crook, M. DeTure et al., "Overexpression of wild-type murine tau results in progressive tauopathy and neurodegeneration," *The American Journal of Pathology*, vol. 175, no. 4, pp. 1598–1609, 2009.

[26] A. Lladó, B. Rodríguez-Santiago, A. Antonell et al., "MAPT gene duplications are not a cause of frontotemporal lobar degeneration," *Neuroscience Letters*, vol. 424, no. 1, pp. 61–65, 2007.

[27] E. B. De Souza, "Corticotropin-releasing factor receptors: physiology, pharmacology, biochemistry and role in central nervous system and immune disorders," *Psychoneuroendocrinology*, vol. 20, no. 8, pp. 789–819, 1995.

[28] Y. Ishitobi, S. Nakayama, K. Yamaguchi et al., "Association of CRHR1 and CRHR2 with major depressive disorder and panic disorder in a Japanese population," *The American Journal of Medical Genetics B*, vol. 159, no. 4, pp. 429–436, 2012.

[29] F. Van Den Eede, T. Venken, J. Del-Favero et al., "Single nucleotide polymorphism analysis of corticotropin-releasing factor-binding protein gene in recurrent major depressive disorder," *Psychiatry Research*, vol. 153, no. 1, pp. 17–25, 2007.

[30] E. Erez, D. Fass, and E. Bibi, "How intramembrane proteases bury hydrolytic reactions in the membrane," *Nature*, vol. 459, no. 7245, pp. 371–378, 2009.

[31] E. R. Smith, C. Cayrou, R. Huang, W. S. Lane, J. Côté, and J. C. Lucchesi, "A human protein complex homologous to the Drosophila MSL complex is responsible for the majority of histone H4 acetylation at lysine 16," *Molecular and Cellular Biology*, vol. 25, no. 21, pp. 9175–9188, 2005.

[32] C. Conrad, C. Vianna, M. Freeman, and P. Davies, "A polymorphic gene nested within an intron of the *tau* gene: implications for Alzheimer's disease," *Proceedings of the National Academy of Sciences of the United States of America*, vol. 99, no. 11, pp. 7751–7756, 2002.

[33] D. A. Koolen, A. J. Sharp, J. A. Hurst et al., "Clinical and molecular delineation of the 17q21.31 microdeletion syndrome," *Journal of Medical Genetics*, vol. 45, no. 11, pp. 710–720, 2008.

[34] C. Shaw-Smith, A. M. Pittman, L. Willatt et al., "Microdeletion encompassing MAPT at chromosome 17q21.3 is associated with developmental delay and learning disability," *Nature Genetics*, vol. 38, no. 9, pp. 1032–1037, 2006.

[35] T. Y. Tan, S. Aftimos, L. Worgan et al., "Phenotypic expansion and further characterisation of the 17q21.31 microdeletion syndrome," *Journal of Medical Genetics*, vol. 46, no. 7, pp. 480–489, 2009.

[36] A. Gregor, M. Krumbiegel, C. Kraus, A. Reis, and C. Zweier, "De novo triplication of the MAPT gene from the recurrent 17q21.31 microdeletion region in a patient with moderate intellectual disability and various minor anomalies," *American Journal of J Medical Genetics A*, vol. 158, no. 7, pp. 1765–1770, 2012.

[37] O. A. Shchelochkov, S. W. Cheung, and J. R. Lupski, "Genomic and clinical characteristics of microduplications in chromosome 17," *The American Journal of Medical Genetics A*, vol. 152, no. 5, pp. 1101–1110, 2010.

26

Intermediate MCAD Deficiency Associated with a Novel Mutation of the *ACADM* Gene: c.1052C>T

Holli M. Drendel,[1] Jason E. Pike,[1] Katherine Schumacher,[1] Karen Ouyang,[1] Jing Wang,[2] Mary Stuy,[1] Stephen Dlouhy,[1] and Shaochun Bai[1]

[1]*Division of Diagnostic Genomics, Department of Medical and Molecular Genetics, Indiana University School of Medicine, 975 West Walnut Street, Indianapolis, IN 46202, USA*
[2]*Department of Molecular and Human Genetics, Baylor College of Medicine, One Baylor Plaza, Houston, TX 77030, USA*

Correspondence should be addressed to Shaochun Bai; bais@iu.edu

Academic Editor: Yoshiyuki Ban

Medium-chain acyl-CoA dehydrogenase deficiency (MCADD) is an autosomal recessive disorder that leads to a defect in fatty acid oxidation. *ACADM* is the only candidate gene causing MCAD deficiency. A single nucleotide change, c.985A>G, occurring at exon 11 of the *ACADM* gene, is the most prevalent mutation. In this study, we report a Caucasian family with multiple MCADD individuals. DNA sequence analysis of the *ACADM* gene performed in this family revealed that two family members showing mild MCADD symptoms share the same novel change in exon 11, c.1052C>T, resulting in a threonine-to-isoleucine change. The replacement is a nonconservative amino acid change that occurs in the C-terminal all-alpha domain of the MCAD protein. Here we report the finding of a novel missense mutation, c.1052C>T (p.Thr326Ile), in the *ACADM* gene. To our knowledge, c.1052C>T has not been previously reported in the literature or in any of the current databases we utilize. We hypothesize that this particular mutation in combination with p.Lys304Glu results in an intermediate clinical phenotype of MCADD.

1. Introduction

Medium-chain acyl-CoA dehydrogenase deficiency (MCADD; OMIM 607008) is an autosomal recessive disorder resulting from a defect of mitochondrial β-oxidation of medium-chain fatty acids [1]. It is one of the most common inborn errors of metabolism with an incidence of $1:15,000$ in 8.2 million newborns worldwide [2]. Metabolic demands that require more energy than available from glycogen stores, such as prolonged fasting, physical exercise, and intercurrent acute illness, may produce symptoms that if are unrecognized could potentially lead to metabolic crisis [3]. The clinical presentation of MCADD may vary from severe, such as hypoglycemia with seizures or death, to a milder form showing precursors of metabolic decompensation only. Intellectual disability and developmental delay are not common in this disorder if individuals are treated in a prospective manner; however, individuals with classic MCADD are at risk of losing developmental milestones

after a metabolic event due to brain injury [1]. Furthermore, approximately 25% of individuals who are undiagnosed will die during the first metabolic crisis while anywhere from 30 to 40% will have some form of intellectual disability or developmental delay [4, 5].

ACADM (NM_000016.4), located at 1p31, is the only candidate gene causing MCAD deficiency. Mutations in the gene may result in reduced or abolished function of the MCAD enzymatic protein. c.985A>G, occurring at exon 11 of the *ACADM* gene is the most prevalent mutation in individuals of European descent. The single-base pair change causes the replacement of a lysine by a glutamate at position 304 of the mature protein, p.Lys304Glu. Approximately 81% of individuals presenting with MCADD will be homozygous for the p.Lys304Glu genotype, while another 18% will be heterozygous for p.Lys304Glu and an additional mutation [6]. Since the introduction of MCADD to the newborn screening (NBS) panel, new mutations continue to be identified. To date, besides the common mutation

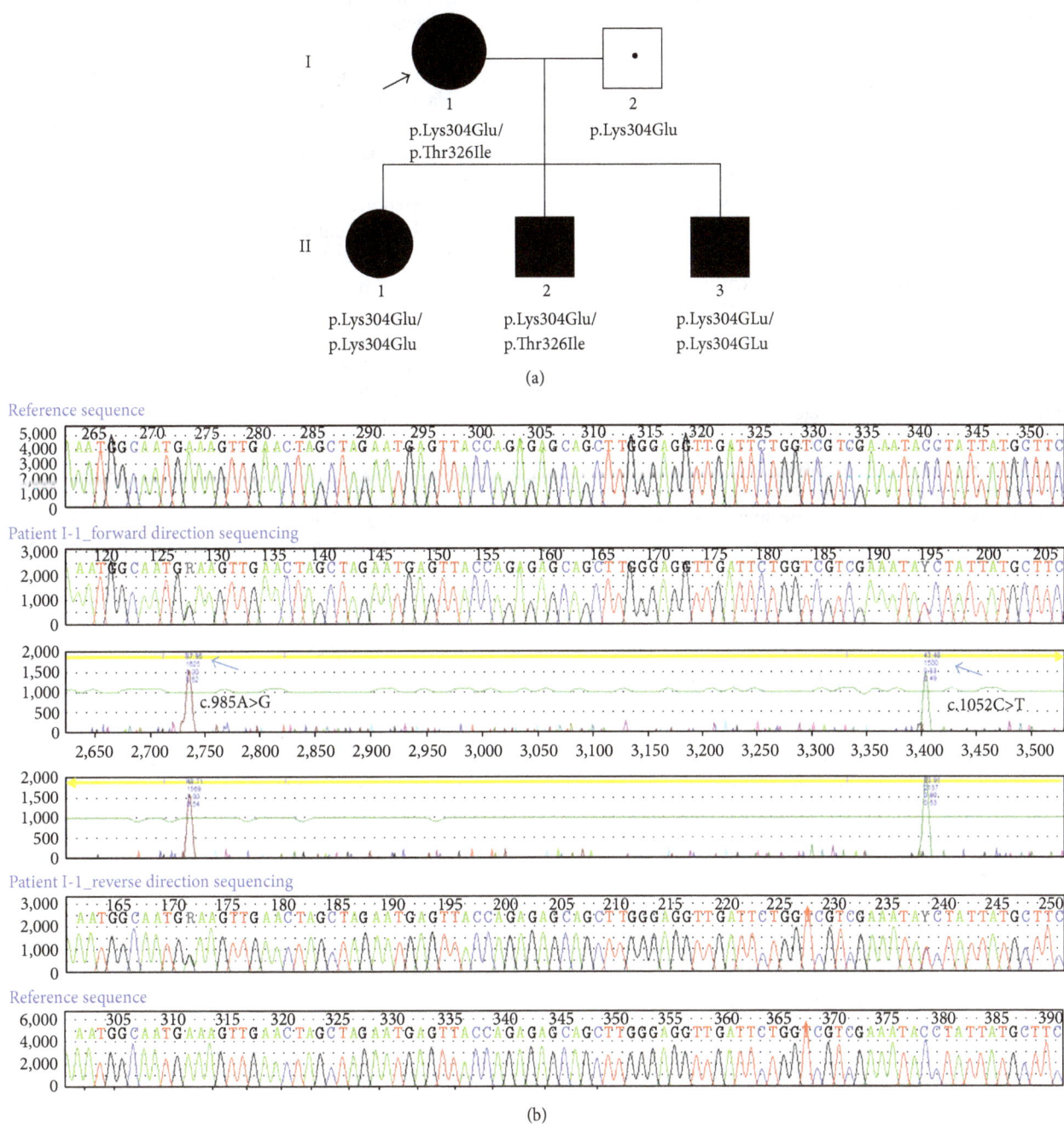

Figure 1: Novel MCADD mutation. (a) MCADD family pedigree. The proband (I-1) is indicated by a black arrow. The father (I-2) is a carrier as indicated by the dot in the center of the square. All affected individuals are indicated by filled circles (females) or squares (males). (b) DNA sequencing results. *ACADM* sequence analysis revealed a heterozygous sequence change of c.1052C>T, p.Thr326Ile in addition to the common mutation p.Lys304Glu in patient I-1. Blue arrows indicate the sequence change in patient I-1.

p.Lys304Glu, more than 90 mutations have been found in the *ACADM* gene (http://www.biobase-international.com/product/hgmd). These mutations are normally found in a compound heterozygous state with p.Lys304Glu and potentially lead to a loss of MCAD enzyme activity.

We report here, for the first time, a novel mutation in the *ACADM* gene, c.1052C>T.

2. Patients and Methods

The proband, a 32-year-old Caucasian female (I-1; Figure 1(a)) with a positive MCADD newborn screening result in her first child, was diagnosed to have MCADD biochemically following her second pregnancy. She generally reports a very mild clinical phenotype with multiple, though

TABLE 1: Plasma concentration of C8 acylcarnitines in the proband and the three children.

Patient	Acylcarnitine profile C8 (μM), first test	Acylcarnitine profile C8 (μM), second test
I-1	3.2 (ref. range 0.02–0.30)	
II-1	13.3 (ref. range < 0.4)	0.36 (ref. range < 0.11)
II-2	4.23 (ref. range < 0.4)	6.76 (ref. range < 0.16)
II-3	9.7 (ref. range < 0.47)	3.58 (ref. range 0.02–0.31)

minor, episodes of hypoglycemia as a child and adolescent. Her firstborn, a daughter (II-1), age 5 years, has a classic MCADD phenotype and, despite early NBS diagnosis and treatment with frequent feedings, L-carnitine and a low fat diet, has required multiple hospitalizations. The proband's second child, a son (II-2), now age 3 years, shares his mother's mild phenotype. The 1-month-old son (II-3) of the proband, also picked up on newborn screening, presented as a less severe phenotype compared to his sister, likely due to the dietary management and carnitine supplementation during the pregnancy. Their biological father (I-2) was also included as part of the family study (Figure 1(a)).

2.1. Sequencing Analysis. Genomic DNA was extracted from peripheral whole blood using a Qiagen Gentra Puregene blood kit (Qiagen, Valencia, CA, USA). All coding exons with exon-intron junctions of *ACADM* were PCR amplified and bidirectionally sequenced using BigDye Terminator v3.1 cycle sequencing (Life Technologies, Grand Island, NY, USA). Products were separated on an ABI PRISM 3130 XL genetic analyzer (Life Technologies, Grand Island, NY, USA). Sequencing data was analyzed by Mutation Surveyor software (SoftGenetics, State College, PA, USA).

2.2. Acylcarnitine Analysis. Plasma acylcarnitines were measured by tandem mass spectrometry [7] at Laboratory Corporation of America for patients I-1, II-2, and II-3. Analysis of patient II-1 acylcarnitine levels was performed at Duke University Hospital, Biochemical Genetics Laboratory.

3. Results and Discussion

Acylcarnitine patterns for MCADD patients display an increase in the levels of hexanoyl-CoA (C6), octanoyl-CoA (C8), decanoyl-CoA (C10), and decenoyl-CoA (C10:1) [8]. Accumulation of levels of C8 > 0.3 μM is potentially considered diagnostic [9]. Plasma acylcarnitines were analyzed in the mother and her three affected children (Table 1). The 5-year-old daughter (II-1) had elevations of C8, C6, and C8/C10 ratios, with overall low carnitine. She was hospitalized in the prenatal intensive care unit at 5 days of age with breathing difficulties, hypoglycemia, and poor breast feeding. She developed elevated liver enzymes. Her symptoms were improved with intravenous glucose and regular infant formula. The proband had her carnitine levels checked at the beginning of the second trimester for her second child (II-2) (Table 1). She was provided carnitine supplementation for the

duration of the pregnancy and was diagnosed biochemically by her acylcarnitine profile demonstrating an elevated C8 species. The second child (II-2) was formula fed. He had no metabolic decompensation. Following his abnormal NBS, plasma carnitine/acylcarnitine profiles were obtained and confirmed diagnostic for MCADD. The proband's third pregnancy began while on carnitine supplementation and was described as the easiest gestation of all three pregnancies, with better consistent nutritional intake and decreased nausea and vomiting. The third child was also identified on NBS and was biochemically diagnosed with MCADD (Table 1).

Sequencing analysis of the *ACADM* gene was performed in the proband (I-1). We detected a heterozygous c.985A>G, p.Lys304Glu mutation and a heterozygous c.1052C>T, p.Thr326Ile mutation (Figure 1(b)). Following these results, targeted mutation analysis of the three children was performed. The daughter (II-1) and the third male child (II-3) were found to be homozygous for p.Lys304Glu mutation. The girl's genotype correlates with her more severe phenotype. At birth, II-3 displayed a C8 profile similar to II-1 (Table 1), although slightly lower due to the mother being supplemented with carnitine for this pregnancy and not the first pregnancy. Patient II-2 was demonstrated to have the same genotype as I-1, p.Lys304Glu and p.Thr326Ile, consistent with his phenotype and the phenotype of his mother. Targeted sequencing analysis was performed for the father and indicated that he is a heterozygous carrier for the p.Lys304Glu mutation (Figure 1(a)).

To date, the p.Thr326Ile missense change has not been reported in MCADD patients. This replacement is a nonconservative amino acid change that occurs in the C-terminal all-alpha domain of the MCAD protein. This domain consists of densely packed α-helices, which appear to be important for the formation of a functional tetramer. Mutations located in this domain (including the common mutation p.Lys304Glu) were reported to affect helix-helix interactions and tetramer assembly and lead to aggregation and loss of function [10, 11]. Utilizing the SIFT Human Protein and Human Coding SNPs database (*Homo sapiens* GrCh37 Ensembl 63) [12, 13], we entered in the region of interest. The results of that analysis provided us with a prediction of a novel, nonsynonymous, and damaging change (SIFT score of 0.04). In addition to SIFT, we used the PolyPhen2 database [14] to determine if the amino acid change is damaging. The results from PolyPhen2 HumDiv and HumVar predicted that the p.Thr326Ile mutation is possibly damaging with a score of 0.922 and 0.623, respectively. Because both databases gave results in concordance with each other and the location in the protein is in the same C-terminal all-alpha domain as p.Lys304Glu, p.Arg309Lys, and p.Ile331Thr [11], it is suggestive that the p.Thr326Ile change is a deleterious mutation. Taken together, it suggests that this novel change is likely to be a disease causing mutation that is associated with a mild MCADD phenotype. It was reported that the mutations associated with the mild phenotype, such as p.Ala27Val, p.Tyr42His, and p.Arg309Lys, have a low risk of metabolic decompensation [15]. To determine the allele frequency of this novel mutation, a survey was performed in the MCADD patient database from Baylor College of Medicine. Five individuals heterozygous for p.Lys304Glu and p.Thr326ILe were identified among 500 patients. Additionally, a search of the ESP6500 database, 1000 Genomes database, and dbSNP concluded that this particular mutation has not been previously classified. Therefore, the allele frequency of p.Thr326Ile is less than 1%. To our knowledge, this is the first report of the c.1052C>T mutation that results in a mild MCADD phenotype.

Conflict of Interests

The authors declare that there is no conflict of interests regarding the publication of this paper.

Authors' Contribution

Holli M. Drendel and Jason E. Pike contributed equally to this work.

References

[1] D. Matern and P. Rinaldo, "Medium-chain acyl-coenzyme A dehydrogenase deficiency," in *GeneReviews*, R. A. Pagon, M. P. Adam, H. H. Ardinger et al., Eds., University of Washington, Seattle, Seattle, Wash, USA, 1993.

[2] W. J. Rhead, "Newborn screening for medium-chain acyl-CoA dehydrogenase deficiency: a global perspective," *Journal of Inherited Metabolic Disease*, vol. 29, no. 2-3, pp. 370–377, 2006.

[3] M. Sturm, D. Herebian, M. Mueller, M. D. Laryea, and U. Spiekerkoetter, "Functional effects of different medium-chain acyl-CoA dehydrogenase genotypes and identification of asymptomatic variants," *PLoS ONE*, vol. 7, no. 9, Article ID e45110, 2012.

[4] B. Wilcken, K. Carpenter, and V. Wiley, "Neonatal screening for medium-chain acyl-CoA dehydrogenase deficiency," *The Lancet*, vol. 359, pp. 627–628, 2002.

[5] E. H. Smith, C. Thomas, D. McHugh et al., "Allelic diversity in MCAD deficiency: the biochemical classification of 54 variants identified during 5 years of ACADM sequencing," *Molecular Genetics and Metabolism*, vol. 100, no. 3, pp. 241–250, 2010.

[6] S. S. Wang, P. M. Fernhoff, W. H. Hannon, and M. J. Khoury, "Medium chain acyl-CoA dehydrogenase deficiency human genome epidemiology review," *Genetics in Medicine*, vol. 1, no. 7, pp. 332–339, 1999.

[7] P. Rinaldo, T. M. Cowan, and D. Matern, "Acylcarnitine profile analysis," *Genetics in Medicine*, vol. 10, no. 2, pp. 151–156, 2008.

[8] D. C. Lehotay, J. LePage, J. R. Thompson, and C. Rockman-Greenberg, "Blood acylcarnitine levels in normal newborns and heterozygotes for medium-chain acyl-CoA dehydrogenase deficiency: a relationship between genotype and biochemical phenotype?" *Journal of Inherited Metabolic Disease*, vol. 27, no. 1, pp. 81–88, 2004.

[9] J. L. K. Van Hove, W. Zhang, S. G. Kahler et al., "Medium-chain ccyl-CoA dehydrogenase (MCAD) deficiency: diagnosis by acylcarnitine analysis in blood," *The American Journal of Human Genetics*, vol. 52, no. 5, pp. 958–966, 1993.

[10] J.-J. P. Kim, M. Wang, and R. Paschke, "Crystal structures of medium-chain acyl-CoA dehydrogenase from pig liver mitochondria with and without substrate," *Proceedings of the National Academy of Sciences of the United States of America*, vol. 90, no. 16, pp. 7523–7527, 1993.

[11] E. M. Maier, S. W. Gersting, K. F. Kemter et al., "Protein misfolding is the molecular mechanism underlying MCADD identified in newborn screening," *Human Molecular Genetics*, vol. 18, no. 9, pp. 1612–1623, 2009.

[12] P. C. Ng and S. Henikoff, "Predicting deleterious amino acid substitutions," *Genome Research*, vol. 11, no. 5, pp. 863–874, 2001.

[13] P. Kumar, S. Henikoff, and P. C. Ng, "Predicting the effects of coding non-synonymous variants on protein function using the SIFT algorithm," *Nature Protocols*, vol. 4, no. 7, pp. 1073–1081, 2009.

[14] I. A. Adzhubei, S. Schmidt, L. Peshkin et al., "A method and server for predicting damaging missense mutations," *Nature Methods*, vol. 7, no. 4, pp. 248–249, 2010.

[15] J. M. Jank, E. M. Maier, D. D. Reib et al., "The domain-specific and temperature-dependent protein misfolding phenotype of variant medium-chain acyl-CoA dehydrogenase," *PLoS ONE*, vol. 9, no. 4, Article ID e93852, 2014.

27

Preaxial Polydactyly of the Foot: Variable Expression of Trisomy 13 in a Case from Central Africa

Sébastien Mbuyi-Musanzayi,[1,2] Aimé Lumaka,[3,4] Bienvenu Yogolelo Asani,[2,5]
Toni Lubala Kasole,[2,6] Prosper Lukusa Tshilobo,[3,4] Prosper Kalenga Muenze,[2,7]
François Tshilombo Katombe,[1] and Koenraad Devriendt[3]

[1] Department of Surgery, University Hospital, University of Lubumbashi, P.O. Box 1825, Lubumbashi, Democratic Republic of Congo
[2] Center for Human Genetics, Faculty of Medicine, University of Lubumbashi, P.O. Box 1825,
  Lubumbashi, Democratic Republic of Congo
[3] Center for Human Genetics, University Hospitals, KU Leuven, UZ Leuven, Campus Gasthuisberg, Herestraat 49,
  P.O. Box 602, 3000 Leuven, Belgium
[4] Department of Pediatrics, University Hospitals, University of Kinshasa, P.O. Box 123, Kin XI, Kinshasa, Democratic Republic of Congo
[5] Department of Ophthalmology, University Hospital, University of Lubumbashi, P.O. Box 1825,
  Lubumbashi, Democratic Republic of Congo
[6] Department of Pediatrics, University Hospital, University of Lubumbashi, P.O. Box 1825, Lubumbashi, Democratic Republic of Congo
[7] Department of Gynecology, University Hospital, University of Lubumbashi, P.O. Box 1825, Lubumbashi, Democratic Republic of Congo

Correspondence should be addressed to Koenraad Devriendt; koenraad.devriendt@uzleuven.be

Academic Editor: Philip D. Cotter

Trisomy 13 is a chromosomal disorder characterized by a severe clinical picture of multiple congenital anomalies. We here describe the clinical and genetic features and prognosis observed in a newborn with trisomy 13 from Central Africa. He presented the rare feature of preaxial polydactyly of the feet.

1. Introduction

Trisomy 13 (also known as Patau syndrome) is the third most common autosomal trisomy [1, 2]. The prevalence is between 1 : 10,000 and 1 : 20,000 live births [3], but it is estimated that the frequency of trisomy 13 is 100 times higher in spontaneous abortions [4, 5]. This chromosomal disorder has a characteristic phenotype consisting of multiple congenital anomalies [6], with a classical clinical triad of microphthalmia or anophthalmia, cleft lip and/or palate, and postaxial polydactyly. However, other anomalies are frequently associated [2, 7]. The objective of this report is to describe the clinical features and prognosis in a Congolese newborn with trisomy 13 and to illustrate the occurrence of a rare manifestation in this syndrome, preaxial polydactyly of the foot.

2. Case Report

The patient, a male, was referred at an age of two days. He was born at 40 weeks of gestation via a normal spontaneous vaginal delivery with birth weight 3250 g (−0.5 SD). His mother was 25 years old and father was 32 years old; both were healthy and unrelated. Family history was unremarkable. Prenatal ultrasound was not performed. He presented median cleft lip and palate, microcephaly (29 cm−−2.6 SD), bilateral anophthalmia, a posterior scalp defect, short neck, micropenis, and bilateral cryptorchidism (Figure 1). He had bilateral postaxial polydactyly of his hands. Of interest, he also had bilateral preaxial polydactyly of the first toes. The child was hypotonic and died at age of 5 days from acute respiratory distress.

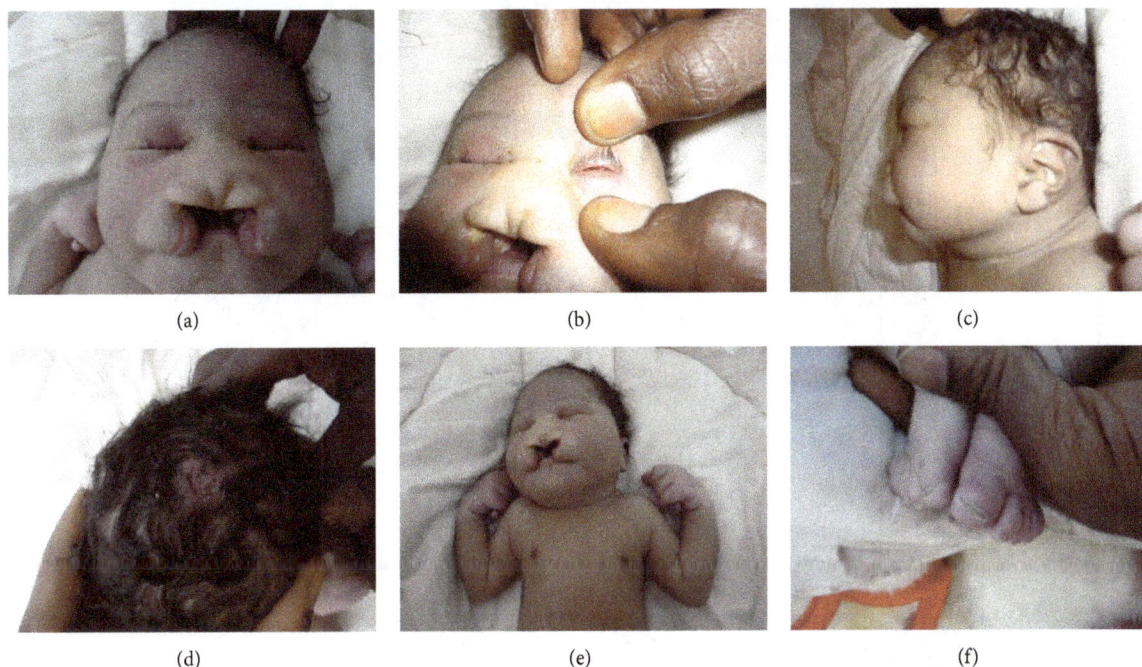

FIGURE 1: Craniofacial abnormalities observed in the patient. Note (a) median cleft lip and palate, (b) anophthalmia, (c) low-set ears, (d) aplasia cutis/scalp defect, (e) postaxial polydactyly on the hands, and (f) preaxial polydactyly of the feet.

3. Methods

Genomic DNA was isolated using standard protocols from the peripheral blood leukocytes and screened for copy number alterations using the Oxford Gene Technology 8 × 60 k Array Platform Custom Design (Catalogue number 027216). Array CGH results were interpreted using Oxford Gene Technology CytoSure Interpret Software_v.3.3.2 (OGT CytoSure, OGT Oxford, UK). All genome coordinates were according to NCBI human genome build 19 (hg19 Feb 2009). We performed array-CGH, which revealed trisomy 13: arr 13q12.11-q34 (20,407,270–115,092,581) ×3 or a duplication of the entire 94.69 Mb of chromosome 13. No additional CNVs were observed. Since karyotyping is not available in this part of the world, we were not able to exclude a Robertsonian translocation.

4. Discussion

We here present the clinical and genetic data in newborn with trisomy 13, diagnosed in the Democratic Republic of Congo. Since its first description by Patau in 1960 [8], trisomy 13 has been recognized as one of the three commonly observed autosomal trisomies observed in live newborns, worldwide. In Central Africa, genetics reports on chromosomal imbalances are scarce, and, to the best of our knowledge, there is only one earlier report on trisomy 13 in the Democratic Republic of Congo, dating from the year 1968 [9]. The case we report here presents the classical triad of cleft lip and palate, postaxial polydactyly, and anophthalmia. Each of these features is observed in 60–80% of cases [6, 10]. The patient had a median cleft lip and palate, with marked hypotelorism, characteristic

of holoprosencephaly, a common finding in trisomy 13. Brain ultrasound scan could not be performed, since the parents could not afford to pay for it. In addition, the patients presented several additional features, commonly observed in trisomy 13, as shown in Table 1. Postaxial polydactyly (especially of the hands) is reported in 52–70% of cases [6, 11–13]. However, the patient presented a very unusual sign: bilateral preaxial polydactyly of the feet. This finding has been reported twice before [6, 14]. While this may be a coincidence, it is tempting to speculate that the expression of this unusual feature in this Congolese boy may be related to its different genetic background. However, we have no firm evidence to support this at present. Postaxial polydactyly, especially of the hands, is a common feature in Africa, with a reported incidence between 10.4/1000 births in South and Central Africa [15, 16] and 22.78/1000 in Nigeria [17]. In contrast to this, preaxial polydactyly is rare in Central Africa as elsewhere (Table 1). The early death of the patient presented here is not unexpected: the median survival of patients with trisomy 13 varies from 2.5 to 10 days [3, 4, 13, 18]. The probability of survival until one month of age is about 28% and only 5–10% survive for one year [1, 3]. The cause of death may be primary apnea, regardless of the presence of a CNS abnormality [1, 5, 19]. Also, recurrent apnea may be related to the common occurrence of a cyanotic heart defect, pulmonary hypertension, congestive heart failure, aspiration pneumonia, gastroesophageal reflux, laryngomalacia, and seizures [20–22]. The case reported here is the first one with trisomy 13 to be reported in Central Africa (with the exception of a report in 1968) [9]. This probably reflects the current lack of teaching and thus interest and knowledge in human genetics and syndromology [23]. Whereas, in most

TABLE 1: Summary of clinical features in trisomy 13.

Study	Taylor [10]	Hodes et al. [11]	Moerman et al. [12]	Lin et al. [13]	Petry et al. [6]	Quelin et al. [14]	Patient
Year	1968	1978	1988	2007	2013	2014	2014
Country	England	USA	Belgium	Taiwan	Brazil	France	DRC
Samples (N)	27	19	12	28	30	3	1
Features	%	%	%	%	%	%	%
Craniofacial							
Abnormal auricles	74	79	25	0	77	0	−
Microphthalmia	70	84	42	54	60	33	−
Anophthalmia	0	11	0	14	10	33	+
Low-set ears	85	0	33	?	47	33	+
Aplasia cutis/scalp defect	0	47	25	29	43	0	+
Microcephaly	59	58	50	61	40	0	+
Cleft palate	67	68	42	?	33	0	+
Cleft lip	56	53	8	?	23	0	+
Short neck	70	16	0	46	30	0	+
Ocular hypotelorism	0	21	17	0	10	0	+
Thorax/abdomen							
Inguinal hernia/umbilical hernia	37	32	−	14	20	0	−
Anogenital							
Cryptorchidism	93	100	50	73	78	0	+
Micropenis	−	5	50	?	30	0	+
Limbs, skin, and neurological							
Postaxial polydactyly hands/feet	70	58	67	64	63	0	+
Single palmar crease	59	0	42	32	33	−	−
Duplicated hallux	−	−	−	−	3	33	+
Capillary hemangioma	56	37	0	14	27	0	−
Mongolian spot	0	0	0	0	0	0	−
Hypertonia/hypotonia	77	16	0	0	33	0	+

industrialized countries, trisomy 13 is diagnosed prenatally, the vast majorities of pregnant women in Central Africa currently do not have access to prenatal ultrasound follow-up and are thus confronted with serious emotional distress when facing an unexpected polymalformed newborn. Early clinical recognition of trisomy 13 at birth remains essential to optimize guidance for care of the child and his family. For instance, one can avoid needless and expensive therapeutic or diagnostic interventions, which is crucial in an environment where access to medical care and investigations is difficult and expensive. Moreover, also in this society, an exact diagnosis offers the opportunity to discuss the cause, refute commonly held mystical and traditional beliefs, and relieve misassigned feelings of guilt [24].

Conflict of Interests

The authors declare that there is no conflict of interests regarding the publication of this paper.

Authors' Contribution

Sébastien Mbuyi-Musanzayi was responsible for clinical examination, treatment of the patient, and redaction of the paper; Aimé Lumaka for analysis of array CGH; Bienvenu Yogolelo Asani for ophthalmological examination; Toni Lubala Kasole for clinical examination; Prosper Lukusa Tshilobo for the paper correction; Prosper Kalenga Muenze for paper correction; François Tshilombo Katombe for clinical examination; Koenraad Devriendt for clinical examination, diagnosis, and paper corrections. All coauthors have read, contributed, and approved the paper.

Acknowledgments

The authors thank the families of the patient for their kind cooperation. The authors thank the Cytogenetics Laboratory of the Center for Human Genetics, KU Leuven, for support. S.M. was supported by a scholarship from Interfaculty Council for Development Cooperation (IRO), KU Leuven and GROS, Holsbeek (Belgium).

References

[1] S. A. Rasmussen, L.-Y. C. Wong, Q. Yang, K. M. May, and J. M. Friedman, "Population-based analyses of mortality in trisomy 13 and trisomy 18," *Pediatrics*, vol. 111, no. 4, pp. 777–784, 2003.

[2] A. C. Duarte, A. I. C. Menezes, E. S. Devens, J. M. Roth, G. L. Garcias, and M. G. Martino-Roth, "Patau syndrome with a long survival. A case report," *Genetics and Molecular Research*, vol. 3, no. 2, pp. 288–292, 2004.

[3] C. M. Brewer, S. H. Holloway, D. H. Stone, A. D. Carothers, and D. R. FitzPatrick, "Survival in trisomy 13 and trisomy 18 cases ascertained from population based registers," *Journal of Medical Genetics*, vol. 39, no. 9, article e54, 2002.

[4] M. J. Parker, J. L. S. Budd, E. S. Draper, and I. D. Young, "Trisomy 13 and trisomy 18 in a defined population: epidemiological, genetic and prenatal observations," *Prenatal Diagnosis*, vol. 23, no. 10, pp. 856–860, 2003.

[5] A. Rios, S. A. Furdon, D. Adams, and D. A. Clark, "Recognizing the clinical features of Trisomy 13 syndrome," *Advances in Neonatal Care*, vol. 4, no. 6, pp. 332–343, 2004.

[6] P. Petry, J. B. Polli, V. F. Mattos et al., "Clinical features and prognosis of a sample of patients with trisomy 13 (Patau syndrome) from Brazil," *The American Journal of Medical Genetics A*, vol. 161, no. 6, pp. 1278–1283, 2013.

[7] J. C. Carey, "Perspectives on the care and management of infants with trisomy 18 and trisomy 13: striving for balance," *Current Opinion in Pediatrics*, vol. 24, no. 6, pp. 672–678, 2012.

[8] K. Patau, D. W. Smith, E. Therman, S. L. Inhorn, and H. P. Wagner, "Multiple congenital anomaly caused by an extra autosome," *The Lancet*, vol. 275, no. 7128, pp. 790–793, 1960.

[9] G. Cornu, J. P. Lintermans, H. van den Berghe, and R. Eeckels, "Trisomy 17-18 and trisomy 13-15 in the African child," *Journal of Tropical Medicine and Hygiene*, vol. 71, no. 4, pp. 105–109, 1968.

[10] A. I. Taylor, "Autosomal trisomy syndromes: a detailed study of 27 cases of Edwards' syndrome and 27 cases of Patau's syndrome," *Journal of Medical Genetics*, vol. 5, no. 3, pp. 227–252, 1968.

[11] M. E. Hodes, J. Cole, C. G. Palmer, and T. Reed, "Trisomy 18 (29 cases) and trisomy 13 (19 cases): a summary," *Birth Defects: Original Article Series Journal*, vol. 14, no. 6, pp. 377–382, 1978.

[12] P. Moerman, J.-P. Fryns, K. van der Steen, A. Kleczkowska, and J. Lauweryns, "The pathology of trisomy 13 syndrome. A study of 12 cases," *Human Genetics*, vol. 80, no. 4, pp. 349–356, 1988.

[13] H.-Y. Lin, S.-P. Lin, Y.-J. Chen et al., "Clinical characteristics and survival of trisomy 13 in a medical center in Taiwan, 1985—," *Pediatrics International*, vol. 49, no. 3, pp. 380–386, 2007.

[14] C. Quelin, E. Spaggiari, S. Khung-Savatovsky et al., "Inversion duplication deletions involving the long arm of chromosome 13: Phenotypic description of additional three fetuses and genotype-phenotype correlation," *The American Journal of Medical Genetics A*, 2014.

[15] J. G. R. Kromberg and T. Jenkins, "Common birth defects in South African Blacks," *South African Medical Journal*, vol. 62, no. 17, pp. 599–602, 1982.

[16] M. A. Sengeyi, K. Tshibangu, R. Tozin et al., "Etiopathogenesis and type of congenital malformations observed in Kinshasa (Zaire)," *Journal de Gynecologie Obstetrique et Biologie de la Reproduction*, vol. 19, no. 8, pp. 955–961, 1990.

[17] A. B. Scott Emuakpor and E. D. N. Madueke, "The study of genetic variation in Nigeria, II: the genetics of polydactyly," *Human Heredity*, vol. 26, no. 3, pp. 198–202, 1976.

[18] H. Goldstein and K. G. Nielsen, "Rates and survival of individuals with trisomy 13 and 18. Data from a 10-year period in Denmark," *Clinical Genetics*, vol. 34, no. 6, pp. 366–372, 1988.

[19] J. P. Wyllie, M. J. Wright, J. Burn, and S. Hunter, "Natural history of trisomy 13," *Archives of Disease in Childhood*, vol. 71, no. 4, pp. 343–345, 1994.

[20] H.-F. Hsu and J.-W. Hou, "Variable expressivity in Patau syndrome is not all related to trisomy 13 mosaicism," *The American Journal of Medical Genetics A*, vol. 143, no. 15, pp. 1739–1748, 2007.

[21] Y. Tunca, J. S. Kadandale, and E. K. Pivnick, "Long-term survival in Patau syndrome," *Clinical Dysmorphology*, vol. 10, no. 2, pp. 149–150, 2001.

[22] B. Zoll, J. Wolf, D. Lensing-Hebben, M. Pruggmayer, and B. Thorpe, "Trisomy 13 (Patau syndrome) with an 11-year survival," *Clinical Genetics*, vol. 43, no. 1, pp. 46–50, 1993.

[23] A. Lumaka, G. Mubungu, C. Nsibu, B. P. Tady, T. Lukusa, and
    K. Devriendt, "X-linked adrenal hypoplasia congenita: a novel
    DAX1 missense mutation and challenges for clinical diagnosis
    in Africa," *European Journal of Pediatrics*, vol. 171, no. 2, pp. 267–
    270, 2012.

[24] C. Haihambo and E. Lightfoot, "Cultural beliefs regarding
    people with disabilities in Namibia: implications for the inclu-
    sion of people with disabilities," *International Journal of Special
    Education*, vol. 25, no. 3, pp. 76–87, 2010.

28

De Novo Trisomy 1q10q23.3 Mosaicism Causes Microcephaly, Severe Developmental Delay, and Facial Dysmorphic Features but No Cardiac Anomalies

Shirley Lo-A-Njoe,[1] Lars T. van der Veken,[2] Clementien Vermont,[1] Louise Rafael-Croes,[1] Vincent Keizer,[1] Ron Hochstenbach,[2] Nine Knoers,[2] and Mieke M. van Haelst[2]

[1]*Department of Pediatrics, Horacio Oduber Hospital, Oranjestad, Aruba*
[2]*Department of Genetics, Wilhelmina Children's Hospital, UMC Utrecht, 3584 EA Utrecht, Netherlands*

Correspondence should be addressed to Shirley Lo-A-Njoe; smloanjoe@yahoo.com

Academic Editor: Philip D. Cotter

Proximal duplications of chromosome 1q are rare chromosomal abnormalities. Most patients with this condition present with neurological, urogenital, and congenital heart disease and short life expectancy. Mosaicism for trisomy 1q10q23.3 has only been reported once in the literature. Here we discuss a second case: a girl with a postnatal diagnosis of a *de novo* pure mosaic trisomy 1q1023.3 who has no urogenital or cardiac anomalies.

1. Introduction

Proximal duplications of chromosome 1q are rare chromosomal abnormalities. Affected patients present with neurological, urogenital, and congenital heart anomalies as reported by Chen et al. [1], Mertens et al. [2], Machlitt et al. [3], Patel et al. [4], and Sifakis et al. [5]. Mosaicism for 1q10q23.3 duplication has only been reported once by Hirshfeld et al. [6]. Here, we report a second case with a postnatal diagnosis of a *de novo* pure mosaic trisomy 1q10q23.3. Although the girl has a developmental delay and similar facial dysmorphism as the previous reported case, she has no cardiac or urogenital anomalies. The absence of cardiac and urogenital anomalies is of importance for prognosis and illustrates the importance of (prenatal) counseling of parents of patients with trisomy 1q10q23.3 mosaicism.

2. Case Report

The proband was the first child of healthy unrelated Caribbean parents. She was born after a term pregnancy with a birth weight of 3120 g. The mother was 19 years old and the father was 22 years old at time of delivery. Apart from her father's sickle cell disease (HbSC), family history is noncontributory. Pregnancy care was performed by a midwife. Because of the uncomplicated pregnancy and the fact that Aruba does not yet have standardized 20-week fetal screening, no additional fetal testing (fetal ultrasound or prenatal genetic testing) was performed. The neonatal period was uncomplicated. At nine months of age she was referred to the pediatrician for evaluation of developmental delay. At that time she had a variable head lag and could not turn or sit independently. Feeding was uneventful and no illnesses, medication, or admissions were noted. On clinical examination, length was 71 cm (75th percentile), weight was 7650 g (10th percentile), and head circumference was 42 cm (<3th percentile). She was microcephalic and had a metopic ridge, small palpebral fissures with epicanthic folds, two naevi on the right side of the face, a wide depressed nasal bridge, a full and long philtrum, retrognathia, creases in the earlobes, a narrow palate, full cheeks, dimples on both elbows, rocker bottom feet, hemangioma on left hallux, and a sacral dimple (Figure 1). Neurological examination revealed axial hypotonia and variable head lag. Additional testing was

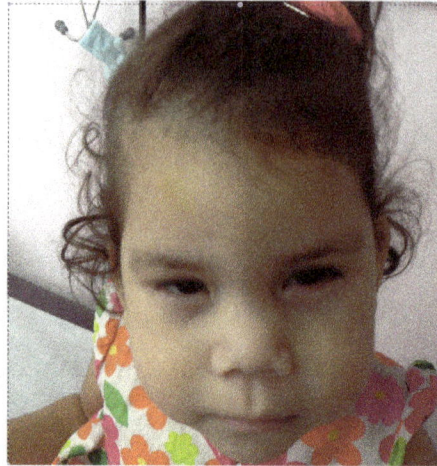

FIGURE 1: Face: note microcephaly; metopic ridge; wide, depressed nasal bridge; long philtrum; full cheeks; and retrognathia.

performed from June 2013 till June 2014. Echocardiography showed a structural and functional normal heart, with a normal aortic arch; there were no signs of (hypertrophic) cardiomyopathy. Electrocardiography showed a normal sinus rhythm, sinus arrhythmia, no preexcitation, and no signs of ventricle hypertrophy, a normal conduction and repolarization. A CT of the brain showed a normal aspect of corpus callosum and normal basal ganglia, and there were no calcifications. MRI of the brain showed subendymal heterotopia towards the right lateral ventricle, without other abnormalities. Sonography of the kidneys showed normal kidneys and urinary tract. Ultrasound of the spine suggested spina bifida; however, MRI of the spine showed only lumbarization of S1 without signs of spina bifida.

Biochemical investigations in blood showed, apart from HbSC, no hematologic, renal, or liver function abnormalities. Cytogenetic analyses on blood lymphocytes showed a mosaic duplication of arm of chromosome 1q10 to 1q23.3. Because the proband was delivered by a midwife after an uneventful pregnancy and delivery she was not seen by a physician, as such no testing was performed at birth of child or placenta. Parental karyotypes were normal.

SNP-array analysis showed a female array profile suggestive of a mosaic copy number gain of ~18.0 Mb in chromosomal region 1q21.1q23.3 (8141 probes) (Figure 2): ISCN 2013 nomenclature, ISCN [7]: arr[hg19] 1q21.1q23.3(144,854,574-162,843,606) × 2~3.

Routine karyotyping confirmed the mosaic copy number gain as suspected by the SNP-array investigation. A supernumerary derivative of chromosome 1 was detected in 4 out of 16 metaphases; analyzing the remaining metaphases showed a normal female karyotype. The derivative consisted of the proximal part of the long arm of chromosome 1 from the centromere to the breakpoint in band 1q23.3 (Figure 3). Follow-up investigation in both parents indicated that the duplication arose *de novo*. The parental origin of the duplicated region was not investigated. The mosaic nature of the duplication probably indicates that the duplication was generated during one of the early postzygotic mitoses.

Thus far there is only one case reported in the literature with mosaicism for overlapping partial trisomy 1q duplication Hirshfeld et al. [6]. This previously reported patient had similar facial dysmorphic features to the present patient (Figure 1). In addition, she had mild bilateral hydronephrosis and hypertrophic cardiomyopathy with left ventricular out flow tract obstruction and Wolff-Parkinson-White syndrome.

Other presented cases with proximal trisomy 1q duplications presented with a wide range of neurological, urogenital, and congenital heart anomalies (Table 1). The authors hypothesize that the cardiac anomalies could be caused by a disruption or increased dosage effect of *TPM3* which is located within the duplicated region. Since cardiac anomalies are absent in the present case and her duplicated chromosomal region harbors (apart from *LMXA1*) the same genes, it is less likely that *TPM3* is a candidate gene for dilated and hypertrophic cardiomyopathy. The cardiac phenotype could thus result from mutations in other sarcomeric genes. The percentage of mosaicism for 1q10q23.3 duplication in the heart can however not be predicted from the performed analysis in blood and could completely differ between the present and previously reported case, possibly explaining the absence of cardiac anomalies in our case. An increased dosage effect of candidate gene *TPM3* could then still result in congenital heart disease in the previous case. Although we did not reveal cardiac abnormalities at the age of 1 year in the present case, a spontaneous closed foramen ovale or patent ductus arteriosus or transient hypertrophy in our case cannot be fully excluded. As yet, no rhythm or conduction disturbances have been noted, but follow-up will occur yearly.

In conclusion, this report suggests that congenital heart disease and urogenital abnormalities are no clear diagnostic features of mosaic trisomy 1q10q23.3. However, as with all mosaic chromosomal anomalies, the severity of affected organs is difficult to predict as it depends on the percentage of mosaicism of the chromosomal abnormality in the specific organ systems. Careful genetic counseling is warranted in case of (prenatal) detection of pure *de novo* trisomy 1q10q23.3 duplication as well as regular cardiac follow-up screening for

TABLE 1: Clinical features in 7 patients, including presented case, with duplication of the proximal long arm of chromosome 1.

	Mertens et al., 1987 [2]	Chen et al., 2008 [1]	Hirshfeld et al., 2001 [6]	Machlitt et al., 2005 [3]	Patel et al., 2009 [4]	Sifakis et al., 2014 [5]	Present case
Karyotype	46,XY,inv dup(1)(q11→q22)	46,XY,dir dup(1)(pter→q25::q12→qpter)	46,XX,dir dup(1)(pter→q23::q12→q23::q23→qter)/46 XX	46,XY,der(1)(lqter→q21::1p36.3→qter)	46,XY,+1,der(1;22)(q10;q10)[25]/46,XY[65]	46,XX,der(1)(pter→q31::q31→q12::q31→qter)	47,XX,+der(1)(::q10→q23.3::)[4]/46,XX[12].ish der(1)(CEP1+,wcp1+)
% mosaic			Amniotic fluid, 100%	Amniotic fluid, 100%	27%	100%	Blood, 25%
Age of Dx	Delivery	Delivery	Delivery	Prenatal	Postmortem	Prenatal	9 months
GA (wk)	37	Term	Term	23	39	22,4	Term
BW (g/percentile)	2800/P25	3260/P25	3100/P25	440/P12	3300/P25	501/P12	3120/P25
Sex	Male	Male	Female	Male	Male	Female	Female
Skull anomalies	+	+	−	+	−	−	+
Brain anomalies	+	+	+	+	+	+	−
Abnormal palate	+	+	+	u	+	−	−
Micro/retrognathia	+	+	+	+	+	+	+
Low set/malrotated ears	+	+	+	+	+	+	−
Eye anomalies	−	−	−	+	u	−	−
Cardiovascular anomalies	+	+	+	+		−	−
Respiratory anomalies	+	+	−	−		−	−
Gastrointestinal anomalies	+	+	+	+		+	−
Kidney anomalies	−	−	+	+		+	−
Genital anomalies	−	+	−	+		−	−
Hand/foot anomalies	+	+	+	+		+	+
Others	Excessive neck skin		Selective deficiency antibody response to polysaccharide antigens	SUA		13 pair ribs, defect vertebra bodies, and collagenopathy	HbSC
Survival	11 months	Dead 2 weeks	15yr	TOP		TOP	2 years

Dx: diagnosis; GA: gestational age; BW: birth weight; SUA: single umbilical artery; HbSC: sickle cell type SC; TOP: termination of pregnancy; + present; −: absent; u: unknown.

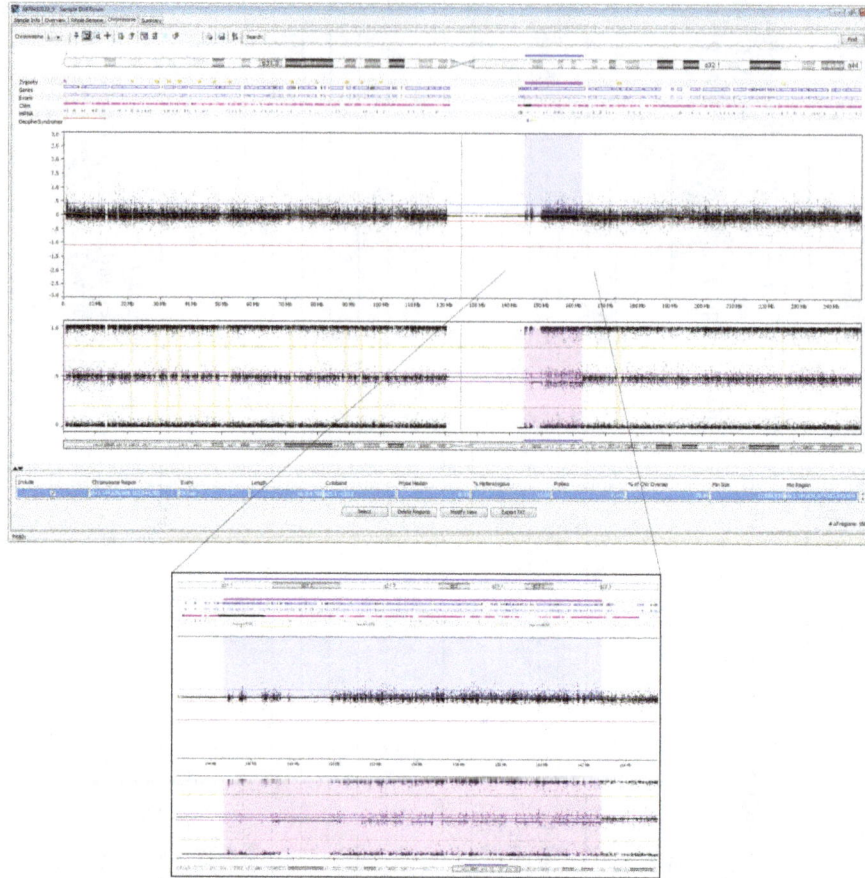

FIGURE 2: SNP-array analysis showed a mosaic duplication of ~18.0 Mb in 1q21.1-1q23.3: arr[hg19] 1q21.1q23.3(144,854,574-162,843,606) × 2~3. The upper y-axis shows the Log2 R ratio and the lower y-axis indicates the B allele frequency.

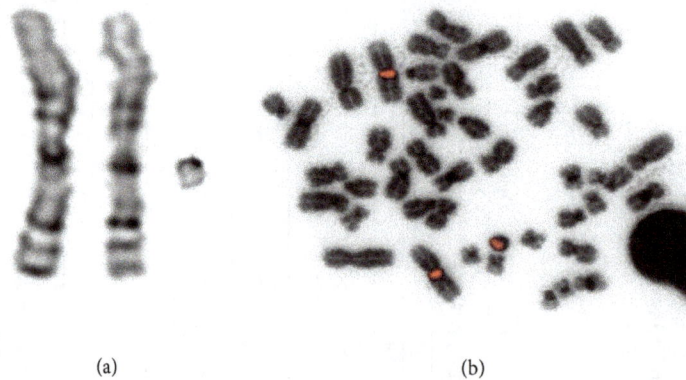

(a)   (b)

FIGURE 3: Partial G-banded karyogram showing both normal chromosomes 1 and the supernumerary der(1)(:q10 → q23.3:) (a) and a metaphase after FISH using a satellite III DNA-probe (Vysis) showing three signals on band 1q12 (b).

similar cases without cardiac anomalies. Since this is only the second report of a mosaic trisomy 1q10q23.3, further cases need to be reported to further delineate the associated phenotype.

Conflict of Interests

The authors declare that there is no conflict of interests regarding the publication of this paper.

References

[1] C.-P. Chen, Y.-J. Chen, S.-R. Chern et al., "Prenatal diagnosis of mosaic 1q31.3q32.1 trisomy associated with occipital encephalocele," *Prenatal Diagnosis*, vol. 28, no. 9, pp. 865–867, 2008.

[2] F. Mertens, B. Johansson, M. Forslund, M. Olsson, and U. Kristoffersson, "Tandem duplication (1) (q11 → q22) in a male infant with multiple congenital malformations," *Clinical Genetics*, vol. 32, no. 1, pp. 46–48, 1987.

[3] A. Machlitt, P. Kuepferling, C. Bommer, H. Koerner, and R. Chaoui, "Prenatal diagnosis of trisomy 1q21-qter: case report and review of literature," *American Journal of Medical Genetics Part A*, vol. 134, no. 2, pp. 207–211, 2005.

[4] C. Patel, G. Hardy, P. Cox, S. Bowdin, C. McKeown, and A. B. Russell, "Mosaic trisomy 1q: the longest surviving case," *American Journal of Medical Genetics Part A*, vol. 149, no. 8, pp. 1795–1800, 2009.

[5] S. Sifakis, M. Eleftheriades, D. Kappou et al., "Prenatal diagnosis of proximal partial trisomy 1q confirmed by comparative genomic hybridization array: molecular cytogenetic analysis, fetal pathology and review of the literature," *Birth Defects Research Part A—Clinical and Molecular Teratology*, vol. 100, no. 4, pp. 284–293, 2014.

[6] A. B. Hirshfeld, W. Reid Thompson, A. Patel, L. B. Boone, and A. M. Murphy, "Proximal trisomy of 1q mosaicism in a girl with hypertrophic cardiomyopathy associated with Wolff-Parkinson-White syndrome and multiple congenital anomalies," *American Journal of Medical Genetics*, vol. 100, no. 4, pp. 264–268, 2001.

[7] ISCN, *An International System for Human Cytogenetic Nomenclature*, edited by L. G. Shaffer, J. McGowan-Jordan and M. Schmid, S. Karger, Basel, Switzerland, 2013.

29

Monosomy 21 Seen in Live Born Is Unlikely to Represent True Monosomy 21: A Case Report and Review of the Literature

Trent Burgess,[1] Lilian Downie,[2] Mark D. Pertile,[1] David Francis,[1] Melissa Glass,[1] Sara Nouri,[1] and Rosalynn Pszczola[2]

[1] *Victorian Clinical Genetics Services, Murdoch Childrens Research Institute, Royal Children's Hospital, Parkville 3052, Melbourne, Australia*
[2] *Sunshine Hospital, Western Health, Sunshine 3020, Melbourne, Australia*

Correspondence should be addressed to Trent Burgess; trent.burgess@vcgs.org.au

Academic Editors: P. D. Cotter, M. Fenger, and C. López Ginés

We report a case of a neonate who was shown with routine chromosome analysis on peripheral blood lymphocytes to have full monosomy 21. Further investigation on fibroblast cells using conventional chromosome and FISH analysis revealed two additional mosaic cell lines; one is containing a ring chromosome 21 and the other a double ring chromosome 21. In addition, chromosome microarray analysis (CMA) on fibroblasts showed a mosaic duplication of chromosome region 21q11.2q22.13 with approximately 45% of cells showing three copies of the proximal long arm segment, consistent with the presence of a mosaic ring chromosome 21 with ring instability. The CMA also showed complete monosomy for an 8.8 Mb terminal segment (21q22.13q22.3). Whilst this patient had a provisional clinical diagnosis of trisomy 21, the patient also had phenotypic features consistent with monosomy 21, such as prominent epicanthic folds, broad nasal bridge, anteverted nares, simple ears, and bilateral overlapping fifth fingers, features which can also be present in individuals with Down syndrome. The patient died at 4.5 months of age. This case highlights the need for additional studies using multiple tissue types and molecular testing methodologies in patients provisionally diagnosed with monosomy 21, in particular if detected in the neonatal period.

1. Introduction

Apparent full monosomy 21 has been reported in ten cases in the pre- and postnatal settings (excluding early pregnancy loss), with most cases being lethal in utero [1–14]. However, many of these cases were reported when cytogenetic techniques were limited and often only single tissues were investigated. Clinical features of monosomy 21 include severe Intrauterine Growth Retardation (IUGR), ear anomalies, clinodactyly (5th finger), seizures, and anteverted nares. Cases of monosomy 21 reported in live born, as was the provisional diagnosis in this case, are unlikely to represent true full monosomy 21. The presence of a second undetected cell line being the most likely explanation for pregnancies reaching term.

The presence of a ring chromosome 21, due to their mitotic instability and propensity for tissue limited mosaicism, provides a plausible explanation for some of the previously reported cases of full monosomy 21. In particular, when detected in the neonatal setting. The associated phenotype in patients with mosaic ring chromosome 21 with monosomy 21 is varied. Features range from apparently normal individuals [15] through to individuals with dysmorphic features and congenital abnormalities [16]. The severity of the phenotype is likely to depend upon the prevalence and tissue distribution of the monosomy 21 cell line, the level of genomic imbalance associated with the formation of the ring chromosome, and the mitotic dynamism of the ring chromosome, also known as "Ring syndrome" [17].

2. Case Presentation

The proband, a female infant was the first of dichorionic-diamniotic (DCDA) twin girls born prematurely at 35 + 3 weeks gestation by elective caesarean section for discordant growth on ultrasound. She had a birth weight of 1650 g; her sister weighed 2510 g. This patient was a result of the sixth pregnancy of a nonconsanguineous couple; all other siblings are alive and well. The 35-year-old mother's past medical history was unremarkable except for latent TB infection; her only pregnancy complication was a finding of vitamin D deficiency. She received standard twin pregnancy antenatal care. Initial fetal morphology scans performed at 17 and 21 weeks gestation showed no abnormalities. Discordant growth was first detected at 26 weeks gestation and monitored with serial ultrasound. At 34+ weeks, ultrasound surveillance showed that the first twin's estimated weight had dropped below the third centile while amniotic fluid index and umbilical artery Doppler flows remained within normal limits; short femur length was also noted for the first time at this scan. Due to increasing growth discordance the decision was made for elective delivery at 35 weeks following betamethasone administration.

The patient required less than one minute of positive pressure ventilation at delivery for poor respiratory effort and was then stabilized on constant positive airway pressure (CPAP). Respiratory support was weaned without complication within the first hour of life. Dysmorphic features were first noted on day 10 of life when she was observed to have prominent epicanthic folds, broad nasal bridge, anteverted nares, simple ears, and bilateral overlapping fifth fingers (Figure 1). Further examinations and imaging were performed to assess for other dysmorphologies and no abnormalities were detected on renal ultrasound, ophthalmology examination, cranial ultrasound, or brain magnetic resolution imaging (MRI). Conventional chromosome analysis on peripheral bloods was requested.

The neonatal course was complicated by seizures occurring on day 22 of life. During these episodes she became pale and inactive and showed jerking movements of all four limbs and had a corresponding decrease in oxygen saturations. Each episode lasted for approximately 20 seconds which self-resolved, but she remained hypotonic for 2-3 minutes following this episode. Treatment was initiated for possible meningitis but colony stimulating factor (CSF) culture and viral studies were negative. No further episodes were noted after this.

A grade 3 systolic cardiac murmur was noted during admission. Subsequent echocardiogram showed a structurally normal heart with a small patent foramen ovale and normal cardiac function.

Persistent thrombocytopenia was documented with platelet nadir of 79×10^9/L on day 25 of life. Blood film analysis was not diagnostic of specific pathology and there was no clinical evidence of bleeding or bruising. All other haematological cell lines were normal.

The patient was discharged on day 63 of life at one month corrected gestational age on full suck feeds with a weight of 2265 grams. On review at 8 weeks corrected age weight gain was very slow with the patient's weight dropping significantly below the 3rd centile in association with poor feeding and decreased caloric. On examination she was markedly hypotonic with significant head lag but demonstrated some antigravity movement in all four limbs. Cardiac murmur was no longer audible.

At 4.5 months the patient died at home after struggling to gain weight. Gavage feeding was discussed but not proceeded with and parents had made a decision not to resuscitate. A postmortem was declined.

3. Results and Discussion

A provisional clinical diagnosis of possible trisomy 21 was made on this patient. However, the patient was shown to have full monosomy 21 on a conventional blood karyotype (60 cells analysed) and interphase FISH analysis (100 cells analysed, using the chromosome 21 specific probe provided in the AneuVysion kit (AneuVysion, Abbott Molecular, Illinois, USA)). True full monosomy 21 is rarely observed and is likely to be lethal in utero [18]. Full monosomy 21 has been reported in the miscarriage and prenatal and postnatal settings; however, the rigor of the testing methods in many cases was not adequate to determine conclusively full nonmosaic monosomy 21 [1–14]. This is due to many factors including a lack of molecular cytogenetic protocols available at the time of testing and the unavailability of multiple tissue types for the exclusion of tissue limited mosaicism. Many of the earlier documented cases of full monosomy 21, through retrospective analyses using molecular techniques, have been shown to represent cryptic unbalanced rearrangements and therefore not to represent true monosomy 21. In particular, there have been several reports of unbalanced derivative chromosomes that have resulted from a cryptic translocation between chromosomes 5p and 21q [19–21]. Other cases of full monosomy 21 diagnosed in live born, where unbalanced derivatives chromosomes have been excluded by molecular techniques, often lack an extensive cytogenetic work-up to exclude tissue limited mosaicism [1, 3, 5, 6, 8, 9, 12, 22, 23]. In these cases, only a single or limited number of tissues have been investigated; therefore a cryptic cell line that would act to reduce the level of genomic imbalance has not been excluded. The presence of an undetected cell line would provide a plausible explanation for apparent nonmosaic monosomy 21 conceptus' surviving to term. The patient described by Mori et al. [12] may represent one of the more rigorously investigated cases of full monosomy 21 detected in the new born period. Here, three different tissues were investigated (fetal blood, kidney, and fibroblasts), with all showing full monosomy 21 with cryptic unbalanced rearrangements being excluded. Our patient shared common features with the patient described by Mori et al. [12] such as IUGR in the prenatal period, ear anomalies, and clinodactyly. Our patient also showed features observed in other reports of monosomy 21 such as anteverted nares and seizures in the neonatal period, which may indicate that the observed phenotype in our patient is primarily due to monosomy 21.

Interphase FISH analysis on buccal cells using the same chromosome 21 specific AneuVysion FISH probe as used on the blood investigation also showed full monosomy 21. However, conventional chromosome analysis on cultured fibroblasts revealed a mosaic karyotype with two cell lines,

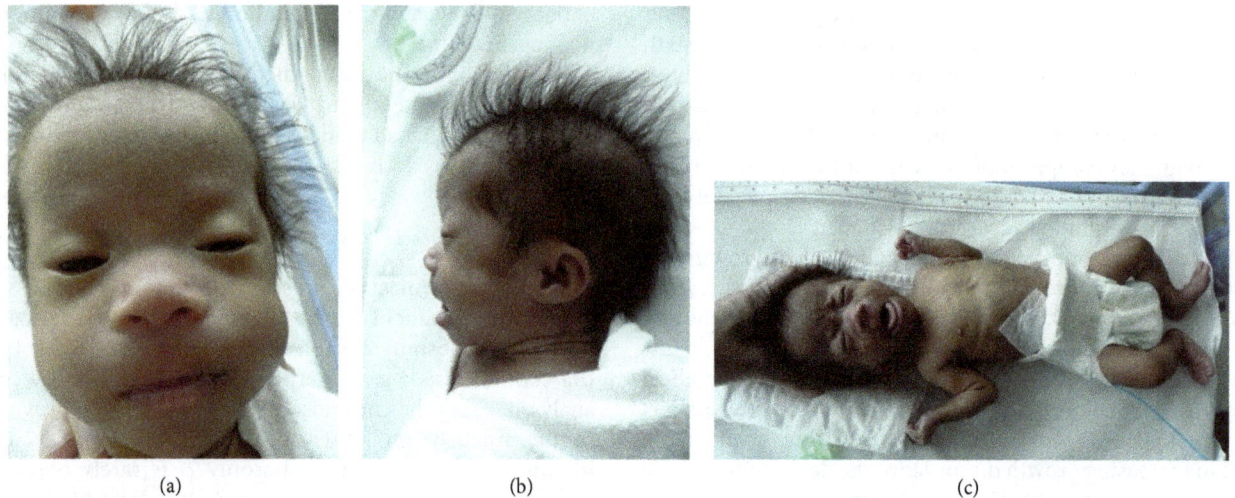

FIGURE 1: (a) demonstrates the observed broad nasal bridge, anteverted nares, and prominent epicanthis folds, (b) simple ears, and (c) bilateral 5th finger clinodactyly.

one with monosomy 21 (8 cells) and the other with a ring chromosome 21 (42 cells). The karyotype is as follows: 45,XX,-21[8]/46,XX,r(21)(p11q?22)[42] (Figure 2(a), only the ring 21 cell line is shown). The detection of this cryptic mosaic ring chromosome 21 cell line is likely to be the reason that our patient survived until 4.5 months of age. The presence of cryptic cell lines that act to reduce the level of genomic imbalance may also provide a plausible explanation for previously reported cases of full monosomy 21 surviving into the neonatal period. Ring chromosomes are known for their mitotic instability and tissue limited mosaicism, so they may not always be detected by investigating a single or small number of tissues. Ring chromosome 21 is a relatively uncommon anomaly and has been described in both the familial and de novo settings [24]. It is associated with a variable phenotype ranging from marked dysmorphism, developmental delay, and death in early infancy to entirely normal growth, development, and appearance [15, 16, 25, 26]. This variability in phenotype is likely to be due to the prevalence and tissue distribution of the monosomy 21 and ring chromosome 21 cell lines, the genomic imbalance (deletions and duplications) associated with ring chromosome formation, and the level of mitotic dynamism "Ring syndrome" observed within the carrier. Investigation of additional tissues (skin fibroblasts and buccal cells) in our patient revealed the presence of a mosaic ring chromosome 21 in the fibroblast cells, highlighting the importance of further investigation in patients who have been found to have full monosomy 21 in a primary tissue sampling.

Further complicating the phenotype of patients with mosaic or nonmosaic ring chromosome 21 is the level of genomic imbalance associated with the ring chromosome formation. Microarray analysis using the Illumina HumanCoreExome v1 (Illumina, San Diego, CA, USA) on cultured skin fibroblasts in our patient confirmed the presence of the mosaic ring chromosome 21 and also showed a terminal long arm deletion of 8.8 Mb (Figure 2(c)). The combined

conventional and molecular karyotypes were determined as 45,XX,-21[8]/46,XX,r(21)(p11q?22)[42].arr 21q11.2q22.13 (15,396,340-39,267,060) x2~3, 21q22.13q22.3 (39,270,074-48,084,247) x1. The deletion, containing approximately 96 genes, resulted in complete monosomy for this region (chr21:39,270,074-48,084,247, UCSC Genome build February 2009 GRCh37/hg19). In a review of terminal chromosome 21 deletions, Lyle et al. [27] suggested that terminal deletions in the range of 5.6 Mb to 11 Mb (comparable to our patient) show a relatively mild phenotype, which includes moderate mental retardation and may or may not include subtle dysmorphisms. It is highly likely that the loss of the 8.8 Mb segment has contributed to our patients phenotype; however, it may be that it has had a milder impact on the phenotype than the loss of the ring chromosome in the monosomy 21 cell line.

In addition, the presence of the relatively large terminal deletion in our case had the potential to cause confusion when investigating the various tissues for monosomy 21. The commercially available and widely used AneuVysion chromosome 21 specific probe, which maps to the proposed Down Syndrome Critical Region (DSCR) at 21q22.13, was contained within the deleted region (by 100 Kb) and would always give the appearance of full monosomy 21 in tissues where the ring chromosome 21 was present. We are confident that the blood sample only contained full monosomy 21 as the microarray performed on DNA extracted from whole blood did not show any evidence of mosaicism for ring chromosome 21 (sensitivity to 5% mosaicism and above as determined by an internal laboratory spiking experiment). However, the presence of the ring chromosome 21 could not be excluded in the buccal sample, which showed full monosomy 21 using FISH (AneuVysion), as no confirmatory testing could be performed. Metaphase FISH using the ETV6/RUNX1 probe (Abbott Molecular, Illinois, USA), which is located outside the deleted region, was performed on cultured fibroblast. This investigation showed 1 copy of RUNX1 (chromosome 21

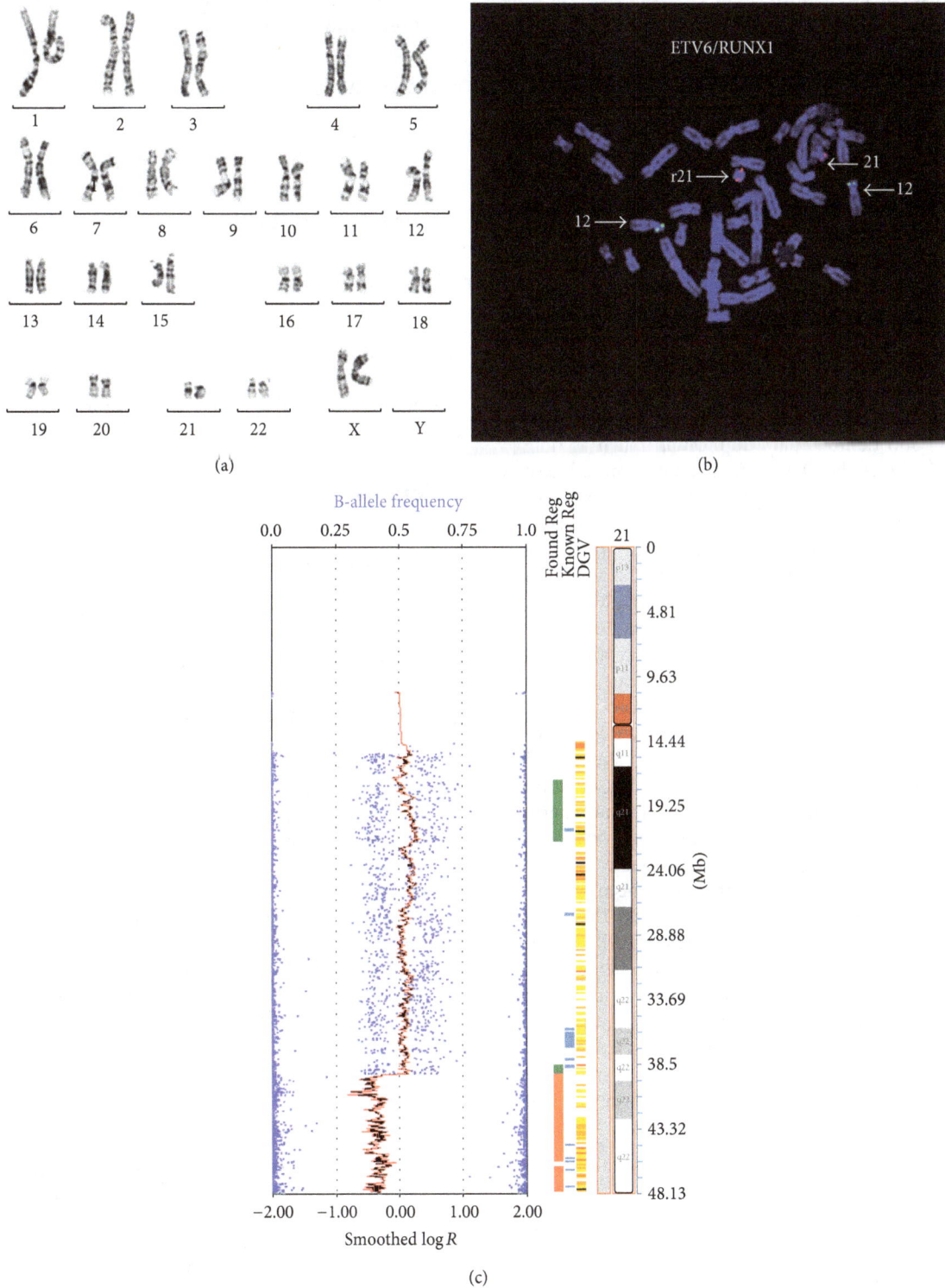

(a)

(b)

(c)

FIGURE 2: The monosomy 21 cell line is not shown. (a) G-banded fibroblast karyotype showing the ring chromosome 21. (b) Metaphase FISH of cultured fibroblasts using the ETV6/RUNX1 probe set indicating the presence of a double ring, that is, 1 copy of RUNX1 on the normal chromosome 21 and 2 copies on the double ring chromosome 21. (c) Chromosome microarray using the Illumina HumanCoreExome v1 performed on cultured fibroblast showing a copy number (Log R) that is consistent with the presence of a monosomic cell line and cell lines with a ring and double ring chromosome 21. The 8.8 Mb terminal deletion is also indicated. The B-allele frequency also confirms the mosaic nature of this finding.

derived) in thirty cells (31%), 2 copies in twenty-nine cells (30%), and 3 copies in thirty-eight cells (39%), indicating the presence of the monosomy cell line, the cell line with the ring chromosome, and an additional cell line with a double sized ring (Figure 2(b), only double ring shown). This highlights one of the many benefits CMA has provided in the investigation of patients suspected of having a chromosome abnormality, allowing for a more accurate evaluation of the genomic imbalance and directing more appropriate follow-up testing protocols.

The mitotic instability observed in our patient resulted in a cell line that contained double rings, meaning there was mosaicism for partial trisomy. In the fibroblast sample the double ring was present in approximately 39% of cells. The high level of double rings in some tissues in our patient may have contributed to the patient's provisional clinical diagnosis of Down syndrome when the ring chromosome 21 is larger in size (i.e., less genomic imbalance due to monosomy) and demonstrates duplication (such as double rings) that includes the DSCR; the patient is more likely to have characteristics consistent with Down syndrome [28]. However, the phenotype of patients previously reported as full monosomy 21 appears to share features common to Down syndrome, such as heart defects, clinodactyly, simian crease, and upslanting palpebral fissures [1–3, 5, 8–10, 12, 13, 23]. As discussed, however, the presence of an additional cell line has not been excluded in many of these previously reported cases.

Ring chromosomes have been observed for all human chromosomes and are well known to be associated with abnormal phenotypes. The impact on phenotype is proposed to be the result of either loss/gain of genetic material during the ring formation (as discussed above) and/or mitotic dynamism of the ring chromosome [17, 29]. The latter can result in cell lines that do not contain the ring (monosomy), cells that contain the ring, and cells with double sized rings (trisomy). Double ring chromosomes have been shown to result from sister chromatid exchange events. This mitotic instability is proposed to lead to increased cell mortality and result in severe growth deficiencies, this being the key feature of "Ring syndrome" [17]. It is difficult to ascertain the significance that "Ring syndrome" may have played in the patient in this case report, especially given the high frequency of the monosomy cell line and the size of the terminal deletion; however it is likely that this has contributed to the evolution of the three cell lines observed.

In conclusion, full monosomy 21 is likely to be lethal in utero. Patients who have been found to have full monosomy 21 in the neonatal period require further investigations using a combination of conventional and molecular cytogenetics techniques to exclude cryptic unbalanced rearrangements. In addition, where available, multiple tissue lineages need to be tested to determine the presence of a cryptic cell line that would act to reduce the level of genomic imbalance. An additional cell line was confirmed in the patient in this case report which constituted a ring chromosome 21. The ring chromosome was shown to have an 8.8 Mb terminal deletion and was shown to be mitotically unstable. CMA provided an important new cytogenetic tool, allowing for the accurate determination of genomic imbalance, the level of mosaicism, and the appropriate selection of FISH probes for interphase FISH examinations, and aided in providing more accurate prognostic information.

Conflict of Interests

The authors declare that there is no conflict of interests regarding the publication of this paper.

Authors' Contribution

Trent Burgess and Lilian Downie contributed equally to this work.

Acknowledgment

The authors would like to thank the family for participating in this study.

References

[1] P. Dziuba, D. Dziekanowska, and H. Hubner, "A female infant with monosomy 21," *Human Genetics*, vol. 31, no. 3, pp. 351–353, 1976.

[2] D. Fisher, A. DiPietro, K. A. Murdison, and C. A. Lemieux, "Full monosomy 21: echocardiographic findings in the third molecularly confirmed case," *Pediatric Cardiology*, vol. 34, no. 3, pp. 733–735, 2013.

[3] J. P. Fryns, F. D'Hondt, P. Goddeeris, and H. van den Berghe, "Full monosomy 21: a clinically recognizable syndrome?" *Human Genetics*, vol. 37, no. 2, pp. 155–159, 1977.

[4] A. Ghidini, S. Fallet, J. Robinowitz, C. J. Lockwood, R. Dische, and J. Willner, "Prenatal detection of monosomy 21 mosaicism," *Prenatal Diagnosis*, vol. 13, no. 3, pp. 163–169, 1993.

[5] U. Gripenberg, J. Elfving, and L. Gripenberg, "A 45,XX,21– child: attempt at a cytological and clinical interpretation of the karyotype," *Journal of Medical Genetics*, vol. 9, no. 1, pp. 110–115, 1972.

[6] K. H. Halloran, W. R. Breg, and M. J. Mahoney, "21 Monosomy in a retarded female infant," *Journal of Medical Genetics*, vol. 11, no. 4, pp. 386–389, 1974.

[7] P. Hardy, J. Bryan, R. Hardy, P. A. Lennon, and K. Hardy, "Is monosomy 21 rare? Seven early miscarriages including one mosaic 45, XX, -21/44, X, -21 in a single study population," *American Journal of Medical Genetics A*, vol. 158, pp. 2050–2052, 2012.

[8] R. Herva, M. Koivisto, and U. Seppanen, "21-Monosomy in a liveborn male infant," *European Journal of Pediatrics*, vol. 140, no. 1, pp. 57–59, 1983.

[9] A. M. S. Jootsen, S. de Vos, D. van Opstal, H. Branderburg, J. L. J. Gaillard, and C. H. Vermeij-Keers, "Full monosomy 21, prenatally diagnosed by fluorescent in situ hybridization," *Prenatal Diagnosis*, vol. 17, no. 3, pp. 271–275, 1997.

[10] A. S. Kulharya, V. S. Tonk, C. Lovell, and D. B. Flannery, "Complete monosomy 21 confirmed by FISH and array-CGH," *American Journal of Medical Genetics A*, vol. 158, no. 4, pp. 935–937, 2012.

[11] E. Manolakos, P. Peitsidis, M. Eleftheriades et al., "Prenatal detection of full monosomy 21 in a fetus with increased nuchal translucency: molecular cytogenetic analysis and review of the

literature," *Journal of Obstetrics and Gynaecology Research*, vol. 36, no. 2, pp. 435–440, 2010.

[12] M. A. Mori, P. Lapunzina, A. Delicado et al., "A prenatally diagnosed patient with full monosomy 21: ultrasound, cytogenetic, clinical, molecular, and necropsy findings," *American Journal of Medical Genetics A*, vol. 127, no. 1, pp. 69–73, 2004.

[13] M. C. Pellissier, N. Philip, and M. A. Voelckel-Baeteman, "Monosomy 21: a new case confirmed by in situ hybridization," *Human Genetics*, vol. 75, no. 1, pp. 95–96, 1987.

[14] M. G. Shah, A. Franco, K. M. Wills, A. S. Kulharya, B. S. Buckler, and J. J. S. Bhatia, "A rare case of complete monosomy 21 with multiple osseous, cardiac, and vascular anomalies," *European Journal of Radiology Extra*, vol. 76, no. 2, pp. e65–e68, 2010.

[15] I. Papoulidis, E. Manolakos, E. Siomou et al., "A fetus with ring chromosome 21 characterized by aCGH shows no clinical findings after birth," *Prenatal Diagnosis*, vol. 30, no. 6, pp. 586–588, 2010.

[16] C.-P. Chen, Y.-H. Lin, S.-Y. Chou et al., "Mosaic ring chromosome 21, monosomy 21, and isodicentric ring chromosome 21: prenatal diagnosis, molecular cytogenetic characterization, and association with 2-Mb deletion of 21q21.1-q21.2 and 5-Mb deletion of 21q22.3," *Taiwanese Journal of Obstetrics and Gynecology*, vol. 51, no. 1, pp. 71–76, 2012.

[17] G. Kosztolanyi, "Does "ring syndrome" exist? An analysis of 207 case reports on patients with a ring autosome," *Human Genetics*, vol. 75, no. 2, pp. 174–179, 1987.

[18] A. Schinzel, "Does full monosomy 21 exist?" *Human Genetics*, vol. 32, no. 1, pp. 105–107, 1976.

[19] P. Gill, S. Uhrich, C. Disteche, and E. Cheng, "Fetal t(5p;21q) misdiagnosed as monosomy 21: a plea for in situ hybridization studies," *American Journal of Medical Genetics A*, vol. 52, no. 4, pp. 416–418, 1994.

[20] M. A. Iqbal, M. Z. Ahmed, D. Wu, and N. Sakati, "A case of presumptive monosomy 21 re-diagnosed as unbalanced t(5p;21q) by FISH and review of literature," *American Journal of Medical Genetics A*, vol. 70, pp. 174–178, 1997.

[21] I. Lopez-Pajares, A. Martin-Ancel, P. Cabello, A. Delicado, A. Garcia-Alix, and C. San Roman, "De novo t(5p;21q) in a patient previously diagnosed as monosomy 21," *Clinical Genetics*, vol. 43, no. 2, pp. 94–97, 1993.

[22] M. C. Phelan, "Additional studies warranted to confirm monosomy 21," *Prenatal Diagnosis*, vol. 22, no. 2, pp. 160–161, 2002.

[23] J. Toral-Lopez, L. M. Gonzalez-Huerta, and S. A. Cuevas-Covarrubias, "Complete monosomy mosaic of chromosome 21: case report and review of literature," *Gene*, vol. 510, no. 2, pp. 175–179, 2012.

[24] M. J. McGinniss, H. H. Kazazian Jr., G. Stetten et al., "Mechanisms of ring chromosome formation in 11 cases of human ring chromosome 21," *American Journal of Human Genetics*, vol. 50, no. 1, pp. 15–28, 1992.

[25] A. R. Melnyk, I. Ahmed, and J. C. Taylor, "Prenatal diagnosis of familial ring 21 chromosome," *Prenatal Diagnosis*, vol. 15, no. 3, pp. 269–273, 1995.

[26] G. Stetten, B. Sroka, V. L. Corson, and C. D. Boehm, "Prenatal detection of an unstable ring 21 chromosome," *Human Genetics*, vol. 68, no. 4, pp. 310–313, 1984.

[27] R. Lyle, F. Béna, S. Gagos et al., "Genotype-phenotype correlations in Down syndrome identified by array CGH in 30 cases of partial trisomy and partial monosomy chromosome 21," *European Journal of Human Genetics*, vol. 17, no. 4, pp. 454–466, 2009.

[28] E. A. Crombez, K. M. Dipple, L. A. Schimmenti, and N. Rao, "Duplication of the Down syndrome critical region does not predict facial phenotype in a baby with a ring chromosome 21," *Clinical Dysmorphology*, vol. 14, no. 4, pp. 183–187, 2005.

[29] G. B. Cote, A. Katsantoni, and D. Deligeorgis, "The cytogenetic and clinical implications of a ring chromosome 2," *Annales de Genetique*, vol. 24, no. 4, pp. 231–235, 1981.

30

Cognitive, Affective Problems and Renal Cross Ectopy in a Patient with 48,XXYY/47,XYY Syndrome

Sefa Resim,[1] **Faruk Kucukdurmaz,**[2] **Nazım Kankılıc,**[1] **Ozlem Altunoren,**[3] **Erkan Efe,**[1] **and Can Benlioglu**[4]

[1]*Department of Urology, Kahramanmaras Sutcu Imam University, Kahramanmaras, Turkey*
[2]*Department of Urology, Nizip State Hospital, Gaziantep, Turkey*
[3]*Department of Psychiatry, Kahramanmaras State Hospital, Kahramanmaras, Turkey*
[4]*Department of Urology, Adiyaman University, Adiyaman, Turkey*

Correspondence should be addressed to Sefa Resim; sefaresim@gmail.com

Academic Editor: Philip D. Cotter

Klinefelter syndrome is the most common sex chromosome abnormality (SCA) in infertile patients and 47,XXY genomic configuration constitutes most of the cases. However, additional Xs and/or Y such as 48,XXYY, 48,XXXY, and 47,XYY can occur less frequently than 47,XXY. Those configurations were considered as variants of Klinefelter syndrome. In this report, we present an infertile man with tall stature and decreased testicular volume. Semen analysis and hormonal evaluation supported the diagnosis of nonobstructive azoospermia. Genetic investigation demonstrated an abnormal male karyotype with two X chromosomes and two Y chromosomes consistent with 48,XXYY(17)/47,XYY (13). Additionally, the patient expressed cognitive and affective problems which were documented by psychomotor retardation and borderline intelligence measured by an IQ value between 70 and 80. Systemic evaluation also revealed cross ectopy and malrotation of the right kidney in the patient. The couple was referred to microtesticular sperm extraction (micro-TESE)/intracytoplasmic sperm injection (ICSI) cycles and preimplantation genetic diagnosis (PGD). To the best of our knowledge, this is the first report of combination of XYY and XXYY syndromes associated with cognitive, affective dysfunction and renal malrotation.

1. Introduction

Sex chromosomal aneuploidy (SCA) is the most common disorder of sex chromosomes in human, with an incidence of 1 in 400 newborns [1]. In Klinefelter syndrome, 47,XXY is the most common SCA, but additional Xs and/or Y such as 48,XXYY, 48,XXXY, and 47,XYY can occur less frequently than 47,XXY [2]. It was reported that the incidence of 48,XXXY and 48,XXYY is 1 in 17.000 and 1 in 50.000 male births, respectively. The frequency of 49,XXXYY karyotype is as rare as 1 in 85.000 to 100.000 boys [3]. Klinefelter syndrome was initially focused on endocrinologic and physical characteristics; however, psychiatric issues and social dysfunction were also reported in this disorder [2, 3]. The addition of more than one extra X and/or Y chromosome to a normal male karyotype is less frequent and has its own distinctive physical and behavioral profile [1–4]. The XXYY syndrome

was previously accepted as a variant of Klinefelter syndrome with hypogenitalism disorders [5]. However, specific clinical features including mental retardation and psychiatric problems have been described. Some neurodevelopmental and psychological disorders are more common and significant in 48,XXYY, 48,XXXY, and 49,XXXXY syndromes and are typically more severe and/or complex when compared with 47,XXY. Developmental dyspraxia may have an effect on the early language and motor deficits [6, 7]. Attention deficit hyperactivity disorder (ADHD) is present in over 70% of males with 48,XXYY, with symptoms of inattention, distractibility, poor organizational skills, hyperactivity, and/or impulsivity affecting daily functioning [8]. This is significantly higher than the 35–45% rate of ADHD in 47,XXY. In addition to ADHD, autism spectrum disorders (ASD) were much more common in 48,XXYY subjects with a rate of 28–50% [8, 9]. The XYY karyotype is rarely diagnosed

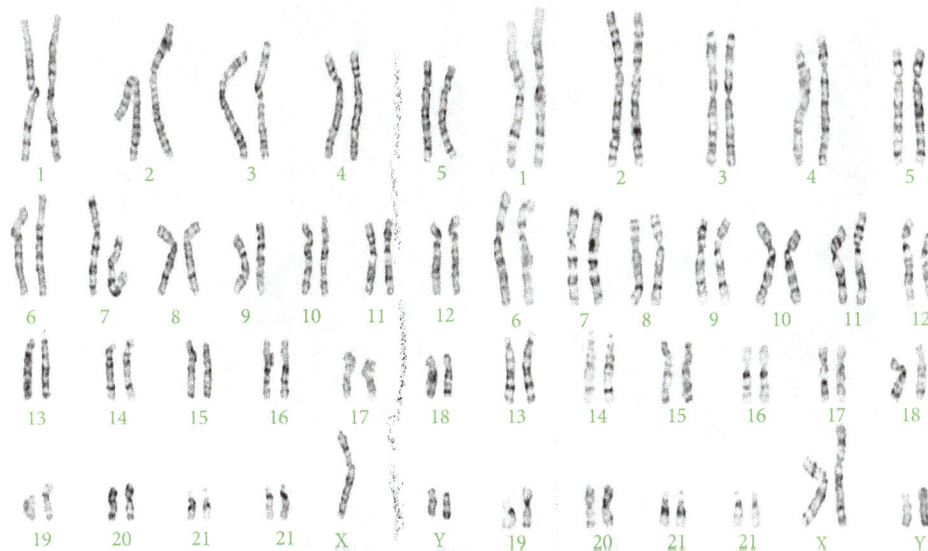

FIGURE 1: Karyotype of the patient.

during childhood or even in the adult [10]. It is now well recognized that the majority of XYY males had normal phenotype; however, variable abnormalities including skeletal, cardiovascular, and genital systems and behavioral problems have been described in the literature and can lead to clinical suspicion of the XYY syndrome. While infertility, various congenital abnormalities, and psychiatric problems were described in XXYY and XYY syndromes, the presence of renal malrotation in 48,XXYY, 47,XYY has not been reported yet. We herein report an infertile man showing XYY/XXYY syndrome associated with cognitive, affective problems and malrotation and cross ectopy of the right kidney.

2. Patient

A couple was referred to our outpatient clinic with the diagnosis of primary infertility. He was 27 years old, illiterate, and unemployed. His physical examination revealed no abnormality except for a decreased testicular volume (12 mL for the right testicle and 8 mm for the left one) and tall stature (1.85 cm and 80 kg). His wife was 24 years old and had normal menstrual cycles. Her gynecological evaluation was also normal. The patient underwent repeated semen analysis, hormonal evaluation, karyotyping of peripheral blood lymphocytes, and molecular tests for Y chromosome microdeletions. Repeated semen analysis showed azoospermia (pellet negative). Hormonal measurements were made by radioimmunoassay. The patient had increased FSH levels (21.9 mUI/mL (normal level (n): 0.7–11.1 mUI/mL)), normal LH (8.73 mUI/mL (n: 0.8–7.6 mUI/mL)), and total testosterone level 474 ng/dL (n: 262–1593 ng/dL). No AZF microdeletion was detected by two different multiplex PCR methods. Chromosomal analysis of peripheral blood lymphocytes was conducted using the standard methods. The proband proved to be a carrier of chromosomal aneuploidy that is mos 48,XXYY(17)/ 47,XYY (13) as seen in Figure 1

[10]. His partner's karyotype was found to be normal. During the examination we determined that the patient expressed cognitive and affective problems with suspected psychomotor retardation. When he was evaluated with Kent EGY test [11] and Porteus Labyrinth test [12], he appeared to have borderline intelligence, with a documented IQ of 70–80. Patient was not able to finish the elementary school. There was no family history of psychiatric or genetic disorders. It was observed that the patient had prominent negative signs which were assessed by PANSS (Positive and Negative Syndrome Scale) [13]. Additionally, systemic evaluation of patient by computerized tomography of the abdomen revealed cross ectopy and malrotation of the right kidney (Figure 2). The couple was referred to an in vitro fertilization center for micro-TESE/ICSI cycles and PGD.

3. Discussion

Klinefelter syndrome presents as XXY in all body cells in 80% of cases and as mosaic (XY/XXY) in the other 20%. Rarely can multiple line mosaicisms be found. The parents' recurrence risk for another chromosomally abnormal live birth is 1% to 2%. The 48,XXYY aneuploidy, first described by Muldal et al. in 1960, was thought for a long time to present as a cytogenetic variant of the Klinefelter syndrome [14]. Most of 48,XXYY cases are thought to result from an aneuploid sperm produced through two consecutive nondisjunction events in both meiosis I and meiosis II in a chromosomally normal father, so a boy with XXYY has one X chromosome from his mother and the additional XYY from his father [15]. In 47,XYY syndrome, the extra Y chromosome results from paternal nondisjunction at meiosis II. Those patients are usually fertile, and their sperm cells mostly contain abnormal karyotype. It has been hypothesized that one of the two Y chromosomes is lost before entering spermatogonia in meiosis. Males with 48,XXYY karyotype display neurodevelopmental disorders (ADHD and ASD), mental retardation,

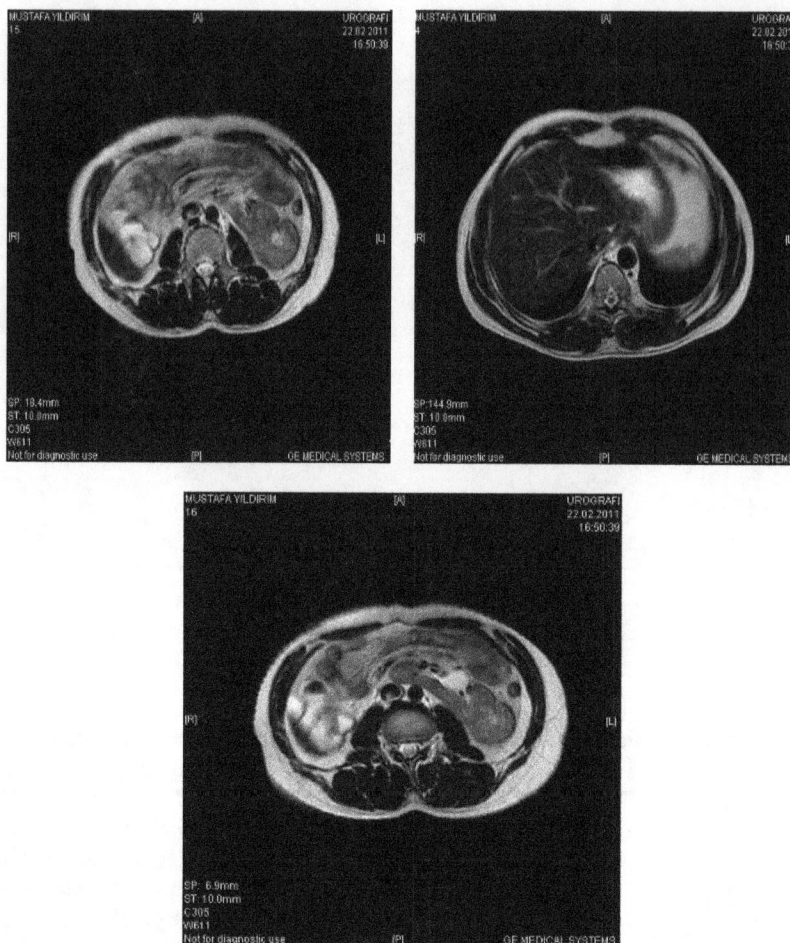

FIGURE 2: Abdominal CT showing cross ectopy and malrotation of the right kidney.

aggressive behavioral problems, hypogonadism, small testes, gynecomastia, and increased rate of varicose veins [16–18]. Males with increased numbers of extra Xs or Ys are at risk of oral language and auditory processing problems that may place them at risk of learning deficits, emotional issues, and school and/or social adjustment difficulties [11]. Males with 48,XXXY have reduced cognitive functions when compared to 48,XXYY, since addition of each X decreases the overall IQ by 15-16 points. It is difficult to precise that these specific features occurred due to the extra X or Y chromosome in these disorders, since additional Y chromosomes are often accompanied by additional X chromosomes (48,XXXY, 49,XXXXY) [9]. The most common clinical features of 47,XYY patients are tall stature, reduced IQ, and poor motor coordination together with numerous nonspecific dysmorphic features associated with minor skeletal abnormalities such as radioulnar synostosis and congenital heart diseases [19]. In the present report, the patient was unable to finish elementary school and had borderline intelligence, with a documented IQ of 70–80. In addition, the patient had negative signs which were assessed by PANSS. Those findings were consistent with the literature. Visootsak et al. suggested that males with 48,XXYY are anxious and easily frustrated

or impatient [3]. In a study of 16 males with 48,XXYY compared to 9 males with 47,XXY between the ages of 5 and 20, findings indicate that 48,XXYY males have verbal and full scale IQs significantly lower than males with 47,XXY [9]. 48,XXYY males are also prone to have problems with hyperactivity, aggression, conduct, and depression compared to males with 47,XXY. Furthermore, 48,XXYY males have significantly lower adaptive functioning than males with 47,XXY [9]. Semen analysis and hormonal measurements of the case provided the diagnosis nonobstructive azoospermia. Similar to other cases with 48,XXYY karyotype, our patient had tall stature and decreased testicular volume [6, 9]. Additionally, systemic evaluation of the patient revealed that he had cross ectopy and malrotation of the right kidney. Abdominal CT showed that the right kidney was located in the left retroperitoneal space over the left kidney and fused with the latter in a narrow area. A slight malrotation of the right kidney was also determined. Previous cases with renal aplasia and ectopy were described in 48,XXYY males; however, cross ectopy and malrotation of the kidney in 48,XXYY/47,XYY patients have not been reported in the literature yet [5, 20].

4. Conclusion

Genetic evaluation should be performed in all nonobstructive azoospermia patients. Our experience confirms that gonosomal aneuploidies with multiple X and Y chromosomes represent a distinct group of disorders that may be recognized at birth or during childhood in relation to their peculiar phenotype and neuropsychiatric profiles. However, the diagnosis of 48,XXYY/47,XYY may be delayed to adulthood. Since various skeletal, cardiac, and renal anomalies associated with this syndrome were reported, systemic evaluation should be performed in all patients.

Conflict of Interests

The authors declare that there is no conflict of interests regarding the publication of this paper.

References

[1] M. G. Linden, B. G. Bender, and A. Robinson, "Sex chromosome tetrasomy and pentasomy," *Pediatrics*, vol. 96, no. 4, part 1, pp. 672–682, 1995.

[2] J. Visootsak and J. M. Graham Jr., "Social function in multiple X and Y chromosome disorders: XXY, XYY, XXYY, XXXY," *Developmental Disabilities Research Reviews*, vol. 15, no. 4, pp. 328–332, 2009.

[3] J. Visootsak, B. Rosner, E. Dykens, N. Tartaglia, and J. M. Graham Jr., "Behavioral phenotype of sex chromosome aneuploidies: 48,XXYY, 48,XXXY, and 49,XXXXY," *American Journal of Medical Genetics, Part A*, vol. 143, no. 11, pp. 1198–1203, 2007.

[4] R. Q. Pasqualini, G. Vidal, and G. E. Bur, "Psychopathology of Klinefelter's syndrome; review of thirtyone cases," *The Lancet*, vol. 270, no. 6987, pp. 164–167, 1957.

[5] P. Katulanda, J. R. Rajapakse, J. Kariyawasam, R. Jayasekara, and V. W. Dissanayake, "An adolescent with 48,xxyy syndrome with hypergonadotrophic hypogonadism, attention deficit hyperactive disorder and renal malformations," *Indian Journal of Endocrinology and Metabolism*, vol. 16, no. 5, pp. 824–826, 2012.

[6] A. L. Gropman, A. Rogol, I. Fennoy et al., "Clinical variability and novel neurodevelopmental findings in 49, XXXXY syndrome," *American Journal of Medical Genetics, Part A*, vol. 152, no. 6, pp. 1523–1530, 2010.

[7] C. Samango-Sprouse and A. Rogol, "XXY: the hidden disability and a prototype for an infantile presentation of developmental dyspraxia (IDD)," *Infants and Young Children*, vol. 15, no. 1, pp. 11–18, 2002.

[8] J. L. Ross, D. P. Roeltgen, H. Kushner et al., "Behavioral and social phenotypes in boys with 47,XYY syndrome or 47,XXY Klinefelter syndrome," *Pediatrics*, vol. 129, no. 4, pp. 769–778, 2012.

[9] N. Tartaglia, S. Davis, A. Hench et al., "A new look at XXYY syndrome: medical and psychological features," *American Journal of Medical Genetics, Part A*, vol. 146, no. 12, pp. 1509–1522, 2008.

[10] L. Mutesa, M. Jamar, A. C. Hellin, G. Pierquin, and V. Bours, "A new 48,XXYY/47,XYY syndrome associated with multiple skeletal abnormalities, congenital heart disease and mental retardation," *Indian Journal of Human Genetics*, vol. 18, no. 3, pp. 352–355, 2012.

[11] H. A. Delp, "Correlations between the Kent EGY and the Wechsler batteries," *Journal of Clinical Psychology*, vol. 9, no. 1, pp. 73–75, 1953.

[12] N. Öner, *Psychologic Tests Used in Turkey*, Bogazici Universitesi Yayinlari, Istanbul, Turkey, 1997.

[13] S. R. Kay, A. Fiszbein, and L. A. Opler, "The positive and negative syndrome scale (PANSS) for schizophrenia," *Schizophrenia Bulletin*, vol. 13, no. 2, pp. 261–276, 1987.

[14] S. Muldal, C. H. Ockey, M. Thompson, and L. L. White, "'Double male'-a new chromosome constitution in the Klinefelter syndrome," *Acta Endocrinologica*, vol. 39, pp. 183–203, 1962.

[15] Genetic Home Reference, XXYY Syndrome, 2010.

[16] M. Borghgraef, J. P. Fryns, and H. Van Den Berghe, "The 48,XXYY syndrome. Follow-up data on clinical characteristics and psychological findings in 4 patients," *Genetic Counseling*, vol. 2, no. 2, pp. 103–108, 1991.

[17] J. Díaz-Atienza and M. P. Blánquez-Rodríguez, "Behavioral and neuropsychological phenotype of the 48,XXYY syndrome: a longitudinal study of a case," *Revista de Neurología*, vol. 29, no. 10, pp. 926–929, 1999.

[18] N. Borja-Santos, B. Trancas, P. S. Pinto et al., "48,XXYY in a general adult psychiatry department," *Psychiatry (Edgemont)*, vol. 7, no. 3, pp. 32–36, 2010.

[19] J. Visootsak, N. Ayari, S. Howell, J. Lazarus, and N. Tartaglia, "Timing of diagnosis of 47,XXY and 48,XXYY: a survey of parent experiences," *American Journal of Medical Genetics, Part A*, vol. 161, no. 2, pp. 268–272, 2013.

[20] B. Zantour, M. H. Sfar, S. Younes et al., "48XXYY syndrome in an adult with type 2 diabetes mellitus, unilateral renal aplasia, and pigmentary retinitis," *Case Reports in Medicine*, vol. 2010, Article ID 612315, 5 pages, 2010.

31

Meningocele in a Congolese Female with Beckwith-Wiedemann Phenotype

Sébastien Mbuyi-Musanzayi,[1,2] Toni Lubala Kasole,[2,3] Aimé Lumaka,[4,5]
Tony Kayembe Kitenge,[6] Leon Kabamba Ngombe,[6] Prosper Kalenga Muenze,[2,7]
Prosper Lukusa Tshilobo,[4,5] François Tshilombo Katombe,[1]
Célestin Banza Lubaba Nkulu,[6] and Koenraad Devriendt[5]

[1]Department of Surgery, University Hospital, University of Lubumbashi, P.O. Box 1825,
Lubumbashi, Democratic Republic of the Congo
[2]Center for Human Genetics, Faculty of Medicine, University of Lubumbashi, P.O. Box 1825,
Lubumbashi, Democratic Republic of the Congo
[3]Department of Pediatrics, University Hospital, University of Lubumbashi, P.O. Box 1825,
Lubumbashi, Democratic Republic of the Congo
[4]Department of Pediatrics, University Hospital, University of Kinshasa, P.O. Box 123, Kin XI,
Kinshasa, Democratic Republic of the Congo
[5]Center for Human Genetics, University Hospital, KU Leuven, Campus Gasthuisberg, Herestraat 49, P.O. Box 602,
3000 Leuven, Belgium
[6]Unit of Toxicology and Environment, School of Public Health, University Hospital, University of Lubumbashi,
P.O. Box 1825, Lubumbashi, Democratic Republic of the Congo
[7]Department of Gynecology, University Hospital, University of Lubumbashi, P.O. Box 1825,
Lubumbashi, Democratic Republic of the Congo

Correspondence should be addressed to Koenraad Devriendt; koenraad.devriendt@uzleuven.be

Academic Editor: Patrick Morrison

Beckwith-Wiedemann syndrome (BWS) is a rare congenital syndrome characterized by an overgrowth, macroglossia, exomphalos, and predisposition to embryonal tumors. Central nervous abnormalities associated with BWS are rare. We describe a one-day-old Congolese female who presented meningocele associated with BWS phenotype.

1. Introduction

Beckwith-Wiedemann syndrome (BWS) is a rare congenital disorder with an incidence of one in 13.700 live births [1, 2]. Initially, its designation was EMG (exomphalos-macroglossia-gigantism syndrome) and was characterized by a triad of an overgrowth, macroglossia, and exomphalos or umbilical hernia [3]. Other features were observed being associated with the triad, such as umbilical hernia, organomegaly (liver, spleen, or kidneys), neonatal hypoglycemia, minor ear anomalies, nevus flammeus, cleft palate, or embryonal tumor development [4, 5]. The clinical features of BWS are variable, and it is accepted that the diagnosis can be established if three major diagnostic findings are present [6]. Its etiology is heterogeneous, arising from dysregulation of one or both imprinting control regions (IC) and/or imprinted growth regulatory genes of the chromosome 11p15.5 [7]. BWS occurs with the same frequency in male and female [8]. Central nervous system anomalies are rare in BWS, but as far as we know not a single case has been described presenting meningocele. Here we present a female newborn who presented meningocele associated with the BWS phenotype.

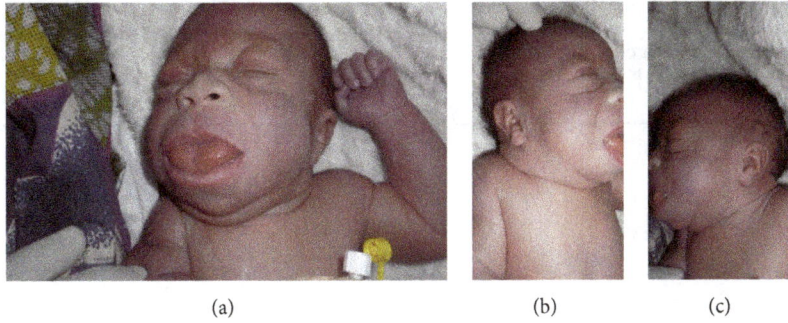

FIGURE 1: Facial signs: note (a) macroglossia and nevus flammeus on the face; (b) crumped helix on her right ear; (c) ear crease on the left lobe.

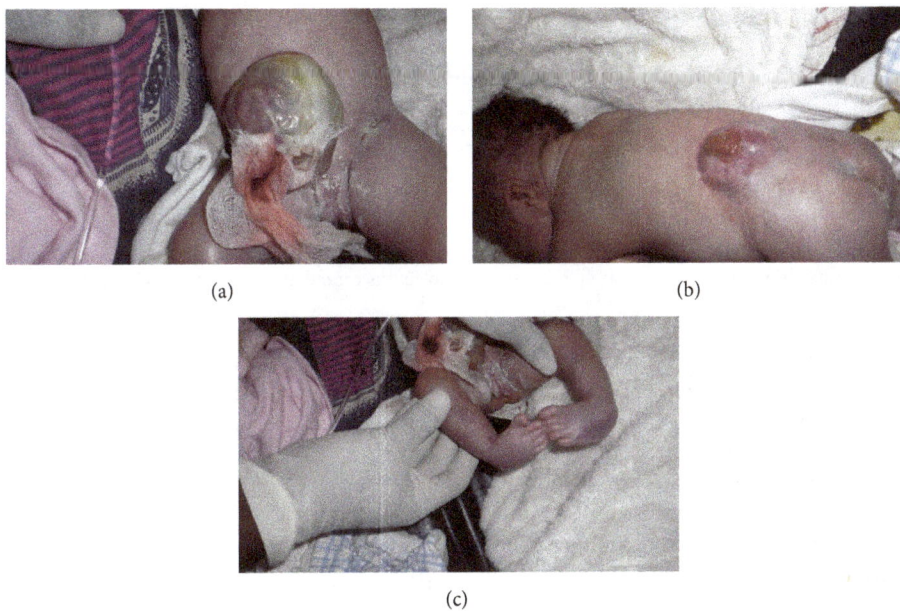

FIGURE 2: Other features: note (a) exomphalos, (b) meningocele, and (c) bilateral club feet.

2. Case Report

The index case is a one-day-old female, born at 39 weeks of gestation via normal spontaneous vaginal delivery with a birth weight of 4400 g (+4 SD, CDC growth charts). Her mother was 27 years, her father was 30 years old, and both were healthy and unrelated. Family history was marked by a primary infertility for 10 years. The mother had many gynecological consultations and medical treatment that she ignored during the last two years. During gestation she had a urinary infection treated with amoxicillin during the first trimester and treatment of threatened miscarriage. She took clay during the entire pregnancy. She received vaccination during the second trimester of gestation. Two prenatal ultrasound scans were performed, one during the first trimester and the second during the second trimester. Both did not show any anomaly. At birth on clinical examination, we observed macroglossia with protruding tongue, nevus flammeus on her face (Figure 1(a)). She presented crumped helix on her right ear

and ear creases on the left lobe (Figures 1(b) and 1(c)). She had an omphalocele containing intestines (Figure 2(a)), a lumbosacral meningocele, and bilateral club feet (Figures 2(b) and 2(c)). She developed acute respiratory distress and died within six hours after birth.

3. Discussion

We present a newborn female, who presented an unusual association, meningocele associated with BWS phenotype. The diagnosis of BWS was based on the classical clinic triad of overgrowth, macroglossia, and exomphalos, associated with some additional minor features such as ear anomalies and frontal hemangioma. The diagnosis could not be confirmed by genetic studies, since the child died prematurely, before DNA could be obtained. The distinctive feature in the present case is lumbosacral meningocele. Central nervous abnormalities associated with BWS are rare, mostly involving

TABLE 1: Central nervous features associated with BWS.

Study Year	Worth et al. [9] 1999	Yamada et al. [10] 1999	Tubbs and Oakes [11] 2005	Russo et al. [12] 2006	Broekman et al. [13] 2008	Kent et al. [14] 2008	Bui et al. [15] 2009	Gardiner et al. [16] 2012	This report 2014
Brain abnormalities									
Abnormal cerebellar vermis	—	—	—	+*	—	—	—	—	—
Arteriovenous malformations	—	+	—	—	—	—	—	—	—
Blake's pouch cyst	—	—	—	—	—	—	—	2/7	—
Chiari malformation	—	—	+	—	—	—	—	—	—
Dandy-Walker malformation	—	—	—	—	—	—	—	3/7	—
Dandy-Walker variant	—	—	—	—	—	—	—	4/7	—
Encephalocele (nasal)	—	—	—	—	+	—	—	—	—
Hydrocephalus	—	—	—	—	—	+	—	—	—
Posterior fossa structures abnormalities	—	—	—	—	—	—	+	—	—
Schizencephaly	+	—	—	—	—	—	—	—	—
Meningocele	—	—	—	—	—	—	—	—	+

*In this case, the associated terminal deletion of chromosome 4p may possibly explain the central nervous system malformation.

the brain (reviewed in Table 1). It is not excluded that this represents a chance association of two pathogenetically unrelated conditions, and the lack of genetic testing is a weakness of this report. Alternatively, given the previous reports of CNS anomalies in other cases with BWS, it is not excluded that the underlying genetic cause of BWS may also predispose to brain malformations (including neural tube defects), especially when imprinting defect involves the imprinting domain 2 at chromosome 11p15.5 [16].

Conflict of Interests

None of the authors has a conflict of interests to disclose in relation to this work.

Authors' Contribution

Sébastien Mbuyi-Musanzayi did clinical examination, treatment of the patient, and redaction of paper. Toni Lubala Kasole did clinical examination. Aimé Lumaka did paper correction. Tony Kayembe Kitenge did clinical examination. Leon Kabamba Ngombe did clinical examination. Prosper Lukusa Tshilobo and Prosper Kalenga Muenze did paper correction. François Tshilombo Katombe did clinical examination. Koenraad Devriendt did clinical examination, diagnosis, and paper corrections. All coauthors have read, contributed to, and approved the paper.

Acknowledgments

The authors thank the family of the patient for their kind cooperation and the Center for Human Genetics, KU Leuven, for support. Sébastien Mbuyi-Musanzayi was supported by a scholarship from interfaculty Council for Development Cooperation (IRO), KU Leuven, and GROS, Holsbeek (Belgium).

References

[1] W. Engstrom, S. Lindham, and P. Schofield, "Wiedemann-Beckwith syndrome," European Journal of Pediatrics, vol. 147, no. 5, pp. 450–457, 1988.

[2] M. J. Thorburn, E. S. Wright, C. G. Miller, and E. H. Smith-Read, "Exomphalos-macroglossia-gigantism syndrome in Jamaican infants," American Journal of Diseases of Children, vol. 119, no. 4, pp. 316–321, 1970.

[3] H. R. Wiedemann, "Familial malformation complex with umbilical hernia and macroglossia—a "new syndrome"?" Journal of Genetics in Human Molecular, vol. 13, pp. 223–232, 1964.

[4] J. R. Engel, A. Smallwood, A. Harper et al., "Epigenotype-phenotype correlations in Beckwith-Wiedemann syndrome," Journal of Medical Genetics, vol. 37, no. 12, pp. 921–926, 2000.

[5] J. Demars, Y. le Bouc, A. El-Osta, and C. Gicquel, "Epigenetic and genetic mechanisms of abnormal 11p15 genomic imprinting in Silver-Russell and Beckwith-Wiedemann syndromes," Current Medicinal Chemistry, vol. 18, no. 12, pp. 1740–1750, 2011.

[6] R. Weksberg, C. Shuman, and A. C. Smith, "Beckwith-Wiedemann syndrome," American Journal of Medical Genetics, vol. 137, no. 1, pp. 12–23, 2005.

[7] K. Delaval, A. Wagschal, and R. Feil, "Epigenetic deregulation of imprinting in congenital diseases of aberrant growth," BioEssays, vol. 28, no. 5, pp. 453–459, 2006.

[8] M. J. Pettenati, J. L. Haines, R. R. Higgins, R. S. Wappner, C. G. Palmer, and D. D. Weaver, "Wiedemann-Beckwith syndrome:

presentation of clinical and cytogenetic data on 22 new cases and review of the literature," *Human Genetics*, vol. 74, no. 2, pp. 143–154, 1986.

[9] L. L. Worth, J. M. Slopis, and C. E. Herzog, "Congenital hepatoblastoma and schizencephaly in an infant with Beckwith-Wiedemann syndrome," *Medical Pediatric Oncology*, vol. 33, no. 6, pp. 591–593, 1999.

[10] K. Yamada, M. Miura, T. Ikeda, H. Miyayama, and Y. Ushio, "Ruptured arteriovenous malformation in a boy with Beckwith-Wiedemann syndrome," *Pediatric Neurosurgery*, vol. 31, no. 3, pp. 163–167, 1999.

[11] R. S. Tubbs and W. J. Oakes, "Beckwith-Wiedemann syndrome in a child with Chiari I malformation: case report," *Journal of Neurosurgery*, vol. 103, no. 2, pp. 172–174, 2005.

[12] S. Russo, P. Finelli, M. P. Recalcati et al., "Molecular and genomic characterisation of cryptic chromosomal alterations leading to paternal duplication of the 11p15.5 Beckwith-Wiedemann region," *Journal of Medical Genetics*, vol. 43, no. 8, p. e39, 2006.

[13] M. L. D. Broekman, E. W. Hoving, K. H. Kho, L. Speleman, K. S. Han, and P. W. Hanlo, "Nasal encephalocele in a child with Beckwith-Wiedemann syndrome: case report," *Journal of Neurosurgery: Pediatrics*, vol. 1, no. 6, pp. 485–487, 2008.

[14] L. Kent, S. Bowdin, G. A. Kirby, W. N. Cooper, and E. R. Maher, "Beckwith Weidemann syndrome: a behavioral phenotype-genotype study," *American Journal of Medical Genetics Part B: Neuropsychiatric Genetics*, vol. 147, no. 7, pp. 1295–1297, 2008.

[15] C. Bui, O. Picone, A. E. Mas et al., "Beckwith-Wiedemann syndrome in association with posterior hypoplasia of the cerebellar vermis," *Prenatal Diagnosis*, vol. 29, no. 9, pp. 906–907, 2009.

[16] K. Gardiner, D. Chitayat, S. Choufani et al., "Brain abnormalities in patients with Beckwith-Wiedemann syndrome," *American Journal of Medical Genetics Part A*, vol. 158, no. 6, pp. 1388–1394, 2012.

32

Rare Manifestation of a c.290 C>T, p.Gly97Glu *VCP* Mutation

Nivedita U. Jerath,[1] Cameron D. Crockett,[1] Steven A. Moore,[1,2] Michael E. Shy,[1]
Conrad C. Weihl,[3] Tsui-Fen Chou,[4] Tiffany Grider,[1] Michael A. Gonzalez,[5]
Stephan Zuchner,[5] and Andrea Swenson[1]

[1]*Department of Neurology, Carver College of Medicine, University of Iowa, Iowa City, IA 52242, USA*
[2]*Department of Pathology, Carver College of Medicine, University of Iowa, Iowa City, IA 52242, USA*
[3]*Department of Neurology, Washington University School of Medicine, St. Louis, MO 63110, USA*
[4]*Division of Medical Genetics, Department of Pediatrics, Harbor-UCLA Medical Centre,*
 Los Angeles Biomedical Research Institute, Torrance, CA 90502, USA
[5]*Dr. John T. Macdonald Foundation Department of Human Genetics and John P. Hussman Institute for Human Genomics,*
 University of Miami Miller School of Medicine, 1501 NW 10 Avenue, Miami, FL 33136, USA

Correspondence should be addressed to Nivedita U. Jerath; njerath@post.harvard.edu

Academic Editor: Patrick Morrison

Introduction. The valosin-containing protein (VCP) regulates several distinct cellular processes. Consistent with this, *VCP* mutations manifest variable clinical phenotypes among and within families and are a diagnostic challenge. *Methods*. A 60-year-old man who played ice hockey into his 50's was evaluated by electrodiagnostics, muscle biopsy, and molecular genetics. *Results*. With long-standing pes cavus and toe walking, our patient developed progressive weakness, cramps, memory loss, and paresthesias at age 52. An axonal sensorimotor neuropathy was found upon repeated testing at age 58. Neuropathic histopathology was present in the quadriceps, and exome sequencing revealed the *VCP* mutation c.290 C>T, p.Gly97Glu. *Conclusions*. Our patient reflects the clinical heterogeneity of VCP mutations, as his neurological localization is a spectrum between a lower motor neuron disorder and a hereditary axonal peripheral neuropathy such as CMT2. Our case demonstrates a rare manifestation of the c.290 C>T, pGly97Glu *VCP* mutation.

1. Introduction

The valosin-containing protein (VCP) has been demonstrated to play a critical role in the maintenance of protein homeostasis through the regulation of protein degradation pathways [1]. Mutations in the gene encoding VCP lead to disruption of autophagy and have been shown to manifest within families as a phenotypically heterogeneous group of presentations including hereditary inclusion body myopathy (IBM), Paget's disease of the bone (PDB), and frontotemporal dementia (FTD), which are known collectively as IBMPFD [2]. More recently, mutations in *VCP* have been implicated as having a role in familial amyotrophic lateral sclerosis (ALS) [3]. Although there is variability in the phenotypic

manifestations of *VCP* mutations within families, *VCP*-related disease is inherited in an autosomal dominant manner [2, 3]. Attempts at determining genotype-phenotype correlations for mutations in the *VCP* gene have been unsuccessful, though analysis of the two most common mutations (p.Arg155Cys and p.Arg155His) showed a significant variation in survival between the groups, suggesting that mutation variants may hold clinical relevance for patients [4].

We report a case of a patient presenting for evaluation of progressive lower extremity weakness and paresthesias in the context of family history of ALS, dementia, and PDB. Exome sequencing revealed a previously reported c.290 C>T, p.Gly97Glu mutation in *VCP*; our patient's phenotype is different from the previously reported case of IBMPFD [5].

(a)

(b)

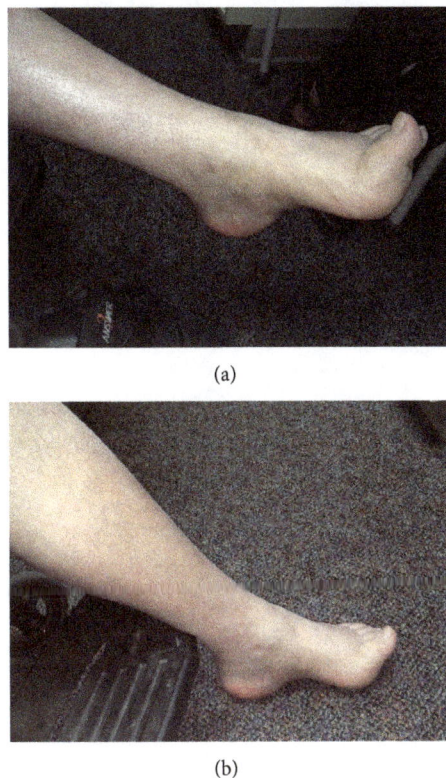

FIGURE 1: Evidence of pes cavus and hammer toes in our patient.

The clinical presentation along a continuum from an axonal sensorimotor polyneuropathy to a lower motor neuronopathy in this patient expands the known clinical phenotypes of *VCP*-related disease.

2. Case Report

The proband is a 60-year-old man of Dutch and Italian descent who was the product of a normal pregnancy and delivery. Although he was a toe walker with high arches and hammertoes, he reached his developmental milestones (including walking) on time. In grade school, he kept up with his peers but was always the slowest runner. He rode a bicycle and played ice hockey until age 52 when he sprained his left ankle and began noticing progressive left greater than right leg weakness. At age 55, he began noticing paresthesias and numbness in his toes with the left side worse than the right. By age 57, holding his trumpet was difficult, although he could still play it well. Three years later, he was unable to climb stairs, had multiple falls, and began to use a walker. He later developed cramps in his hands and trouble with fine finger dexterity. Additionally, he noticed memory and word-finding difficulties.

Upon neurological examination in our clinic at age 60, he presented with bilateral scapular winging, lumbar lordosis, pes cavus, hammer toes, and tight heel cords (Figure 1). Strength exam (MRC scale) demonstrated proximal upper and proximal/distal lower extremity weakness. There was weakness in trapezius (R/L) 3/3 with scapular winging as well

as weakness in the iliopsoas 4+/4+, quadriceps 4+/5, knee flexion 4/4, foot dorsiflexion 1/4, and foot plantar flexion 4+/5. Vibratory sense and pinprick were decreased distally in the lower extremities. Deep tendon reflexes were depressed throughout the upper and lower extremities with absent ankle jerks and downgoing toes. There was no tremor. Cerebellar testing was normal. Gait was wide-based with bilateral steppage; he was unable to walk 25 feet independently due to the weakness in his lower extremities. Speech and language were intact. Cranial nerves were normal including facial strength, facial sensation, and tongue strength. No fasciculations were noted on exam. Of note, he did not develop any upper motor neuron signs over the years including hyperreflexia, dysphagia, dysarthria, or dyspnea.

Laboratory testing included creatine kinase level of 930 u/L (normal 40–200 u/L) and a normal alkaline phosphatase level.

2.1. Electrodiagnostic Exam. Although the abnormalities on the EMG remained constant, nerve conduction studies (NCS) changed over time.

At age 56, needle EMG revealed fibrillations, positive sharp waves, fasciculations, and large amplitude motor unit potentials with reduced recruitment in bilateral tibialis anterior, bilateral vastus lateralis, left gastrocnemius, left deltoid, left first dorsal interosseous, and left thoracic paraspinal musculature. Nerve conduction studies of the left ulnar, sural, and tibial nerves were normal. At this time, the impression was a lower motor neuron syndrome.

At age 58, although the EMG remained the same, sensory and motor nerve conduction studies were now abnormal. The left median, ulnar, and peroneal motor nerve conduction velocities were normal. Compound muscle action potentials (CMAPs) of the left median, ulnar, and peroneal nerves were normal. Sensory nerve action potentials (SNAPs) of the left median, radial, and superficial peroneal nerves were normal; right ulnar SNAP had reduced amplitude (13 uV). The left sural and superficial peroneal sensory responses were absent; right sural sensory responses had reduced amplitude (4 uV). Left median and ulnar distal motor latencies were prolonged (5.5 ms and 4.2 ms, resp.); left median sensory distal latency was mildly prolonged at 4.0 ms. At this time, the impression was an axonal sensorimotor neuropathy.

The axonal sensorimotor neuropathy was worked up for acquired causes. Laboratory testing included normal thyroid stimulating hormone, serum protein electrophoresis, serum immunofixation, vitamin B-12, and fasting glucose.

2.2. Muscle Biopsy. Muscle biopsy of the quadriceps at age 60 revealed chronic, active neurogenic atrophy. Paraffin and frozen H&E sections, NADH, and trichrome staining revealed skeletal muscle with moderate variation in fiber size due to the presence of angulated, atrophic fibers in small groups (Figure 2(a)). Immunoperoxidase stains for slow and fast myosin heavy chains revealed small fiber type groups (Figures 2(b) and 2(c)). Rare targetoid fibers were seen (not shown here). Some muscle fascicles had end stage muscle pathology (Figure 2(d)), likely the result of longstanding

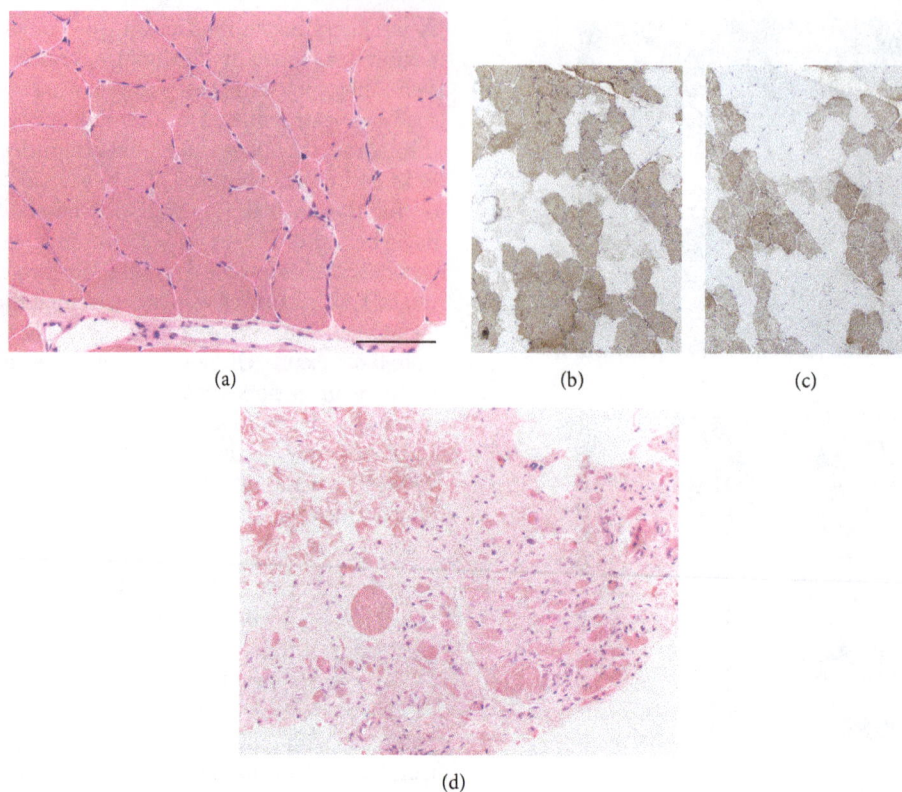

FIGURE 2: Muscle biopsy of the quadriceps revealed chronic active neurogenic atrophy ((a), H&E). Fiber type grouping is seen in immunoperoxidase staining for both slow myosin (b) and fast myosin (c). Some muscle fascicles are much more severely affected and show features of end stage muscle (d). Scale bar = 100 μm in panels (a) and (d); 150 μm in panels (b) and (c).

neuropathic disease. No inflammation, myonecrosis, regeneration, endomysial fibrosis, inclusion bodies, rimmed vacuoles, or ragged-red fibers were identified. All fibers stained positively for cytochrome C oxidase.

2.3. Neuropsychological Testing. Neuropsychological testing revealed only mild impairments as he was noted to have high average to superior baseline functioning. He had only mild weakness in speed of information processing, problem solving, fine motor dexterity, speed in visual motor sequencing, rapid cognitive shifting, verbal memory, and short-term memory for simple geometric designs. He had an otherwise normal performance in all other areas (verbal, nonverbal intellectual skills, single word reading, and language). He was diagnosed with cognitive deficits, not otherwise specified.

2.4. Family History. Further investigation into the patient's family history disclosed his father's diagnoses of ALS, dementia, and PDB (Figure 3(a)). Muscle biopsy results from the father are not available. One sister had flat, narrow feet. The patient's teenage daughter has high arches and was a toe walker as a child; she has not had a neurological evaluation and further evaluation has been declined at this time. His other teenage daughter is currently asymptomatic. There is no family history of IBM.

2.5. Genetic Testing. Exome sequencing was performed and revealed the *VCP* mutation c.290 C>T, p.Gly97Glu, G97E. This same mutation resulting in the same amino acid substitution has been reported in five family members with PDB. All five affected individuals had varying degrees of muscle weakness diagnosed as inclusion body myopathy, and none have FTD [5].

3. Discussion

Phenotypic variability is a hallmark of VCP-related disease. VCP is a member of the type II AAA+ ATPase family mapped to 9p13.3 that is ubiquitously expressed at high levels and exerts an influence on a variety of cellular activities including cell cycle progression, DNA damage repair, the ubiquitin-proteasome system, and autophagic processes [7–9]. This variation in physiological activity allows for an equally impressive range of pathological manifestations to arise from mutations in the *VCP* gene, including IBM, PDB, FTD, and ALS [10]. We believe the *VCP* mutation c.290 C>T, p.Gly97Glu, G97E mutation is pathogenic because the mutation in our patient shows increased ATPase activity, similar to other *VCP* mutations (Figure 3(b)).

Our patient's presentation is not straightforward clinically. It is not simply a hereditary axonal sensorimotor polyneuropathy (given the asymmetry and bilateral scapular

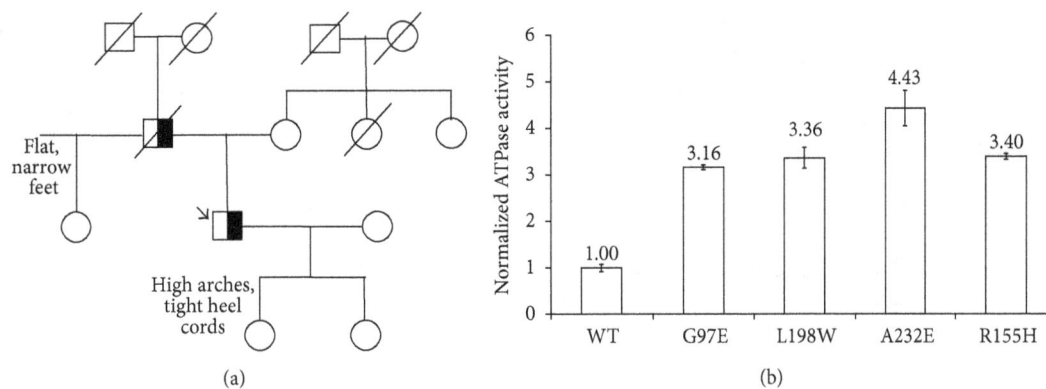

(a)

(b)

FIGURE 3: (a) Family Pedigree. Squares indicate men; circles, women; diagonal lines, deceased; black, VCP mutation. An arrow indicates the proband. (b) ATPase activity data that shows that the G97E (Gly97Glu mutation) has increased ATPase activity similar to other mutants. The detailed method was described previously [6]. Purified human p97 proteins (25 nM monomer final concentration) were used in Assay Buffer (50 mM Tris pH 7.4, 20 mM MgCl$_2$, 1 mM EDTA, and 0.5 mM TCEP) containing 0.01% Triton X-100 and 200 μM ATP. ATPase activity was determined by addition of Biomol Green Reagent (Enzo Life Sciences). Absorbance at 635 nm was measured after 4 min on the Synergy Neo Microplate Reader (BioTek).

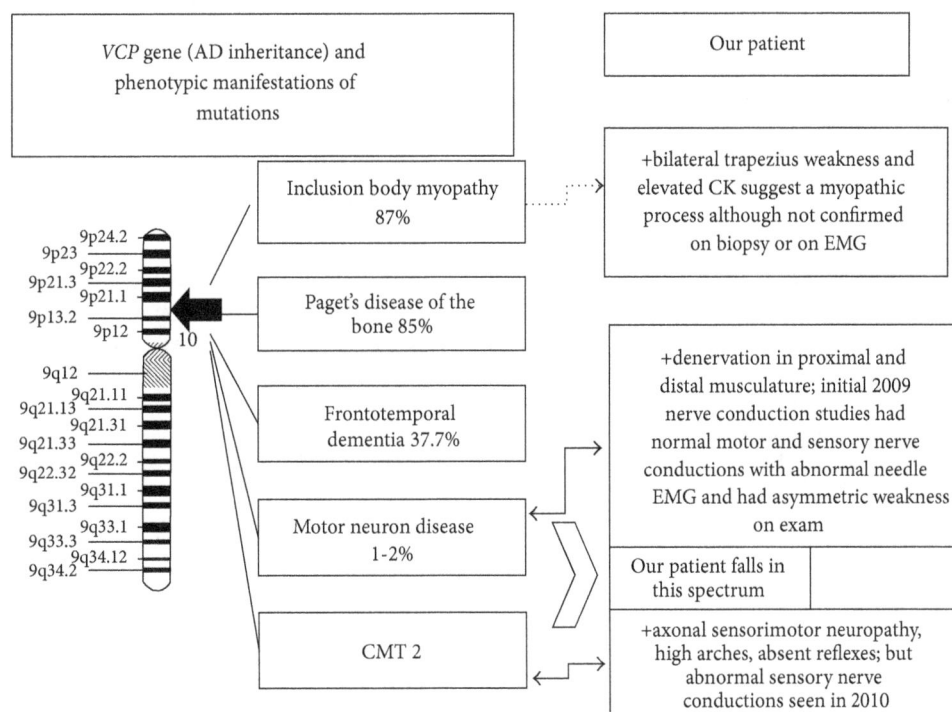

FIGURE 4: Spectrum of phenotypic manifestations seen in our patient with a VCP mutation.

winging), a purely lower motor neuron syndrome (given the bilateral scapular winging and sensory nerve conduction abnormality) nor a myopathy (despite elevated CK and scapular winging, there were no myopathic features on quadriceps muscle biopsy). We propose that our patient presents along a spectrum of a lower motor neuron syndrome and axonal neuropathy (Figure 4). The difficulty in diagnosing a VCP-related condition is due to this extreme heterogeneity in clinical presentations. A recent study demonstrates that a VCP mutation can result in CMT 2 further validating

the phenotypic variability seen in patients with a VCP mutation [11]. Of note, exome sequencing was negative for other genetic variants that are known to cause CMT and a lower motor neuron disease phenotype; this included the HSPB, BSCL2, GARS, DCTN1, SLC5A7, FBX038, IGHMBP2, ATP7A, and SETX genes.

Of those individuals reported with VCP mutations, 87.7% presented with IBM, 45% with PDB, and 37.7% with FTD [12]. VCP mutations are also estimated to be the cause of 1-2% of familial ALS cases [3]. Further complicating this clinical scenario is the incomplete penetrance of phenotypes of IBM, PDB, and FTD as well as the variability in presentation for *VCP*-related ALS [12, 13]. The Gly97Glu mutation was previously reported in both affected and unaffected members of one family, suggesting that the mutation may not be fully penetrant [5]. *VCP* mutations have also been demonstrated to manifest with variable upper motor neuron signs or bulbar findings. EMG results can be neuropathic or myopathic, with many displaying mixed morphology [13]. Other features have been observed less frequently in VCP disease, including dilated cardiomyopathy, cataracts, and axonal sensorimotor polyneuropathy [10].

Because of the variability in clinical presentations, the family history is critical. Mutations in *VCP* are transmitted in an autosomal dominant fashion. Obtaining a pedigree that includes IBM, PDB, FTD, or ALS throughout multiple family members may lead to the consideration of *VCP* sequencing as a diagnostic step. Furthermore, repeated electrodiagnostic testing can be critical to evaluate the progression of the disease. Our case demonstrates how the electrodiagnostic testing changed over the years from the initial electrodiagnostic diagnosis of a lower motor neuron syndrome to the later diagnosis of motor neuron disease plus a sensorimotor axonal neuropathy. Although the neuropathy could be a manifestation of CMT 2 given his long-standing toe walking and pes cavus, the appearance of the neuropathy on electrodiagnostic testing was late. Basic testing for acquired neuropathies was unrevealing, and thus the electrodiagnostic changes could possibly reflect a late onset hereditary neuropathy like CMT 2.

Here we present a case with variable phenotypic manifestations ranging from an axonal sensorimotor polyneuropathy to a lower motor neuron syndrome or even a myopathy all arising from a mutation in the gene encoding *VCP*. This novel presentation further expands the clinical phenotype associated with *VCP* mutations and suggests that sequencing for this gene should be considered for any patients presenting with these symptoms who have family history positive for IBM, PDB, FTD, or ALS.

Consent

Informed consent was obtained from the patient.

Conflict of Interests

The authors declare that there is no conflict of interests regarding the publication of this paper.

Acknowledgments

Michael E. Shy would like to acknowledge support from the National Institute of Neurological Disorders and Stroke (NINDS) and Office of Rare Diseases (U54, NS065712) as well as grants from the Muscular Dystrophy Association (MDA) and Charcot Marie Tooth Association (CMTA). Nivedita U. Jerath would like to acknowledge support from an MDA Clinical Research Training grant and a University of Iowa Internal Funding Initiatives award. Cameron D. Crockett received funding by NIH through the Iowa Wellstone Muscular Dystrophy Cooperative Research Center (U54, NS053672). Steven A. Moore is supported in part by NIH through the Iowa Wellstone Muscular Dystrophy Cooperative Research Center (U54, NS053672). Tsui-Fen Chou is supported by the National Center for Advancing Translational Sciences through UCLA CTSI Grant UL1TR000124 and the LA BioMed Seed Grant program (20826-01) and is a member of UCLA Johnson Comprehensive Cancer Center.

References

[1] J.-S. Ju, R. A. Fuentealba, S. E. Miller et al., "Valosin-containing protein (VCP) is required for autophagy and is disrupted in VCP disease," *The Journal of Cell Biology*, vol. 187, no. 6, pp. 875–888, 2009.

[2] G. D. J. Watts, J. Wymer, M. J. Kovach et al., "Inclusion body myopathy associated with Paget disease of bone and frontotemporal dementia is caused by mutant valosin-containing protein," *Nature Genetics*, vol. 36, no. 4, pp. 377–381, 2004.

[3] J. O. Johnson, J. Mandrioli, M. Benatar et al., "Exome sequencing reveals VCP mutations as a cause of familial ALS," *Neuron*, vol. 68, no. 5, pp. 857–864, 2010.

[4] S. G. Mehta, M. Khare, R. Ramani et al., "Genotype-phenotype studies of VCP-associated inclusion body myopathy with Paget disease of bone and/or frontotemporal dementia," *Clinical Genetics*, vol. 83, no. 5, pp. 422–431, 2013.

[5] J.-M. Gu, Y.-H. Ke, H. Yue et al., "A novel VCP mutation as the cause of atypical IBMPFD in a Chinese family," *Bone*, vol. 52, no. 1, pp. 9–16, 2013.

[6] T.-F. Chou, S. L. Bulfer, C. C. Weihl et al., "Specific inhibition of p97/VCP ATPase and kinetic analysis demonstrate interaction between D1 and D2 ATPase domains," *Journal of Molecular Biology*, vol. 426, no. 15, pp. 2886–2899, 2014.

[7] F. Bartolome, H.-C. Wu, V. S. Burchell et al., "Pathogenic VCP mutations induce mitochondrial uncoupling and reduced ATP levels," *Neuron*, vol. 78, no. 1, pp. 57–64, 2013.

[8] J.-S. Ju and C. C. Weihl, "Inclusion body myopathy, Paget's disease of the bone and fronto-temporal dementia: a disorder of autophagy," *Human Molecular Genetics*, vol. 19, no. 1, pp. R38–R45, 2010.

[9] Y. Iguchi, M. Katsuno, K. Ikenaka, S. Ishigaki, and G. Sobue, "Amyotrophic lateral sclerosis: an update on recent genetic insights," *Journal of Neurology*, vol. 260, no. 11, pp. 2917–2927, 2013.

[10] A. Nalbandian, S. Donkervoort, E. Dec et al., "The multiple faces of valosin-containing protein-associated diseases: inclusion body myopathy with Paget's disease of bone, frontotemporal dementia, and amyotrophic lateral sclerosis," *Journal of Molecular Neuroscience*, vol. 45, no. 3, pp. 522–531, 2011.

[11] M. A. Gonzalez, S. M. Feely, F. Speziani et al., "A novel mutation in VCP causes charcot-marie-tooth type 2 disease," *Brain*, vol. 137, no. 11, pp. 2897–2902, 2014.

[12] V. E. Kimonis, E. Fulchiero, J. Vesa, and G. Watts, "VCP disease associated with myopathy, Paget disease of bone and frontotemporal dementia: review of a unique disorder," *Biochimica et Biophysica Acta*, vol. 1782, no. 12, pp. 744–748, 2008.

[13] M. Benatar, J. Wuu, C. Fernandez et al., "Motor neuron involvement in multisystem proteinopathy: implications for ALS," *Neurology*, vol. 80, no. 20, pp. 1874–1880, 2013.

33

Identification of *SLC22A5* Gene Mutation in a Family with Carnitine Uptake Defect

Hatice Mutlu-Albayrak,[1] **Judit Bene,**[2,3] **Mehmet Burhan Oflaz,**[4] **Tijen Tanyalçın,**[5] **Hüseyin Çaksen,**[1] **and Bela Melegh**[2,3]

[1]*Division of Pediatric Genetics, Department of Pediatrics, Meram Medical Faculty, University of Necmettin Erbakan, Meram, 42080 Konya, Turkey*
[2]*Department of Medical Genetics, University of Pécs, Pécs, Hungary*
[3]*Szentagothai Research Centre, University of Pécs, Pécs, Hungary*
[4]*Division of Pediatric Cardiology, Department of Pediatrics, Meram Medical Faculty, University of Necmettin Erbakan, Meram, 42080 Konya, Turkey*
[5]*Tanyalcin Medical Laboratory, Selective Screening and Metabolism Unit, Izmir, Turkey*

Correspondence should be addressed to Hatice Mutlu-Albayrak; haticemutlu@gmail.com

Academic Editor: Patrick Morrison

Primary systemic carnitine deficiency is caused by homozygous or compound heterozygous mutation in the *SLC22A5* gene on chromosome 5q31. The most common presentations are in infancy and early childhood with either metabolic decompensation or cardiac and myopathic manifestations. We report a case of 9-year-old boy with dysmorphic appearance and hypertrophic cardiomyopathy. Tandem MS spectrometry analysis was compatible with carnitine uptake defect (CUD). His sister had died due to sudden infant death at 19 months. His second 4-year-old sister's echocardiographic examination revealed hypertrophic cardiomyopathy, also suffering from easy fatigability. Her tandem MS spectrometry analyses resulted in CUD. We sequenced all the exons of the *SLC22A5* gene encoding the high affinity carnitine transporter OCTN2 in the DNA. And one new mutation (c.1427T>G → p.Leu476Arg) was found in the boy and his sister in homozygous form, leading to the synthesis of an altered protein which causes CUD. The parent's molecular diagnosis supported the carrier status. In order to explore the genetic background of the patient's dysmorphic appearance, an array-CGH analysis was performed that revealed nine copy number variations only. Here we report a novel *SLC22A5* mutation with the novel hallmark of its association with dysmorphologic feature.

1. Introduction

Primary systemic carnitine deficiency (PCD) is caused by homozygous or compound heterozygous mutation in the *SLC22A5* gene (MIM # 603377) on chromosome 5q31. PCD is caused by defective activity of the OCTN2 carnitine transporter, resulting in urinary carnitine wasting, low serum carnitine levels, and decreased intracellular carnitine accumulation. Carnitine is a water-soluble quaternary amine that serves as an essential cofactor in transport of long-chain fatty acids across the inner mitochondrial membrane for subsequent beta oxidation. The lack of carnitine (due to OCTN2 transporter deficiency) impairs the ability to use fat as energy source during periods of fasting or stress [1]. OCTN2 transporter deficiency is a lethal, autosomal recessive disorder characterised by early childhood onset cardiomyopathy, with or without weakness and hypotonia, recurrent hypoglycemic hypoketotic seizures and/or coma, failure to thrive, and extremely low plasma and tissue carnitine concentrations (<%5 of normal) [2]. The clinical manifestations of PCD can vary widely with respect to age of onset, organ involvement, and severity of symptoms. The most common presentations are in infancy and early childhood with either metabolic decompensation or cardiac and myopathic manifestations, respectively. Half of the patients typically present in later childhood around the age of 4

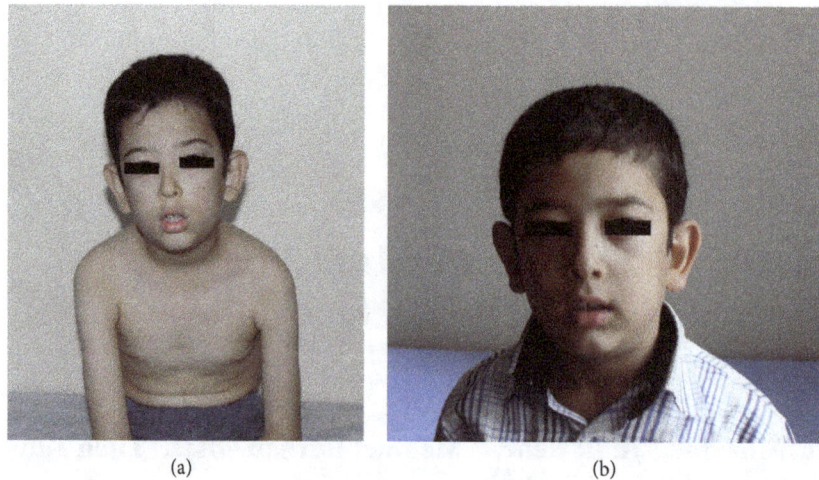

(a)   (b)

FIGURE 1: (a) The boy, before carnitine treatment with significant mask face and dysmorphic findings (protruding large ears, hypertelorism, epicanthal folds, swollen eyelids, narrow columella, and small nose). (b) The boy, 2 months after carnitine treatment.

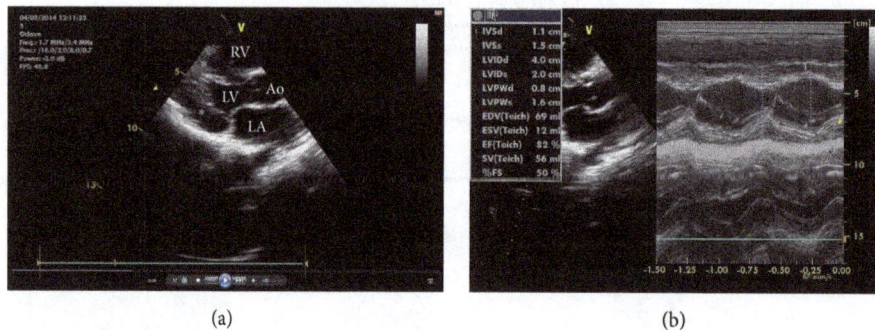

(a)   (b)

FIGURE 2: (a) Parasternal long-axis view depicting abnormally small left ventricular end-diastolic cavity, concentric left ventricular hypertrophy (∗), and normal regional wall motion; (b) M-mode tracing across the interventricular septum demonstrating prominent wall hypertrophy. LA: left atrium; LV: left ventricle; RV: right ventricle; Ao: aorta; IVSd: interventricular septum diastolic diameter; IVSs: interventricular systolic diameter; LVIDd: left ventricular end-diastolic diameter; LVISd: left ventricular end systolic diameter; LVPWd: left ventricular posterior wall thicknesses diastolic diameter; LVPWs: left ventricular posterior wall thicknesses systolic diameter; EF: ejection fraction; FS: fractional shortening.

years (range: 1 year to 7 years) with dilated cardiomyopathy, hypotonia, muscle weakness, and elevated creatine kinase [3]. Following the finding of low plasma carnitine levels on a screening assay, in a symptomatic individual, or in an asymptomatic at-risk relative, the diagnosis of PCD can be confirmed by SLC22A5 gene analysis. One molecular genetic testing strategy is sequence analysis of SLC22A5. If biallelic pathogenic variants are identified, the diagnosis of PCD is confirmed [4].

2. Case Presentation

We report a case of 9-year-old boy referred to Pediatric Genetics Clinic because of his dysmorphic appearance and hypertrophic cardiomyopathy. He was suffering from easy fatigability until he started walking. He was the first child of a consanguineous (mother and father were first degree cousins) family. He was born at 35th gestational week, 1500 g and there was not any pre- or postnatal complication. He could hold his head at 3-4 months, sat without being supported at 12th

month, and was able to walk at the age of 18 months. On his examination his weight and height were on 50th percentile. His frontooccipital head measurement was below the −2 SD. He had a long, mask face and protruding large ears, hypertelorism, epicanthal folds, swollen eyelids, narrow columella, and small nose (Figure 1(a)). His shoulders were inclined forward while sitting. His muscle strength was 5/5 for four limbs and deep tendon reflexes were depressed. Creatine kinase level was 150 u/L (30–200) and electromyography revealed a myopathic pattern. Tandem MS spectrometry analyses found very low (0.92 uM) free carnitine (>3.8 uM normal) and low (0.13 uM) C3 + C16 acylcarnitines (>2 normal). Carnitine uptake defect (CUD) score was found 244, where 65 or more is interpreted as severe carnitine deficiency. A transthoracic echocardiography was performed revealing abnormally small left ventricular end-diastolic cavity, concentric left ventricular hypertrophy with an ejection fraction of 82%, and normal regional wall motion (Figure 2(a)). The M-mode image shows the increased septal and left ventricular posterior wall thickness more than two standard deviations from

TABLE 1: Detected CNVs, genomic position, and genes concerned based on hg19 (GRCh37).

Chromosome region	Type of variation	Genomic position	Length	OMIM genes involved (OMIM number)
2p21	Duplication	45,172,033–45,172,359	327	*SIX3* (603714)
2q21.1	Duplication	131,280,135–131,280,852	718	*CFC1* (605194)
6p25.3	Deletion	259,911–279,697	19,787	No genes
6q24.2	Duplication	144,328,772–144,328,954	184	*PLAGL1* (603044)
8p23.1	Deletion	7,187,789–7,410,327	222,540	*DEFB4A* (602215), *DEFB103A* (606611), *SPAG11* (606560)
10q11.22	Deletion	46,550,833–47,776,322	1,225,490	*PTPN20A* (610630), *PTPN20B* (610631), *SYT15* (608081), *GPRIN2* (611240), *PPYR1* (601790), *ANXA8* (602396)
10q11.22	Deletion	48,879,347–49,262,377	383,031	No genes
14q32.33	Duplication	106,405,733–107,209,400	803,668	No genes
Xp22.33	Deletion	77,270–161,183	83,914	No genes

CNV = copy number variation.

the mean (Figure 2(b)). His second sister had died due to sudden infant death at the age of 19 months. His third 4-year-old sister was also suffering from easy fatigability. She was examined by Pediatric Cardiology Clinic and diagnosed as hypertrophic cardiomyopathy. Her tandem MS spectrometry analyses resulted in CUD. Carnitine supplementation (100 mg/kg/daily) was started orally and both cases urinary carnitine levels increased after treatment. During the follow-up the dosage of carnitine was increased to 200 mg/kg for the boy. No adverse reactions were seen. Both of the siblings showed clinical improvement (Figure 1(b)). CUD was not detected on the mother and fathers' tandem MS spectrometry analysis. Their echocardiographic evaluations were normal. The boy and his sister's molecular genetic test revealed a homozygous *SLC22A5* c.1427 T>G mutation leading to an abnormal protein synthesis; therefore it supported the diagnoses of OCTN2 carnitine transporter deficiency. We sequenced all the 10 exons of the *SLC22A5* gene encoding the high affinity carnitine transporter OCTN2 both in the father's and the mother's DNA using a previously described method [5]. Compared to the reference sequence one mutation (c.1427T>G → p.Leu476Arg) was found in heterozygous form and three already known variants (rs 2631365, rs 274558, and rs 274557) were detected in heterozygous form in the mother's DNA and homozygous form in the father's DNA. The protein coding mutation has not been described so far. Software analysis (PolyPhen-2) predicted that the detected mutation is possibly damaging. Molecular diagnosis supports the carrier status.

An array-CGH analysis was performed on the DNA extracted from whole blood of the proband using the Agilent CytoChip ISCA SurePrint 8 × 60 K oligo-array (Agilent Technologies, USA) to explore the genetic background of the patient's dysmorphic appearance. Nine CNVs (copy number variations) were detected in six chromosomes (Table 1); none of them were proved to be pathogenic based on our in-house database and the publicly available databases such as DECIPHER (Database of Chromosomal Imbalance and Phenotype in Humans using Ensembl Resources) [6], DGV

(the Database of Genomic Variants) [7], and Ensembl [8]. Moreover, none of them was found to be associated with dysmorphic feature.

3. Discussion

PCD is an autosomal recessive disorder that impairs fatty acid oxidation. It has a frequency of ranging from 1 : 40,000 to 1 : 120,000 newborns in different parts of the world [9–11] and is possibly the second most frequent disorder of fatty acid oxidation after medium chain acyl CoA dehydrogenase deficiency [4]. In the heart, carnitine is essential for normal fatty acid β-oxidation and even partial deficiency could lead to organ dysfunction.

Cardiomyopathy is the most common clinical manifestation in children with PCD, which include dilated cardiomyopathy and hypertrophic cardiomyopathy [12]. In patients with PCD dilated cardiomyopathy is more frequently found [13] while cardiac hypertrophy can be seen in heterozygotes for this condition [9]. Heterozygotes for PCD may have mildly reduced plasma carnitine levels [14]. Over time, heterozygotes develop benign cardiac hypertrophy and it is unclear whether they have a higher incidence of cardiomyopathy or heart disease [9, 15]. Newborn screening with tandem mass spectrometry is not routine in our country so our patients are diagnosed late. The cases presented with cardinal symptoms of easy fatigability. Hypertrophic cardiomyopathy was detected by echocardiography. The mother and father who determined heterozygous mutation of *SLC22A5* were screened by tandem mass and no carnitine deficiency was revealed. Their echocardiographic screening was normal as well. No association between genotype and phenotype in PCD was found in previous studies [16]. Patients with identical mutations can have different ages of onset and different types of clinical presentations [17]. Even siblings with the same mutation have different ages of onset and different progressions of disease pointing to the presence of clinical heterogeneity [18]. Affected children, between the ages of 3 months and 2 years, can present episodes of

TABLE 2: Sequence analysis of the *SLC22A5* gene.

Patient	Gene tested	Genotype
Siblings		c.285T>C homozygous sequence change (p.Leu95Leu) c.807A>G homozygous sequence change (p.Leu269Leu) c.824+13T>C homozygous sequence change **c.1427 T>G homozygous sequence change (p.Leu476Arg)**
Mother	*SLC22A5*	c.285T>C heterozygous sequence change (p.Leu95Leu) c.807A>G heterozygous sequence change (p.Leu269Leu) c.824+13T>C heterozygous sequence change **c.1427 T>G heterozygous sequence change (p.Leu476Arg)**
Father		c.285T>C homozygous sequence change (p.Leu95Leu) c.807A>G homozygous sequence change (p.Leu269Leu) c.824+13T>C homozygous sequence change **c.1427 T>G heterozygous sequence change (p.Leu476Arg)**

metabolic decompensation triggered by fasting or common illnesses such as upper respiratory tract infection or gastroenteritis. These episodes are characterized clinically by poor feeding, irritability, lethargy, and hepatomegaly. Laboratory evaluations usually reveal hypoketotic hypoglycemia (hypoglycemia with minimal or no ketones in urine), hyperammonemia, and elevated liver transaminases [4]. Both the boy and his elder sister had skeletal and cardiac myopathic signs. However, his little sister died due to sudden infant death. It seems likely that her carnitine deficiency was more severe and she had died with episode of hypoglycemia.

The boy had facial dysmorphia and microcephaly. The chromosomal analysis of this case was normal and this case could not be related to another dysmorphic syndrome. Kilic et al. [18] reported one case CUD with facial dysmorphic findings; however the dysmorphic status of that patient clearly differs from that of our case. Meanwhile, dysmorphic status cannot be explained with known function of carnitine [19–23]. The array-CGH analysis of the proband revealed known benign CNVs only, which are not affected by any genes involved in the carnitine homeostasis and these CNVs are not associated with dysmorphic feature.

More than 60 mutations in the *SLC22A5* gene have been found to cause primary carnitine deficiency. A total of four genetic mutations in the *SLC22A5* gene were identified in this study (Table 2), which of one was described as novel.

Limitation of this study was that the supposed carnitine uptake defect was not confirmed with the investigation of the uptake by fibroblast.

4. Conclusion

A new homozygous mutation of c.1427T>G → p.Leu476Arg was identified in these cases. Carnitine uptake defect is one of the rare treatable etiologies of metabolic cardiomyopathies. It should be suspected and searched for by measuring the levels of free and total carnitine in plasma and urine from such patients. The diagnosis of primary systemic carnitine deficiency should be confirmed by identification of biallelic pathogenic variants of *SLC22A5* by molecular genetic testing.

Conflict of Interests

The authors declare that there is no conflict of interests regarding the publication of this paper.

Authors' Contribution

Hatice Mutlu-Albayrak and Judit Bene equally contributed to the paper.

Acknowledgments

The study was supported by the Hungarian Scientific Research Fund (OTKA) K103983 grant to Bela Melegh and János Bolyai Research Scholarship of the Hungarian Academy of Sciences to Judit Bene. The authors also thank Marta Czako and Balazs Duga for performing array-CGH analysis.

References

[1] N. Longo, C. Amat di San Filippo, and M. Pasquali, "Disorders of carnitine transport and the carnitine cycle," *American Journal of Medical Genetics—Seminars in Medical Genetics*, vol. 142, no. 2, pp. 77–85, 2006.

[2] S. E. Olpin, "Fatty acid oxidation defects as a cause of neuromyopathic disease in infants and adults," *Clinical Laboratory*, vol. 51, no. 5-6, pp. 289–306, 2005.

[3] A. W. El-Hattab, F.-Y. Li, J. Shen et al., "Maternal systemic primary carnitine deficiency uncovered by newborn screening: clinical, biochemical, and molecular aspects," *Genetics in Medicine*, vol. 12, no. 1, pp. 19–24, 2010.

[4] R. A. Pagon, M. P. Adam, H. H. Ardinger et al., Eds., *Systemic Primary Carnitine Deficiency*, GeneReviews, University of Washington, Seattle, DC, USA, 1993–2014.

[5] B. Melegh, J. Bene, G. Mogyorósy et al., "Phenotypic manifestations of the OCTN2 V295X mutation: sudden infant death and carnitine-responsive cardiomyopathy in Roma families," *American Journal of Medical Genetics A*, vol. 131, no. 2, pp. 121–126, 2004.

[6] Decipher, http://decipher.sanger.ac.uk.

[7] The Database of Genomic Variants, http://projects.tcag.ca/variation.

[8] Ensembl, http://www.ensembl.org.

[9] A. Koizumi, J.-I. Nozaki, T. Ohura et al., "Genetic epidemiology of the carnitine transporter OCTN2 gene in a Japanese population and phenotypic characterization in Japanese pedigrees with primary systemic carnitine deficiency," *Human Molecular Genetics*, vol. 8, no. 12, pp. 2247–2254, 1999.

[10] B. Wilcken, V. Wiley, K. G. Sim, and K. Carpenter, "Carnitine transporter defect diagnosed by newborn screening with electrospray tandem mass spectrometry," *Journal of Pediatrics*, vol. 138, no. 4, pp. 581–584, 2001.

[11] B. Wilcken, V. Wiley, J. Hammond, and K. Carpenter, "Screening newborns for inborn errors of metabolism by tandem mass spectrometry," *The New England Journal of Medicine*, vol. 348, no. 23, pp. 2304–2312, 2003.

[12] L. Fu, M. Huang, and S. Chen, "Primary carnitine deficiency and cardiomyopathy," *Korean Circulation Journal*, vol. 43, no. 12, pp. 785–792, 2013.

[13] Y. Wang, M. A. Kelly, T. M. Cowan, and N. Longo, "A missense mutation in the OCTN2 gene associated with residual carnitine transport activity," *Human Mutation*, vol. 15, no. 3, pp. 238–245, 2000.

[14] F. Scaglia, Y. Wang, R. H. Singh et al., "Defective urinary carnitine transport in heterozygotes for primary carnitine deficiency," *Genetics in Medicine*, vol. 1, no. 1, pp. 34–39, 1998.

[15] C. Amat di San Filippo, M. R. G. Taylor, L. Mestroni, L. D. Botto, and N. Longo, "Cardiomyopathy and carnitine deficiency," *Molecular Genetics and Metabolism*, vol. 94, no. 2, pp. 162–166, 2008.

[16] Y. Wang, S. H. Korman, J. Ye et al., "Phenotype and genotype variation in primary carnitine deficiency," *Genetics in Medicine*, vol. 3, no. 6, pp. 387–392, 2001.

[17] U. Spiekerkoetter, G. Huener, T. Baykal et al., "Silent and symptomatic primary carnitine deficiency within the same family due to identical mutations in the organic cation/carnitine transporter OCTN2," *Journal of Inherited Metabolic Disease*, vol. 26, no. 6, pp. 613–615, 2003.

[18] M. Kilic, R. K. Özgül, T. Coşkun et al., "Identification of mutations and evaluation of cardiomyopathy in Turkish patients with primary carnitine deficiency," in *JIMD Reports—Case and Research Reports, 2011/3*, vol. 3 of *JIMD Reports*, pp. 17–23, Springer, Berlin, Germany, 2012.

[19] B. Melegh, B. Sumegi, and A. D. Sherry, "Preferential elimination of pivalate with supplemental carnitine via formation of pivaloylcarnitine in man," *Xenobiotica*, vol. 23, no. 11, pp. 1255–1261, 1993.

[20] B. Melegh, M. Pap, E. Morava, D. Molnar, M. Dani, and J. Kurucz, "Carnitine-dependent changes of metabolic fuel consumption during long-term treatment with valproic acid," *The Journal of Pediatrics*, vol. 125, no. 2, pp. 317–321, 1994.

[21] B. Melegh, J. Kerner, A. Sándor, M. Vincellér, and G. Kispál, "Effects of oral L-carnitine supplementation in low-birth-weight premature infants maintained on human milk," *Biology of the Neonate*, vol. 51, no. 4, pp. 185–193, 1987.

[22] B. Melegh, J. Kerner, G. Acsadi, J. Lakatos, and A. Sandor, "L-carnitine replacement therapy in chronic valproate treatment," *Neuropediatrics*, vol. 21, no. 1, pp. 40–43, 1990.

[23] F. M. Vaz, B. Melegh, J. Bene et al., "Analysis of carnitine biosynthesis metabolites in urine by HPLC-electrospray tandem mass spectrometry," *Clinical Chemistry*, vol. 48, no. 6, part 1, pp. 826–834, 2002.

34

Incidental Finding of a Homozygous p.M348K Asymptomatic Italian Patient Confirms the Many Faces of Cystic Fibrosis

Rossana Molinario, Sara Palumbo, Paola Concolino, Sandro Rocchetti, Roberta Rizza, Giovanni Luca Scaglione, Angelo Minucci, and Ettore Capoluongo

Laboratory of Clinical Molecular and Personalized Diagnostics, Department of Laboratory Medicine, University Hospital "A. Gemelli", 8 Largo A. Gemelli, 00168 Rome, Italy

Correspondence should be addressed to Rossana Molinario; rossanamolinario@libero.it

Academic Editor: Philip D. Cotter

Cystic fibrosis (CF; OMIM number 219700) is an autosomal recessive disease caused by mutations in the *CFTR* (cystic fibrosis transmembrane conductance regulator) gene, which results in abnormal viscous mucoid secretions in multiple organs and whose main clinical features are pancreatic insufficiency, chronic endobronchial infection, and male infertility. We report the case of a 47-year-old apparently normal male resulting in homozygosity for the mutation p.M348K from nonconsanguineous parents. The proband was screened using a standard panel of 70 different tested on NanoChip 400 platform. The massive parallel pyrosequencing on 454 JS machine allowed the second level analysis. The patient was firstly screened with two different platforms available in our laboratory, obtaining an ambiguous signal for the p.R347P mutation. For this reason we decided to clarify the discordant result of *CFTR* status by Next Generation Sequencing (NGS) using 454 Junior instrument. The patient is resulted no carrier of the p.R347P mutation, but NGS highlighted a homozygous substitution from T>A at position 1043 in the coding region, causing an amino acid substitution from methionine to lysine (p.M348K). Casual finding of p.M348K homozygote mutation in an individual, without any feature of classical or nonclassical CF form, allowed us to confirm that p.M348K is a benign rare polymorphism.

1. Introduction

Cystic fibrosis (CF; OMIM number 219700) is an autosomal recessive disease caused by mutations in the *CFTR* (cystic fibrosis transmembrane conductance regulator) gene, which results in abnormal viscous mucoid secretions in multiple organs and whose main clinical features are pancreatic insufficiency, chronic endobronchial infection, and male infertility [1]. In recent years it has been acknowledged that a wide clinical spectrum of diseases is associated with *CFTR* mutations. About 10% of the patients present with a mild form of CF, mild respiratory symptoms, pancreatic sufficiency associated to normal, or borderline sweat test results [2]. Since the clinical features of CF are highly variable, the diagnosis of the CFTR-related disorders (CFTR-RD) may be very complex.

Until now more than 1900 different mutations have been reported, with distributions varying among populations (http://www.genet.sickkids.on.ca/app). In Italy, the CF incidence is approximately 1 : 2,700 individuals indicating a rate of carrier individuals of about 1 : 25 [3].

We report the case of a 47-year-old Italian male who was addressed to our department for being submitted to *CFTR* mutation screening, preliminary to an in vitro fertilization procedure, since his partner presented a personal history of reduced ovarian reserve.

The patient was screened using two different platforms available in our laboratory, obtaining an equivocal result for the p.R347P mutation. For this reason we decided to verify the CFTR status by Next Generation Sequencing (NGS). This innovative molecular approach revealed the homozygosity for the nucleotide substitution (c.1043T>A), causing the amino acid change of methionine to lysine at position 348 (p.Met348Lys). This sequence variation is not included in the current *CFTR* mutation screening panel recommended by the American College of Medical Genetics and American College of Obstetricians and Gynecologists. During the subsequent posttest counseling the patient did not report any specific clinical sign associated with CF.

In this study, NGS allowed us to identify for the first time an Italian patient with homozygous amino acid substitution, p.M348K. In addition, in this context, we underline that the use of the NGS for the molecular analysis of the *CFTR* gene can help to expand the spectrum of the *CFTR* mutations facilitating the identification of known, rare, or novel mutations causing the disease, as well as genomic variants that require functional characterization. NGS 454 Junior allowed an accurate and cost-effective approach for the CF genetic testing, suitable for routine clinical practice and ready to be a valid alternative to Sanger sequencing.

2. Case Report

A 47-year-old male was referred to our hospital for a checkup before assisted conception. His clinical history was completely negative for (a) consanguinity; (b) infertility, since he is father of a daughter from a previous marriage; (c) pancreatic or acute pulmonary infection; (d) congenital bilateral aplasia of the vas deferens (CBAVD), mild pulmonary expression with bronchiectasis, idiopathic chronic pancreatitis, steatorrhea, hyperbilirubinemia, sinusitis, allergic bronchopulmonary, and asthma. Besides, semen investigation is completely normal. This individual refused to undergo sweat-test since he is often involved in training programs that do not allow performing this type of biochemical evaluation.

Genomic DNA was isolated from peripheral blood by a commercially available CE-IVD kit (High Pure PCR Template Preparation Kits, Roche Diagnostics, USA, http://www.roche.com/index.htm) and the DNA concentration and purity were spectrophotometrically measured (NanoPhotometer, Implen, München, Germany, http://www.implen.de/). Furthermore, the DNA integrity was verified by 0.8% agarose electrophoresis. Initially, the patient was screened using a standard panel of 59 different CF mutations, by reverse dot blots INNO-LiPA *CFTR* 19, *CFTR* 17+ IVS 8 polyT Update, and *CFTR* Italian Regional (Innogenetics, Ghent, Belgium). Dubious INNO-LiPA *CFTR* result was tested with CF70 kit (Nanogen, CA, USA) on NanoChip 400 machine.

NanoChip technology is basically a forward allele-specific oligonucleotide (ASO) based assay which is placed in an electronically controlled microarray format. Each NanoChip consists of 400 spots attached to platinum wire connections. DNA negatively charged is electronically guided to a test site where biotinylated samples bind streptavidin in the site. After denaturation, the CF 70 Data Analysis Spreadsheet indicates the genotype through the Green-to-Red signal ratio for each mutation fluorescent probes (green and red) and signal is detected after stringent washing procedures [4]. For the presence of two discordant results, full coding sequence and exon/intron junctions of the *CFTR* gene were performed by NGS. In particular, we used *CFTR* MASTR v2 assay (Multiplicom, Molecular Diagnostics), following the manufacturer's instructions. Amplicons were purified separately using Agencourt Ampure XP kit (Beckman Coulter) and subsequently quantified with Light Cycler 480 (Roche Diagnostics) by

means of the Quant-iT PicoGreen dsDNA Assay kit (Invitrogen). The equimolar pool was amplified to generate an amplicon library using the GS Junior Titanium emPCR Kit (Roche Diagnostics) following the manufacturer's instructions. Four hundred fifty-four sequencing were subsequently performed on a 454 GS Junior v 2.7 system (Roche) using the GS Junior Titanium Sequencing kit (Roche Diagnostics). We employed a new in-house bioinformatics tool, named "*Amplicon Suite*," able to automatically analyze each single GS Junior Sequencing run. The analysis included different steps: (a) quality control check of sequencing ("coverage" for each *CFTR* amplicon), (b) identification of variants (pathogenic or not), and (c) evaluation of functional effect of variants of uncertain significance (VUS) by processing them with several prediction tools (such as SIFT and PolyPhen). Several filters were applied to discard sequencing errors and to discriminate between polymorphisms and mutations. To confirm the p.M348K mutation, identified by NGS, Sanger sequencing of the *CFTR* exon 8 was carried out. Therefore, DNA sample was amplified using specific primers *CFTR* E8F: 5′-CTCAGGGTTCTTTGTGGTGT-3′ and CFTR E8R: 5′-AATGCCACTCTCATCCATCA-3′. Cycle sequencing reaction was carried out using same primers and Big Dye Termination Kit v. 3.1 (Applied Biosystems). Sequencing PCR products were analyzed using ABI3500 Genetic Analyzer (Applied Biosystems) and aligned to the reference sequences NG_016465.1 of the *CFTR* gene.

Preliminary analysis was collected by the Sequencing Software and performed by SeqScape Software v. 3 (Applied Biosystems).

CFTR screening by Inno-LiPA kit showed the presence of a weak wild-type band for p.R347P mutation. Since this result was also confirmed on a reextracted DNA sample, the patient was genotyped with an extensive 70 mutation panel through NanoChip technology. In this case NanoChip technology showed a green signal criteria for all *CFTR* markers with a G : R scaled value > 5. This finding highlighted the wild-type genotype for p.R347P mutation. Although this result could be reassuring, the discrepancy between the two technologies suggested a complete screening of *CFTR* gene to detect the possible alteration or mutation due to aberrant reaction found by Inno-LiPA assay.

The emerging NGS allowed us to analyze the full *CFTR* coding region and exon/intron junctions. "*CFTR* scanning" showed a homozygous replacement from T>A at position 1043 in the coding region. Codon 348 (ATG) changed to AAG, causing an amino acid substitution from methionine to lysine (p.M348K) (Figure 1(a)), which is not conservative, since methionine (an apolar amino acid) was replaced by the lysine (a polar amino acid). This result was then confirmed by Sanger sequencing (Figure 1(b)).

3. Discussion

To date, over 1900 *CFTR* mutations and 300 polymorphisms have been reported (http://www.genet.sickkids.on.ca/app). As widely reported in the literature, the frequencies of *CFTR* mutations are very different depending on the geographical area [5]. The simplest and rapid approach for mutational

(a)

(b)

(c)

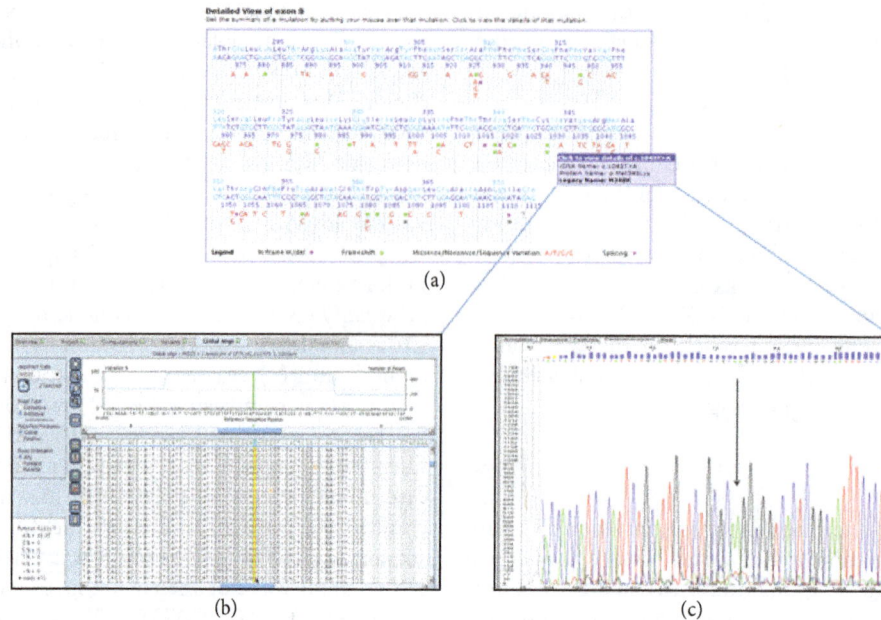

FIGURE 1: (a) Sequence reference by Cystic Fibrosis Mutation Database (http://www.genet.sickkids.on.ca/app). (b) Amplicon Variant Analyzer v 2.7 (AVA) aligns the sequencing reads to the reference sequences NG_016465.1 for *CFTR* gene (Reads = 470; % A = 99.36%). (c) Sequencing electropherograms of patient showing the substitution of T to A at nucleotide 1043 at exon 8 (the arrow indicates the mutant nucleotide).

research involves usage of a defined panel of mutations, able to cover more than 80% of disease risk in the population. However, high *CFTR* genetic heterogeneity is a limiting factor when this approach is used. In fact, mutation panels included in various commercially available kits cannot completely cover all geographical worldwide areas. Therefore, the low detection rate can provide not highly informative first level cystic fibrosis screening assay, above all in absence of family risk situations, such as in case of patients who require CFTR genetic testing before IVD procedure. In these conditions the probability of a CFTR missing test is very high. In fact, since 2003, we have screened more than 9,000 individuals (90% of which was evaluated only in the context of sterility or IVD screening programs): the great part of them (about 96%) resulted as negative at first level *CFTR* testing. Although the large amount of negative CFTR results may be justified by a preventive approach before IVD procedures, we should also take into account that all these individuals were analyzed with commercial kit able to cover a risk ratio close to 85%. Therefore, we cannot exclude the presence of other variants or mutations, not included in the kit employed, within about 8100 individuals screened since 2003. Consequently, in order to provide a complete *CFTR* gene scanning, we analyze the full coding region and exon/intron junctions by Sanger sequencing. Moreover, massive parallel sequencing (MPS) is a novel and efficient strategy that can replace other current low-throughput and time-consuming molecular methods. In fact, MPS approach allows simultaneous complete molecular analysis of different genes in the same run, reducing costs and turnaround time. In this context, our laboratory workflow is able to analyze *BRCA1/2*, *CFTR*, and familiar hypercholesterolemia genes in the same 454

Junior run. For this reason, we decided to introduce NGS as a valid alternative method to *CFTR* gene Sanger sequencing. Further advantage of NGS technology is its flexibility, since it can be coupled also with homemade bioinformatics tools, thus strongly reducing the cost of commercial software: therefore, in our experience, MPS represents reliable and robust approach for the molecular diagnostics of CF and CFTR-RD [6].

Through NGS, we identify the first Italian patient homozygous for the p.M348K *CFTR* mutation. This amino acidic substitution in M6 domain of CFTR protein is nonconservative: methionine is replaced by lysine. This mutation was previously identified: (a) as innocuous polymorphism in a cystic fibrosis at-risk family [7]; (b) in compound heterozygosis with L346P in a Cypriot male individual [8]; and (c) in homozygote boy with respiratory symptoms and failure to thrive [9]. As reported by Hentschel et al. [9], clinical relevance of p.M348K mutation remains unclear. In this regard, the clinical and functional translation of *CFTR* (CFTR2) project represents a novel approach for clinical and functional annotation of mutations identified in disease-causing genes [10]. In fact, CFTR2 will help interpretation of individual genotype-phenotype correlation as for p.M348K, confirming the hypothesis of nonpathogenic role of this variant, although it is still classified as a disease-causing mutation in the Human Genome Mutation Database.

Furthermore, we underline that p.M348 amino acidic residue is completely conserved in 7 species analyzed suggesting evolutionary pressure (data not shown). Since 348 residues are located in the transmembrane M6 domain, which have an important role in the regulation of pore function, the structure of the CFTR protein might be altered, possibly determining a pathological effect due to replacement of the methionine to lysine. Since the transmembrane M6 domain consists of only 3 polar and 16 nonpolar amino acids, amino acid change from methionine to lysine (from polar-to-nonpolar) could not affect chloride channel structure because the other 15 amino acid residues could guarantee the functional structure of the hydrophobic M6 domain: we speculate that this mechanism could explain neutral effect of this mutation on CFTR protein.

In conclusion, based on the clinical features of the patient, we can confirm the data published by D'Apice et al. and Hentschel et al. who considered p.M348K as nonpathogenic variant. In fact our individual did not show any feature of CF or other symptoms related to mild CF form and/or CF-related disorders.

Considering the phenotype and the clinical feature of our proband, we can be able to answer to question addressed by Hentschel et al. in the title of their paper responding that p.M348K is not a disease-causing mutation but a benign rare polymorphism.

Conflict of Interests

The authors declare that there is no conflict of interests regarding the publication of this paper.

References

[1] P. B. Davis, M. Drumm, and M. W. Konstan, "Cystic fibrosis," *American Journal of Respiratory and Critical Care Medicine*, vol. 154, no. 5, pp. 1229–1256, 1996.

[2] E. Kerem, "Atypical CF and CF related diseases," *Paediatric Respiratory Reviews*, vol. 7, supplement 1, pp. S144–S146, 2006.

[3] G. Mastella, *Cystic Fibrosis*, CE.D.RI.M., 1998.

[4] C. S. Richards and W. W. Grody, "Prenatal screening for cystic fibrosis: past, present and future," *Expert Review of Molecular Diagnostics*, vol. 4, no. 1, pp. 49–62, 2004.

[5] J. L. Bobadilla, M. Macek Jr., J. P. Fine, and P. M. Farrell, "Cystic fibrosis: a worldwide analysis of *CFTR* mutations—correlation with incidence data and application to screening," *Human Mutation*, vol. 19, no. 6, pp. 575–606, 2002.

[6] D. Trujillano, M. D. Ramos, J. González et al., "Next generation diagnostics of cystic fibrosis and CFTR-related disorders by targeted multiplex high-coverage resequencing of CFTR," *Journal of Medical Genetics*, vol. 50, no. 7, pp. 455–462, 2013.

[7] M. R. D'Apice, S. Gambardella, S. Russo et al., "Segregation analysis in cystic fibrosis at-risk family demonstrates that the M348K *CFTR* mutation is a rare innocuous polymorphism," *Prenatal Diagnosis*, vol. 24, no. 12, pp. 981–983, 2004.

[8] C. C. Deltas, K. Boteva, A. Georgiou, E. Papageorgiou, and C. Georgiou, "Description of a symptomless cystic fibrosis L346P/M348K compound heterozygous Cypriot individual," *Molecular and Cellular Probes*, vol. 10, no. 4, pp. 315–318, 1996.

[9] J. Hentschel, G. Riesener, H. Nelle et al., "Homozygous *CFTR* mutation M348K in a boy with respiratory symptoms and failure to thrive. Disease-causing mutation or benign alteration?" *European Journal of Pediatrics*, vol. 171, no. 7, pp. 1039–1046, 2012.

[10] C. Castellani, G. Cutting, P. Sosnay et al., "CFTR2: how will it help care?" *Paediatric Respiratory Reviews*, vol. 14, supplement 1, pp. 2–5, 2013.

35

Progressive Lower Extremity Weakness and Axonal Sensorimotor Polyneuropathy from a Mutation in *KIF5A* (c.611G>A;p.Arg204Gln)

Nivedita U. Jerath, Tiffany Grider, and Michael E. Shy

Department of Neurology, Carver College of Medicine, University of Iowa, 200 Hawkins Drive, Iowa City, IA 52242, USA

Correspondence should be addressed to Nivedita U. Jerath; njerath@post.harvard.edu

Academic Editor: Jose Luis Royo

Introduction. Hereditary Spastic Paraplegia (HSP) is a rare hereditary disorder that primarily involves progressive spasticity of the legs (hamstrings, quadriceps, and calves). *Methods.* A 27-year-old gentleman was a fast runner and able to play soccer until age 9 when he developed slowly progressive weakness. He was wheelchair-bound by age 25. He was evaluated by laboratory testing, imaging, electrodiagnostics, and molecular genetics. *Results.* Electrodiagnostic testing revealed an axonal sensorimotor polyneuropathy. Genetic testing for HSP in 2003 was negative; repeat testing in 2013 revealed a mutation in KIF5A (c.611G>A;p.Arg204Gln). *Conclusions.* A recent advance in neurogenetics has allowed for more genes and mutations to be identified; over 76 different genetic loci for HSP and 59 gene products are currently known. Even though our patient had a sensorimotor polyneuropathy on electrodiagnostic testing and a 2003 HSP genetic panel that was negative, a repeat HSP genetic panel was performed in 2013 due to the advancement in neurogenetics. This revealed a mutation in *KIF5A*.

1. Introduction

Hereditary Spastic Paraplegia (HSP) is a rare hereditary disorder that involves progressive spasticity of the legs (hamstrings, quadriceps, and calves). Pathophysiology of HSP involves a length dependent degeneration of the corticospinal tract, degeneration of longest ascending sensory fibers, degeneration of spinocerebellar fibers, and neuronal cell bodies.

Previous classifications of HSP included age, mode of inheritance, or symptoms. Classifying by age, type 1 HSP is earlier (age < 35 years old) with slower progression; weakness, sensory loss, and urinary symptoms are less marked. Type 2 HSP (age > 35) is later with a more rapidly progressive disease, muscle weakness, sensory loss, and marked urinary involvement. These individuals lose the ability to walk by the age of 60–70. HSP can be inherited AD, AR, or X-linked recessive. HSP can be pure (spasticity in lower limbs alone) or complicated with additional symptoms (peripheral neuropathy, epilepsy, ataxia, optic neuropathy, retinopathy, dementia, ichthyosis, mental retardation, deafness, and problems with speech/swallowing).

Recent classifications of HSP have focused on abnormal cellular function. A recent advance in neurogenetics over the past 10 years has allowed for more genes and mutations to be identified; over 76 different genetic loci and 59 gene products are currently known [1].

We report a case of HSP in a patient who required repeat genetic testing for this rare condition. This case reflects the marked advancement in diagnosis of genetic disorders and the need for repeat genetic testing if prior genetic testing has been outdated. Even though our patient had a sensorimotor polyneuropathy on electrodiagnostic testing and a 2003 HSP genetic panel that was negative, a repeat HSP genetic panel performed in 2013 revealed a mutation in KIF5A resulting in his clinical presentation.

2. Case Report

A 27-year-old man presented with progressive weakness in his lower extremities and a slowly developing inability to walk. He was the product of a normal pregnancy and delivery. He reached his developmental milestones on time; he walked at around 1 year of age. He was able to play soccer as a child and was a fast runner until age 9, when he stopped playing soccer. He developed lower extremity weakness after a 2-3-day flu-like illness. His symptoms slowly progressed ever since. For example, he was able to run (although slowly) at age 15 but unable to do so at age 21. He continued to walk until age 25 when he had to use a wheelchair. At age 18, he developed attention deficit hyperactivity syndrome (ADHD) and was started on Dexedrine. He was morbidly obese and developed obstructive sleep apnea for which he was started on a BiPAP (bilevel positive airway pressure).

Review of systems was positive for occasional muscle cramps and muscle stiffness. He had no loss of sensation in the lower extremities, no problems with fine motor function of his hands, no bowel or bladder incontinence, no diabetes, and no scoliosis.

Examination at age of 27 years was significant for distal lower extremity weakness: MRC grade 4/5 strength in the tibialis anterior muscle, gastrocnemii, foot eversion, right foot inversion, and right toe dorsi/plantar flexion. Sensory examination was significant for mild decrease in vibration in toes, but the rest of the sensory exam was normal. Deep tendon reflexes were brisk in his lower extremities with sustained clonus at both ankles. He had bilateral Babinski signs and a brisk brachioradialis reflex on the left. Hoffman's sign was absent. Jaw jerk reflex was normal. He had increased tone and spasticity in both legs.

2.1. Laboratory Testing. Vitamin B-12, folic acid, ceruloplasmin, homocysteine, vitamin E, arylsulfatase A, methylmalonic acid, peroxisomal panel, VDRL, HTLV-1, and thyroid testing were normal.

2.2. Imaging. Brain and spine MRI were normal.

2.3. Electrodiagnostic Testing. Electrodiagnostic testing was performed and results were significant for an axonal sensorimotor polyneuropathy.

2.4. Pedigree. A family pedigree was unrevealing except for mom with possible "Charcot Marie Tooth Disease" and being in a wheelchair; the patient's sister had "walking trouble," which was attributed to previous infection with polio (see Figure 1). Mom and sister chose not to undergo genetic testing.

2.5. Genetic Testing in 2003. Genetic testing from a tertiary referral center in 2003 came back with a normal frataxin gene (for Friedreich's ataxia) and normal SPG3A and SPG4 (for Autosomal Dominant Hereditary Spastic Paraplegia 3A and Spastic Paraplegia 4), and the patient was left with no diagnosis.

2.6. Genetic Testing in 2013. Given the strong clinical suspicion of Hereditary Spastic Paraplegia (HSP) with predominantly lower extremity spasticity, further genetic testing for HSP was performed via a commercial lab. He had an updated panel of genes for HSP that were tested and came back normal: BSCL2 (Spastic Paraplegia 17), KIAA0196 (Spastic Paraplegia 8), NIPA1 (Spastic Paraplegia 6), and REEP1 (Spastic Paraplegia 31), plus a negative deletion analysis of SPAST and REEP1. Genetic testing results for the KIF5A gene showed a heterozygous missense mutation—"a variant of unknown significance" (c.611G>A;p.Arg204Gln) per report. Upon more detailed review of the literature, however, this variant was responsible for SPG 10 (Spastic Paraplegia type 10) and axonal CMT type 2 disease [2, 3].

3. Discussion

The prevalence of HSP is rare (2–6/100,000). Presentation can occur at any age from infancy to late adulthood (there have been cases reported at age of 85 years). Most patients, however, will experience onset between second and fourth decades of life. Patients with HSP (who have corticospinal tract, dorsal column, and spinocerebellar degeneration) may present with a hereditary motor and/or sensory neuropathy; our patient was found to have an axonal sensorimotor polyneuropathy on electrodiagnostic testing as well as diminished vibration sense on exam.

Our patient presented with lower extremity weakness and spasticity that progressed steadily since childhood. There were upper motor neuron signs (increased muscle tone, brisk reflexes, and upgoing toes) as well as mild sensory loss in lower extremities. Differentials for our patient's presentation include HSP (the official abbreviation is SPG), MTHR deficiency, multiple sclerosis, spinocerebellar ataxia, cervical/lumbar spondylosis, arginase deficiency, vitamin B-12/vitamin E/copper deficiency, lathyrism, HTLV-1, Friedrich's ataxia, Krabbe's disease, ALS, PLS, metachromatic leukodystrophy, or adrenoleukodystrophy (see Table 1). Important negative findings that led to our patient's diagnosis include normal cranial nerve function, no corticobulbar involvement, no autonomic disturbances, no bladder dysfunction, no ataxia, and normal upper extremity function.

Clinically, individuals with HSP will have difficulty walking, increased muscle tone, weakness in the legs (more commonly in iliopsoas, tibialis anterior muscle, and hamstrings), reduced sensation in legs, urinary incontinence, and fatigue due to increased effort or poor sleep from cramps.

Examination features include increased muscle tone, weakness, mild loss of vibratory sensation, and upper motor neuron signs in the lower extremities distinguishing HSP from other diseases. High arched feet are prominent in older patients. MRI of the spinal cord can show atrophy of the spinal cord. Cortical evoked potentials show a reduced conduction velocity and reduced amplitude of the evoked potential of the corticospinal tract. Lower extremity somatosensory evoked potentials (SSEPs) show a conduction delay in the dorsal column fibers. Upper extremity SSEPs are usually normal. CSF protein can be mildly elevated.

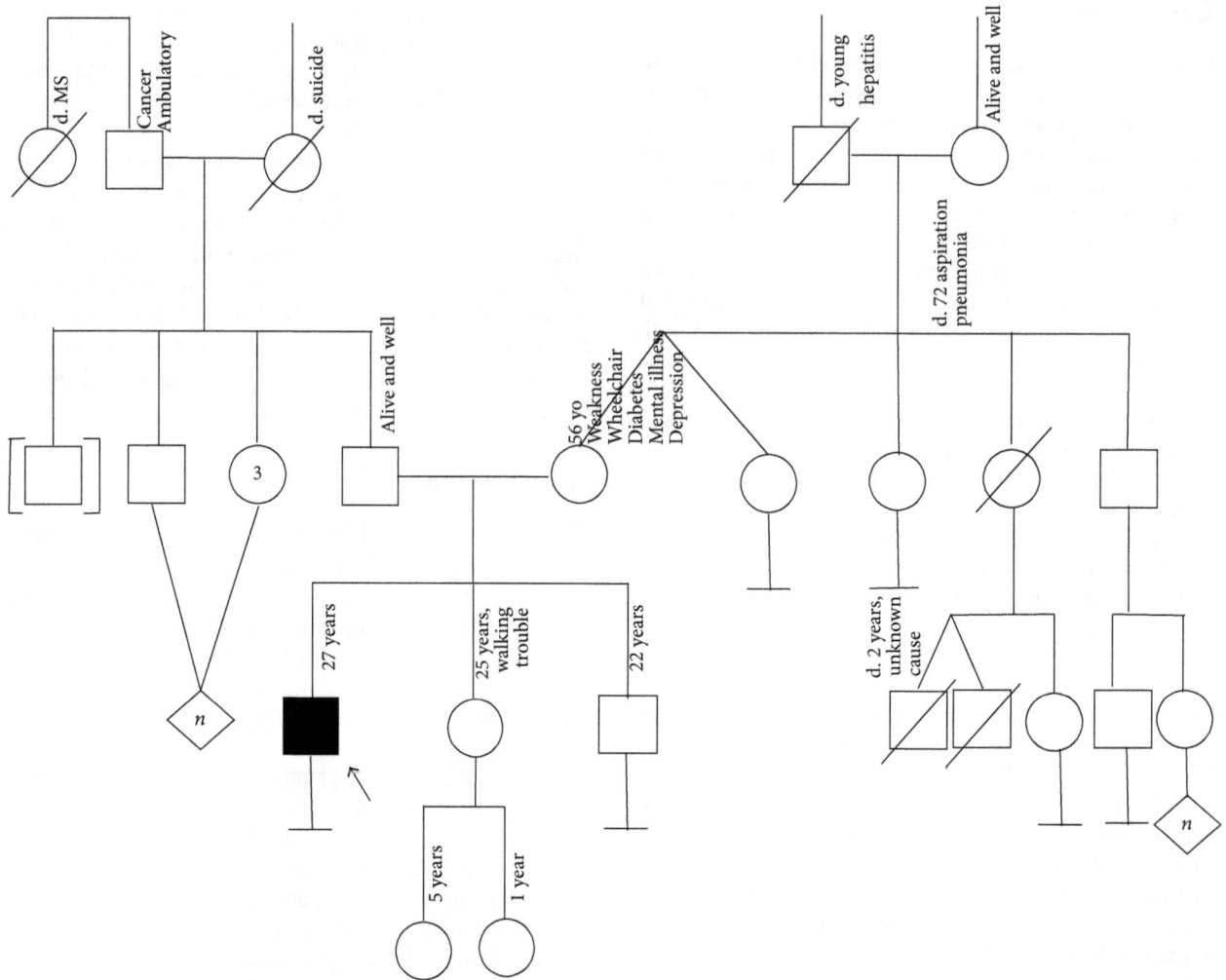

FIGURE 1: Family pedigree. Squares indicate men; circles indicate women; diagonal lines indicate deceased; black indicates *KIF5A* mutation. An arrow indicates the proband. "*n*" stands for number of unaffected relatives.

Our patient had a mutation in *KIF5A* resulting in SPG 10; this leads to a mutation in kinesin, a two-headed motor protein in eukaryotic cells resulting in abnormal movement along microtubule filaments [4]. Kinesin uses energy derived from ATP hydrolysis to transport diverse types of intracellular cargo towards the ends of microtubules within axons [5]. Kinesin is powered by ATP and supports mitosis, meiosis, and axonal transport. It is involved in anterograde axonal transport (cell body to the periphery), whereas dynein is responsible for retrograde transport. Mutated kinesin decreases the efficiency of cargo transport to the distal axon because the mutated kinesin is slower and has a reduced microtubule binding affinity. The mutation is hypothesized to act in a dominant-negative manner by competing with wild-type motors for cargo binding [6].

Clinical features of SPG 10 have been described in a 2009 paper from France illustrating 17 patients from eight families. 7 out of the 8 families had a complex phenotype with peripheral neuropathy, severe upper limb amyotrophy, mental impairment, Parkinsonism, deafness, and/or retinitis pigmentosa [3]. A study performed in 2014 confirmed that

KIF5A mutations can involve both the peripheral and central nervous system, resulting in variable phenotypes ranging from HSP to Charcot Marie Tooth Disease type 2 [7]. As discussed in the paper, there were three patients who had CMT2 as the predominant phenotype, but only one had classical CMT2, whereas the other two had some pyramidal tract involvement. The other three discussed in this paper had Spastic Paraplegia with two of them having a peripheral neuropathy; our patient is similar to the ones with Spastic Paraplegia as the predominant phenotype. Additional features of the six previously reported patients included cognitive dysfunction, learning difficulties, and cerebellar ataxia; our patient had ADHD [7].

Treatment of HSP involves physical therapy (exercise and muscle flexibility), orthotics, orthopedic surgical interventions, Botox, dorsal rhizotomy, and baclofen for treatment of spasticity. Further knowledge of kinesin-1 movement and its influence on axon generation may result in therapies for diseases such as SPG 10.

Our case illustrates that clinical findings are crucial and given our patient's significant lower extremity spasticity, the

TABLE 1: Differential diagnosis of lower extremity weakness and spasticity.

Disease	Upper motor neuron signs	Peripheral neuropathy	Cognitive dysfunction	Cerebellar ataxia	Other
HSP (Hereditary Spastic Paraparesis)	•	•			Bilateral symmetric lower extremity spasticity, gait disturbance, urinary urgency, sparing of craniobulbar function, and abnormal SSEP's
MTHR (methylene tetrahydrofolate reductase) deficiency	•	•	•		Behavior changes, seizures, and leukoencephalopathy
Multiple sclerosis	•			•	Wide range: dysarthria, dysphagia, optic neuritis, nystagmus, chronic pain, fatigue, weakness, and bladder/bowel difficulties
Spinocerebellar ataxia				•	Dysarthria, nystagmus, intentional tremor, and hyporeflexia
Cervical or lumbar spondylosis	•				Neck or back pain, leg or arm weakness, abnormal gait, loss of bowel/bladder control, and MRI imaging of the spine will be abnormal
Arginase deficiency	•		•	•	Seizures and tremor, usually evident by age 3
Vitamin B-12 deficiency	•	•	•		Macrocytic anemia
Vitamin E deficiency		•		•	Retinitis pigmentosa
Copper deficiency	•	•			Optic neuropathy, anemia, and neutropenia
Lathyrism	•				From excessive consumption of the chickling pea; restricted to India, Bangladesh, and Ethiopia; it results in an irreversible, nonprogressive spastic paraparesis
HTLV-1 (human T lymphocytic virus-1)	•	•			More frequent in IV drug users, weakness, nocturia, arthralgia, gingival bleeding, dry oral mucosa, and erectile dysfunction
Friedreich's ataxia		•		•	Usually no spasticity (although it can develop later); pes cavus, scoliosis, cardiomyopathy, and arrhythmias
Krabbe's disease	•	•	•	•	Loss of vision is also seen.
ALS (amyotrophic lateral sclerosis)	•				ALS is typically more rapidly progressive and not limited to legs as seen in HSP. Symptoms include upper and lower motor neuron signs, weakness, fasciculations, cramps, dysarthria, dysphagia, dyspnea, muscle spasms, sialorrhea, emotional lability, and cognitive difficulties.
PLS (primary lateral sclerosis)	•				Not limited to legs as seen in HSP; weakness, dysarthria, dysphagia, emotional lability, and bladder urgency can be seen.
Metachromatic leukodystrophy	•		•		Seizures, optic atrophy, and tremors can be seen.
Adrenal leukodystrophy	•		•	•	Vision loss, seizures, adrenal insufficiency, dysphagia, dysarthria, deafness, weakness, vomiting, or aggression can be seen.

diagnosis of Hereditary Spastic Paraplegia (HSP) was still in favor despite initial negative genetic testing for HSP. Furthermore, it has been discovered that *KIF5A* mutations can involve both the peripheral and central nervous system, resulting in variable phenotypes ranging from HSP to Charcot Marie Tooth Disease type 2.

Given the recent advancement in neurogenetics over the past 10 years, it is important to repeat genetic testing that has been outdated. The initial genetic testing was done in 2003 when the "complete" HSP panel included *SPG3A* and *SPG4*; genetic testing for HSP was repeated in 2013 at a time when many new genes for HSP have been discovered. Additional genetic testing for HSP confirmed the diagnosis of a *KIF5A* mutation in our patient; with strong clinical skills and suspicion and knowledge of appropriate genetic testing, elusive diagnoses are becoming more readily apparent.

Conflict of Interests

The authors declare that there is no conflict of interests regarding the publication of this paper.

Authors' Contribution

All the authors contributed to design and conceptualization of the study, analysis and interpretation of the data, and drafting and revising of the paper.

Acknowledgments

Dr. Michael E. Shy would like to acknowledge support from the National Institute of Neurological Disorders and Stroke (NINDS) and Office of Rare Diseases (U54NS065712) as well as grants from the Muscular Dystrophy Association (MDA) and Charcot Marie Tooth Association (CMTA). Dr. Nivedita U. Jerath would like to acknowledge support from an MDA Clinical Research Training grant and a University of Iowa Internal Funding Initiatives award.

References

[1] S. Klebe, G. Stevanin, and C. Depienne, "Clinical and genetic heterogeneity in hereditary spastic paraplegias: from SPG1 to SPG72 and still counting," *Revue Neurologique*, vol. 171, no. 6-7, pp. 505–530, 2015.

[2] C. Crimella, C. Baschirotto, A. Arnoldi et al., "Mutations in the motor and stalk domains of KIF5A in spastic paraplegia type 10 and in axonal Charcot-Marie-Tooth type 2," *Clinical Genetics*, vol. 82, no. 2, pp. 157–164, 2012.

[3] C. Goizet, A. Boukhris, E. Mundwiller et al., "Complicated forms of autosomal dominant hereditary spastic paraplegia are frequent in SPG10," *Human Mutation*, vol. 30, no. 2, pp. E376–E385, 2009.

[4] C. Blackstone, "Cellular pathways of hereditary spastic paraplegia," *Annual Review of Neuroscience*, vol. 35, pp. 25–47, 2012.

[5] M. Fichera, M. Lo Giudice, M. Falco et al., "Evidence of kinesin heavy chain (KIF5A) involvement in pure hereditary spastic paraplegia," *Neurology*, vol. 63, no. 6, pp. 1108–1110, 2004.

[6] B. Ebbing, K. Mann, A. Starosta et al., "Effect of spastic paraplegia mutations in KIF5A kinesin on transport activity," *Human Molecular Genetics*, vol. 17, no. 9, pp. 1245–1252, 2008.

[7] Y.-T. Liu, M. Laurá, J. Hersheson et al., "Extended phenotypic spectrum of *KIF5A* mutations: from spastic paraplegia to axonal neuropathy," *Neurology*, vol. 83, no. 7, pp. 612–619, 2014.

36

Pheochromocytoma in a Twelve-Year-Old Girl with SDHB-Related Hereditary Paraganglioma-Pheochromocytoma Syndrome

Daryl Graham,[1] **Megan Gooch,**[2] **Zhan Ye,**[3] **Edward Richer,**[4] **Aftab Chishti,**[1] **Elizabeth Reilly,**[5] **and John D'Orazio**[1,5]

[1] *Department of Pediatrics, University of Kentucky College of Medicine, Lexington, KY 40536, USA*
[2] *University of Kentucky College of Medicine, Lexington, KY 40536, USA*
[3] *Department of Pathology, University of Kentucky College of Medicine, Lexington, KY 40536, USA*
[4] *Department of Radiology, University of Kentucky College of Medicine, Lexington, KY 40536, USA*
[5] *Markey Cancer Center, University of Kentucky College of Medicine, Combs Research Building, 800 Rose Street, Lexington, KY 40536-0096, USA*

Correspondence should be addressed to John D'Orazio; jdorazio@uky.edu

Academic Editor: Soo-Cheon Chae

A twelve-year-old girl presented with a history of several weeks of worsening headaches accompanied by flushing and diaphoresis. The discovery of markedly elevated blood pressure and tachycardia led the child's pediatrician to consider the diagnosis of a catecholamine-secreting tumor, and an abdominal CT scan confirmed the presence of a pheochromocytoma. The patient was found to have a mutation in the succinyl dehydrogenase B (SDHB) gene, which is causative for SDHB-related hereditary paraganglioma-pheochromocytoma syndrome. Herein, we describe her presentation and medical management and discuss the clinical implications of SDHB deficiency.

1. Case Presentation

A previously healthy 12-year-old girl presented with worsening headaches of six-month duration, described as diffuse, throbbing, and intense, occurring daily and lasting up to eight hours or more. They were not associated with time of day, posture, activity, and prodromal visual, auditory, or gustatory symptoms, and there were no associated neurologic abnormalities. Headaches were occasionally accompanied by lightheadedness, nausea, palpitations, and flushing. She had lost roughly 25% of her preillness body weight, had been fatigued and "warm," and noted polydipsia and polyuria for several days prior to admission. The patient's mother, an experienced cardiology nurse, reported that the patient's blood pressure had been as high as 200/160 mmHg. The patient had a history of prematurity, being born at 27-week gestation and requiring intubation and mechanical ventilation for prematurity-induced respiratory distress. However,

aside from exercise-induced reactive airways disease, she had no other ongoing medical problems. The patient had normal growth and development and was doing well in school. Family history was noncontributory for oncologic or endocrine diseases.

At her primary care physician's office, the patient's blood pressure was 205/160 mmHg, and the heart rate was 120 beats per minute. An abdominal CT scan, ordered to investigate the possibility of a neuroendocrine tumor, revealed a large right-sided suprarenal mass, which prompted a referral to our institution for further workup and management. The patient was referred to our service with the presumptive diagnosis of malignant hypertension secondary to a catecholamine-secreting pheochromocytoma (PCC) of the right adrenal gland. On arrival, the patient was alert, well-appearing, and in no distress. She was well-developed and nondysmorphic. The height was 152 cm (25th percentile for age) and weight was 54 kg (75th percentile for age). She was afebrile, the

TABLE 1: Presenting serum and urine catecholamine levels.

Test	Patient result	Normal range
Plasma		
(i) Total catecholamines	>8,705 pg/mL	123–1,125 pg/mL
(ii) Norepinephrine	>8,000 pg/mL	112–1,109 pg/mL
(iii) Dopamine	653 pg/mL	10–20 pg/mL
(iv) Epinephrine	52 pg/mL	50–95 pg/mL
Urine		
(i) Total metanephrines	9,907 mcg	110–714 mcg
(ii) Normetanephrine	9,828 mcg	67–503 mcg
(iii) Homovanillic acid	66.1 mg	<6.8 mg
(iv) Metanephrine	79 mcg	<275 mcg

respiratory rate was 20 breaths per minute, the heart rate was 124 beats per minute and regular, and the blood pressure was 157/107 mmHg (the 95th percentile for a girl her age and height is 123/80 mmHg). Oxygen saturation was >95% on room air. She was mildly diaphoretic but had normal skin turgor and perfusion. Capillary refill was brisk and she was slightly flushed in her cheeks. Skin examination revealed no rashes, abnormal lesions, growths, café-au-lait spots, or axillary freckling. Cardiac examination revealed a hyperdynamic precordium and a grade II/VI systolic murmur best heard at the upper left sternal border. Peripheral pulses were 2+ throughout and all extremities were warm and well-perfused. The abdomen was soft, nontender, and nondistended without palpable masses or organomegaly. The patient was alert and oriented to person, place, and time. The neurologic and musculoskeletal exams were nonfocal.

The patient's CBC, differential, peripheral blood smear, electrolytes, and liver function tests were all normal except for serum glucose of 125 mg/dL (normal 60–99 mg/dL). Serum uric acid was mildly elevated at 7.0 mg/dL (2.3–5.9 mg/dL), and serum lactate dehydrogenase (LDH) fell within the normal range (201 U/L; normal 110–293 U/L). Ionized calcium, serum cortisol, and thyroid stimulating hormone (TSH) were normal. Serum and urine catecholamines were markedly abnormal, especially plasma norepinephrine and urine normetanephrine (Table 1). Radiographic imaging confirmed a large right-sided suprarenal mass (Figure 1). The patient was diagnosed with malignant hypertension secondary to PCC. She was placed on telemetry and was started on intravenous fluids and α-blockade with phenoxybenzamine; headaches, flushing, diaphoresis, and nausea resolved within 24 hours. The patient was treated with progressive α and β catecholamine blockade (Table 2); the patient's medication history and vital findings are summarized (Figure 2). The tumor was completely resected on the fifteenth day of catecholamine blockade. The patient tolerated anesthesia well, and the blood pressure and heart rate remained stable. The patient's postoperative course was complicated by rebound hypotension requiring robust fluid support which led to pulmonary edema and respiratory failure requiring mechanical ventilation and pressor support. The patient recovered and was discharged 10 days after tumor resection. Histologic examination of the resected tumor confirmed that it was a PCC (Figure 3).

Currently, the patient is well now nine months after diagnosis. She is symptom-free and has normal blood pressure and plasma catecholamines. Because of the strong association between PCC and inherited cancer syndromes, the patient was evaluated for known genetic mutations associated with PCC and PGL (paraganglioma). The NF1, RET, TMEM127, VHL, MAX, and succinate dehydrogenase (SDHx) genes were sequenced, revealing a p.R27* point mutation in SDHB (c.79C>T) resulting in the change of a cytosine to a thymine and creating a premature stop codon in exon 2. This mutation, known to predispose to PGLs and PCCs, also increases risk for renal cell carcinoma [1–8].

Because of the risk of relapse and/or development of a secondary malignancy, we have educated the patient and her family about signs/symptoms that might indicate disease recurrence (e.g., headache, hypertension, flushing, diaphoresis, etc.). Following National Comprehensive Cancer Network (NCCN) guidelines, our surveillance plan includes a careful history and physical, blood pressure measurement, and urine and plasma catecholamine assessment every three months through the first year and every 6–12 months thereafter through 10 years. We will incorporate abdominal ultrasonography and/or MRI at her clinic visits as well as yearly FDG-PET scans. Critically, we have referred her immediate family for formal genetic evaluation to screen for SDHB mutations and to provide genetic counseling regarding the implications of the patient's identified cancer syndrome.

2. Discussion

PCCs and PGLs are neuroendocrine tumors that arise from chromaffin cells in the adrenal gland (PCC) or in extra-adrenal sympathetic nerve ganglia (PGL). Because of their chromaffin cell origin, PCCs secrete catecholamines, which explains the underlying sympathetic paraneoplastic symptoms many patients exhibit. However, unlike normal chromaffin cells which are innervated by sympathetic neurons and release catecholamines only when initiated by an appropriate neural impulses, PCCs produce and release catecholamines in an unregulated and markedly exaggerated way. As with our patient, PCCs frequently come to medical attention because of symptoms of catecholamine excess rather than because

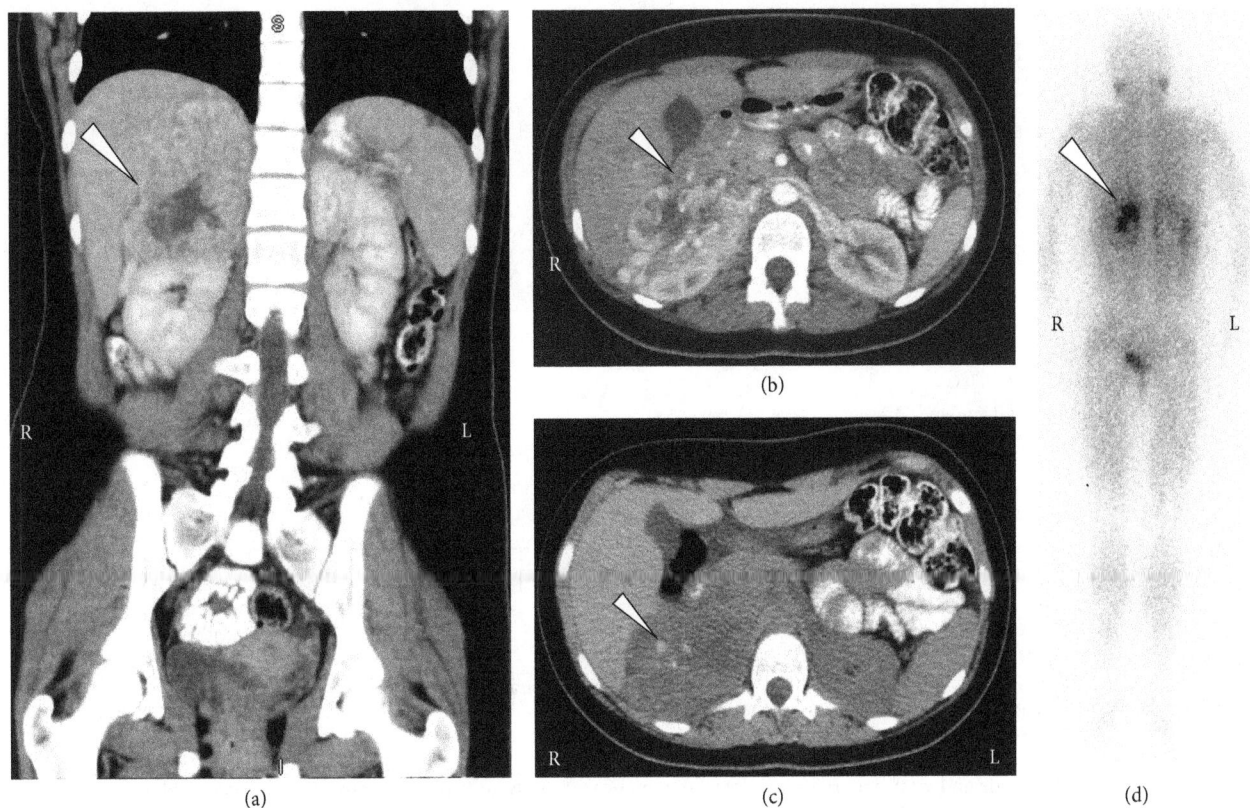

FIGURE 1: Radiologic imaging of the patient at presentation. (a, b, c) Computed tomography images showing a right-sided contrast-enhancing suprarenal mass (white arrows) displacing both the kidney and the liver. Note calcifications in the mass (arrow; image (c)), which is typical for pheochromocytoma. (d) MIBG nuclear scan showing uptake by the adrenal mass (arrow) and no evidence of other sites of disease.

TABLE 2: Suggested algorithm for preoperative catecholamine blockade for PCC/PGL. Patients are best managed first with a pure alpha adrenergic blockade to relax arteriolar smooth muscles and reduce catecholamine-induced blood vessel constriction. Once the blood pressure is well-controlled, beta blockers can be added to treat tachycardia.

Medication	Recommended dose	Notes
Phenoxybenzamine	(i) Days 1-2: 0.2 mg/kg (max 10 mg) q12h (ii) Days 3-4: 0.2 mg/kg q8h (iii) Days 5-6: 0.2 mg/kg q6h (iv) Days 7-8: 0.4 mg/kg (max 20 mg) q6h (v) Days 9-10: 0.4 mg/kg qid (vi) Days 11-12: 0.6 mg/kg (max 30 mg/dose) q6h (vii) Days 13-14: 0.6–0.8 mg/kg q6h	(i) Goal is low normal blood pressure, at least below 50th percentile but preferably below 25th percentile (ii) Side effects: congestion, tachycardia, hypotension, dizziness, especially when standing up (and true orthostatic hypotension), malaise, anorexia, and very rare allergic reactions (iii) Simultaneously load the patient with salt and water to allow maximum blockade
Beta blockade	Propranolol 0.5 mg/kg/dose tid and advanced as necessary to keep HR <110	(i) Should never be used as a first agent (ii) Helpful for symptomatic tachycardia (iii) Begin 5–7 days after phenoxybenzamine

Notes that if the timetable for surgery must be compressed (so that surgical resection is planned 7-8 days after diagnosis), we consider advancing catecholamine blockade daily and using metyrosine to reduce amount of catecholamines produced by the tumor.

of problems caused by the tumor itself. Most PCCs, including those presenting in childhood, preferentially secrete norepinephrine but they can also secrete epinephrine and dopamine. Catecholamines mediate their effects through α-adrenergic and β-adrenergic receptors. Alpha effects include arteriolar constriction causing hypertension and diminished insulin secretion and enhanced gluconeogenesis and glycogenolysis all of which promote hyperglycemia. Beta stimulation, on the other hand, enhances cardiac contractility and rate. The most common presenting signs and symptoms, therefore, include tachycardia, hypertension, palpitations, diaphoresis, flushing, and headache. Weight loss is common because of a chronic hypermetabolic state. Early identification is critical to prevent secondary complications including myocardial infarction, cerebrovascular accident, renal injury, and arterial aneurysms. Other conditions to consider in the differential diagnosis include neuroblastoma, coarctation of the aorta, and other causes of hypertension.

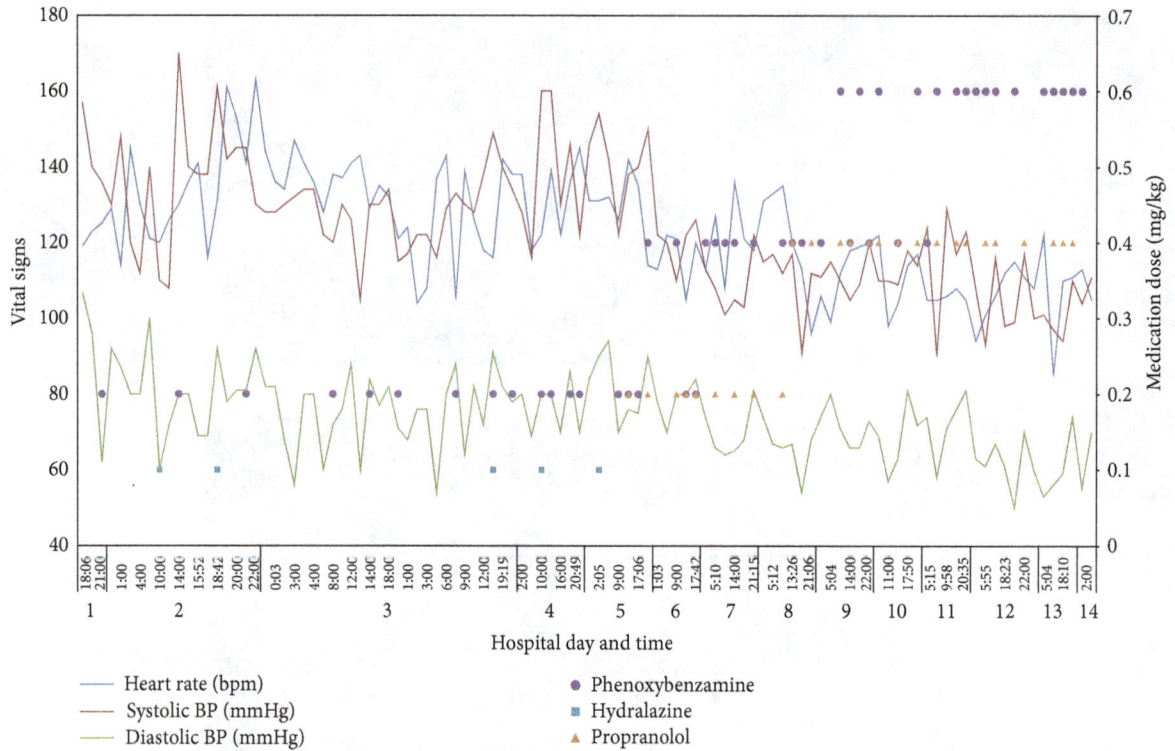

FIGURE 2: Sympathetic blockade and vital signs. Clinical data showing heart rate, systolic blood pressure, and diastolic blood pressure from admission until the time of tumor resection. Also shown are anticatecholamine medications and their doses over time. Note the progressive decreases in hypertension and tachycardia over the patient's hospital course.

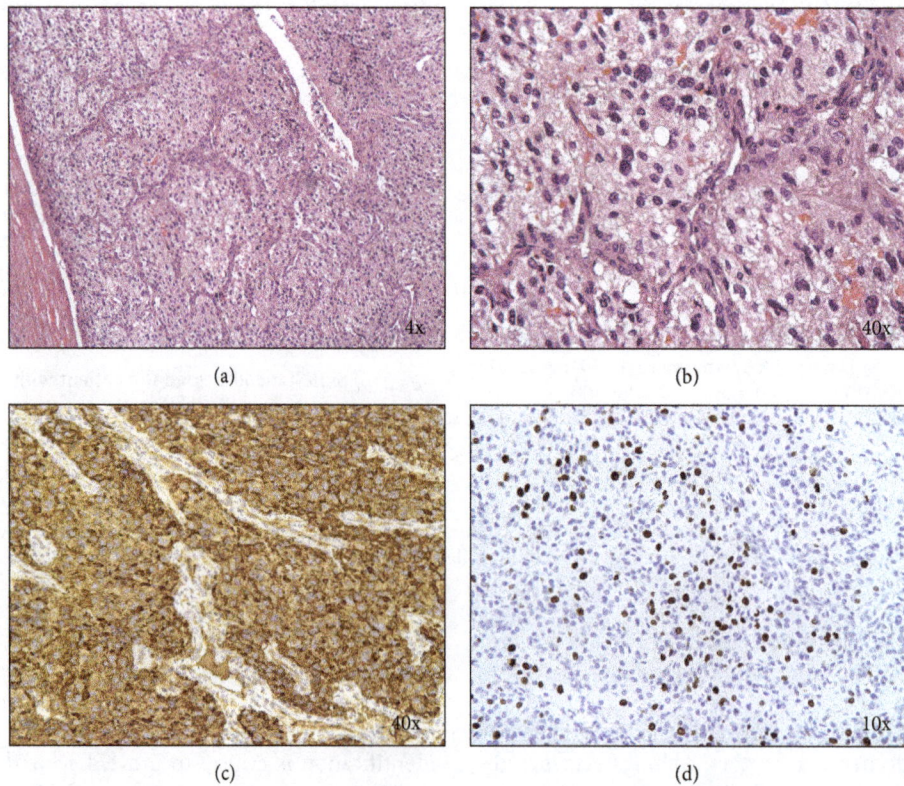

FIGURE 3: Pathologic images of resected tumor. (a, b) H & E-stained sections of the tumor showing tumor cells with abundant eosinophilic cytoplasm arranged in a nested and trabecular pattern and surrounded by fibrovascular stroma. (c) Chromogranin A staining demonstrating strong positivity of tumor cells. (d) Ki67 (MIB-1) immunostaining confirmed a high proliferation index (>10%) of the tumor cell population.

Diagnosis of PCCs relies on detection of elevations of catecholamines and metanephrines in plasma and/or the urine. Plasma metanephrine testing is preferred to urine testing. Radiologic imaging localizes and confirms tumor presence. Beside conventional imaging modalities such as computed tomography (CT) or magnetic resonance imaging (MRI), nuclear medicine approaches such as FDG-PET scanning can be helpful in tumor localization and staging. DOPA-PET scanning is highly specific to catecholamine-producing tumors and therefore can be useful in differentiating PCC/PGL from other metabolically active lesions such as inflammatory or infectious lymph nodes [9, 10]. Alternatively, because cells in sympathetic neurons preferentially take up metaiodobenzylguanidine, MIBG scanning is used in certain centers to determine anatomic sites of PCC involvement.

The annual incidence rate for PCCs and PGLs is roughly 1 in 100,000 persons, with up to 20% occurring in the pediatric age range. Among affected children, 70% of cases are unilateral, are localized to the adrenal gland, and are presenting between the ages of 6 and 14 years with a mean of 11 years. The majority of PCCs diagnosed in children are benign, with tumors remaining localized to their site of origin and cured by surgical resection alone [11]. Because of unregulated sympathetic release, PCCs can precipitate serious comorbid conditions; therefore, timely diagnosis and management are important [12]. Caution must be taken in preparing patients with PCCs for tumor resection because of the risk of dramatic blood pressure swings. Catecholamine blockade before surgery is critical to avoid unpredictable and exaggerated catecholamine release at the time of tumor resection [13]. Perioperative mortality has dropped from as high as 40% to under 3% over the last several decades because of more effective preoperative catecholamine blockade, better diagnostic accuracy in localization, improved surgical skills, and better perioperative medical management [14, 15]. In general, preoperative medical management is accomplished by sequential α-blockade followed by β-blockade along with restoration of adequate circulating volume to replenish intravascular volume reduced from catecholamine-induced vasoconstriction. The most widely used alpha antagonist for PCCs is phenoxybenzamine, a nonselective alpha adrenergic blocker. In general dose is titrated to effect, up to 1 mg/kg/day [16]. Major side effects include reflex tachycardia and sedation, and the long half-life of the drug can lead to sustained hypotension after tumor resection. Selective alpha-1 antagonists such as prazosin and doxazosin may be associated with less reflex tachycardia; however, clinical studies comparing either to phenoxybenzamine have not been conclusive. Beta blockers, typically metoprolol or propranolol, are effective at preventing or treating catecholamine-induced tachyarrhythmias; however, their use as front-line agents is contraindicated until effective α-blockade has been established due to unopposed α-adrenergic stimulation by catecholamine excess [17].

PCCs and PGLs can occur sporadically or as part of an inherited predisposition syndrome, most notably multiple endocrine neoplasia (MEN) syndromes 2A and 2B, neurofibromatosis (NF) type 1, and von Hippel-Lindau (VHL) disease [18–22]. More recently, genes that encode proteins in the mitochondrial complex II, particularly the succinyl dehydrogenase components SDHD, SDHB, and SDHC, have been identified as causative for PCC-PGL syndromes [1, 23–27]. Roughly a third of PCCs occur in the setting of an inherited cancer syndrome and the likelihood of a global predisposition syndrome underlying a PCC or PGL is higher for children than adults [28, 29]. Our patient was found to harbor a p.R27* point mutation in SDHB (c.79C>T) creating a premature stop codon in exon 2 and establishing the diagnosis of SDHB-related hereditary paraganglioma-pheochromocytoma syndrome [30]. SDHB mutations, known to predispose to PGLs and PCCs, also increase risk of renal cell carcinoma [31]. Letouzé and coworkers recently reported that SDHx mutations lead to excess methylation and epigenetic silencing of key genes involved in neuroendocrine differentiation, thereby contributing to malignant degeneration of cells [32]. In one series studying patients with SDHB mutations, the mean age at diagnosis was 33.7 years with most patients presenting with extra-adrenal tumors [30]. On reviewing the literature, we found that PCC/PGLs associated with SDHB mutations have been described in children as young as eight years old; however, most pediatric SDHB-associated PCC/PGLs present in adolescence [33–35]. SDHB mutations are known to be highly penetrant, with lifetime risk of PGL/PCC as high as 77–100% and lifetime risk of renal cell carcinoma estimated to be 10–20% [35].

Overall, children with PCC have an excellent long-term prognosis. In one large-scale study, mean life expectancy was 62 years among patients with hereditary PCC/PGL; however, SDHB mutations are associated with more aggressive disease in terms of early age at diagnosis, higher metastatic potential, recurrence, and the development of other primary malignancies (PCC, PGL, and renal cell carcinomas) [36, 37]. As a result, our patient will be monitored closely including every three-month history and physical clinic visits accompanied by plasma chromogranin A and metanephrine testing along with abdominal ultrasonography. We plan yearly FDG-PET or DOPA-PET scans [38]. Perhaps most importantly, we have instructed the patient and her family to report signs of catecholamine excess (diaphoresis, tachycardia, flushing, headache, and hypertension) to us as rapidly as possible should they develop between clinic visits. Thus far, the patient is well, now almost nine months since her initial presentation, without evidence of disease. Genetic evaluation of other family members for SDHB mutations is in progress, along with genetic counseling regarding the implications of the patient's identified cancer syndrome. It is critical to evaluate patients for inherited cancer predisposition syndromes in order to understand what tumor(s) and other conditions the patient may be at risk for, to develop an appropriate surveillance plan to monitor the patient for sequelae specific to the particular genotype, to provide genetic counseling to the patient, and to offer genetic testing and counseling to the patient's family [39, 40].

Conflict of Interests

The authors declare that there is no conflict of interests regarding the publication of this paper.

Acknowledgments

Sources of support are The University of Kentucky College of Medicine and the Markey Cancer Center.

References

[1] H. P. Neumann, B. Bausch, and S. R. McWhinney, "Germline mutations in nonsyndromic pheochromocytoma," *The New England Journal of Medicine*, vol. 346, no. 19, pp. 1459–1466, 2002.

[2] H. P. Neumann, C. Pawlu, M. Peczkowska et al., "Distinct clinical features of paraganglioma syndromes associated with SDHB and SDHD gene mutations," *The Journal of the American Medical Association*, vol. 292, no. 8, pp. 943–951, 2004.

[3] S. Vanharanta, M. Buchta, S. R. McWhinney et al., "Early-onset renal cell carcinoma as a novel extraparaganglial component of SDHB-associated heritable paraganglioma," *The American Journal of Human Genetics*, vol. 74, no. 1, pp. 153–159, 2004.

[4] C. M. McDonnell, D. E. Benn, D. J. Marsh, B. G. Robinson, and M. R. Zacharin, "K40E: a novel succinate dehydrogenase (SDH)B mutation causing familial phaeochromocytoma and paraganglioma," *Clinical Endocrinology*, vol. 61, no. 4, pp. 510–514, 2004.

[5] A. Cascón, Í. Landa, E. López-Jiménez et al., "Molecular characterisation of a common SDHB deletion in paraganglioma patients," *Journal of Medical Genetics*, vol. 45, no. 4, pp. 233–238, 2008.

[6] J. P. Bayley, M. M. Weiss, A. Grimbergen et al., "Molecular characterization of novel germline deletions affecting SDHD and SDHC in pheochromocytoma and paraganglioma patients," *Endocrine-Related Cancer*, vol. 16, no. 3, pp. 929–937, 2009.

[7] M. Naito, T. Usui, T. Tamanaha et al., "R27X nonsense mutation of the *SDHB* gene in a patient with sporadic malignant paraganglioma," *Endocrine*, vol. 36, no. 1, pp. 10–15, 2009.

[8] H. Kodama, M. Iihara, S. Nissato et al., "A large deletion in the succinate dehydrogenase B gene (SDHB) in a Japanese patient with abdominal paraganglioma and concomitant metastasis," *Endocrine Journal*, vol. 57, no. 4, pp. 351–356, 2010.

[9] F. Imani, V. G. Agopian, M. S. Auerbach et al., "18F-FDOPA PET and PET/CT accurately localize pheochromocytomas," *Journal of Nuclear Medicine*, vol. 50, no. 4, pp. 513–519, 2009.

[10] P. Santhanam and D. Taïeb, "Role of ^{18}F-FDOPA PET/CT imaging in Endocrinology," *Clinical Endocrinology*, 2014.

[11] S. Edmonds, D. M. Fein, and A. Gurtman, "Pheochromocytoma," *Pediatrics in Review*, vol. 32, no. 7, pp. 308–310, 2011.

[12] K. Pacak, "Preoperative management of the pheochromocytoma patient," *Journal of Clinical Endocrinology and Metabolism*, vol. 92, no. 11, pp. 4069–4079, 2007.

[13] S. Hariskov and R. Schumann, "Intraoperative management of patients with incidental catecholamine producing tumors: a literature review and analysis," *Journal of Anaesthesiology Clinical Pharmacology*, vol. 29, no. 1, pp. 41–46, 2013.

[14] V. Apgar and E. M. Papper, "Pheochromocytoma. Anesthetic management during surgical treatment.," *A.M.A. Archives of Surgery*, vol. 62, no. 5, pp. 634–648, 1951.

[15] E. G. Grubbs, T. A. Rich, C. Ng et al., "Long-term outcomes of surgical treatment for hereditary pheochromocytoma," *Journal of the American College of Surgeons*, vol. 216, no. 2, pp. 280–289, 2013.

[16] A. N. A. van der Horst-Schrivers, M. N. Kerstens, and B. H. R. Wolffenbuttel, "Preoperative pharmacological management of phaeochromocytoma," *Netherlands Journal of Medicine*, vol. 64, no. 8, pp. 290–295, 2006.

[17] R. M. Crago, J. W. Eckholdt, and J. G. Wismell, "Pheochromocytoma. Treatment with alpha- and beta-adrenergic blocking drugs," *The Journal of the American Medical Association*, vol. 202, no. 9, pp. 870–874, 1967.

[18] S. Kirmani and W. F. Young, "Hereditary paraganglioma-pheochromocytoma syndromes," in *GeneReviews*, R. A. Pagon, M. P. Adam, H. H. Ardinger et al., Eds., University of Washington, Seattle, Wash, USA, 1993.

[19] J. Welander, P. Söderkvist, and O. Gimm, "Genetics and clinical characteristics of hereditary pheochromocytomas and paragangliomas," *Endocrine-Related Cancer*, vol. 18, no. 6, pp. R253–R276, 2011.

[20] L. Fishbein and K. L. Nathanson, "Pheochromocytoma and paraganglioma: understanding the complexities of the genetic background," *Cancer Genetics*, vol. 205, no. 1-2, pp. 1–11, 2012.

[21] K. Kolačkov, K. Tupikowski, and G. Bednarek-Tupikowska, "Genetic aspects of pheochromocytoma," *Advances in Clinical and Experimental Medicine*, vol. 21, no. 6, pp. 821–829, 2012.

[22] P. J. Mazzaglia, "Hereditary pheochromocytoma and paraganglioma," *Journal of Surgical Oncology*, vol. 106, no. 5, pp. 580–585, 2012.

[23] D. Astuti, F. Latif, A. Dallol et al., "Gene mutations in the succinate dehydrogenase subunit SDHB cause susceptibility to familial pheochromocytoma and to familial paraganglioma," *The American Journal of Human Genetics*, vol. 69, no. 1, pp. 49–54, 2001.

[24] A. Cascón, A. Cebrián, S. Ruiz-Llorente, D. Tellería, J. Benítez, and M. Robledo, "SDHB mutation analysis in familial and sporadic phaeochromocytoma identifies a novel mutation," *Journal of Medical Genetics*, vol. 39, no. 10, p. E64, 2002.

[25] A. Gimenez-Roqueplo, J. Favier, P. Rustin et al., "Mutations in the SDHB gene are associated with extra-adrenal and/or malignant phaeochromocytomas," *Cancer Research*, vol. 63, no. 17, pp. 5615–5621, 2003.

[26] J. Bayley, P. Devilee, and P. E. M. Taschner, "The SDH mutation database: an online resource for succinate dehydrogenase sequence variants involved in pheochromocytoma, paraganglioma and mitochondrial complex II deficiency," *BMC Medical Genetics*, vol. 6, article 39, 2005.

[27] B. Pasini and C. A. Stratakis, "SDH mutations in tumorigenesis and inherited endocrine tumours: lesson from the phaeochromocytoma-paraganglioma syndromes," *Journal of Internal Medicine*, vol. 266, no. 1, pp. 19–42, 2009.

[28] R. R. De Krijger, B. J. Petri, F. H. Van Nederveen et al., "Frequent genetic changes in childhood pheochromocytomas," *Annals of the New York Academy of Sciences*, vol. 1073, pp. 166–176, 2006.

[29] R. Armstrong, M. Sridhar, K. L. Greenhalgh et al., "Phaeochromocytoma in children," *Archives of Disease in Childhood*, vol. 93, no. 10, pp. 899–904, 2008.

[30] H. J. L. M. Timmers, A. Kozupa, G. Eisenhofer et al., "Clinical presentations, biochemical phenotypes, and genotype-phenotype correlations in patients with succinate dehydrogenase subunit B-associated pheochromocytomas and paragangliomas," *Journal of Clinical Endocrinology and Metabolism*, vol. 92, no. 3, pp. 779–786, 2007.

[31] C. Ricketts, E. R. Woodward, P. Killick et al., "Germline SDHB mutations and familial renal cell carcinoma," *Journal of the National Cancer Institute*, vol. 100, no. 17, pp. 1260–1262, 2008.

[32] E. Letouzé, C. Martinelli, C. Loriot et al., "SDH mutations estab-
      lish a hypermethylator phenotype in paraganglioma," *Cancer
      Cell*, vol. 23, no. 6, pp. 739–752, 2013.

[33] R. Renella, J. Carnevale, K. A. Schneider, J. L. Hornick, H.
      Q. Rana, and K. A. Janeway, "Exploring the association of
      succinate dehydrogenase complex mutations with lymphoid
      malignancies," *Familial Cancer*, 2014.

[34] S. Norbedo, S. Naviglio, F. M. Murru et al., "A boy with sudden
      headache," *Pediatric Emergency Care*, vol. 30, no. 3, pp. 182–184,
      2014.

[35] B. Bausch, U. Wellner, D. Bausch et al., "Long-term prognosis of
      patients with pediatric pheochromocytoma," *Endocrine-Related
      Cancer*, vol. 21, no. 1, pp. 17–25, 2014.

[36] K. S. King, T. Prodanov, V. Kantorovich et al., "Metastatic
      pheochromocytoma/paraganglioma related to primary tumor
      development in childhood or adolescence: significant link to
      SDHB mutations," *Journal of Clinical Oncology*, vol. 29, no. 31,
      pp. 4137–4142, 2011.

[37] K. S. King and K. Pacak, "Familial pheochromocytomas and
      paragangliomas," *Molecular and Cellular Endocrinology*, vol.
      386, no. 1-2, pp. 92–100, 2014.

[38] S. Zuber, R. Wesley, and T. Prodanov, "Clinical utility of
      chromogranin A in SDHx-related paragangliomas," *European
      Journal of Clinical Investigation*, vol. 44, no. 4, pp. 365–371, 2014.

[39] S. R. Bornstein and A. P. Gimenez-Roqueplo, "Genetic testing
      in pheochromocytoma: increasing importance for clinical deci-
      sion making," *Annals of the New York Academy of Sciences*, vol.
      1073, pp. 94–103, 2006.

[40] L. Fishbein, S. Merrill, D. L. Fraker, D. L. Cohen, and K. L.
      Nathanson, "Inherited mutations in pheochromocytoma and
      paraganglioma: why all patients should be offered genetic
      testing," *Annals of Surgical Oncology*, vol. 20, no. 5, pp. 1444–
      1450, 2013.

37

Early Morphokinetic Monitoring of Embryos after Intracytoplasmic Sperm Injection with Fresh Ejaculate Sperm in Nonmosaic Klinefelter Syndrome: A Different Presentation

Ali Sami Gurbuz,[1] Ahmet Salvarci,[2] Necati Ozcimen,[3] and Ayse Gul Zamani[4]

[1]*Department of Obstetrics and Gynecology, Novafertil IVF Center, Meram Yeni Yol No. 75, Meram, 42090 Konya, Turkey*
[2]*Department of Urology, Novafertil IVF Center and Konya Hospital, Meram Yeni Yol No. 75, Meram, 42090 Konya, Turkey*
[3]*Medicana Konya IVF Center, Medicana Konya Feritpaşa Mah., Gurz Sok. No. 1, Selçuklu, 42060 Konya, Turkey*
[4]*Department of Medical Genetic, Meram Tip Faculty, Necmettin Erbakan Universıty, Yunus Emre Mah., Meram, 42060 Konya, Turkey*

Correspondence should be addressed to Ahmet Salvarci; drsalvarci@hotmail.com

Academic Editor: Balraj Mittal

The patient was diagnosed with nonmosaic 47, XXY Klinefelter Syndrome with the AZF deletion absent and SRY+. The nonmosaic 47, XXY karyotype was confirmed on a skin biopsy chromosomal analysis. Using only ejaculate motile sperms, 11 oocytes underwent ICSI and were placed rapidly in a time lapse (Embryoscope ©) with a specific culture dish. Biopsies were performed on six embryos on the 3rd day, and numerical chromosomal abnormalities were observed using the FISH test before transfer. PGS results were normal in only two embryos with normal morphokinetics in the Embryoscope. For clinical confirmation of pregnancy, ultrasonographic examination was performed during the 7th week of pregnancy, and two gestational sacs and fetal heart beat were observed.

1. Introduction

Eighty percent of KS cases have 47, XXY karyotypes, termed the classical form, while 20% have the 46, XY/47, XXY mosaic form, a high degree of aneuploidy, and X chromosome structural abnormalities [1, 2]. In the nonmosaic type, viable births have been reported following intracytoplasmic sperm injection (ICSI) with ejaculate and testis sperm [3]. In various studies, increased chromosomal anomaly rates in embryos obtained from males with KS have been reported with aneuploidy screening (PGS). It was also noted that, in the follow-up of these embryos, results indicative of unfavorable prognosis were obtained from pronuclear morphology evaluation, suggesting that the children will be born with KS [4]. It was suggested that some previously unknown characteristics during incubation may be the decisive criteria for the prospect of pregnancy in studies on embryo development. Therefore, procedures following early development have been initiated to increase the chance of pregnancy in IVF-ICSI cycles using a time lapse imaging incubator system (time lapse = Embryoscope) [5, 6]. This system can be used to determine whether irregularly or rapidly dividing embryos with impaired morphokinetics can occur. Time lapse imaging can be used to monitor embryos without removing them from the incubator. It was suggested that time lapse is used as an alternative to PGS in young patients and those at a low risk of aneuploidy, since it can be used to track early embryo morphokinetics [5, 6].

In the present case of nonmosaic KS, pregnancy and live viable birth were obtained with fresh ejaculate sperm. As an initial example of KS, early embryo development was followed by a time lapse system and embryo morphokinetics were controlled. In addition, preimplantation genetic diagnosis (PGS) was performed on embryos prior to transfer, and PGS and time lapse techniques were compared for the detection of chromosome number abnormalities.

TABLE 1: Result of PGS by FISH examination.

Embryo	13	18	21	XY	Result
1	2	1	1	N	Monosomy 18, monosomy 21
2	2	2	2	N	Normal
3	3	2	3	XXY	Trisomy 13, 21, XXY
4	3	2	2	N	Trisomy 13
5	2	1	2	XXX	Monosomy 18, XXX
6	2	2	2	N	Normal

PGS method: multicolor FISH; material used: blastomere; protocol number: PGT14-18; probes used: Vysis MultiVysion PGS FISH.

2. Case

Our patient was 34 years old. He had been married for 9 years. Based on semen analysis, the volume was determined to be 3.4 cc, with a concentration of 2×10^6/mL, 73% immotility, and 99% sperm with head and neck anomalies. The patient was diagnosed with nonmosaic 47, XXY, KS (based on peripheral blood culture) with the AZF deletion absent and SRY+ (Figure 3). The nonmosaic 47, XXY karyotype was confirmed on a skin biopsy chromosomal analysis. His spouse was a 30-year-old healthy female. Her karyotype was normal (46XX). According to ISCN, 20 metaphases were analyzed with HRB banding technique [7].

The couple attempted pregnancy twice with no success at another IVF center with IVF-ICSI using fresh ejaculate sperm and classical embryo monitorization.

The family was counseled regarding the probability of chromosomal number and structural abnormalities in an infant with KS, and embryonic monitorization and PGS were recommended. The family was also educated on the study and informed consent was obtained. Using only motile sperms, 11 oocytes underwent ICSI and were placed rapidly in an Embryoscope with a specific culture dish. Vitrolife sequential media were used for embryo culture, with embryos being cultured in G1 plus medium from days 0 to 3. Early morphokinetics of each embryo were followed by images obtained every 20 min with time lapse after ICSI [6, 8]. On the 2nd day of time lapse, pathological findings were observed in early embryo morphokinetics of seven embryos. In one embryo, total fertilization failure was observed. In the other two embryos, morphokinetics were normal. The time lapse until six embryos divided from 3 cells to 4 and 5 cells was 49 and 53 h, respectively, while the division times of two embryos with normal morphokinetics were found to be 24 and 31 h, respectively. Using the Vysis MultiVysion FISH probe, chromosome aneuploidy screening was performed on blastomeres using the multicolor FISH method (Figure 2). Biopsies were performed on six embryos on the 3rd day, and numerical chromosomal abnormalities were observed using the FISH test before transfer (monosomy 18, monosomy 21, trisomy 13, trisomy 21, XXY, and XXX) (Table 1). PGS results were normal in only two embryos with normal morphokinetics in the Embryoscope (Figure 1) and were transferred on the 5th day of oocyte retrieval. Twelve days following embryo transfer, hCG levels were measured as 782.75 pg/mL in blood. For clinical confirmation of pregnancy, ultrasonographic examination was performed

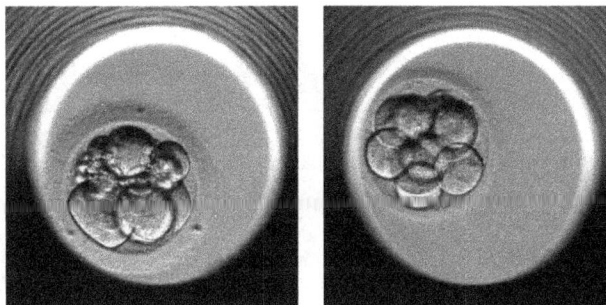

FIGURE 1: Two embryos: with normal morphokinetics in Embryoscope and with normal PGS (2nd and 6th embryos).

during the 7th week of pregnancy, and two gestational sacs and fetal heart beat were observed. On the 37th week, a boy with a weight of 2,425 g and length of 48 cm and a girl with a weight of 2,812 g and length of 50 cm were delivered via Cesarean section. Peripheral leukocyte chromosome analysis of the infants revealed 46, XX and 46, XY karyotypes.

3. Discussion

In 1959 it was shown that KS is a chromosomal disease, and an extra X chromosome leads to this clinical presentation [1]. Between 1997 and 2013 pregnancy and births were reported in nonmosaic KS cases following ICSI with testicular sperm [4, 9]. Based on sperm analysis of nonmosaic KS patients, haploid sperms were observed at rates of 76.47% and 92.25% [4]. Based on FISH analysis, 91.38% of sperms had a haploid structure. PGS is recommended in IVF-ICSI on patients with KS using testicular or ejaculate sperms due to the higher rate of aneuploid chromosome abnormalities caused by gametes. In addition, it is believed that embryo scoring and selection should be performed according to PGS chromosome abnormality and pronuclear morphology, so that the chance of pregnancy is increased [4, 9]. In 1996 and 2000, Staessen and Bielanska et al., respectively, performed and recommended embryo biopsy for X and Y chromosomes in ICSIs with sperms obtained from patients with KS and suggested that, in the embryos of these patients, chaotic chromosome patterns would be present at a rate of 70% [9].

The time lapse imaging system is used for early embryo morphokinetics to select high quality embryos and increase the pregnancy rate to 0.22. Since the time lapse imaging

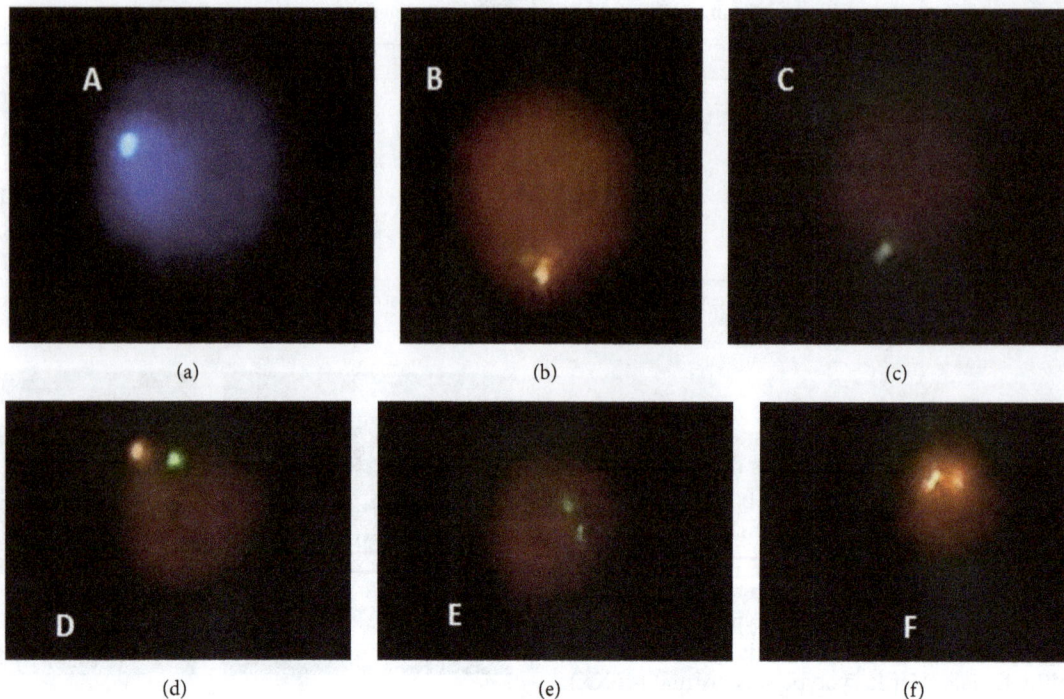

FIGURE 2: Different images of the patient's sperm FISH: (a) (18), (b) (Y), (c) (X) normal gametes, (d) (XY), (e) (XX), and (f) (YY) disomic gametes.

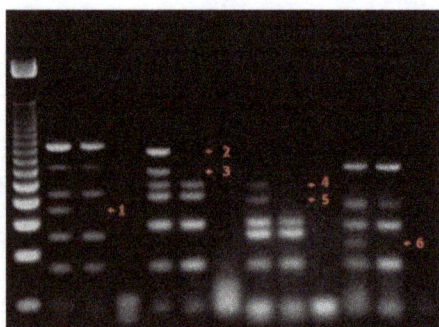

FIGURE 3: Agar gel, AZF with no deletions, and SRY (+).

system is a noninvasive method, it was proposed that it can be used in young patients and those at a low risk of aneuploidy instead of PGS to avoid embryo biopsy [6, 8]. We evaluated all embryos with time lapse and PGS. It was possible to see the embryos with the best morphokinetics with the contribution of time lapse which is currently believed to follow up early embryo development most objectively. If the family had not wanted PGS and if we had not decided to perform PGS, we would have used the embryos with the best morphokinetics observed with time lapse in the transfer.

4. Conclusion

Twin pregnancy and viable live birth were obtained in a patient with nonmosaic KS with embryos of sound structure and number using fresh ejaculate sperm. We have not decided

relying only time lapse. Time lapse is a new application. The outcome even in the normal patients is still a wonder. Time lapse is currently the most objective method for monitoring embryo. We believe that there should be larger case studies including the monitoring of PGS and time lapse of both normal patients and patients with KS. Klinefelter group should be followed up so that healthy embryos can be selected by time lapse.

Ethical Approval

In case humans are involved informed consent was obtained from all individual participants included in the study.

Conflict of Interests

The authors declare no conflict of interests or financial interests.

Acknowledgment

The English in this document has been checked by at least two professional editors; both are native speakers of English. For a certificate, please see http://www.textcheck.com/certificate/2sZsCK.

References

[1] F. Lanfranco, A. Kamischke, M. Zitzmann, and P. E. Nieschlag, "Klinefelter's syndrome," *The Lancet*, vol. 364, no. 9430, pp. 273–283, 2004.

[2] A. Bojesen, S. Juul, and C. H. Gravholt, "Prenatal and postnatal prevalence of Klinefelter syndrome: a national registry study," *Journal of Clinical Endocrinology and Metabolism*, vol. 88, no. 2, pp. 622–626, 2003.

[3] G. Fullerton, M. Hamilton, and A. Maheshwari, "Should non-mosaic Klinefelter syndrome men be labelled as infertile in 2009?" *Human Reproduction*, vol. 25, no. 3, pp. 588–597, 2010.

[4] S. Kahraman, N. Findikli, H. Berkil et al., "Results of preimplantation genetic diagnosis in patients with Klinefelter's syndrome," *Reproductive BioMedicine Online*, vol. 7, no. 3, pp. 346–352, 2003.

[5] J. E. Swain, "Could time-lapse embryo imaging reduce the need for biopsy and PGS?" *Journal of Assisted Reproduction and Genetics*, vol. 30, no. 8, pp. 1081–1090, 2013.

[6] T. Freour, J. Lammers, C. Splingart, M. Jean, and P. Barriere, "Time lapse (Embryoscope) as a routine technique in the IVF laboratory: a useful tool for better embryo selection?" *Gynecologie Obstetrique Fertilite*, vol. 40, no. 9, pp. 476–480, 2012.

[7] A. Simons, L. G. Shaffer, and R. J. Hastings, "Cytogenetic nomenclature: changes in the ISCN 2013 compared to the 2009 edition," *Cytogenetic and Genome Research*, vol. 141, no. 1, pp. 1–6, 2013.

[8] M. Meseguer, J. Herrero, A. Tejera, K. M. Hilligsøe, N. B. Ramsing, and J. Remoh, "The use of morphokinetics as a predictor of embryo implantation," *Human Reproduction*, vol. 26, no. 10, pp. 2658–2671, 2011.

[9] E. Greco, F. Scarselli, M. G. Minasi et al., "Birth of 16 healthy children after ICSI in cases of nonmosaic Klinefelter syndrome," *Human Reproduction*, vol. 28, no. 5, pp. 1155–1160, 2013.

38

Alsin Related Disorders: Literature Review and Case Study with Novel Mutations

Filipa Flor-de-Lima,[1,2] **Mafalda Sampaio,**[3] **Nahid Nahavandi,**[4] **Susana Fernandes,**[5] **and Miguel Leão**[3,5]

[1] *Department of Pediatrics, Hospital Pediátrico Integrado, Centro Hospitalar de São João, Alameda Prof. Hernâni Monteiro, 4200-319 Porto, Portugal*

[2] *Faculty of Medicine, University of Porto, Alameda Prof. Hernâni Monteiro, 4200-319 Porto, Portugal*

[3] *Unit of Pediatric Neurology, Hospital Pediátrico Integrado, Centro Hospitalar de São João, Alameda Prof. Hernâni Monteiro, 4200-319 Porto, Portugal*

[4] *Centogene AG, Schillingallee 68, 18057 Rostock, Germany*

[5] *Department of Genetics, Faculty of Medicine, University of Porto, Alameda Prof. Hernâni Monteiro, 4200-319 Porto, Portugal*

Correspondence should be addressed to Filipa Flor-de-Lima; filipa.flordelima@gmail.com

Academic Editor: Patrick Morrison

Mutations in the *ALS2* gene cause three distinct disorders: infantile ascending hereditary spastic paraplegia, juvenile primary lateral sclerosis, and autosomal recessive juvenile amyotrophic lateral sclerosis. We present a review of the literature and the case of a 16-year-old boy who is, to the best of our knowledge, the first Portuguese case with infantile ascending hereditary spastic paraplegia. Clinical investigations included sequencing analysis of the ALS2 gene, which revealed a heterozygous mutation in exon 5 (c.1425_1428del p.G477Afs*19) and a heterozygous and previously unreported variant in exon 3 (c.145G>A p.G49R). We also examined 42 reported cases on the clinical characteristics and neurophysiological and imaging studies of patients with known ALS2 gene mutations sourced from PubMed. This showed that an overlap of phenotypic manifestations can exist in patients with infantile ascending hereditary spastic paraplegia, juvenile primary lateral sclerosis, and juvenile amyotrophic lateral sclerosis.

1. Introduction

Three apparently distinct disorders involving retrograde degeneration of the upper motor neurons of the pyramidal tracts seem to be caused by mutations in the ALS2 gene, which provides instructions for making a protein called Alsin. They comprise a clinical continuum from infantile ascending hereditary spastic paraplegia (IAHSP) (OMIM number 607225), to juvenile forms without lower motor neuron involvement, namely, juvenile primary lateral sclerosis (JJPLS) (OMIM number 606353), and to forms with lower motor neuron involvement, namely, autosomal recessive juvenile amyotrophic lateral sclerosis (JALS) (OMIM number 205100) [1, 2]. There is no available data on the prevalence of ALS2 related disorders. However, they are probably currently underdiagnosed, even if they have been described in individuals from a variety of ethnic backgrounds, mainly from the Mediterranean [1].

All the patients are homozygous or heterozygous compounds for ALS2 mutations [1]. To date, a total of 45 patients with known mutations in the ALS2 gene have been described, but the phenotype-genotype correlation remains unclear [2]. In the present study, we describe the clinical and genetic features of a 16-year-old boy with IAHSP from Northern Portugal (Table 1).

2. Case Report

The patient was born after a twin pregnancy from nonconsanguineous parents and the pregnancy included maternal hemorrhage in the second trimester. Delivery was at the

TABLE 1: Mutations in ALS2 related disorders.

Patient	Exon/intron	Mutation	Predicted protein	Phenotypic classification	References
1	Intron 24	c.3836+1G>T	p.k1234fs*3	IAHSP	Racis et al., 2014 [5]
2	Intron 9	c.2000-2A>T	p.E724fs*32	IAHSP	Herzfeld et al., 2009 [6]
3	Exon 9	c.1825_1826ins5	p.E609fs*9	IAHSP	Sztriha et al., 2008 [7]
4	Exon 13	c.2529G>T	p.G1177*	IAHSP	
5, 6	Exon 10	c.2143C>T	p.Q715*	IAHSP	Verschuuren-Bemelmans et al., 2008 [8]
7, 8	Exon 4	c.467G>A	p.C156Y	IAHSP	Eymard-Pierre et al., 2006 [9]
9, 10	Exon 18	c.2992C>T	p.R998*	IAHSP	Devon et al., 2003 [10]
11	Exon 32	c.4844delT	p.I331fs335	IAHSP	Gros-Louis et al., 2003 [11]
12–17	Exon 4	c.1130delAT	p.I331fs335	IAHSP	Eymard-Pierre et al., 2002 [12]
	Exon 13	c.2660delAT	p.N845fs858	IAHSP	
	Exon 6	c.1471_1480del10	p.V491Gfs*3	IAHSP	
	Exon 22	c.3742delA	p.M1206*	IAHSP	
18–20	Exon 5	C.1548delAG	p.T475Tfs*70	IAHSP	Hadano et al., 2001 [4]
21	Exon 3	c.1427_1428del	p.G477Afs*19	IAHSP	Our study
	Exon 3	c.145G>A	p.G49R		
22-23	Exon 4	c.299G>T	p.S100I	JALS	Luigetti et al., 2013 [13]
	Exon 14	c.2580-2A>G		JALS	
24-25	Exon 22	c.3565delG	p.V1189WfsX19	JALS	Shirakawa et al., 2009 [2]
26	Exon 4	c.553delA	p.T185LfsX5	JALS	Kress et al., 2005 [14]
27–38	Exon 3	c.138delA	p.A46AfsX5	JALS	Hadano et al., 2001 [4]
39–41	Intron 17	c.2980-A>G	p.T993fs*7	JPLS	Mintchev et al., 2009 [15]
42	Exon 6	c.1619G	p.G540E	JPLS	Panzeri et al., 2006 [16]

36th week of gestation by Cesarean section. The twins were dizygotic twins and the patient's twin sibling is healthy. His 42-year-old mother is healthy and his father died at the age of 35 after a car accident, without any signs of a neurological disorder. The boy acquired cephalic control at three months and started to sit unaided at six months, crawl at nine months, and walk with support at 10 to 11 months. Stiffness of the lower limbs and tiptoeing with hyperactive deep tendon reflexes were noticed at the age of three and scissoring gait started during his fourth year. He was never able to walk without support and underwent Achilles tenotomy at the ages of three and five. An ascending progression of motor difficulties was observed, with spasticity becoming evident in the upper extremities after the age of six. Muscle atrophy in the lower limbs was evident after the age of seven and he was wheelchair bound at the age of eight. Sphincter incontinence started at the same time and he developed supranuclear bulbar palsy, with progressive dysarthria. MRI, electromyography, and nerve conduction studies at that age were normal. Anarthria was evident at the age of 13. At the age of 14, there was clinical worsening and since then he has had bilateral limitation of horizontal eye movements, dysphagia when drinking liquids, chewing difficulties, severe drooling, and paroxysms of laughter. Cognitive function is still normal at the age of 16.

3. Material and Methods

DNA was extracted from a peripheral blood sample from the patient, his mother, and twin brother. All 34 exons of the ALS2 gene were analysed by PCR and sequencing of both DNA strands of the entire coding region was carried out, including the highly conserved exon-intron splice junctions.

We also reviewed all cases of ALS2 related disorders with known ALS2 gene mutations and detailed clinical, neurophysiological, and imaging data that have so far been reported in PubMed. Continuous variables with asymmetric distribution are described by medians (minimum to maximum) and categorical variables are described by absolute and relative frequencies. To compare the three phenotypes (IAHSP, JALS, and JPLS) we used the Kruskal-Wallis test if the variables were continuous and the Monte Carlo test if they were categorical. The statistical analysis was performed using SPSS v.20 (IBM, USA) and P values of less than 0.05 were considered significantly different.

4. Results and Discussion

Our patient displays a clinical picture that is highly suggestive of ALS2 related disorder. This case study presents evidence of previously unreported heterozygous variants in

TABLE 2: Summary of the characteristics of 42 patients with known ALS2 gene mutations.

Patient	Age	Origin	Motor development by 1 year	Age at onset	Loss of walking	Upper limb involvement	Bulbar involvement	Speech impairment	Ocular movements	Wheelchair bound	EMG	Evoked potentials	Brain imaging	Phenotypic classification	References
1	17 y	Italy	Ab	12 mo	NA	8 y	8 y	Disyrthria at 8 y; Anarthria at 11 y		8 y	Ab	SSEP ab	Ab	IAHSP	Racis et al., 2014 [5]
2	7 y	Germany	Ab	18 mo	<7 y	<7 y	7 y		N	7 y	Ab		Ab	IAHSP	Herzfeld et al., 2009 [6]
3	11 y	Hungary	Ab	10 mo	NA	2 y	5 y	No	N	11 y	N	Motor ab	N	IAHSP	Sztriha et al., 2008 [7]
4	6 y	Hungary	Ab	<1 y	NA	No	5 y	No	N	5 y			N	IAHSP	
5	13 y	The Netherlands	Ab	8 mo	NA	3 y	5 y	Anarthria at 13 y	N	13 y	N	MEP Unobtainable	N	IAHSP	Verschuuren-Bemelmans et al., 2008 [8]
6	8 y	The Netherlands	Grossly N	18 mo	NA	Yes	4 y	No	N	No	N	MEP Unobtainable	N	IAHSP	
7	22 y	Turkey	Ab	1 y	12 y	12 y	16 y	No		12 y	N		Ab	IAHSP	Eynard-Pierre et al., 2006 [9]
8	20 y	Turkey	Ab	1 y	10 y		12 y	No		10 y		Motor ab	Ab	IAHSP	
9	9 y	Bukhari Jewish	N	1-2 y	NA	2 y	3 y	Dysarthria at 9 y		No				IAHSP	Devon et al., 2003 [10]
10	6 y	Bukhari Jewish	N	14 mo	6 y	6 y	6 y	Dysarthria at 6 y		No	N		N	IAHSP	
11	12 y	Pakistan	Ab	18 mo	12 y		<12 y	Anarthria at 12 y		12 y		MEP and SSEP abnormal		IAHSP	Gros-Louis et al., 2003 [11]
12	36 y	Algeria		1 y	NA	<7 y	13 y	Dysarthria at 13 y	N		N	MEP and SSEP abnormal	Ab	IAHSP	Eynard-Pierre et al., 2002 [12]
13	31 y	Algeria		1 y	NA	<7 y	13 y	Dysarthria at 13 y	N		N	MEP and SSEP abnormal		IAHSP	
14	24 y	Algeria		1 y	NA	<7 y	13 y	Dysarthria at 13 y	N		N	MEP and SSEP abnormal	Ab	IAHSP	
15	18 y	France		1.5 y	4 y	6 y	8 y	Dysarthria at 4 y; anarthria at 12 y	Ab		N	MEP and SSEP abnormal	Ab	IAHSP	
16	23 y	Italy		14 y	5 y	10 y	12 y	Dysarthria at 10 y; anarthria at 16 y	Ab		N	MEP and SSEP abnormal	Ab	IAHSP	
17	20 y	Italy		1.5 y	4 y	9 y	13 y	Dysarthria at 11 y; anarthria at 18 y	Ab		N	MEP and SSEP abnormal	Ab	IAHSP	
18	14 y	Kuwait	N	14 mo	2 y	9 y	4 y	Dysarthria at 4 y, 14 y	N		N	N	Ab	IAHSP	Hadano et al., 2001 [4]
19	6 y	Kuwait	Ab	11 mo	NA		5 y	Dysarthria at 5 y;	N	No		N	Ab	IAHSP	
20	2 y	Kuwait	Ab	9 mo	NA									IAHSP	
21	16 y	Portugal	N	3 y	NA	6 y	8 y	Dysarthria at 8 y; anarthria at 13 y	Ab	8 y	N	N	N	IAHSP	Our study

TABLE 2: Continued.

Patient	Age	Origin	Motor development by 1 year	Age at onset	Loss of walking	Upper limb involvement	Bulbar involvement	Speech impairment	Ocular movements	Wheelchair bound	EMG	Evoked potentials	Brain imaging	Phenotypic classification	References
22	27 y	Italy	N	3 y				Dysarthria at 7 y; anarthria at 14 y			Ab	SSEP N	N	JALS	Luigetti et al., 2013 [13]
23	21 y	Italy	N	6 y				Dysarthria at 11 y; anarthria at 14 y			Ab	SSEP N	N	JALS	
24	32 y	Japan	N	13 mo	No		11 y	Dysarthria		No	Ab		N	JALS	Shirakawa et al., 2009 [2]
25	23 y	Japan	N	3 y	No			Dysarthria		No				JALS	
26	32 y	Turkey	Ab	22 mo	16 y	12 y	15 y	18 y		16 y	Ab	Motor ab, SSEP N		JALS	Kress et al., 2005 [14]
27	60 y	Tunisia	N	10 y			10 y				N	Motor N		JALS	Hadano et al., 2001 [4]
28	36 y	Tunisia	N	6.5 y			6.5 y				N			JALS	
29	27 y	Tunisia	N	3.5 y			Yes				N	Motor N, SSEP ab		JALS	
30	22 y	Tunisia	N	6.5 y			6.5 y				N	Motor N		JALS	
31	21 y	Tunisia	N	9 y			9 y				N			JALS	
32	14 y	Tunisia	N	6.5 y			6.5 y				N	Motor N		JALS	
33	23 y	Tunisia	N	6.5 y			6.5 y				N			JALS	
34	28 y	Tunisia	N	3.5 y			Yes				N	Motor N		JALS	
35	32 y	Tunisia	N	7.5 y			Yes				N			JALS	
36	22 y	Tunisia	N	6.5 y			Yes				N	Motor N		JALS	
37	21 y	Tunisia	N	10 y			Yes				N	Motor N, SSEP ab		JALS	
38	7 y	Tunisia	N	6 y			Yes				N			JALS	
39	55 y	Cyprus	N	2 y	50 y	Yes	3 y		Ab	50 y		SSEP N	N	JPLS	Mintchev et al., 2009 [15]
40	42 y	Cyprus	N	2 y	2 y	Yes	2 y		Ab	2 y				JPLS	
41	16 y	Cyprus	N	2 y	No	Yes	2 y		Ab	No	Ab			JPLS	
42	34 y	Italy	N	2 y	19 y	2 y	6 y	Dysarthria at 6 y; anarthria at 20 y	Ab	34 y	Ab	Motor ab	N	JPLS	Panzeri et al., 2006 [16]

EMG: electromyography; N: normal; Ab: abnormal; NA: not achieved; y: years; mo: months; MEP: motor evoked potentials; SSEP: somatosensory evoked potentials.

exon 5 (c.1425_1428del p.G477Afs*19) and exon 3 (c.145G>A p.G49R).

To date, case studies of 45 patients with ALS mutations have been reported. Four patients with JALS were excluded because a detailed clinical description was not available [3]. The clinical characteristics and neurophysiological and imaging studies of the remaining 41 cases, plus our case study, are summarized in Table 2. Of these, 21 (50%) of the patients were classified as having an IAHSP phenotype, 17 (40.5%) had a JALS phenotype, and four (9.5%) had a JPLS phenotype. Median age at onset of walking loss, upper limb involvement, speech impairment, and becoming wheelchair bound was similar between the three groups.

The heterozygous variant in exon 5 (c.1425_1428del p.G477Afs*19) creates a shift in the reading frame, starting at codon 477. The new reading frame ends in a stop codon 18 positions downstream, which is very likely to result in truncated protein or loss of protein production. Therefore, it is very likely to be a disease causing mutation. A small deletion in this region (c.1427_1428delAG), which also causes a frameshift, has previously been described as disease causing for ALS2 [4]. The other unreported heterozygous variant was found in exon 3 (c.145G>A p.G49R), which is located in a moderately conserved amino acid, with moderate physio-chemical differences between the amino acids glycine and arginine. Polyphen-2, SIFT, and MutationTaster predict that this variant is probably damaging. This variant in exon 3 was also found in our patient's twin brother and their mother, who were both healthy. It was impossible to test his father because he was dead.

Despite the limited number of patients reported in the literature with known ALS2 mutations and considering the bias related to the age, the majority of clinical characteristics were similar between both groups. Because all the families reported to date have had different ALS2 mutations, it is impossible to draw any genotype-phenotype correlation.

5. Conclusions

Despite the limited information about clinical characteristics, patients with IAHSP, JALS, and JPLS may present with different phenotypes that overlap.

Conflict of Interests

The authors declare that there is no conflict of interests regarding the publication of this paper.

References

[1] R. A. Pagon, T. D. Bird, C. R. Dolan et al., *ALS2-Related Disorders*, University of Washington, Seattle, Wash, USA, 1993.

[2] K. Shirakawa, H. Suzuki, M. Ito et al., "Novel compound heterozygous als2 mutations cause juvenile amyotrophic lateral sclerosis in Japan," *Neurology*, vol. 73, no. 24, pp. 2124–2126, 2009.

[3] Y. Yang, A. Hentati, H. X. Deng et al., "The gene encoding alsin, a protein with three guanine-nucleotide exchange factor domains, is mutated in a form of recessive amyotrophic lateral sclerosis," *Nature Genetics*, vol. 29, pp. 160–165, 2001.

[4] S. Hadano, C. K. Hand, H. Osuga et al., "A gene encoding a putative GTPase regulator is mutated in familial amyotrophic lateral sclerosis 2," *Nature Genetics*, vol. 29, pp. 166–173, 2001.

[5] L. Racis, A. Tessa, M. Pugliatti, E. Storti, V. Agnetti, and F. M. Santorelli, "Infantile-onset ascending hereditary spastic paralysis: a case report and brief literature review," *European Journal of Paediatric Neurology*, vol. 18, no. 2, pp. 235–239, 2014.

[6] T. Herzfeld, N. Wolf, P. Winter, H. Hackstein, D. Vater, and U. Müller, "Maternal uniparental heterodisomy with partial isodisomy of a chromosome 2 carrying a splice acceptor site mutation (IVS9-2A>T) in ALS2 causes infantile-onset ascending spastic paralysis (IAHSP)," *Neurogenetics*, vol. 10, no. 1, pp. 59–64, 2009.

[7] L. Sztriha, C. Panzeri, R. Kálmánchey et al., "First case of compound heterozygosity in *ALS2* gene in infantile-onset ascending spastic paralysis with bulbar involvement," *Clinical Genetics*, vol. 73, no. 6, pp. 591–593, 2008.

[8] C. C. Verschuuren-Bemelmans, P. Winter, D. A. Sival, J. W. Elting, O. F. Brouwer, and U. Müller, "Novel homozygous ALS2 nonsense mutation (p.Gln715X) in sibs with infantile-onset ascending spastic paralysis: The first cases from northwestern Europe," *European Journal of Human Genetics*, vol. 16, no. 11, pp. 1407–1411, 2008.

[9] E. Eymard-Pierre, K. Yamanaka, M. Haeussler et al., "Novel missense mutation in ALS2 gene results in infantile ascending hereditary spastic paralysis," *Annals of Neurology*, vol. 59, no. 6, pp. 976–980, 2006.

[10] R. S. Devon, J. R. Helm, G. A. Rouleau et al., "The first nonsense mutation in alsin results in a homogeneous phenotype of infantile-onset ascending spastic paralysis with bulbar involvement in two siblings," *Clinical Genetics*, vol. 64, no. 3, pp. 210–215, 2003.

[11] F. Gros-Louis, I. A. Meijer, C. K. Hand et al., "An ALS2 gene mutation causes hereditary spastic paraplegia in a Pakistani kindred," *Annals of Neurology*, vol. 53, no. 1, pp. 144–145, 2003.

[12] E. Eymard-Pierre, G. Lesca, S. Dollet et al., "Infantile-onset ascending hereditary spastic paralysis is associated with mutations in the alsin gene," *The American Journal of Human Genetics*, vol. 71, no. 3, pp. 518–527, 2002.

[13] M. Luigetti, S. Lattante, A. Conte et al., "A novel compound heterozygous *ALS2* mutation in two Italian siblings with juvenile amyotrophic lateral sclerosis," *Amyotrophic Lateral Sclerosis and Frontotemporal Degeneration*, vol. 14, no. 5-6, pp. 470–472, 2013.

[14] J. A. Kress, P. Kühnlein, P. Winter et al., "Novel mutation in the ALS2 gene in juvenile amyotrophic lateral sclerosis," *Annals of Neurology*, vol. 58, no. 5, pp. 800–803, 2005.

[15] N. Mintchev, E. Zamba-Papanicolaou, K. A. Kleopa, and K. Christodoulou, "A novel ALS2 splice-site mutation in a Cypriot juvenile-onset primary lateral sclerosis family," *Neurology*, vol. 72, no. 1, pp. 28–32, 2009.

[16] C. Panzeri, C. de Palma, A. Martinuzzi et al., "The first *ALS2* missense mutation associated with JPLS reveals new aspects of alsin biological function," *Brain*, vol. 129, no. 7, pp. 1710–1719, 2006.

39

Mandibuloacral Dysplasia Caused by *LMNA* Mutations and Uniparental Disomy

Shaochun Bai,[1] Anthony Lozada,[1] Marilyn C. Jones,[2] Harry C. Dietz,[3] Melissa Dempsey,[1] and Soma Das[1,4]

[1] *University of Chicago, 5841 South Maryland Avenue, Chicago, IL 60637, USA*
[2] *University of California and Children's Hospital of San Diego, San Diego, CA 92123, USA*
[3] *Johns Hopkins University School of Medicine and Howard Hughes Medical Institute, Baltimore, MD 21287, USA*
[4] *Department of Human Genetics, University of Chicago, 5841 South Maryland Avenue, Chicago, IL 60637, USA*

Correspondence should be addressed to Soma Das; sdas@bsd.uchicago.edu

Academic Editors: C.-W. Cheng and A. Sazci

Mandibuloacral dysplasia (MAD) is a rare autosomal recessive disorder characterized by postnatal growth retardation, craniofacial anomalies, skeletal malformations, and mottled cutaneous pigmentation. Hutchinson-Gilford Progeria Syndrome (HGPS) is characterized by the clinical features of accelerated aging in childhood. Both MAD and HGPS can be caused by mutations in the *LMNA* gene. In this study, we describe a 2-year-old boy with overlapping features of MAD and HGPS. Mutation analysis of the *LMNA* gene revealed a homozygous missense change, p.M540T, while only the mother carries the mutation. Uniparental disomy (UPD) analysis for chromosome 1 showed the presence of maternal UPD. Markers in the 1q21.3–q22 region flanking the *LMNA* locus were isodisomic, while markers in the short arm and distal 1q region were heterodisomic. These results suggest that nondisjunction in maternal meiosis followed by loss of the paternal chromosome 1 during trisomy rescue might result in the UPD1 and homozygosity for the p.M540T mutation observed in this patient.

1. Introduction

Mandibuloacral dysplasia (MAD) is a rare autosomal recessive disorder characterized by postnatal growth retardation, craniofacial anomalies, skeletal malformations, and mottled cutaneous pigmentation [1, 2]. Hutchinson-Gilford Progeria Syndrome (HGPS) is an autosomal dominant disorder demonstrating varying symptoms including short stature, hair loss, joint degeneration, and atherosclerosis [3]. Pathogenic mutations in the *LMNA* gene on chromosome 1q22 and encoding the Lamin A/C protein have been reported in both MAD and HGPS. To date, the majority of cases of MAD are caused by missense mutations in exons 8–10 of the *LMNA* gene [4, 5] that codes for the LAP2 and emerin-binding domain of the Lamin A/C protein.

Recently, we encountered a two-year-old boy with overlapping features of MAD and HGPS. *LMNA* sequence analysis was performed to determine the genetic cause of his clinical phenotype. With the aim of identifying the molecular etiology of this boy's phenotype, a comprehensive study was performed on the patient and parents.

2. Materials and Methods

2.1. LMNA Sequence Analysis. The 12 coding exons plus exon-intron boundaries of the *LMNA* gene were amplified by polymerase chain reaction (PCR). The purified PCR products were sequenced in both directions using ABI Big Dye terminator mix (Life Technologies, Foster City, CA). Data were analyzed using Mutation Surveyor 3.20 software (SoftGenetics, LLC, PA).

2.2. LMNA Deletion Analysis by Real-Time Quantitative-PCR. Real-time quantitative-PCR (RT-qPCR) was performed using 3 different primer pairs specific to exon 10 of the *LMNA* gene and detected using Power SYBR Green (Life Technologies) following manufacturer instructions. The relative copy

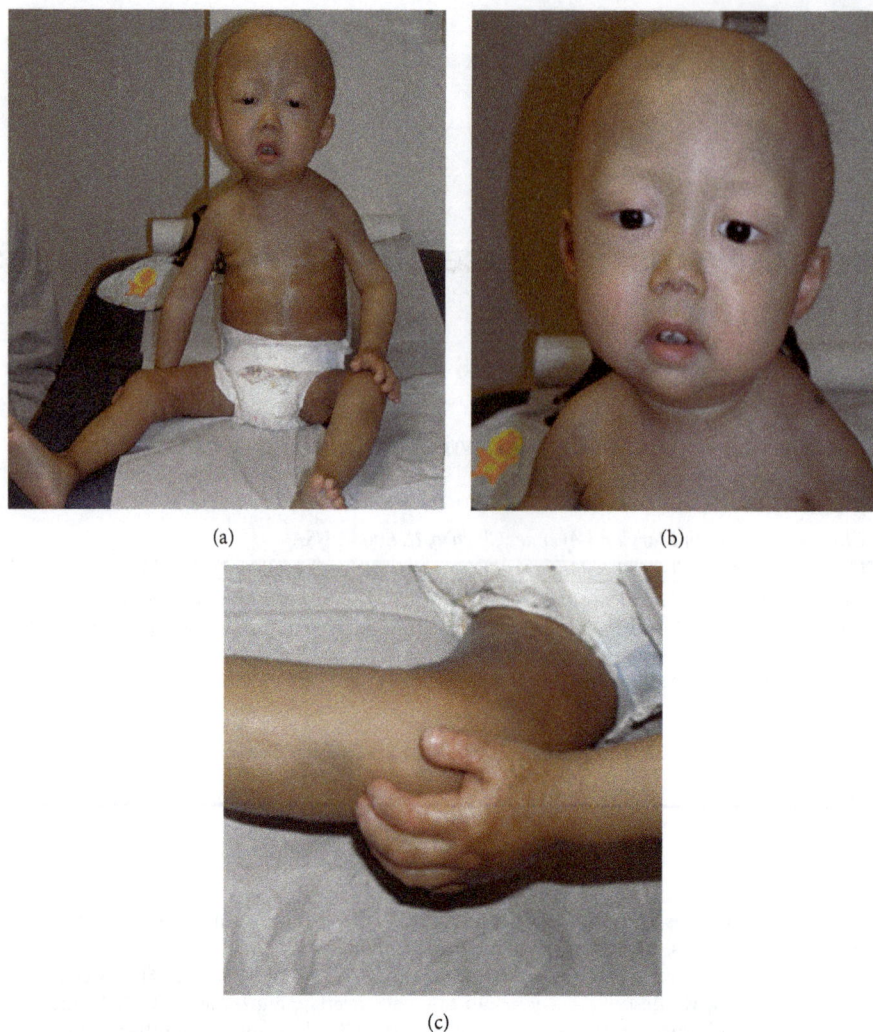

FIGURE 1: Clinical features of the patient with a homozygous mutation p.M540T. (a) presents proband's hyperpigmented and thickened skin (especially on his truck and thighs) and thin clavicles. (b) depicts patient's prominent cranium and the loss of hair. (c) demonstrates his small contracted hands with bulbous distal tips.

number was calculated based on the standard curve method and compared to *PMP22* gene, which was used as an internal control. A ratio of 0.8–1.2 was indicative of no deletion/duplication.

2.3. Microsatellite Analysis. Genotyping of microsatellite markers on chromosomes 1, 6, and 15 was performed on the patient and both parental samples. Microsatellite markers were amplified and separated on an ABI PRISM 3130xl Genetic Analyzer (Life Technologies). The PCR fragments were analyzed using ABI PRISM GeneScan and Genotyper software (Life Technologies).

This study was approved by the University of Chicago Institutional Review Board (IRB protocol number 11-0151).

3. Results

3.1. Clinical Phenotype. The patient is a two-year-old boy from a nonconsanguineous family of Chinese descent. At 3 months of age, he started presenting with progressive hair loss. Thickening of the skin on his knees developed at 6 months of age followed by progressive joint contractures and hyperpigmentation with sclerosis of the skin. By 1 year of age, his weight was reduced to below the 3rd percentile; he also developed stiffness and blunting of the fingertips. Osteoporosis was noted on radiographs. At 18 months of age, his head circumference, height, and weight were 50th, 25th, and below the 3rd percentiles, respectively. He was cognitively normal with physical restrictions related to joint contractures. He had striking alopecia, prominent scalp veins, limited jaw mobility, and dental crowding. His hands were small and contracted with bulbous distal tips and purplish discoloration over the extensor surfaces. Contractures were present in all major joints. His skin was diffusely thick. At 2 years of age, radiographs showed striking acroosteolysis in the clavicles, hands and feet, wormian bones, and osteopenia. His phenotype shared features of both MAD and HGPS (Figure 1). Molecular genetic testing was requested to make the molecular

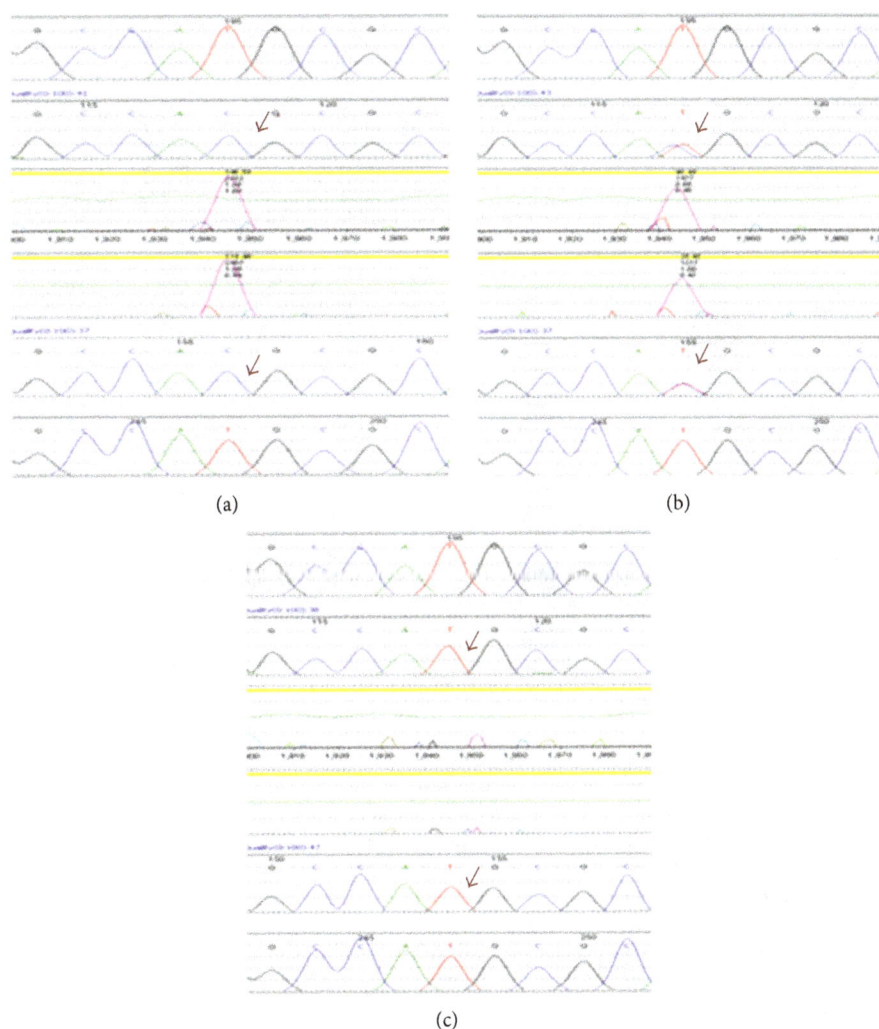

FIGURE 2: DNA sequencing results. (a) DNA sequencing revealed a homozygous mutation of c.1619T>C, p.M540T in the patient. (b) Mother is a carrier. (c) Father is not a carrier. The c.1619 nucleotide residue is depicted by an arrow in forward and reverse sequence traces for the patient and both parents. The sequence of a normal control sample is shown for each case for comparison.

diagnosis. Over time, the patient suffered continued growth failure with progressive skin thickening and stiffness that was partially relieved by topical pimecrolimus. He had a pathological fracture of his radius at the age of 3. Progressive acroosteolysis of the jaw resulted in premature dental loss. Stamina has decreased.

3.2. Molecular Analysis. DNA sequencing revealed a homozygous c.1619T>C, p.M540T mutation in exon 10 of the *LMNA* gene in this patient (Figure 2(a)). Subsequent analysis of the parental samples revealed that the mother was a heterozygous carrier of the same mutation but the father was not (Figures 2(b) and 2(c)). This result was confirmed by repeat PCR/sequence analysis using different sets of PCR primers to rule out the possibility of an SNP interfering with PCR amplification. Nonpaternity was excluded by genotyping of 13 microsatellite markers across chromosomes 6 and 15 (data not shown). The presence of a deletion of one copy of the *LMNA* gene in the patient (which would make the p.M540T mutation appear homozygous) and the patient's father was

investigated by RT-qPCR of exon 10 of the *LMNA* gene and two copies of the gene were identified (data not shown).

In order to investigate whether uniparental disomy (UPD) involving chromosome 1 may be present in this patient, microsatellite analysis was performed using markers spanning chromosome 1, with increased density in the 1q22 region, where the *LMNA* gene resides. Analysis of 11 informative microsatellite markers showed that the genotype of the patient matched that of the mother with complete absence of the paternal chromosome 1, indicating maternal UPD (Figure 3(a)). Furthermore, the microsatellite data demonstrated that the proband has a minimal region of isodisomy between markers *D1S498* and *D1S3792*, a 27.2 Mb segment in the 1q21.3–q22 region where *LMNA* is located, with the rest of chromosome 1 being heterodisomic (Figure 3(b)).

4. Discussion

MAD is a rare, autosomal recessive disorder with clinical manifestation involving skin, skeleton, and adipose tissue.

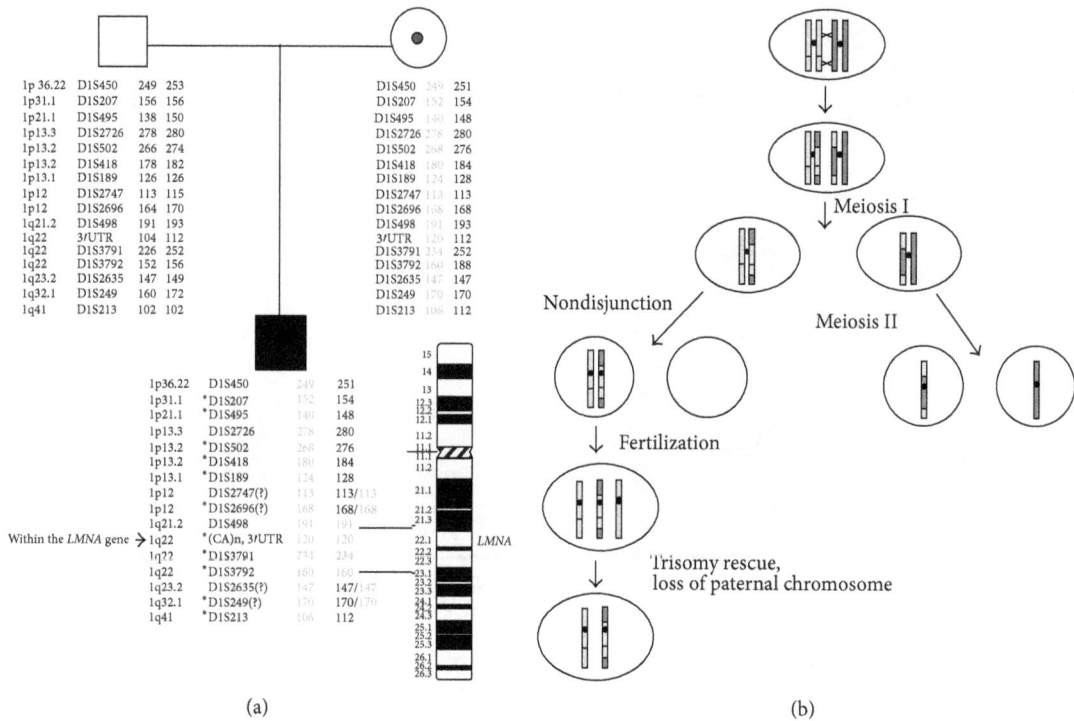

1p 36.22	D1S450	249	253
1p31.1	D1S207	156	156
1p21.1	D1S495	138	150
1p13.3	D1S2726	278	280
1p13.2	D1S502	266	274
1p13.2	D1S418	178	182
1p13.1	D1S189	126	126
1p12	D1S2747	113	115
1p12	D1S2696	164	170
1q21.2	D1S498	191	193
1q22	3'UTR	104	112
1q22	D1S3791	226	252
1q22	D1S3792	152	156
1q23.2	D1S2635	147	149
1q32.1	D1S249	160	172
1q41	D1S213	102	102

	D1S450	249	251
	D1S207	152	154
	D1S495	140	148
	D1S2726	278	280
	D1S502	268	276
	D1S418	180	184
	D1S189	124	128
	D1S2747	113	113
	D1S2696	168	168
	D1S498	191	193
	3'UTR	129	112
	D1S3791	234	252
	D1S3792	160	188
	D1S2635	147	147
	D1S249	170	170
	D1S213	106	112

1p36.22	D1S450	249	251
1p31.1	*D1S207	152	154
1p21.1	*D1S495	140	148
1p13.3	D1S2726	278	280
1p13.2	*D1S502	268	276
1p13.2	*D1S418	180	184
1p13.1	D1S189	124	128
1p12	D1S2747(?)	113	113/113
1p12	*D1S2696(?)	168	168/168
1q21.2	D1S498	191	
Within the LMNA gene → 1q22	*(CA)n, 3'UTR	120	120	LMNA
1q??	*D1S3791	234	234
1q22	*D1S3792	160	160
1q23.2	D1S2635(?)	147	147/147
1q32.1	*D1S249(?)	170	170/170
1q41	*D1S213	106	112

(a)   (b)

FIGURE 3: Uniparental disomy analysis of chromosome 1 and schematic representation of the generation of the homozygous p.M540T mutation. (a) Markers around the region of the LMNA gene in 1q22 show maternal isodisomy. Allele sizes for each marker are indicated. Informative markers for maternal UPD are denoted with an asterisk (*). Based on the results, one recombination event could have occurred proximal to D1S189 at 1p13.1 and a second recombination event could have occurred proximal to D1S213 at 1q41 resulting in maternal isodisomy for the 1q21-q22 region where the LMNA resides. Due to the uninformative nature of markers D1S2747, D1S2696, D1S2635, and D1S249 in the mother, it is unclear whether these regions are isodisomic or heterodisomic. The uninformative markers are indicated with question marks. (b) Schematic representation of the generation of the homozygous p.M540T mutation in the patient by the process of recombination and nondisjunction in maternal meiosis followed by trisomy rescue. Nondisjunction is shown as occurring in meiosis II in this figure, but it could also have occurred in meiosis I; the microsatellite markers used could not distinguish between these two possibilities. The p.M540T mutation is indicated by the red bar on one of the maternal chromosome 1's. Paternal chromosome 1 is indicated by the blue colored. LMNA gene is indicated by the red bar.

The pathogenesis of this rare disorder remains incompletely understood. The majority of MAD patients are caused by point mutations in the LMNA gene [6–8]. Patients with overlapping features of MAD and HGPS have also been reported with mutations in the LMNA gene [9–12]. In this study, we report a patient with MAD clinical features, with some overlapping features of HGPS, who presented with a homozygous p.M540T mutation in the LMNA gene. This mutation has previously been identified in the compound heterozygous state with another missense mutation in a patient with HGPS in whom atypical pathological findings on fibroblast were observed [13]. The p.M540T mutation affects a conserved region within the C-terminal globular domain of A-type lamins and affects a highly evolutionarily conserved amino acid residue. The observation of this mutation in the homozygous state is the likely cause of the disease phenotype in this patient.

Subsequent analysis of the patient's parents demonstrated only the patient's mother to be a carrier of the p.M540T mutation and the presence of maternal UPD for chromosome 1 as the cause of the homozygosity in the patient. Previous studies have reported UPD as one of the causes leading to the

homozygous mutations in several autosomal recessive disorders [14–17]. In fact, UPD involving the LMNA gene was identified in some of the first molecularly characterized patients with HGPS [18]. Our patient demonstrated isodisomy for the region encompassing the LMNA gene, flanked by heterodisomy. We speculate that during maternal meiosis two recombination events, proximal and distal to the LMNA gene, followed by nondisjunction resulted in a gamete with two copies of chromosome 1 both containing the p.M540T mutation. The further loss of paternal chromosome 1 through trisomy rescue after fertilization led to homozygosity of the p.M540T mutation in the patient (Figure 3(b)).

In conclusion, we have identified a patient with MAD and some overlapping features of HGPS in whom a homozygous p.M540T mutation in the LMNA gene was identified. The homozygosity of the LMNA mutation in this patient was due to maternal UPD of chromosome 1. While UPD involving the LMNA gene has previously been identified in patients with HGPS, our patient represents the first case of UPD1 concomitant with LMNA mutation in MAD. This observation adds to the growing list of autosomal recessive conditions where UPD contributes to the clinical phenotype.

Abbreviations

MAD: Mandibuloacral dysplasia
HGPS: Hutchinson-Gilford Progeria Syndrome
UPD: Uniparental disomy.

Conflict of Interests

The authors declare that there is no conflict of interests regarding the publication of this paper.

Authors' Contribution

Dr. Shaochun Bai designed and performed the study, drafted the initial paper, and reviewed the final paper as submitted. Mr. Anthony Lozada performed the sequence in the study. Dr. Marilyn C. Jones performed the clinical evaluation of the patient. Dr. Harry C. Dietz was involved in the initial identification of the mutation in this patient. Ms. Melissa Dempsey helped with the revision of the manuscript. Dr. Soma Das helped in designing the study, revising, reviewing and approving the final paper as submitted.

References

[1] B. Burke and C. L. Stewart, "Life at the edge: the nuclear envelope and human disease," *Nature Reviews Molecular Cell Biology*, vol. 3, no. 8, pp. 575–585, 2002.

[2] V. Simha, A. K. Agarwal, E. A. Oral, J.-P. Fryns, and A. Garg, "Genetic and phenotypic heterogeneity in patients with mandibuloacral dysplasia-associated lipodystrophy," *Journal of Clinical Endocrinology and Metabolism*, vol. 88, no. 6, pp. 2821–2824, 2003.

[3] R. C. M. Hennekam, "Hutchinson-Gilford progeria syndrome: review of the phenotype," *American Journal of Medical Genetics A*, vol. 140, no. 23, pp. 2603–2624, 2006.

[4] A. Garg, O. Cogulu, F. Ozkinay, H. Onay, and A. K. Agarwal, "A novel homozygous Ala529Val LMNA mutation in Turkish patients with mandibuloacral dysplasia," *Journal of Clinical Endocrinology and Metabolism*, vol. 90, no. 9, pp. 5259–5264, 2005.

[5] T. Kosho, J. Takahashi, T. Momose et al., "Mandibuloacral dysplasia and a novel LMNA mutation in a woman with severe progressive skeletal changes," *American Journal of Medical Genetics A*, vol. 143, no. 21, pp. 2598–2603, 2007.

[6] B. C. Capell and F. S. Collins, "Human laminopathies: nuclei gone genetically awry," *Nature Reviews Genetics*, vol. 7, no. 12, pp. 940–952, 2006.

[7] F. Lombardi, F. Gullotta, M. Columbaro et al., "Compound heterozygosity for mutations in LMNA in a patient with a myopathic and lipodystrophic mandibuloacral dysplasia type A phenotype," *Journal of Clinical Endocrinology and Metabolism*, vol. 92, no. 11, pp. 4467–4471, 2007.

[8] G. Novelli, A. Muchir, F. Sangiuolo et al., "Mandibuloacral dysplasia is caused by a mutation in LMNA-encoding lamin A/C," *American Journal of Human Genetics*, vol. 71, no. 2, pp. 426–431, 2002.

[9] M. Al-Haggar, A. Madej-Pilarczyk, L. Kozlowski et al., "A novel homozygous p.Arg527Leu LMNA mutation in two unrelated Egyptian families causes overlapping mandibuloacral dysplasia and progeria syndrome," *European Journal of Human Genetics*, vol. 20, pp. 1134–1140, 2012.

[10] A. K. Agarwal, I. Kazachkova, S. Ten, and A. Garg, "Severe mandibuloacral dysplasia-associated lipodystrophy and progeria in a young girl with a novel homozygous Arg527Cys LMNA mutation," *Journal of Clinical Endocrinology and Metabolism*, vol. 93, no. 12, pp. 4617–4623, 2008.

[11] A. Garg, L. Subramanyam, A. K. Agarwal et al., "Atypical progeroid syndrome due to heterozygous missense LMNA mutations," *Journal of Clinical Endocrinology and Metabolism*, vol. 94, no. 12, pp. 4971–4983, 2009.

[12] B. Zirn, W. Kress, T. Grimm et al., "Association of homozygous LMNA mutation R471C with new phenotype: mandibuloacral dysplasia, progeria, and rigid spine muscular dystrophy," *American Journal of Medical Genetics A*, vol. 146, no. 8, pp. 1049–1054, 2008.

[13] V. L. R. M. Verstraeten, J. L. V. Broers, M. A. M. van Steensel et al., "Compound heterozygosity for mutations in LMNA causes a progeria syndrome without prelamin A accumulation," *Human Molecular Genetics*, vol. 15, no. 16, pp. 2509–2522, 2006.

[14] L. Pulkkinen, F. Bullrich, P. Czarnecki, L. Weiss, and J. Uitto, "Maternal uniparental disomy of chromosome 1 with reduction to homozygosity of the LAMB3 locus in a patient with Herlitz junctional epidermolysis bullosa," *American Journal of Human Genetics*, vol. 61, no. 3, pp. 611–619, 1997.

[15] B. D. Gelb, J. P. Willner, T. M. Dunn et al., "Paternal uniparental disomy for chromosome 1 revealed by molecular analysis of a patient with pycnodysostosis," *American Journal of Human Genetics*, vol. 62, no. 4, pp. 848–854, 1998.

[16] C. L. S. Turner, D. J. Bunyan, N. S. Thomas et al., "Zellweger syndrome resulting from maternal isodisomy of chromosome 1," *American Journal of Medical Genetics A*, vol. 143, no. 18, pp. 2172–2177, 2007.

[17] W.-Q. Zeng, H. Gao, L. Brueton et al., "Fumarase deficiency caused by homozygous P131R mutation and paternal partial isodisomy of chromosome 1," *American Journal of Medical Genetics*, vol. 140, no. 9, pp. 1004–1009, 2006.

[18] M. Eriksson, W. T. Brown, L. B. Gordon et al., "Recurrent de novo point mutations in lamin A cause Hutchinson-Gilford progeria syndrome," *Nature*, vol. 423, no. 6937, pp. 293–298, 2003.

40

Rhabdomyolysis and Cardiomyopathy in a 20-Year-Old Patient with CPT II Deficiency

M. Vavlukis,[1] **A. Eftimov,**[2] **P. Zafirovska,**[1] **E. Caparovska,**[1] **B. Pocesta,**[1] **S. Kedev,**[1] **and A. J. Dimovski**[2]

[1] *University Clinic of Cardiology, Medical Faculty, Ss. Cyril and Methodius University, Mother Teresa 17, 1000 Skopje, Macedonia*
[2] *Faculty of Pharmacy, Ss. Cyril and Methodius University, Mother Teresa 47, 1000 Skopje, Macedonia*

Correspondence should be addressed to A. J. Dimovski; adimovski@ff.ukim.edu.mk

Academic Editors: D. J. Bunyan, P. D. Cotter, C. Julier, and B. Melegh

Aim. To raise the awareness of adult-onset carnitite palmitoyltransferase II deficiency (CPT II) by describing clinical, biochemical, and genetic features of the disease occurring in early adulthood. *Method.* Review of the case characteristics and literature review. *Results.* We report on a 20-year-old man presenting with dyspnea, fatigue, fever, and myoglobinuria. This was the second episode with such symptoms (the previous one being three years earlier). The symptoms occurred after intense physical work, followed by a viral infection resulting in fever treated with NSAIDs. Massive rhabdomyolysis was diagnosed, resulting in acute renal failure necessitating plasmapheresis and hemodialysis, acute hepatic lesion, and respiratory insufficiency. Additionally, our patient had cardiomyopathy with volume overload. After a detailed workup, CPT II deficiency was suspected. We did a sequencing analysis for exons 1, 3, and 4 of the CPT II gene and found that the patient was homozygote for Ser 113 Leu mutation in exon 3 of the CPT II gene. The patient recovery was complete except for the cardiomiopathy with mildly impaired systolic function. *Conclusion.* Whenever a patient suffers recurrent episodes of myalgia, followed by myoglobinuria due to rhabdomyolysis, we should always consider the possibility of this rare condition. The definitive diagnose of this condition is achieved by genetic testing.

1. Introduction

Carnitine palmitoyltransferase (CPT) deficiencies are genetic disorders of mitochondrial fatty acid oxidation. Long-chain fatty acids are required for fueling the skeletal muscles and are only able to cross mitochondrial membrane after esterification with carnitine in a reaction with the enzyme CPT I. Inside the mitochondria, the fatty acid is reactivated to acyl-CoA from acylcarnitine and CoA with the help of CPT II in order to enter the β-oxidation cycle [1–3].

The CPT II deficiency presents in three different forms: lethal neonatal form; severe infantile hepatocardiomuscular form, and adult-myopathic form [1–8].

The adult-myopathic form is the most prevalent type of the disease with about 300 cases reported. The first description was made in 1973 by the brothers Di Mauro. The first symptoms most often occur between 6 and 20 years of age but the age of onset may be over 50 years and as early as 8 months

of life [9, 10]. The symptomatology usually consists of recurrent attacks of rhabdomyolysis presenting as myalgias, muscle stiffness and weakness, and myoglobinuria. In rare situations, rhabdomyolysis may result in life-threatening complications such as acute renal failure and respiratory insufficiency secondary to respiratory muscles involvement [11, 12].

We are describing such a clinical case.

2. Case Presentation

We report a case of a 20-year-old man transferred to our clinic under suspicion of myocarditis. He presented with dyspnea, fatigue, myalgia, fever, and myoglobinuria. The patient reported those three days before becoming symptomatic, he was subjected to a more intense physical work (unloading a truck). The next day he felt like coming down with a cold, he felt weak and had muscle pains. Later that day, he was admitted to the ER with fever (40°C) where he received

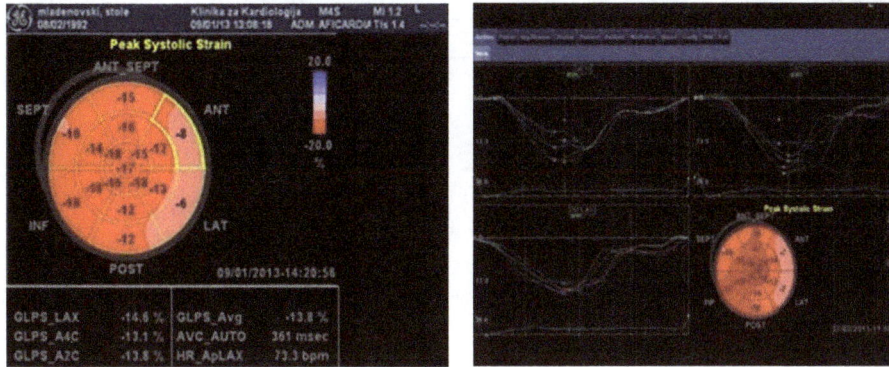

FIGURE 1: Strain analysis of the left ventricle.

a parenteral therapy with NSAIDs. After the parenteral therapy, he complained of worsening of the symptoms with strong myalgia, dyspnea, fatigue, sweating, and myoglobinuria.

Influenza B was identified, and increased markers of inflammation-fibrinogen, CRP, leukocytosis, plasma levels of CPK up to 114000 IU, CK-MB 5400 IU, and myoglobin up to 33000 IU were detected, resulting in acute renal failure (necessitating plasmapheresis and hemodialysis treatments), respiratory insufficiency (necessitating a noninvasive ventilation support), and a mild to moderate hepatic lesion.

During the whole period, the blood glucose levels were in the range of 3, 4-5, 4 mmol/L (lower normal limit), and no significant hypoglycemia was registered.

Muscle biopsy identified exacerbated chronic vasculitis with atrophy of certain muscle cells. The immunologic markers and hemoculture were negative. The pneumoslide was only positive to IgM for Influenza B.

The echocardiographic examination revealed enlarged left ventricle (LVEDd 65; LVEDs 48) with EF of 47% by the Simpson method. Strain analysis using speckle tracking identified GLPS average of −13.8% (Figure 1).

After one-month hospitalization period, the patient was stabilized and discharged from the hospital. During the nine-month follow-up period he was stable, completely recovered, and asymptomatic, except for a mildly impaired left ventricular systolic function.

His prior history revealed that the patient used to feel cramps and pain in the legs after prolonged walking in the childhood. He experienced a similar episode three years earlier after prolonged exercise (body building for several hours), exposure to a cold temperature, and infection (febrile illness), when he was hospitalized in another institution with severe signs of rhabdomyolysis (creatinine phosphokinase up to 42000 IU) and hepatic lesion (AST, ALT up to ×10 over the upper limit) and was diagnosed with cardiomyopathy with increased LV dimensions LVEDd > 60 mm, EF 45%. There were no signs of renal impairment at that time. He was stabilized and discharged from hospital. During attack-free periods, the patient was asymptomatic.

The patient had a deceased father from heart failure of unknown origin and a sister that died at the age of 18 months in unclear circumstances after "being sick all the time" when she received an injection for fever.

During hospitalization, the diagnosis of CPT II deficiency was suspected and the patient was referred for genetic analyses. Sequencing analysis of exons 1, 3, and 4 of the CPT II gene revealed that the patient was homozygote for Ser 113 Leu mutation (Figure 2). Diagnosis of adult myopathic form of carnitine palmitoyltransferase II deficiency was made based on the genetic findings and signs and symptoms as well as the age of onset.

3. DNA Sequencing

DNA was extracted from a peripheral blood sample using QiAmp DNA Blood Mini Kit (Qiagen). Exons 1, 3, and 4 of the CPT II gene were amplified by PCR using the following oligonucleotide primer pairs: CPT2 Ex 1 F: 5′-ACTCCA-GAACTCCCCACTTG-3′/CPT2 Ex 1 R: 5′- CGGGTTCAC-TAGAGGAGTCA-3′ (299 bp PCR fragment); CPT2 Ex 3 F: 5′-CCTCGCCATGAACCTAAAAA-3′/CPT2 Ex 3 R: 5′-TTCATTATGGAGGGCTCTGG-3′ (231 bp PCR fragment); CPT2 Ex 4 F: 5′-CCCATTAAGGACCTTGTCCA-3′, CPT2 Ex 4 R: 5′-GCCTCAGAGCACCTCTTTGT-3′ (564 bp PCR fragment). Direct sequencing was performed at 3500 Series AB Genetic Analyzer (Applied Biosystems, Foster City, CA, USA).

4. Discussion

Carnitine palmitoyltransferase (CPT) CPT I deficiency is a very rare condition and is recognized in three different forms, of which the last two have not been identified in humans yet (might be incompatible with life): liver type CPT I deficiency; muscle-type and brain-type CPT I deficiency [1–3].

The CPT II deficiency presents in three different forms:

  (i) lethal neonatal form,

 (ii) severe infantile hepatocardiomuscular form, and

(iii) adult-myopathic form [1–6].

The lethal neonatal form is characterized by episodes of liver failure, hypoketotic hypoglycemia, cardiomyopathy, cardiac arrhythmias, seizures and coma after fasting or infection, and facial and structural abnormalities [4]. This presentation is fatal; the CPT II activity is barely detectable in any of the tissues, leading to death in the neonatal period [2, 7].

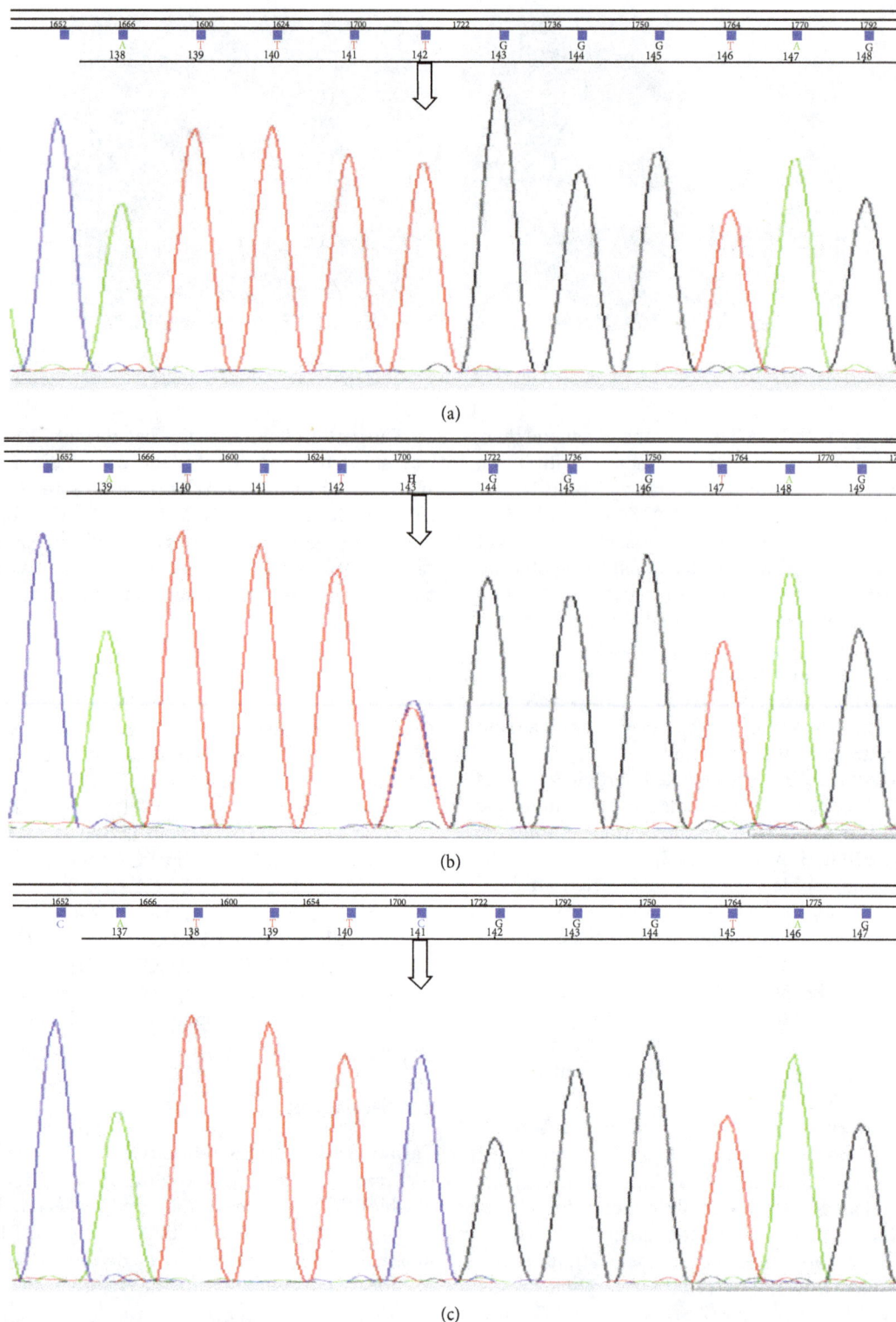

FIGURE 2: Sequencing analysis demonstrating the detection of TCG > TTG or S113L mutation in exon 3 of the CPT II gene (a: patient; b: mother of the patient; c: normal control).

The severe infantile hepatocardiomuscular form is characterized by liver failure, cardiomyopathy, seizures, hypoketotic hypoglycemia, peripheral myopathy, and attacks of abdominal pain. The onset is more often before one-year of age and usually ends with a sudden death secondary to paroxysmal heart beat disorders [2, 4, 8].

The adult-myopathic form is the most prevalent type of the disease with about 300 cases reported. The majority of the patients are males (~80%) and it is inherited in an autosomal recessive manner. The first description was made in 1973 by the brothers Di Mauro. The first symptoms most often occur between 6 and 20 years of age but the age of onset may be over 50 years and as early as 8 months of life [9, 10]. The symptomatology usually consists of recurrent attacks of rhabdomyolysis presenting as myalgias, muscle stiffness and weakness, and myoglobinuria. The frequency of the symptoms is highly variable and they resolve within hours to days with clinically symptom-free periods between attacks. The rhabdomyolysis may occasionally be complicated by three kinds of life-threatening events, that is, acute renal failure due to myoglobinuria, respiratory insufficiency secondary to respiratory muscles involvement, and paroxysmal heart arrhythmias [11, 12]. The symptoms are usually provoked by prolonged exercise, fasting, high fat intake, exposure to cold, infections accompanied by fever, and general anesthesia and drugs such as ibuprofen, diazepam, and valproic acid. In general, the patients have normal life expectancy with complications such as acute kidney failure in massive rhabdomyolysis, usually sparing other organs. In our patient we observed cardiac complications.

Our patient presented with all the typical signs and symptoms, including a respiratory failure combined with heart failure, probably worsened by volume overload during the uric period of the disease. The findings of the echocardiography examinations done three years earlier and at present time identify dilated cardiomyopathy with a reduced ejection fraction. The strain analysis using speckle tracking showed average GLPS decrease of 13.8%. These findings could be prescribed to the nature of the disease and consequence of lipid storage in the myocardium even though unspecific for this form of disease. Could myocardial biopsy help us with our hypothesis? Comparisons with the results obtained three years ago showed a relatively stable course of heart failure (no significant progression of the left ventricle dimension or reduction of the ejection fraction).

Diagnosing CPT II deficiency can be done by acylcarnitine analysis using tandem mass spectrometry (peak at C16 is indicative of the condition). Measurement of the CPT II activity can be performed as well as many laboratory findings, such as low carnitine levels, increased serum creatinine kinase, and transaminase, which can be associated with the disease. For a definitive diagnosis, sequencing of the CPT II gene for a mutation analysis is recommended. The CPT II gene has been assigned to chromosome 1p32. It contains five exons and more than 25 mutations have been described [3]. The S113L is the most common mutation in the myopathic form. There is evidence that the S113L mutation leads to a thermolabile CPT II protein whose activity is reduced when the body temperature is high, as with exercise, fever, or heat stress [13].

Definitive diagnosis in our patient was established with the CPT II gene sequencing for mutation analysis, and the Ser 113 Leu mutation in exon 3 of the CPT II gene was identified (Figure 2). Genetic analyses were performed on the patient's family (mother and two siblings). We found that his mother, brother, and sister are carriers for the mutation, but none of them described any myalgia or symptoms suggestive of rhabdomyolysis.

The treatment of this condition consists of hygiene-dietary changes that would prevent attacks and symptomatic treatment of myoglobinuria and possible renal complications. Patients are advised to reduce the intake of long-chain dietary fat and increase the consumption of meals rich in carbohydrates. They should have more frequent meals and avoid fasting. Other things that should be avoided include prolonged exercise as well as some drugs (ibuprofen, diazepam, valproic acid, and general anesthesia). During intercurrent infections infusion of glucose can be administered. Oral carnitine supplementation can be considered as an adequate therapy. The medium-chain fatty acid triheptanoin may be effective in the adult-onset CPT II deficiency.

At present, nine months after this episode, our patient is clinically stable and no episodes of rhabdomyolysis have been registered. He is on heart failure treatment medications, and he is following the advice given to him concerning his life style modification. He does not work as a lorry driver anymore.

Consent

The patient gave informed consent for publishing of this paper.

Conflict of Interests

There is no conflict of interests.

References

[1] K. J. Hogan and G. D. Vladutiu, "Malignant hyperthermia-like syndrome and carnitine palmitoyltransferase II deficiency with heterozygous R503C mutation," *Anesthesia and Analgesia*, vol. 109, no. 4, pp. 1070–1072, 2009.

[2] J.-P. Bonnefont, F. Djouadi, C. Prip-Buus, S. Gobin, A. Munnich, and J. Bastin, "Carnitine palmitoyltransferases 1 and 2: biochemical, molecular and medical aspects," *Molecular Aspects of Medicine*, vol. 25, no. 5-6, pp. 495–520, 2004.

[3] E. Sigauke, D. Rakheja, K. Kitson, and M. J. Bennett, "Carnitine palmitoyltransferase II deficiency: a clinical, biochemical, and molecular review," *Laboratory Investigation*, vol. 83, no. 11, pp. 1543–1554, 2003.

[4] R. A. Pagon, T. D. Bird, C. R. Dolan et al., "Carnitine palmytoil-transferase II deficiency," in *GeneReviews [Internet]*, pp. 1993–2013, University of Washington, Seattle, Wash, USA, 2004.

[5] M. Deschauer, T. Wieser, and S. Zierz, "Muscle carnitine palmitoyltransferase II deficiency: clinical and molecular genetic features and diagnostic aspects," *Archives of Neurology*, vol. 62, no. 1, pp. 37–41, 2005.

[6] S. Albers, D. Marsden, E. Quackenbush, A. R. Stark, H. L. Levy, and M. Irons, "Detection of neonatal carnitine palmitoyltransferase II deficiency by expanded newborn screening with tandem mass spectrometry," *Pediatrics*, vol. 107, no. 6, article E103, 2001.

[7] O. N. Elpeleg, C. Hammerman, A. Saada, A. Shaag, and E. Golzand, "Antenatal presentation of carnitine palmitoyltransferase II deficiency," *American Journal of Medical Genetics*, vol. 102, no. 2, pp. 183–187, 2001.

[8] F. Demaugre, J.-P. Bonnefont, M. Colonna, C. Cepanec, J.-P. Leroux, and J. M. Saudubray, "Infantile form of carnitine palmitoyltransferase II deficiency with hepatomuscular symptoms and sudden death. Physiopathological approach to carnitine palmitoyltransferase II deficiencies," *Journal of Clinical Investigation*, vol. 87, no. 3, pp. 859–864, 1991.

[9] K. Gempel, C. Von Praun, J. Baumkötter et al., "'Adult' form of muscular carnitine palmitoyltransferase II deficiency: manifestation in a 2-year-old child," *European Journal of Pediatrics*, vol. 160, no. 9, pp. 548–551, 2001.

[10] H. Hurvitz, A. Klar, I. Korn-Lubetzki, R. J. A. Wanders, and O. N. Elpeleg, "Muscular carnitine palmitoyltransferase II deficiency in infancy," *Pediatric Neurology*, vol. 22, no. 2, pp. 148–150, 2000.

[11] L. Thuillier, C. Sevin, F. Demaugre et al., "Genotype/phenotype correlation in carnitine palmitoyl transferase II deficiency: lessons from a compound heterozygous patient," *Neuromuscular Disorders*, vol. 10, no. 3, pp. 200–205, 2000.

[12] K. H. Smolle, P. Kaufmann, and R. Gasser, "Recurrent rhabdomyolysis and acute respiratory failure due to carnitine palmityltransferase deficiency," *Intensive Care Medicine, Supplement*, vol. 27, no. 1, article 1235, 2001.

[13] A. M. Lamhonwah, S. E. Olpin, R. J. Pollitt et al., "Novel OCTN2 mutations: no genotype-phenotype correlations: early carnitine therapy prevents cardiomyopathy," *American Journal of Medical Genetics*, vol. 111, no. 3, pp. 271–284, 2002.

41

3p14 De Novo Interstitial Microdeletion in a Patient with Intellectual Disability and Autistic Features with Language Impairment: A Comparison with Similar Cases

Ana Belén de la Hoz,[1,2] **Hiart Maortua,**[2,3] **Ainhoa García-Rives,**[2,4]
María Jesús Martínez-González,[2,4] **Maitane Ezquerra,**[1,3] **and María-Isabel Tejada**[2,3]

[1]*Plataforma de Genética Genómica, Instituto de Investigación Sanitaria BioCruces (IIS BioCruces), Hospital Universitario Cruces, Barakaldo, 48903 Bizkaia, Spain*
[2]*GCV-CIBER de Enfermedades Raras (CIBERER-ISCIII), 28029 Madrid, Spain*
[3]*Laboratorio de Genética Molecular, Servicio de Genética, IIS BioCruces, Hospital Universitario Cruces, Barakaldo, 48903 Bizkaia, Spain*
[4]*Sección de Neuropediatría del Servicio de Pediatría, IIS BioCruces, Hospital Universitario Cruces, Barakaldo, 48903 Bizkaia, Spain*

Correspondence should be addressed to María-Isabel Tejada; mariaisabel.tejadaminguez@osakidetza.net

Academic Editor: Anton M. Jetten

To date, few cases of 3p proximal interstitial deletions have been reported and the phenotype and genotype correlation is not well understood. Here, we report a new case of a 3p proximal interstitial deletion. The patient is an 11-year-old female with speech and social interaction difficulties, learning disability, and slight facial dysmorphism, but no other major malformations. An 8 Mb de novo interstitial deletion at 3p14.2-p14.1, from position 60.461.316 to 68.515.453, was revealed by means of array comparative genomic hybridization and confirmed using quantitative reverse-transcription polymerase chain reaction assays. This region includes six genes: *FEZF2, CADPS, SYNPR, ATXN7, PRICKLE,* and *MAGII,* that are known to have a role in neurodevelopment. These genes are located on the proximal side of the deletion. We compare our case with previously well-defined patients reported in the literature and databases.

1. Introduction

It has previously been reported that interstitial deletions of chromosome 3p are rather rare and there are no well-defined breakpoints. However, since the first report of this condition in 1979 by Kogame and Kudo [1], various heterozygous overlapping deletions involving the short arm of chromosome 3 have been found in patients with global developmental delay, intellectual disability, language impairment, and autistic features, but without any other major malformations [2–6]. Some other features have also been correlated with this alteration, namely, defective lymphopoiesis [7] and defective cardiac development [8]. All of the aforementioned authors believed that *FOXP1* was responsible for these features.

Recently, various authors [9–11] have published studies in which they characterized proximal deletions in 3p in a total of

six patients, accurately defining their phenotypical features. None of those overlapping deletions affected the *FOXP1* gene. All of the patients had intellectual disabilities, gross motor delay, slight facial dysmorphism, nonexpressive language, and autistic features. After comparing their patients with four individuals with 3p14-deletions reported with full clinical descriptions in the Database of Chromosomal Imbalance and Phenotype in Humans using Ensembl Resources (DECI-PHER) database, they concluded that all these deletions in 3p14 were associated with very similar features, namely, intellectual disability, autistic features, developmental delay, and often speech impairment but only mild facial dysmorphism. The lack of external features characteristic in these patients makes it difficult to reach a correct diagnosis without array CGH analysis. In addition, the shortage of cases in the literature makes it difficult to identify the gene or the core region responsible for these phenotypes. Here, we report a new case of 3p14 deletion, because we consider it extremely important to share information on cases of deletions that involve this genomic region in order to identify the gene or genes associated with these disorders.

2. Case Presentation

The child is a female first-born of healthy nonconsanguineous parents. There is no family history of congenital abnormalities or intellectual disability and the pregnancy was unremarkable. She was born at term (39 weeks of gestation) by normal delivery, with a weight of 2400 g (<p3) and head circumference of 33.5 cm (<p25). Her Apgar score was 7/10 at 1 and 5 minutes and there were no remarkable observations in the perinatal period. She was first evaluated by our neuropediatric team at the age of 6 months because of poor response to stimuli and lack of a social smile. Clinical examination revealed significant motor developmental delay; a cranial ultrasound, an electroencephalogram, and auditory evoked potentials testing were requested, with results being normal in all cases.

During the first year of life, moderate psychomotor impairment became evident and, therefore, from the age of 12 months, she has received cognitive stimulation therapy. At 20 months, despite motor clumsiness, the patient was able to walk without support but had speech difficulties with a marked expressive language disorder and global learning problems. She had some autistic features including stereotypic movements and difficulties with eye contact. In a psychometric assessment at 7 years of age, she obtained an intelligence quotient of 40. Cranial magnetic resonance imaging, at 9 years of age, did not reveal any abnormalities. On recent assessment, at 11 years of age, her motor skills had improved significantly but she still had speech and social interaction difficulties, as well as learning disability. From the point of view of phenotype, she has been growing proportionately with age without any strong phenotypic features. As can be observed in Figure 1, she presents only slight facial dysmorphism, having a long face with a prominent chin, broad forehead, and a broad, large mouth with widely spaced upper front teeth and slightly large and detached ears.

2.1. Genetic Analysis. With written informed consent from the parents, we carried out initial genetic studies, including karyotyping and molecular analysis of *MECP2* by means of MLPAs and Sanger sequencing. After that, we decided to perform array comparative genomic hybridization (array CGH) in samples from the patient and her parents, and results were confirmed with quantitative reverse-transcription polymerase chain reaction (qRT-PCR) assays, using applied biosystems real-time PCR instruments and software.

Firstly, DNA was purified from peripheral blood according to standard protocols and a Perkin Elmer CGX Oligo Array 8x60K was used to perform genome-wide copy number analysis. This microarray covers over 245 cytogenetically relevant regions, as well as genes involved in development,

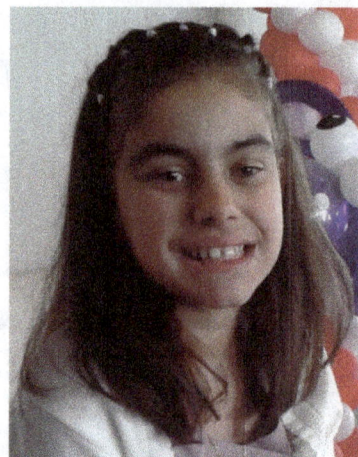

FIGURE 1: The facial photograph of the patient does not show any remarkable phenotypic features. Only slight facial dysmorphism could be observed: a long face with a prominent chin; broad forehead; and a broad, large mouth with widely spaced upper front teeth. Although not visible in this photograph, she has slightly protruding prominent ears.

pericentromeric regions, and subtelomeres. The Agilent Sure-Scan microarray scanner and Agilent Feature Extraction 11.0.1.1 software were used according to the manufacturer's instructions. Results were analyzed with CytoGenomics v.2.7 (Agilent) and Genoglyphix (Signature Genomics) software.

To validate the results, qRT-PCR was performed in a final volume of 20.0 μL using SYBR Green real-time PCR Master Mix Kit and the 7900HT fast real-time PCR System (both from Life Technologies), in accordance with the manufacturer's instructions. Three pairs of primers were designed using Primer 3 Plus software.

2.2. Genetic Results. The karyotype was normal, as was the *MECP2* gene. However, array CGH analysis revealed an 8 Mb proximal deletion at 3p14.2-p14.1, from position 60.461.316 to 68.515.453 (Figure 2) (GRCh37/hg19). Among the genes mapped to this region, six are known or believed to have a role in neurodevelopment: *FEZF2* (OMIM# 607414), *CADPS* (OMIM# 604667), *SYNPR* (no OMIM entry), *TXN7* (OMM# 607640), *PRICKLE2* (OMIM# 608501), and *MAGI1* (OMIM# 602625). The deletion was confirmed to be de novo, on the basis of a comparative study with the parental DNA by qRT-PCR (Table 1).

3. Discussion

Several microdeletions and microduplications mapped to 3p have been identified in patients with developmental disorders, autistic features, and/or global developmental delay. However, the lack of characteristic facial dysmorphisms or other distinct external features in these patients makes it very difficult to diagnose without array CGH technology. Nevertheless, it is known that a correct diagnosis is important to estimate recurrence risk for genetic counseling and may

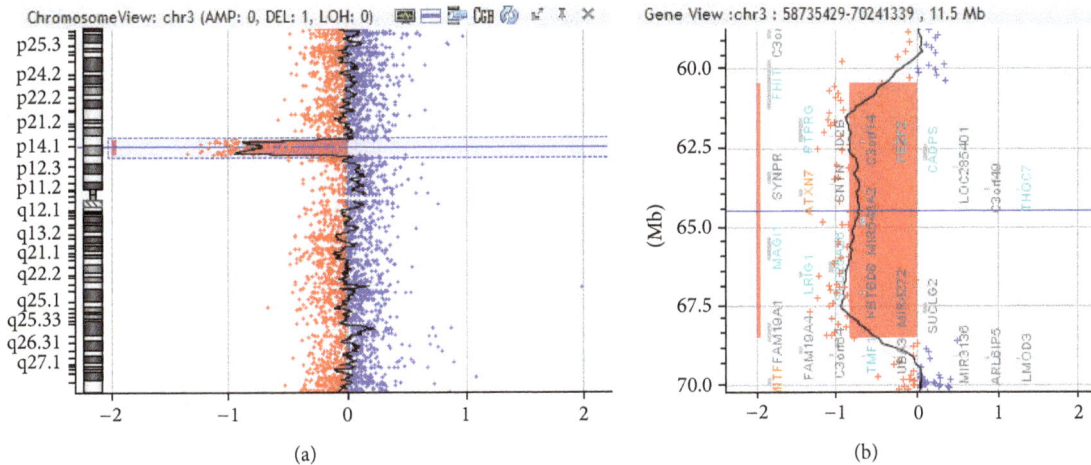

FIGURE 2: The array comparative genomic hybridization (CGH) profile of chromosome 3 showing an interstitial deletion. (a) View of chromosome 3 and (b) the enlarged view of the rearrangement as generated by CytoGenomics v.2.7 (Agilent Technologies). The deletion breakpoint was between 60.461.316 and 68.515.453 (3p14.2-p14.1). The size of the deletion was ~8 Mb

TABLE 1: Validation with quantitative reverse-transcription polymerase chain reaction (qRT-PCR) assays. This table shows the values obtained by means of qRT-PCR in the patient analyzed and her mother. Two amplicons were amplified by qRT-PCR; they were located in the deleted region (3p14.2-p14.1), in the FAM19A1 and ATXN7 genes. The control gene used to normalize the data was RPP30, located at 10q23.31. The $2^{-\Delta\Delta Ct\pm SD}$ values of the patient were less than half the values of her mother, who was used as the normal control.

	$2^{-\Delta\Delta Ct\pm SD}$	
	Patient	Mother
FAM19A1	0.480	1.06
ATXN7	0.450	1.06

$\Delta\Delta Ct = (Ct_{target} - Ct_{Ref})DNA_{test} - (Ct_{target} - Ct_{Ref})DNA_{Ref}$.

$SD_{DNA\,test} = (sd1^2 + sd2^2)^{1/2}$.

$2^{-\Delta\Delta Ct\pm SD}$.

also play an essential role in improving the clinical management of these patients. Here, we have reported a case of a de novo 8 Mb microdeletion of 3p14 in an 11-year-old girl with speech and social interaction difficulties, as well as mild facial dysmorphisms.

Table 2 summarizes the clinical features of patients reported previously [9–11], as well as seven other 3p14 carriers listed with full clinical descriptions in DECIPHER. The DNA sequence between 60.461.316 and 68.515.453 points in chromosome 3 (Figure 3) contains 19 genes, 6 of which encode proteins that could be responsible for the phenotypes observed in these patients. These candidate genes are FEZF2, CADPS, SYNPR, ATXN7, PRICKLE2, and MAGI1. The FEZF2 gene encodes a transcription factor that is required for the specification of corticospinal neuron identity and connectivity [12, 13], and the SYNPR gene encodes a protein that is an integral membrane component of synaptic vesicles [14]. The CADPS gene is expressed in the fetal and adult brain and it is an essential regulator of synaptic vesicle and large dense core vesicle priming in mammalian neurons

and neuroendocrine cells [15]. Expansions in ATXN7 cause spinocerebellar ataxia type 7, but the role of other kinds of mutations (nonsynonymous substitutions or deletions) in this gene in nervous system disorders is not yet well understood [9]. The fifth gene is PRICKLE2, which encodes a postsynaptic Wnt/planar cell polarity pathway component required for the normal development of synapses [16] and whose disruption in mouse hippocampal neurons leads to reductions in dendrite branching, synapse number, and postsynaptic density. It has recently been shown that disruption in PRICKLE2 is associated with behavioral abnormalities including altered social interaction, learning abnormalities, and behavioral inflexibility [17]. On the other hand, though Okumura et al. [9] propose PRICKLE2 as the most likely causative gene of autistic features observed in their cases, this is not consistent with earlier findings by other authors [11, 18]. Finally, MAGI1 is a protein of membrane-associated guanylate kinase (MAGUK) complexes that act as key scaffolds in surface complexes containing receptors, adhesion proteins, and various signaling molecules, playing key roles in cell-to-cell communication. MAGUK proteins are present in neuronal synapses and they help to organize the postsynaptic structure via associations with other scaffolding proteins [19]. Previous studies have demonstrated an association of MAGI1 copy number variation with bipolar affective disorder [20].

Regarding the study conducted by Schwaibold et al. [10], the deletion found in monozygotic twins was around 6.32 Mb long, with breakpoints between 3p14.1 and 3p14.3 (58.244.794–64.571.699), and in the adult patient, the deletion was approximately 4.76 Mb long, with breakpoints between 3p14.1 and 3p14.2 (59.443.171–64.162.112). The three patients had very similar features, namely, intellectual disabilities, gross-motor delay, slight facial dysmorphism, nonexpressive language, and autistic features, although the adult started to show friendly behavior in adolescence. The phenotypes of the cases reported by Tao et al. [11] with microdeletions from 62.665.527 to 64.890.116 and by Okumura et al. [9]

TABLE 2: Summary of patients with overlapping deletions in 3p14.

Patient	Deletion breakpoints	Developmental delay/ID	Speech impairment	Autistic features	Ear anomalies	Facial dysmorphisms	Limb anomalies	Other distinctive features
Present Study	60.461.316–68.515.453	Severe	Yes	Yes, lack of a social smile, difficulties with eye contact, stereotypic movements	Slightly large and detached ears	Long face, prominent chin, broad forehead, wide mouth, widely spaced upper front teeth	None	motor developmental delay
Okumura et al., [9] Twins A/B	60.472.496–67.385.119	Severe	No expressive language until the last follow-up at 49 months of age.	Yes	Low-set, posterior rotated	Arched down-slanting eyebrow, prominent forehead, epicanthic folds, micrognathia, hypertelorism, broad nasal brige, short philtrum	Camptodactyly	Twin 2: intestinal malrotation, ventriculomegaly
Schwaibold et al., [10] Twins 1/2	58.224.794–64.571.699	Extend no specified	Undirected double syllables at 2 10/12 years of age	Yes (stereotypic movements)	Low-set, slightly posterior rotated	Arched, downslanting eyebrows, positional plagiocephaly, Twin B: cowlicks	Twin B: Thick left thumb with sites for two nails	Severe feeding problems, small stature, Twin B: hydrocephalus, hypoplasia of corpus callosum
Schwaibold et al., [10] Patient 3	59.443.171–64.162.112	Extend no specified	No active speech, he follows simple orders at 18 years of age	Yes, in his adolescence he started to develop eye contact	None	Broad mouth, prominent chin, widely spaced teeth, deep-set eyes, long slender face, flat occiput	High tonicity in lower limbs	Brain anomalies in MRI
Tao et al., [11] Patient 6	62.665.527–64.890.116	Severe	N/M	Yes	N/M	N/M	N/M	Epilepsy
D2250	54.452.525–65.609.348	Extend no specified	None	N/M	Extend no specified	Wide mouth, high palate, broad forehead, epicanthus, thick eyebrows	Camptodactyly, talipes equinovalgus, valgus, ulnar deviation of hands	High palate, strabismus
D250453	58.717.185–61.696.115	Extend no specified	Extend no specified	N/M	Low-set, posterior rotated, abnormality of the pinna	Low anterior hairline, mandibular prognathism, widely spaced teeth	N/M	Nevi, lentigines
D255918	62.749.576–63.021.934	Extend no specified	N/M	N/M	N/M	Plagiocephaly	2-3 toe syndactyly	Scrotal hypoplasia

TABLE 2: Continued.

Patient	Deletion breakpoints	Developmental delay/ID	Speech impairment	Autistic features	Ear anomalies	Facial dysmorphisms	Limb anomalies	Other distinctive features
D260004	59.813.606–65.296.648	Extend no specified	Severe	N/M	Low-set, posterior rotated	Prominent forehead/fontal bossing	Clinodactyly	None
nssv1605032	57.416.265–64.870197	Extend no specified	N/M	N/M	N/M	N/M	N/M	Muscular hypotonia
nssv577904	61.956.521–68.514.983	Extend no specified	N/M	N/M	N/M	N/M	N/M	N/M
nssv577902	54.079.045–66.046.136	Extend no specified	N/M	N/M	N/M	N/M	N/M	Failure to thrive, microcephaly

N/M: Not mentioned.

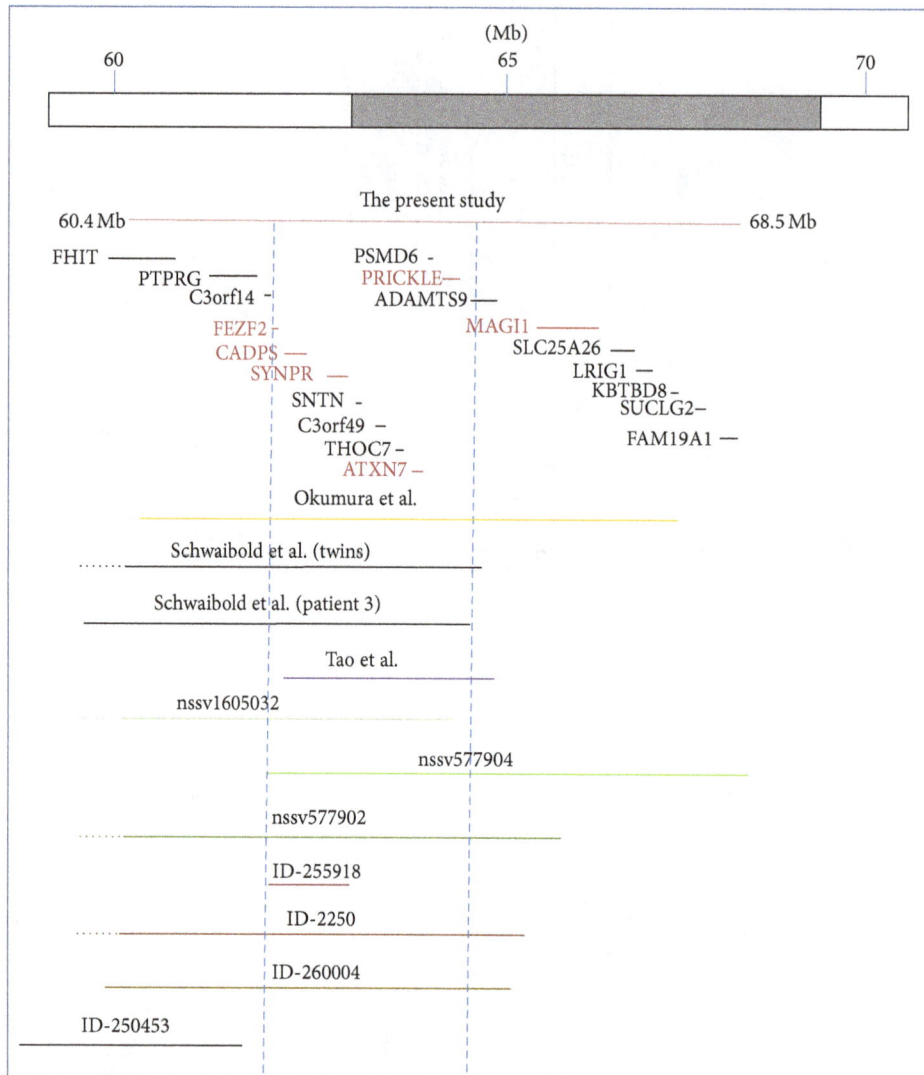

FIGURE 3: Schematic representation of the 3p14 deletions. The orange line represents the deletion in our patient. The deletions found by Okumura et al., Schwaibold et al., and Tao et al. are represented by lines in yellow, blue, and purple, respectively. The green and brown lines are deletions described previously in ISCA Consortium and DECIPHER databases, respectively. The thin red and black horizontal lines indicate the genes that are located in the 3p14 deleted region, the red ones being those that might be responsible for the phenotypic features given their known biological functions. The blue vertical dashed lines indicate the region in which the candidate genes are located and the overlapping deleted regions in 10 of the 11 cases.

with breakpoints between 60.472.496 and 67.385.119 were also quite similar.

Although the deletion found in our patient is considerably longer and extends further toward the centromere, especially compared to deletions described by Schwaibold et al. [10] and Tao et al. [11], respectively, the phenotypic features are quite similar to those in the previously described patients with deletions in 3p14. Moreover, none of the additional genes deleted in our patient seems to play an important role in brain development; with the exception of MAGI1, which was also deleted in Okumura et al.'s twins [9] (Figure 3). Therefore, we believe that our findings support the conclusions of previous authors who have indicated that the candidate gene(s) for these common features may well be among those located in the region distal to the centromere, between breakpoints 62.3 and 64.5 Mb (the left part of the deletion in Figure 3), and

a combination of genes in this region involved in brain or cognitive development might be responsible. Apart from the patients reported in the literature [9–11, 18] and the cases mentioned by Schwaibold et al. [10] which are reported in the DECIPHER database, we are aware of another three patients, reported in the International Standards for Cytogenomic Arrays (ISCA) Consortium database with their phenotypes, that have overlapping deletions in 3p14 (Figure 3). All these patients have similar features and also showed global developmental delay.

4. Conclusion

Our results support the hypothesis that a novel 3p14.2 core region in 3p proximal deletions is associated with neurodevelopmental disorders. We were not able to identify a single gene responsible for the phenotypes associated with microdeletions in 3p14, but we rather believe that several candidate genes located in this region could be the cause of these disorders. In consequence, we consider it very important to report new cases with overlapping deletions in the 3p segment to more precisely identify the genotype-phenotype correlation.

The characteristic lack of external features in these patients makes it difficult to reach a correct diagnosis without high-resolution molecular cytogenetic techniques such as array CGH.

Conflict of Interests

The authors declare that there is no conflict of interests regarding the publication of this paper.

Acknowledgments

The authors would like to thank the patient and her family for agreeing to the publication of this study. This work was financially supported by grants 2007111045 and 2011111090 from the Department of Health of the Government of the Basque Country and a grant from the Jesús Gangoiti Barrera Foundation. Data discussed in this paper were obtained from the ISCA Consortium database (http://www.iscaconsortium.org/), with this information having been generated using NCBI's database of genomic structural variation (http://www.ncbi.nlm.nih.gov/dbvar/), study nstd37. Samples and associated phenotype data were provided by ISCA Consortium member laboratories.

References

[1] K. Kogame and H. Kudo, "Interstitial deletion 3p associated with t(3p−;18q+) translocation," *The Japanese Journal of Human Genetics*, vol. 24, no. 4, pp. 245–252, 1979.

[2] C. W. Carr, D. Moreno-De-Luca, C. Parker et al., "Chiari i malformation, delayed gross motor skills, severe speech delay, and epileptiform discharges in a child with *FOXP1* haploinsufficiency," *European Journal of Human Genetics*, vol. 18, no. 11, pp. 1216–1220, 2010.

[3] F. F. Hamdan, H. Daoud, D. Rochefort et al., "De novo mutations in FOXP1 in cases with intellectual disability, autism, and language impairment," *American Journal of Human Genetics*, vol. 87, no. 5, pp. 671–678, 2010.

[4] D. Horn, J. Kapeller, N. Rivera-Brugués et al., "Identification of FOXP1 deletions in three unrelated patients with mental retardation and significant speech and language deficits," *Human Mutation*, vol. 31, no. 11, pp. E1851–E1860, 2010.

[5] O. Palumbo, L. D'Agruma, A. F. Minenna et al., "3p14.1 de novo microdeletion involving the *FOXP1* gene in an adult patient with autism, severe speech delay and deficit of motor coordination," *Gene*, vol. 516, no. 1, pp. 107–113, 2013.

[6] M. J. Pariani, A. Spencer, J. M. Graham Jr., and D. L. Rimoin, "A 785 kb deletion of 3p14.1p13, including the *FOXP1* gene, associated with speech delay, contractures, hypertonia and blepharophimosis," *European Journal of Medical Genetics*, vol. 52, no. 2-3, pp. 123–127, 2009.

[7] H. Hu, B. Wang, M. Borde et al., "Foxp1 is an essential transcriptional regulator of B cell development," *Nature Immunology*, vol. 7, no. 8, pp. 819–826, 2006.

[8] B. Wang, J. Weidenfeld, M. M. Lu et al., "Foxp1 regulates cardiac outflow tract, endocardial cushion morphogenesis and myocyte proliferation and maturation," *Development*, vol. 131, no. 18, pp. 4477–4487, 2004.

[9] A. Okumura, T. Yamamoto, M. Miyajima et al., "3p interstitial deletion including PRICKLE2 in identical twins with autistic features," *Pediatric Neurology*, vol. 51, no. 5, pp. 730–733, 2014.

[10] E. M. Schwaibold, B. Zoll, P. Burfeind et al., "A 3p interstitial deletion in two monozygotic twin brothers and an 18-year-old man: further characterization and review," *American Journal of Medical Genetics Part A*, vol. 161, no. 10, pp. 2634–2640, 2013.

[11] H. Tao, J. R. Manak, L. Sowers et al., "Mutations in prickle orthologs cause seizures in flies, mice, and humans," *The American Journal of Human Genetics*, vol. 88, no. 2, pp. 138–149, 2011.

[12] M. Kmet, C. Guo, C. Edmondson, and B. Chen, "Directed differentiation of human embryonic stem cells into corticofugal neurons uncovers heterogeneous Fezf2-expressing subpopulations," *PLoS ONE*, vol. 8, no. 6, Article ID e67292, 2013.

[13] S. Shim, K. Y. Kwan, M. Li, V. Lefebvre, and N. Šestan, "Cis-regulatory control of corticospinal system development and evolution," *Nature*, vol. 486, no. 7401, pp. 74–79, 2012.

[14] T. Sun, H. S. Xiao, P.-B. Zhou, Y. J. Lu, L. Bao, and X. Zhang, "Differential expression of synaptoporin and synaptophysin in primary sensory neurons and up-regulation of synaptoporin after peripheral nerve injury," *Neuroscience*, vol. 141, no. 3, pp. 1233–1245, 2006.

[15] I. Brunk, C. Blex, D. Speidel, N. Brose, and G. Ahnert-Hilger, "Ca^{2+}-dependent activator proteins of secretion promote vesicular monoamine uptake," *Journal of Biological Chemistry*, vol. 284, no. 2, pp. 1050–1056, 2009.

[16] T. Nagaoka, R. Ohashi, A. Inutsuka et al., "The Wnt/planar cell polarity pathway component Vangl2 induces synapse formation through direct control of N-cadherin," *Cell Reports*, vol. 6, no. 5, pp. 916–927, 2014.

[17] L. P. Sowers, L. Loo, Y. Wu et al., "Disruption of the non-canonical Wnt gene PRICKLE2 leads to autism-like behaviors with evidence for hippocampal synaptic dysfunction," *Molecular Psychiatry*, vol. 18, no. 10, pp. 1077–1089, 2013.

[18] A. C. Țuțulan-Cuniță, S. M. Papuc, A. Arghir et al., "3p interstitial deletion: novel case report and review," *Journal of Child Neurology*, vol. 27, no. 8, pp. 1062–1066, 2012.

[19] C.-Y. Zheng, G. K. Seabold, M. Horak, and R. S. Petralia, "MAGUKs, synaptic development, and synaptic plasticity," *Neuroscientist*, vol. 17, no. 5, pp. 493–512, 2011.

[20] R. Karlsson, L. Graae, M. Lekman et al., "MAGI1 copy number variation in bipolar affective disorder and schizophrenia," *Biological Psychiatry*, vol. 71, no. 10, pp. 922–930, 2012.

42

Complex Variant of Philadelphia Translocation Involving Chromosomes 9, 12, and 22 in a Case with Chronic Myeloid Leukaemia

F. Malvestiti,[1] C. Agrati,[1] S. Chinetti,[1] A. Di Meco,[1] S. Cirrincione,[2]
M. Oggionni,[2] B. Grimi,[1] F. Maggi,[1] G. Simoni,[1] and F. R. Grati[1]

[1] *Research and Development, Cytogenetics and Molecular Biology, TOMA Advanced Biomedical Assays S.p.A.,*
   25/27 Francesco Ferrer Street, 21052 Busto Arsizio, Varese, Italy
[2] *Treviglio Caravaggio Hospital, 1 Pittori Cavenaghi Square, 24043 Caravaggio, Bergamo, Italy*

Correspondence should be addressed to F. Malvestiti; fmalvestiti@tomalab.com

Academic Editor: Gopalrao Velagaleti

Chronic myeloid leukemia (CML) is a hematopoietic stem cell disorder included in the broader diagnostic category of myeloproliferative neoplasms, associated with fusion by BCR gene at chromosome 22q11 to ABL1 gene at chromosome 9q34 with the formation of the Philadelphia (Ph) chromosome. In 2–10% of CML cases, the fusion gene arises in connection with a variant translocation, involving chromosomes 9, 22, and one or more different chromosomes; consequently, the Ph chromosome could be masked within a complex chromosome rearrangement. In cases with variant Ph translocation a deletion on der(9) may be more frequently observed than in cases with the classical one. Herein we describe a novel case of CML with complex variant Ph translocation involving chromosomes 9, 12, and 22. We present the hematologic response and cytogenetic response after Imatinib treatment. We also speculated the mechanism which had originated the chromosome rearrangement.

1. Introduction

Chronic myeloid leukemia (CML) is a hematopoietic stem cell disease included in the broader diagnostic category of myeloproliferative neoplasms [1] that is characterized by neoplastic overproduction of mainly granulocytes. CML is consistently associated with fusion by chromosome translocation of the breakpoint cluster region gene (*BCR*) at chromosome 22q11 to the Abelson gene (*ABL1*) at chromosome 9q34. This fusion gene BCR/ABL1 encodes for an oncoprotein (P210, more rarely P190 or P230) with a strong constitutive activated tyrosine kinase activity inducing several downstream signals causing the transformation of hemopoietic stem cells [2]. The translocation t(9;22) may be detected by routine karyotype as Philadelphia (Ph) chromosome, although in 2–10% of the cases, the fusion gene arises from a variant translocation [3]. Two variant subgroups have been recognized: the simple variant group with the 22q segment translocated on chromosome other than 9 and the complex variant translocation involving chromosomes 9, 22, and one or more additional chromosome/s. Consequently, the Ph chromosome could be masked within a complex chromosome rearrangement. Although all chromosomes could be involved in these variant translocations, there is a marked clustering to specific chromosomal bands suggesting that specific regions are particularly prone to breakage. In addition, in variant cases a deletion on der(9) may be more frequent than in cases with the classical Ph translocation (40% versus 14%) [4]. Prognostic evaluation of different complex variants was attempted in a limited number of CML cases giving controversial and inconclusive results [5]. Herein we describe a novel CML case with complex variant Ph translocation involving chromosomes 9, 12, and 22. We evaluated the response to the Imatinib treatment and speculated the molecular events underlying this chromosome rearrangement.

2. Case Report

The patient, a 72-year-old woman, had a clinical history of immune-mediated thrombocytopenia. During routine laboratory analysis, an unexpected increase of white blood count (WBC) was found and a CML was suspected. The laboratory data showed a WBC count of 39.2×10^3/mcL, with 60% of neutrophils, 21% of lymphocytes, 10% of monocytes, 2% of eosinophils, 2% of basophils, 4% of myelocytes, and 1% of metamyelocytes. Hemoglobin concentration of 13.5 g/dL was within the normal range, while the platelet count was low (101×10^3/mcL). Cytogenetic analysis on bone marrow and RT-PCR on peripheral blood were carried out. Conventional cytogenetic analysis was performed on unstimulated 24- and 48-hour bone marrow cultures. Cells were cultured and processed by standard methods [6] and chromosomes were stained by QFQ-banding. The analysis was performed according to the Italian and European Acquired Cytogenetics and the ESMO (European Society of Medical Oncology) clinical practice guidelines [7–9]. FISH analysis using BCR/ABL1 t(9;22) Triple-Color and Dual-Fusion probe and Sub-Telomere 9qter probe (Kreatech Diagnostics Vlierweg 20, 1032 LG Amsterdam, The Netherlands) was done following the manufacturer procedures. Karyotype result was described according to the ISCN 2013 [10]. Reverse-transcription quantitative polymerase chain reaction (RT-PCR) for chimeric BCR-ABL1 transcript on peripheral blood was performed with Philadelphia p210 Q-PCR Alert kit (Nanogen Inc., San Diego, CA, USA), based on TaqMan technology. RNA extraction and RT-PCR were performed following the insert kit instructions (Nanogen Inc., San Diego, CA, USA). The measurement of the cDNA of P210 was normalized to the cDNA of ABL1 gene. Conventional cytogenetic analysis on bone marrow showed on 22 metaphases a reciprocal translocation involving the long arm of chromosomes 12 and 22, t(12;22), without the involvement of chromosome 9 (Figure 1(a)). The presence of a cryptic BCR/ABL1 fusion transcript was detected by RT-PCR and subsequently by interphase FISH analyses on bone marrow. Quantitative RT-PCR analysis for BCR/ABL1 on peripheral blood revealed the major chimeric transcript, with a BCR-ABL1(P210)/ABL1 ratio of 14.95% (International Scale). FISH analysis with BCR/ABL1 t(9;22) Triple-Color and Dual-Fusion probe was performed to characterize the t(12;22) translocation and to detect the localization of the fusion gene. The probe set is a mixture of ASS-ABL1 probe labeled in red and of BCR probe with the proximal BCR region labeled in blue and the distal one in green. FISH on 200 metaphases and nuclei showed the following: (i) one purple (blue/red) fusion signal representing the fusion gene (BCR/ABL1) on der(22), (ii) one green signal of 3′ BCR sequences on chromosome 12 involved in translocation t(12;22), (iii) a green/blue signal on normal chromosome 22, and (iv) a red signal on normal chromosome 9 (Figures 1(b) and 1(c)). The reciprocal fusion ABL1/BCR signal was not detected. FISH analysis on 200 nuclei and metaphases using the subtelomeric 9qter probe was performed to further investigate the involvement of chromosome 9 in the complex rearrangement: it showed a normal signal pattern.

In summary, FISH disclosed the deletion of the 5′ ABL1 sequences, including the ASS gene, on der(9), and allowed to map the breakpoint of t(12;22) within the sequences distal to BCR gene. The BCR probe gave a splitted signal on der(22) and on der(12), respectively. The ISCN karyotype was 46,XX,der(9)del(9)(q34q34)ins(22;9)(q11.2;q34q34),der(12)t(12;22)(q13;q11.2),der(22)ins(22;9)t(12;22)[22]. All these results were consistent with the CML diagnosis and the patient started the treatment with Imatinib mesylate (Glivec). After three months of therapy, the WBC count was 5.1×10^3/mcL, with 49.7% of neutrophils, 37.8% of lymphocytes, 7.6% of monocytes, 4.3% of eosinophils, 0.6% of basophils, the hemoglobin concentration was 12.4 g/dL, and platelets count was 211×10^3/mcL. The molecular cytogenetic followup by interphase FISH with BCR/ABL1 probe on 200 nuclei, after 4 and 6 months of therapy, showed a normal signal pattern, while the chromosome analysis at six months revealed a new abnormal clone detected in the 5% (2 out of 5 metaphases and 10 out of 200 interphase nuclei analyzed by FISH with chromosomes 8 and 9 centromeric probes) of the sample with trisomies 8 and 9 (48,XX,+8,+9).

3. Discussion

We describe a patient with CML associated with a novel cryptic complex variant t(9;22), involving chromosome 12 besides chromosomes 9 and 22, which was unmasked and characterized by RT-PCR and FISH analyses. In agreement with ESMO clinical practice guidelines, this case report proves the role of these molecular approaches in detecting cryptic fusion gene in some types of variant translocations with masked Ph and der(9) chromosomes. As previously reported, the breakpoints location of complex variant t(9;22) is nonrandom with a marked clustering to specific chromosome bands suggesting that some regions are more prone to breakage. This finding could be explained by the presence of a specific genomic structure mediating the recombination. Indeed a significant clustering was described for high CG content regions, Alu repeats, LINE, genes, and miRNA explaining the presence of recombination hotspots [11, 12]. The 12q13 chromosome region, involved in our case, was described by Costa et al. [13] in association with complex Philadelphia translocation and in some cases of three-way translocation t(9;22) [11]. In addition, this region is involved both in other chromosomal translocations, originating chimeric genes related to different subtypes of leukemia as reported in Mitelman et al. [14] and in Atlas of chromosome in cancer databases [15], and in the fragile site, FRA12A, which is caused by an expanded CGG repeat in the 5-prime untranslated region of the DIP2B gene (OMIM 611379) [16]. Combining all these data we can speculate that the presence of specific genomic motif in 12q13, such as CGG repeats, could have caused the variant t(9;22) observed in our patient. To the best of our knowledge, this is the first case with this type of variant translocation in a CML patient.

We can also hypothesize that this chromosomal rearrangement was arisen by one-step mechanism with at least four simultaneous breaks and joints because (i) at

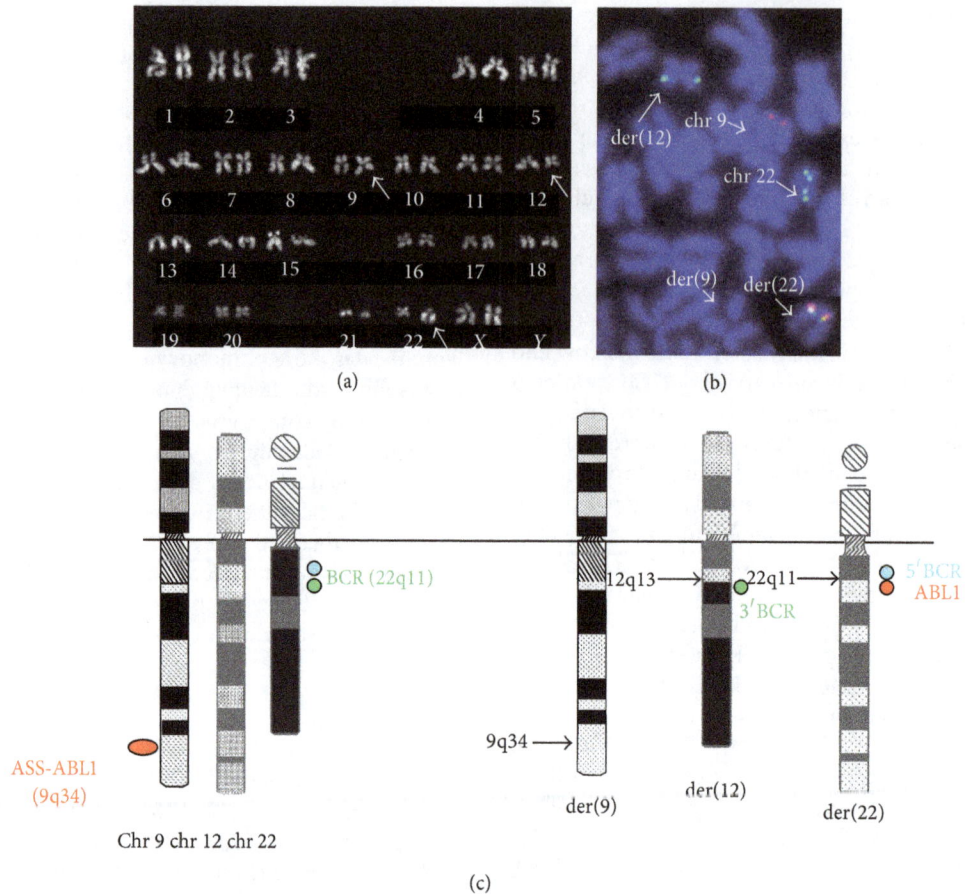

FIGURE 1: (a) QFQ karyotype derived from bone marrow cells. The arrows indicate the derivative chromosomes involved in the rearrangement. (b) BCR/ABL1 FISH signal pattern on metaphase. The arrows indicate the rearranged chromosomes and the normal chromosomes 9 and 22. (c) Ideogram of the rearrangement identified in our CML case with the schematic representation of the FISH probe signals.

diagnosis we did not detect additional clonal abnormalities and (ii) on der(22) only one breakpoint occurred, which is located within the BCR gene and that originated both the fusion gene and the t(12;22). Conversely other cases showed the coexistence of standard and complex translocation in the same patient suggesting that two or more consecutive translocations caused the formation of the complex variant translocation [4].

Prognostic data on response to Imatinib in cases with complex Philadelphia translocation are contradictory and the poor prognostic outcome in some patient of this group was explained by an increased frequency of the concomitant deletion on der(9) rather than to the type of chromosome rearrangement [5]. Our patient has been treated with Imatinib, and at 3 months of therapy she achieved the hematological and cytogenetics responses despite the presence of the deletion on der(9), while at six months of therapy she developed a clone with trisomies 8 and 9. These trisomies have apparently no prognostic significance in CML. In more detail trisomy 8 may arise after interferon and/or Imatinib treatment with unknown significance and trisomy 9 is assumed to represent a gain-of-function mechanism with respect to the JAK2 gene on 9p24 coding for the JAK2 kinase

with no prognostic impact according to follow-up studies of limited sample sizes [17].

Up to now our patient showed a good response to Imatinib treatment, but further studies are needed to confirm this finding.

Conflict of Interests

The authors declare that there is no conflict of interests regarding the publication of this paper.

References

[1] J. W. Vardiman, J. Thiele, D. A. Arber et al., "The 2008 revision of the World Health Organization (WHO) classification of myeloid neoplasms and acute leukemia: Rationale and important changes," *Blood*, vol. 114, no. 5, pp. 937–951, 2009.

[2] A. Quintás-Cardama, H. Kantarjian, and J. Cortes, "Tyrosine kinase inhibitors for chronic myelogenous leukemia," *The New England Journal of Medicine*, vol. 357, no. 15, pp. 1557–1558, 2007.

[3] B. Johansson, T. Fioretos, and F. Mitelman, "Cytogenetic and molecular genetic evolution of chronic myeloid leukemia," *Acta Haematologica*, vol. 107, no. 2, pp. 76–94, 2002.

[4] A. G. Reid, B. J. P. Huntly, C. Grace, A. R. Green, and E. P. Nacheva, "Survival implications of molecular heterogeneity in variant Philadelphia-positive chronic myeloid leukaemia," *British Journal of Haematology*, vol. 121, no. 3, pp. 419–427, 2003.

[5] M. M. T. El-Zimaity, H. Kantarjian, M. Talpaz et al., "Results of imatinib mesylate therapy in chronic myelogenous leukaemia with variant Philadelphia chromosome," *British Journal of Haematology*, vol. 125, no. 2, pp. 187–195, 2004.

[6] A. Babu and R. S. Verma, *Human Chromosomes Principles and Techniques*, McGraw Hill, Texas, Tex, USA, 2nd edition, 1995.

[7] "Citogenetica delle neoplasie oncoematolofiche," http://www.sigu.net/.

[8] R. Hastings, R. Howell, D. Betts et al., *Guidelines and Quality Assurance for Acquired Cytogenetics*, E.C.A. European Cytogeneticists Association Newsletter No. 31, 2013, http://e-c-a.eu/files/downloads/NL31_Acquired_Guidelines.pdf.

[9] M. Baccarani, S. Pileri, J.-L. Steegmann, M. Muller, S. Soverini, and M. Dreyling, "Chronic myeloid leukemia: ESMO clinical practice guidelines for diagnosis, treatment and follow-up," *Annals of Oncology*, vol. 23, no. 7, Article ID mds228, pp. vii72–vii77, 2012.

[10] L. G. Shaffer, J. McGowan-Jordan, and M. Schmid, *International System for Human Cytogenetic Nomenclature*, Karger, Basel, Switzerland, 2013.

[11] F. Albano, L. Anelli, A. Zagaria et al., "Non random distribution of genomic features in breakpoint regions involved in chronic myeloid leukemia cases with variant t(9;22) or additional chromosomal rearrangements," *Molecular Cancer*, vol. 9, article 120, 2010.

[12] A. M. Fisher, P. Strike, C. Scott, and A. V. Moorman, "Breakpoints of variant 9;22 translocations in chronic myeloid leukemia locate preferentially in the CG-richest regions of the genome," *Genes Chromosomes and Cancer*, vol. 43, no. 4, pp. 383–389, 2005.

[13] D. Costa, A. Carrió, I. Madrigal et al., "Studies of complex Ph translocations in cases with chronic myelogenous leukemia and one with acute lymphoblastic leukemia," *Cancer Genetics and Cytogenetics*, vol. 166, no. 1, pp. 89–93, 2006.

[14] F. Mitelman, B. Johansson, and F. Mertens, *The Mitelman Database of Chromosome Aberrations in Cancer*, http://www.cgap.nci.nih.gov/Chromosomes/Mitelman.

[15] *Atlas of Chromosome in Cancer*, http://atlasgeneticsoncology.org/index.html.

[16] OMIM, http://www.ncbi.nlm.nih.gov/omim/?term=OMIM.

[17] U. Bacher, T. Haferlach, W. Hiddemann, S. Schnittger, W. Kern, and C. Schoch, "Additional clonal abnormalities in Philadelphia-positive ALL and CML demonstrate a different cytogenetic pattern at diagnosis and follow different pathways at progression," *Cancer Genetics and Cytogenetics*, vol. 157, no. 1, pp. 53–61, 2005.

43

A New Case of 13q12.2q13.1 Microdeletion Syndrome Contributes to Phenotype Delineation

Giorgia Mandrile,[1,2] **Eleonora Di Gregorio,**[3,4] **Alessandro Calcia,**[3] **Alessandro Brussino,**[3] **Enrico Grosso,**[4] **Elisa Savin,**[4] **Daniela Francesca Giachino,**[1,2] **and Alfredo Brusco**[3,4]

[1] *Medical Genetics Unit, "San Luigi Gonzaga" University Hospital, University of Torino, Regione Gonzole 10, 10143 Orbassano, Italy*
[2] *Department of Clinical & Biological Sciences, University of Torino, 10143 Orbassano, Italy*
[3] *Department of Medical Sciences, University of Torino, Via Santena 19, 10126 Torino, Italy*
[4] *Medical Genetics, "Città della Salute e della Scienza" University Hospital, 10126 Torino, Italy*

Correspondence should be addressed to Giorgia Mandrile; giorgia.mandrile@unito.it and Alfredo Brusco; alfredo.brusco@unito.it

Academic Editor: Evica Rajcan-Separovic

A recently described genetic disorder has been associated with 13q12.3 microdeletion spanning three genes, namely, *KATNAL1*, *LINC00426*, and *HMGB1*. Here, we report a new case with similar clinical features that we have followed from birth to 5 years old. The child carried a complex rearrangement with a double translocation: 46,XX,t(7;13)(p15;q14),t(11;15)(q23;q22). Array-CGH identified a *de novo* microdeletion at 13q12.2q13.1 spanning 3–3.4 Mb and overlapping 13q12.3 critical region. Clinical features resembling those reported in the literature confirm the existence of a distinct 13q12.3 microdeletion syndrome and provide further evidence that is useful to characterize its phenotypic expression during the 5 years of development.

1. Introduction

Array-CGH has gained increased recognition as a first-tier technique to identify and characterize the genetic determinants of intellectual disability (ID) syndromes. Following its introduction, the detection rate of molecular cytogenetic alterations has increased by up to 15% in unselected patients with ID [1, 2]. The possibility of comparing patient phenotypes with overlapping rearrangements has led to the identification of several novel microdeletion/microduplication syndromes [2]. A 13q12.3 microdeletion syndrome has recently been described involving a ~300 kb critical region spanning only three genes, namely, *KATNAL1*, *HMGB1*, and the noncoding RNA *LINC00426* [3].

Here, we describe a Caucasian patient with a *de novo* complex chromosomal rearrangement [t(7;13) and t(11;15)] including a 3–3.4 Mb microdeletion on 13q12.2q13.1, overlapping with the 13q12.3 microdeletion syndrome region. This

subject displays the characteristic dysmorphic features highlighted in the recently reported cases, as well as psychomotor developmental delay and markedly delayed speech.

2. Clinical Report

The proband was the third daughter of a 41-year-old mother and a 42-year-old father. Both parents and siblings were healthy. Prenatal ultrasounds did not reveal any foetal malformations. Prenatal karyotype analysis by standard GTG banding, performed due to advanced maternal age, showed a *de novo* double translocation [46,XX,t(7;13)(p15;q14),t(11;15)(q23;q22)] (Figure 1(a)); UPD was ruled out for chromosomes 7, 11, and 15. Birth occurred through elective caesarean section at the 38th week of gestation (APGAR 7/8). Birth parameters were at the 50th centile according to the Italian growth curves (length: 50 cm (50th cent); weight: 2.79 kg (50th cent); head circumference: 34.5 cm (50th cent)).

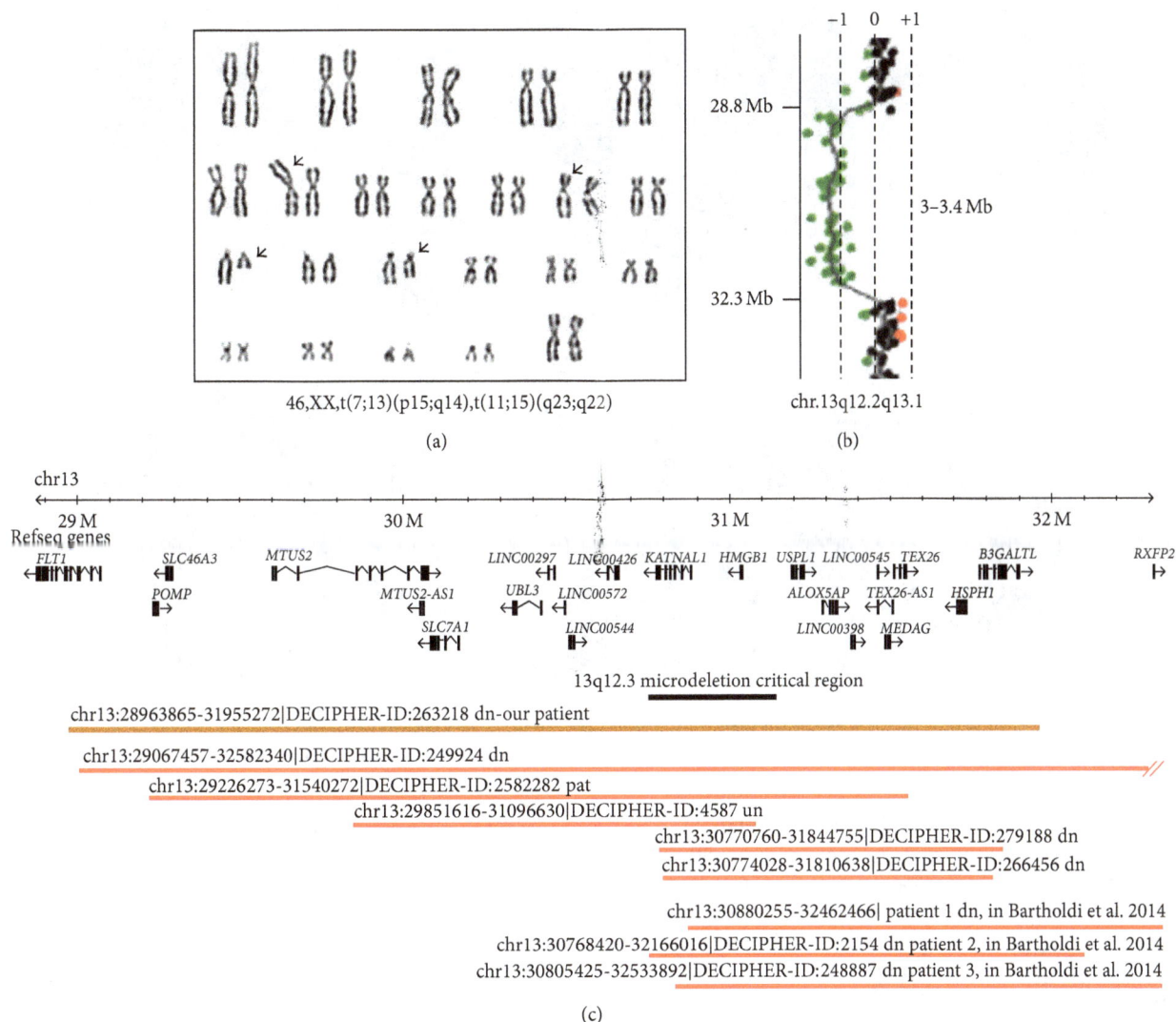

FIGURE 1: Karyotype, array-CGH analysis and schematic representation of the deleted region with reported DECIPHER cases. (a) The G-band karyotype of the patient. Black arrows indicate translocated chromosomes. (b) Chromosome 13 array-CGH results [arr 13q12.2q13.1 (28,875,081x2, 28,963,865-31,955,272x1, 32,313,799x2)dn]. (c) A scheme of the deleted region with distances in Mb and the Refseq genes are reported (GRCh37/hg19). The region deleted in our patient (code: 263218, orange bar) and the overlapping reported deletions (red bars) as shown by the Decipher database (http://decipher.sanger.ac.uk/, version 5.1) are reported. Above each bar the extension of the rearrangement and the mode of inheritance is reported (dn: *de novo*; pat: paternal origin, and un: unknown).

We excluded cerebral malformations by brain ultrasound analysis and ocular defects by carrying out a *fundus oculi* exam. ECG examination showed a long QT (QTc: 470 ms), which was not reconfirmed at 17 days. Dysmorphisms included large wide set eyes, long philtrum, thin upper lip, and large ears (Figure 2). An angioma was present on the thorax and another was found on the top of the head.

From infancy to the last follow-up at 5 years old, growth parameters were consistently below target levels. At 5 years, the measured parameters of the child were as follows: height: 100 cm (3rd cent); weight: 13 kg (<3rd cent/−2.8 SD); head circumference: 49 cm (10th cent). She displayed psychomotor delay: at 8 months she was unable to sit unsupported and at 18 months, after physiotherapy treatment, she still required

support for walking. Lallation began at 16 months and language development was markedly impaired (at 5 years she pronounced very few words that included phonological alterations). The Griffiths test performed at 20 months old revealed a mental age of 14.4 months.

Examination at 2 years old revealed a normal EEG but brain MRI showed mild hypomyelination of the subcortical regions and thinning of the *corpus callosum*. Urinary and plasmatic aminoacid screenings were normal.

Postnatal array-CGH 44 K (Agilent, Santa Clara, CA) performed at 1 year old identified a 3–3.4 Mb microdeletion on chromosome 13q12.2q13.1, close to the translocation breakpoint on chromosome 13 (Figure 1(b)). The deletion was shown to span from position 28,963,865 to 31,955,272

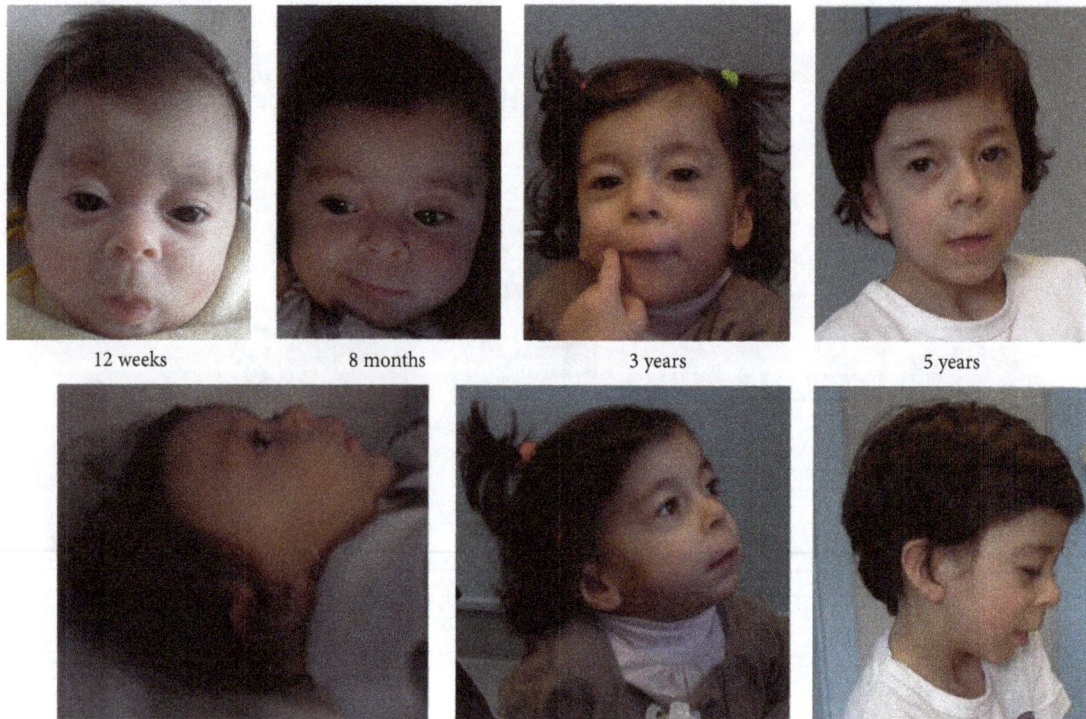

FIGURE 2: Proposita at 12 weeks, 8 months, 3 years, and 5 years old.

(minimal region) (NCBI Build 37/hg19), to contain 20 transcripts (15 coding genes), and did not overlap with common copy number variants (Database of Genomic Variants, http://projects.tcag.ca/variation/) (Figure 1(c)). The deletion was confirmed by real-time quantitative PCR assay designed to target exon 4 of the microtubule-associated tumour suppressor candidate 2 gene (*MTUS2*, NM_001033602.2). The same assay was used to confirm the *de novo* origin of this rearrangement.

3. Discussion

The 13q12.3 microdeletion syndrome was recently described in three patients presenting with intellectual disability, microcephaly, and eczema/atopic dermatitis [3]. Here, we describe a fourth patient with strikingly similar dysmorphic features, confirming the presence of a recognizable phenotype.

Common clinical features included reduced head circumference, triangular face, high frontal hairline, large ears, wide set eyes, fullness of eyelids, malar flattening, a prominent nose with underdeveloped *alae nasi* and low insertion columella, thin upper lip vermilion, and a pointed chin. Our patient had one episode of cutaneous rash, but a specific diagnosis of atopic dermatitis was not made. All patients have shown delayed speech development and moderate intellectual deficit. In three out of four patients recurrent upper airway respiratory infections were reported. Other features shared by the described patients (namely, recurrent vomiting, failure to thrive, allergies, abnormal vision, oligodontia, or truncal obesity) were not observed in our proband.

Several other deletions and duplications that partially or totally overlap the present one, which are associated with a particular phenotype, are reported in the Decipher database (https://decipher.sanger.ac.uk/) (Figure 1(c) and Table 1). In particular, four deletions are partially or totally included in the deletion of this case study (DECIPHER cases numbers 249924, 282282, 4587, 266456, and 279188) and these patients show intellectual disability, language delay, microcephaly, and facial dysmorphisms. Moreover, behavioural abnormalities similar to the ones described by Bartholdi et al. were reported in two cases (Table 1). The minimal shared region between these deletions and the deletion reported in our patient includes the three genes *KATNAL1* (MIM 614764), *LOC100188949*, and *HMGB1* (MIM 163905) [3]. A causal role can be easily suggested for *HMGB1* only, which encodes a ubiquitous nonhistone chromosomal protein expressed in brain (Allen Mouse Brain Atlas, http://mouse.brain-map.org/). This is a possible dosage-sensitive gene involved in the inflammatory response that may contribute to neuronal excitability and seizures [4, 5].

Three other genes within the deleted region in our patient, but not found to be involved in the patients investigated by Bartholdi et al., are associated with OMIM phenotypes: (i) UDP-Gal:beta-GlcNAc beta-1,3-galactosyltransferase-like (*B3GALTL*, MIM 610308), which is mutated in the autosomal recessive Peters plus syndrome (MIM 261540), characterized by anterior eye-chamber abnormalities, disproportionate short stature, and developmental delay [6]; (ii) arachidonate 5-lipoxygenase-activating protein (*ALOX5AP*, MIM 603700) gene, whose sequence variants confer increased susceptibility to stroke (MIM 603700) [7]; (iii) proteasome maturation

TABLE 1: Phenotypic features of Decipher patients with a deletion that overlaps with our case.

Decipher code	263218 (our case)	249924	282282	4587	266456	279188	Patient 1 [3]	2154 Patient 2 [3]	248887 Patient 3 [3]
From (bp)	28,963,865	29,067,457	29,226,273	29,851,616	30,774,028	30,770,760	30,880,255	30,768,420	30,805,425
To (bp)	31,955,272	32,582,340	31,540,272	31,096,830	31,810,638	31,841,755	32,462,46	32,166,016	32,533,8
Size (Mb)	(3.4)	(3.51)	(2.31)	(1.25)	(1.04)	(1.07)	(1.58)	(1.4)	(1.73)
Inheritance	De novo	De novo	Paternal*	Unknown	De novo	De novo	De novo	De novo	De novo
Age (yrs)	5	15	11	?	2	0	19	12	12,5
Height	3rd cent					Growth ret.	3rd–10th cent	25th–50th cent	<3rd cent
Weight			Obesity				25th–50th cent	25th–50th cent	<3rd cent
Microcephaly	OFC: 10th cent		+	+		+	n.a.	OFC: 25th cent	–
Ears	Large			Large					Hearing loss
Wide set, large eyes	+			–			+	+	+
Puffy eyelids	+						+	+	+
Eyes, others	Normal vision					D.p.f	Hypermetropia	Hypermetropia	Hypermetropia
Narrow nasal bridge	+			+			+	+	+
Underdeveloped alae nasi	+						+	+	+
Low insertion columella	+			+			+	+	+
Thin vermilion upper lip	+						+	+	+
Oligodontia	–						+	–	+
Thorax	Mild pectus excavatum			Pectus excavatum					
Atopic dermatitis	One episode of cutaneous rash								
Skin	Two haemangiomas			Spotty hyperpigm					
Others			Metatarsus adductus; hypogonadism	2–3 toe syndactyly	Cutaneous finger syndactyly		Hip dysplasia; cryptorchidism	Congenital hernia of diaphragm	Asymmetry legs
Intellectual deficit	+		+	+	+	+	+	+	+
Language delay	+		+		+	+	+	+	+
Behavioural abnormalities	–		ADHD	Hyperactivity			Hyperactivity	Hyperactivity	Hyperactivity
Hypotonia	+								
Neurological features			Hyperreflexia						

Note: ADHD: attention deficit hyperactivity disorder. n.a.: not available. del: deletion. Asterisk indicates that the father of patient 282282 was affected. hyperpigm: hyperpigmentation. D.p.f.: Downslent palpebral fissures; Phanotype of 249924 was not available; Growth ret.: growth retardation.

protein (*POMP*, MIM 613386) gene, which is associated with the recessive phenotype keratosis linearis with ichthyosis congenita and sclerosing keratoderma (MIM 601952) [8]. The clinical features of these diseases are not clearly related to our patient's phenotype, in line with the recessive nature of the associated syndromes. Comparison of our patient with the four reported in Decipher did not suggest any phenotypic effect of the additional deleted genes in the 13q12.2q13.1 region. Moreover, we cannot exclude the occurrence of position effect or gene disruption at any of the breakpoints of this complex karyotype and the deletion span may contribute to the phenotypic differences. Thus, the gene(s) responsible for the phenotypic differences with reference to the individuals in the study of Bartholdi et al. presently remains elusive.

The relevance of the 13q12q13 deletion, currently supported by the phenotypic similarity and *de novo* deletion origin of the three DECIPHER cases, the three individuals reported by Bartholdi et al., and our affected subject will be confirmed by identifying additional cases, in particular those carrying point mutations in *HMGB1* or another gene in this region.

Abbreviations

CGH: Comparative genome hybridization
CCR: Complex chromosomal rearrangements
UPL: Universal probe library
UPD: Uniparental disomy
ECG: Electrocardiogram
EEG: Electroencephalogram
MRI: Magnetic resonance imaging.

Conflict of Interests

The authors declare that there is no conflict of interests regarding the publication of this paper.

Acknowledgments

The authors are grateful to the patient and her family for agreeing to take part in this study. This work was supported by the Regione Piemonte Ricerca Sanitaria Finalizzata and MURST60%. This study makes use of data generated by the DECIPHER Consortium. A full list of centres who contributed to the generation of the data is available from http://decipher.sanger.ac.uk/ and via email from decipher@sanger.ac.uk. Funding for the project was provided by the Wellcome Trust. Dissemination of information. The case reported here has been entered in the "DECIPHER" database (http://decipher.sanger.ac.uk/) with the code number 263218.

References

[1] D. T. Miller, M. P. Adam, S. Aradhya et al., "Consensus statement: chromosomal microarray is a first-tier clinical diagnostic test for individuals with developmental disabilities or congenital anomalies," *The American Journal of Human Genetics*, vol. 86, no. 5, pp. 749–764, 2010.

[2] L. E. L. M. Vissers, B. B. A. de Vries, and J. A. Veltman, "Genomic microarrays in mental retardation: from copy number variation to gene, from research to diagnosis," *Journal of Medical Genetics*, vol. 47, no. 5, pp. 289–297, 2010.

[3] D. Bartholdi, A. Stray-Pedersen, S. Azzarello-Burri et al., "A newly recognized 13q12.3 microdeletion syndrome characterized by intellectual disability, microcephaly, and eczema/atopic dermatitis encompassing the *HMGB1* and *KATNAL1* genes," *American Journal of Medical Genetics Part A*, vol. 164, no. 5, pp. 1277–1283, 2014.

[4] M. Maroso, S. Balosso, T. Ravizza et al., "Toll-like receptor 4 and high-mobility group box-1 are involved in ictogenesis and can be targeted to reduce seizures," *Nature Medicine*, vol. 16, no. 4, pp. 413–419, 2010.

[5] L. Apetoh, F. Ghiringhelli, A. Tesniere et al., "Toll-like receptor 4-dependent contribution of the immune system to anticancer chemotherapy and radiotherapy," *Nature Medicine*, vol. 13, no. 9, pp. 1050–1059, 2007.

[6] S. A. J. L. Oberstein, M. Kriek, S. J. White et al., "Peters Plus syndrome is caused by mutations in *B3GALTL*, a putative glycosyltransferase," *The American Journal of Human Genetics*, vol. 79, no. 3, pp. 562–566, 2006.

[7] R. Ji, J. Jia, X. Ma, J. Wu, Y. Zhang, and L. Xu, "Genetic variants in the promoter region of the ALOx5AP gene and susceptibility of ischemic stroke," *Cerebrovascular Diseases*, vol. 32, no. 3, pp. 261–268, 2011.

[8] J. Dahlqvist, J. Klar, N. Tiwari et al., "A single-nucleotide deletion in the POMP 5' UTR causes a transcriptional switch and altered epidermal proteasome distribution in KLICK genodermatosis," *The American Journal of Human Genetics*, vol. 86, no. 4, pp. 596–603, 2010.

44

Osteoporosis-Pseudoglioma in a Mauritanian Child due to a Novel Mutation in *LRP5*

Noura Biha,[1,2] **S. M. Ghaber,**[2,3] **M. M. Hacen,**[4] **and Corinne Collet**[5]

[1] *Rheumatology Department, Nouakchott Military Hospital, Mauritania*
[2] *Faculté de Médecine de Nouakchott, Mauritania*
[3] *Service des Laboratoires, Centre Hospitalier National de Nouakchott, Mauritania*
[4] *Service de Chirurgie Orthopédique, Hôpital Militaire de Nouakchott, Mauritania*
[5] *Assistance Publique-Hôpitaux de Paris, Hôpital Lariboisière, Laboratoire de Biochimie et de Biologie Moléculaire, Paris, France*

Correspondence should be addressed to Noura Biha; nourabiha80@gmail.com

Academic Editor: Shoji Ichikawa

Osteoporosis-pseudoglioma (OPPG) syndrome is a very rare autosomal recessive disorder, caused by mutations in the low-density lipoprotein receptor-related protein 5 (LRP5) gene. It manifests by severe juvenile osteoporosis with congenital or infancy-onset visual loss. We describe a case of OPPG due to novel mutation in LRP5 gene, occurring in a female Mauritanian child. This 10-year-old female child was born blind, and after then multiple fragility fractures appeared. PCR amplification and sequencing revealed a novel homozygous nonsense mutation in exon 10 of the LRP5 gene (c.2270G>A; pTrP757*); this mutation leads to the production of a truncated protein containing 757 amino acids instead of 1615, located in the third β-propeller domain of the LRP5 protein. Both parents were heterozygous for the mutation. This is the first case of the OPPG described in black Africans, which broadens the spectrum of LRP5 gene mutations in OPPG.

1. Introduction

Osteoporosis-pseudoglioma (OPPG) syndrome (OPPG, OMIM 259770) is a very rare autosomal recessive disorder. It combines severe juvenile osteoporosis with congenital blindness. This serious disease is caused by loss-of-function mutations in the low-density lipoprotein receptor-related protein 5 (LRP5) gene [1]. The LRP5 is a coreceptor of *Wnt*, situated on the osteoblast cell; it located between two other receptors named Frizzled (Fz) and Kremen family that plays a central role in *Wnt/-catenin* canonical pathway [2].

OPPG was first described in 1931 [3]. Gong et al. [4] had first identified loss of function mutation of the LRP5 gene leading to osteoporosis pseudoglioma (OPPG). To date, thirty mutations have been described in OPPG including fourteen homozygous mutations, principally located in the second and third beta-propeller domains of LRP5 [1, 2], which have a high affinity with *wnt* ligand [5].

Besides, gain-function mutations of LRP5 lead to high bone mass (HBM) (Familial High Bone Mass Syndrome) [6],

osteopetrosis autosomal dominant type 1 [7], and osteosclerosis [8]. low-density lipoprotein receptor-related protein *5* (*LRP5*), located on chromosome 11q13, has 23 coding exons. LRP5 cDNA which contains 4845 base pairs encodes a 1615-amino acid protein [9]. To date, only sixty OPPG cases were identified [2]. Here we describe a case of OPPG due to a novel LRP5 mutation occurring in a female Mauritanian child.

2. Case

This report concerns a ten-year-old Mauritanian female child, who was referred by orthopedics service for assessment of fragility fractures. She was born to consanguineous parents. Congenital blindness was diagnosed at birth. She then presented with five broken limbs (humerus, wrist, ankle, and femur) after a fall from standing height, which premiered at the age of 5 years. Since femur fracture, she did not walk again. On clinical examination, we observed microphthalmia, corneal opacity (Figure 1), dorsal kyphosis, and incurvation of tibias and lower limb length inequality

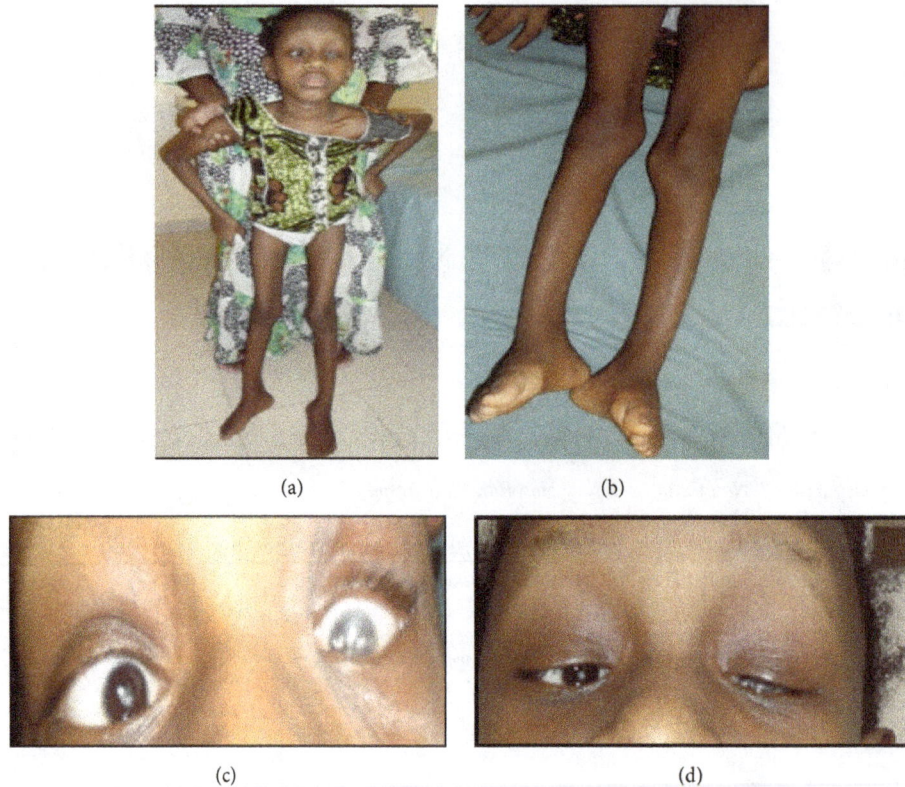

(a)   (b)

(c)   (d)

FIGURE 1: Photograph of child with OPPG showing corneal opacity, microphthalmia (c, d), and incurvation of Tibia (a, b).

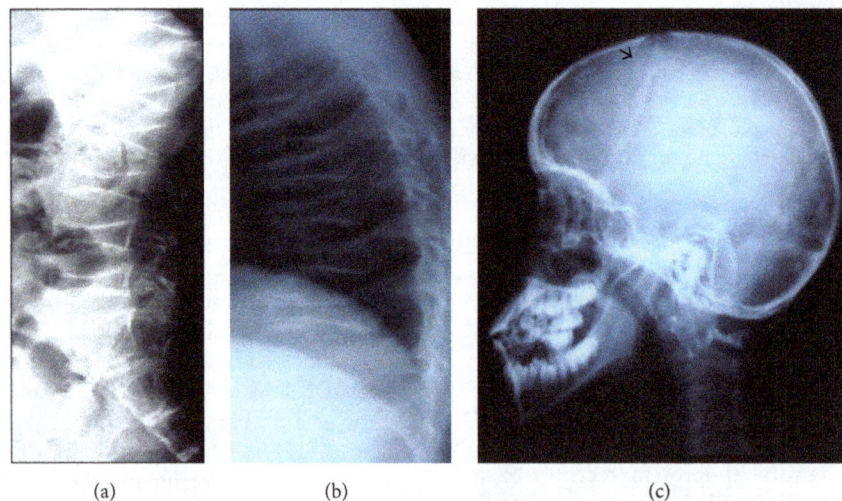

(a)   (b)   (c)

FIGURE 2: Lateral spine radiographs showing severe osteopenia, platyspondyly (a, b), Skull X-ray revealed wormian bone ↘ (c).

(Summarized Figure 1). Her weight was 15 kg and size was 117 cm, both far below the second percentile for her age. Neurological examination was normal. Serum calcium, phosphate, alkaline phosphatase, creatinine, and 25 OH vitamin D3 were all normal. Radiographs showed diffuse bone demineralization, multiple vertebral fractures, and platyspondyly (Figure 2). Bone mineral density (BMD) revealed a Z score of −5.5 at the spine.

3. Sequencing Analysis

Written informed consent was obtained from her parents. Genomic DNA was extracted from the patient peripheral blood leukocytes using QIAamp DNA blood midi kit (QIA-GEN). We screened all the 23 coding exons of *LRP5* for the case and for her parents. The PCR products were sequenced on both strands with ABI Prism 3130 Genetic Analyzer (Life

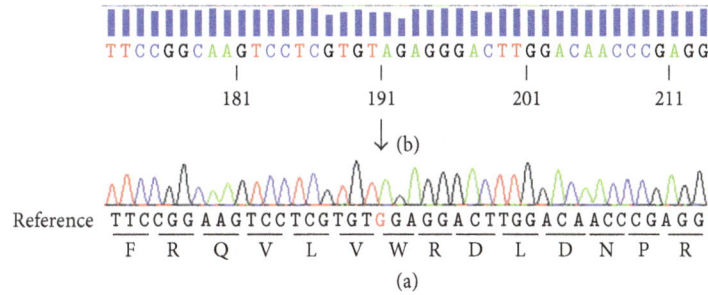

FIGURE 3: *c.2270G>A, p.Trp757* mutation in the LRP5 gene. (a) cDNA reference sequence for LRP5. (b) cDNA of the proband revealed a G----A substitution at nucleotide 2270, resulting in a trp757-to-stop codon.

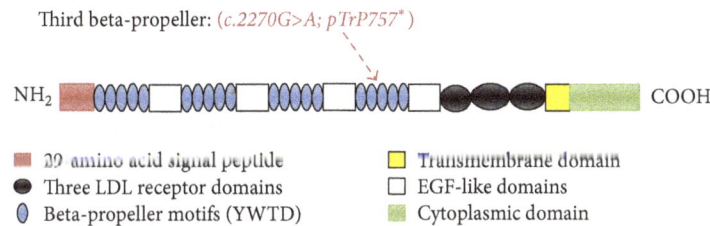

FIGURE 4: Schematic presentation of the protein structure and domain organization of LRP5. The novel LRP5 mutation is described here (shown in the schematic protein).

Technologies, Saint-Aubin, France). Sequences were analyzed using SeqScape 4.0 software (Life Technologies) and compared with the genomic reference sequence (NG_015835.1) for *LRP5*. Mutation nomenclature was based on HGVS nomenclature guidelines [http://www.hgvs.org/mutnomen/] and exonic numbering was based on genomic reference (Figure 3).

4. Results

PCR amplification and sequencing revealed a novel nonsense mutation in exon 10 of the LRP5 gene (c.2270G>A; pTrP757*). It produces a truncated protein containing 757 amino acids instead of 1615. This mutation is located in the third beta-propeller domain (YWTD repeat) in the extracellular domain of the receptor. Both parents were heterozygous for the mutation.

5. Discussion

OPPG syndrome is extremely rare genetic disorders, transmitted by autosomal recessive, associating congenital or infancy-onset visual loss with early-onset severe osteoporosis [6]. Other clinical manifestations can be observed like a muscular hypotonia, ligamentous laxity, mental retardation, and obesity [10]. Ocular abnormalities is due to persistence of the fetal ocular fibrovascular system, which seems due to a failure of macrophage-induced endothelial cell apoptosis (which needs *wnt* protein) [11].

We described here the case of a 10-year-old Mauritanian female child, who had a clinical OPPG phenotype. Molecular analysis identified a novel homozygous nonsense mutation

in the LRP5 gene, leading to the substitution of G-to-A at nucleotide 2270 in exon 10, resulting in a trp757-to-stop codon (c.2270G>A; p.Trp757*). This mutation, never described in the literature, permitted us to confirm the diagnosis of OPPG and it is the first case of OPPG among black Africans [9, 10, 12–14].

The mutation in the proband led to the production of a truncated protein containing 757 amino acids instead of 1615. In accord with previous studies [15, 16], the novel nonsense mutations reported here were equally located in the third β-propeller domain of the LRP5 protein.

To simplify, the LRP5 protein contains a large extracellular domain (ECD), membrane-spanning domain, and an intracellular domain. The amino terminus of the extracellular domain (ECD) is followed by alternating beta-propeller motifs (YWTD), epidermal growth factor (EGF), and three LDL receptor domains [17]. The spanning domain is followed by a short intracellular domain (as shown in Figure 4). The YWTD is a binding domain that has a high affinity with *wnt* ligand [4, 5].

The p. Trp757* truncated protein containing the signal peptide, the first and second propeller (YWTD) domain, the first and second EGF-like domain, and a part of third β propeller domain (YWTD) (as shown in Figure 4), but lacking the transmembrane and cytoplasmic domains, which are crucial LRP5 protein regions [1], leading to degradation of truncated protein by the proteasome [6, 18].

For at least 14 different homozygous mutations and 16 compounds, heterozygous mutations have been described [1], with no phenotypic difference between homozygotes and heterozygotes in the literature [16, 19]. However, some heterozygous patients have been reported to have milder bone phenotype and normal eye phenotype [16]. The sever phenotype described in this report suggests that this novel mutation (c.2270G>A; pTrP757*) is more pathogenic.

The pathogenic mechanism of OPPG is well understood: when wnt binds to Fz and LRP5, this allows beta-catenin stabilization, which interacts with gene transcription regulators. The above interactions lead to bone formation activation [16, 20]. Therefore, a mutation that prevents the connection between LRP5 and wnt will cause loss of function of the receptor, which results in OPPG syndrome [4, 19].

The function of LRP5 in eye development is complex [16]; however, many studies suggest that Lrp5 is also necessary for the normal regression of embryonic vasculature in the eye [11].

Several studies have shown the role of LRP5 gene in the acquisition of peak bone mass during growth [21, 22]. In addition to this, common polymorphisms of LRP5 have been associated with fracture risk and variations in BMD [23, 24]. Thus, thorough knowledge of OPPG can help us understand the physiology of bone tissue and therapeutic targets for osteoporosis.

In conclusion, we described the clinical and molecular features of a female Mauritanian child with OPPG due to a novel *nonsense* mutation in the LRP5. Our case expands the spectrum of LRP5 gene mutations in OPPG and highlights the important role of LRP5 in bone formation.

Conflict of Interests

The authors declare that there is no conflict of interests regarding the publication of this paper.

Acknowledgments

The authors thank the child's parents for their courage and support. They would especially like to acknowledge Mrs Habi ly (KISSI clinic Hospital) and Maurilab laboratory staff.

References

[1] A. Marques-Pinheiro, R. Levasseur, C. Cormier et al., "Novel LRP5 gene mutation in a patient with osteoporosis-pseudoglioma syndrome," *Joint Bone Spine*, vol. 77, no. 2, pp. 151–153, 2010.

[2] C. M. Laine, B. D. Chung, M. Susic et al., "Novel mutations affecting LRP5 splicing in patients with osteoporosis-pseudoglioma syndrome (OPPG)," *European Journal of Human Genetics*, vol. 19, no. 8, pp. 875–881, 2011.

[3] B. V. Pellathy, "V. Ablatio retinae und Uveitis congenita bei drei Geschwistern," *Z Augenheilkd*, vol. 73, no. 4-5, pp. 249–254, 1931.

[4] Y. Gong, R. B. Slee, N. Fukai et al., "LDL receptor-related protein 5 (LRP5) affects bone accrual and eye development," *Cell*, vol. 107, no. 4, pp. 513–523, 2001.

[5] J. Takagi, Y. Yang, J. H. Liu, J. H. Wang, and T. A. Springer, "Complex between nidogen and laminin fragments reveals a paradigmatic β-propeller interface," *Nature*, vol. 424, no. 6951, pp. 969–974, 2003.

[6] R. Levasseur, D. Lacombe, and M. C. De Vernejoul, "LRP5 mutations in osteoporosis-pseudoglioma syndrome and high-bone-mass disorders," *Joint Bone Spine*, vol. 72, no. 3, pp. 207–214, 2005.

[7] M. L. Johnson, "LRP5 and bone mass regulation: where are we now?" *BoneKEy Reports*, vol. 1, article 1, 2012.

[8] L. Van Wesenbeeck, E. Cleiren, J. Gram et al., "Six novel missense mutations in the LDL receptor-related protein 5 (LRP5) gene in different conditions with an increased bone density," *The American Journal of Human Genetics*, vol. 72, no. 3, pp. 763–771, 2003.

[9] Y. Gong, M. Vikkula, L. Boon et al., "Osteoporosis-pseudoglioma syndrome, a disorder affecting skeletal strength and vision, is assigned to chromosome region 11q12-13," *The American Journal of Human Genetics*, vol. 59, no. 1, pp. 146–151, 1996.

[10] H. Somer, A. Palotie, M. Somer, V. Hoikka, and L. Peltonen, "Osteoporosis-pseudoglioma syndrome: clinical, morphological, and biochemical studies," *Journal of Medical Genetics*, vol. 25, no. 8, pp. 543–549, 1988.

[11] M. Kato, M. S. Patel, R. Levasseur et al., "Cbfa1-independent decrease in osteoblast proliferation, osteopenia, and persistent embryonic eye vascularization in mice deficient in Lrp5, a Wnt coreceptor," *Journal of Cell Biology*, vol. 157, no. 2, pp. 303–314, 2002.

[12] N. Alonso, D. C. Soares, E. V. McCloskey, G. D. Summers, S. H. Ralston, and C. L. Gregson, "Atypical femoral fracture in osteoporosis pseudoglioma syndrome associated with two novel compound heterozygous mutations in *LRP5*," *Journal of Bone and Mineral Research*, vol. 30, no. 4, pp. 615–620, 2015.

[13] E. R. Barros, M. R. Dias da Silva, I. S. Kunii, O. M. Hauache, and M. Lazaretti-Castro, "A novel mutation in the LRP5 gene is associated with osteoporosis-pseudoglioma syndrome," *Osteoporosis International*, vol. 18, no. 7, pp. 1017–1018, 2007.

[14] A. S. Teebi, S. A. Al-Awadi, M. J. Marafie, R. A. Bushnaq, and S. Satyanath, "Osteoporosis-pseudoglioma syndrome with congenital heart disease: a new association," *Journal of Medical Genetics*, vol. 25, no. 1, pp. 32–36, 1988.

[15] W. Balemans and W. Van Hul, "Minireview: the genetics of low-density lipoprotein receptor-related protein 5 in bone: a story of extremes," *Endocrinology*, vol. 148, no. 6, pp. 2622–2629, 2007.

[16] E. A. Streeten, D. McBride, E. Puffenberger et al., "Osteoporosis-pseudoglioma syndrome: description of 9 new cases and beneficial response to bisphosphonates," *Bone*, vol. 43, no. 3, pp. 584–590, 2008.

[17] Z. A. Zhong and B. O. Williams, "LRP5(low density lipoprotein receptor-related protein 5)," *Atlas of Genetics and Cytogenetics in Oncology and Haematology*, vol. 15, no. 3, pp. 270–275, 2011.

[18] V. S. Spiegelman, T. J. Slaga, M. Pagano, T. Minamoto, Z. Ronai, and S. Y. Fuchs, "Wnt/beta-catenin signaling induces the expression and activity of betaTrCP ubiquitin ligase receptor," *Molecular Cell*, vol. 5, no. 5, pp. 877–882, 2000.

[19] M. Ai, S. Heeger, C. F. Bartels, D. K. Schelling, and M. L. Warman, "Clinical and molecular findings in osteoporosis-pseudoglioma syndrome," *The American Journal of Human Genetics*, vol. 77, no. 5, pp. 741–753, 2005.

[20] R. Baron and G. Rawadi, "Targeting the Wnt/β-catenin pathway to regulate bone formation in the adult skeleton," *Endocrinology*, vol. 148, no. 6, pp. 2635–2643, 2007.

[21] M. A. Koay, J. H. Tobias, S. D. Leary, C. D. Steer, C. Vilariño-Güell, and M. A. Brown, "The effect of LRP5 polymorphisms on

bone mineral density is apparent in childhood," *Calcified Tissue International*, vol. 81, no. 1, pp. 1–9, 2007.

[22] D. L. Koller, S. Ichikawa, M. L. Johnson et al., "Contribution of the LRP5 gene to normal variation in peak BMD in women," *Journal of Bone and Mineral Research*, vol. 20, no. 1, pp. 75–80, 2005.

[23] S. L. Ferrari, S. Deutsch, U. Choudhury et al., "Polymorphisms in the low-density lipoprotein receptor-related protein 5 (LRP5) gene are associated with variation in vertebral bone mass, vertebral bone size, and stature in white," *American Journal of Human Genetics*, vol. 74, no. 5, pp. 866–875, 2004.

[24] R. Sassi, H. Sahli, C. Souissi et al., "Association of LRP5 genotypes with osteoporosis in Tunisian post-menopausal women," *BMC Musculoskeletal Disorders*, vol. 15, no. 1, article 144, 2014.

45

A Novel Nonsense Mutation of the AGL Gene in a Romanian Patient with Glycogen Storage Disease Type IIIa

Anca Zimmermann,[1] Heidi Rossmann,[2] Simona Bucerzan,[3] and Paula Grigorescu-Sido[3]

[1]*Department of Endocrinology and Metabolic Diseases, 1st Clinic of Internal Medicine, University of Mainz, Langenbeckstrasse 1, 55131 Mainz, Germany*
[2]*Institute for Clinical Chemistry and Laboratory Medicine, University of Mainz, Langenbeckstrasse 1, 55131 Mainz, Germany*
[3]*Center of Genetic Diseases, Emergency Children's Hospital, University of Medicine and Pharmacy, Motilor Street 68, 400370 Cluj, Romania*

Correspondence should be addressed to Anca Zimmermann; zimmeran@uni-mainz.de

Academic Editor: Shoji Ichikawa

Background. Glycogen storage disease type III (GSDIII) is a rare metabolic disorder with autosomal recessive inheritance, caused by deficiency of the glycogen debranching enzyme. There is a high phenotypic variability due to different mutations in the *AGL* gene. *Methods and Results.* We describe a 2.3-year-old boy from a nonconsanguineous Romanian family, who presented with severe hepatomegaly with fibrosis, mild muscle weakness, cardiomyopathy, ketotic fasting hypoglycemia, increased transaminases, creatine phosphokinase, and combined hyperlipoproteinemia. GSD type IIIa was suspected. Accordingly, genomic DNA of the index patient was analyzed by next generation sequencing of the AGL gene. For confirmation of the two mutations found, genetic analysis of the parents and grandparents was also performed. The patient was compound heterozygous for the novel mutation c.3235C>T, p.Gln1079* (exon 24) and the known mutation c.1589C>G, p.Ser530* (exon 12). c.3235 >T, p.Gln1079* was inherited from the father, who inherited it from his mother. c.1589C>G, p.Ser530* was inherited from the mother, who inherited it from her father. *Conclusion.* We report the first genetically confirmed case of a Romanian patient with GSDIIIa. We detected a compound heterozygous genotype with a novel mutation, in the context of a severe hepatopathy and an early onset of cardiomyopathy.

1. Introduction

Glycogen storage disease type III (GSDIII), sometimes referred to as Cori-Forbes disease (OMIM 232400), is a metabolic disorder with autosomal recessive inheritance, caused by glycogen debranching enzyme (GDE) deficiency, with accumulation of an intermediate glycogen form called limit-dextrin (LD) in affected tissues [1].

GDE contains two catalytic sites with two different functions: 4-alpha-glucanotransferase (EC 2.4.1.25) and amylo-1,6-glucosidase (EC 3.2.1.33) [2–4].

AGL (amylo-alpha-1, 6-glucosidase, 4-alpha-glucano-transferase), the gene encoding GDE, spans 85 kb of genomic DNA, contains 35 exons [3], and is located on chromosome 1p21.2 [5]. Bao et al. recognized the presence of six different isoforms of GDE that differ in the 5′ end [6]. Transcript variant 1 of the *AGL* gene (NM_000642.2), which is mainly expressed in liver and kidney, consists of 34 exons, 33 of which are coding. Tissue-specific alternative splicing may contribute to the wide range of enzymatic and clinical variability described for GSDIII mutations (Human Gene AGL (uc001dsi.1); https://genome.ucsc.edu/). The glycogen binding site is encoded by exons 31 and 32 and the active site is encoded by exons 6, 13, 14, and 15 [7].

GDE deficiency leads to storage of LD in affected tissues (liver, skeletal muscles, and myocardium), with morphological and functional consequences. There are four subtypes of GSDIII, depending on the type of enzymatic deficiency and its location. The most frequent two subtypes are caused by the deficiency of both catalytical GDE functions, with involvement of liver and muscle in GSDIIIa (85% of patients) or only of liver in GSDIIIb (15% of patients) [8].

The clinical picture varies according to age. In infants, hepatomegaly, keto-hypoglycemic episodes, muscular hypotonia, and growth retardation occur, accompanied by highly increased transaminases, combined hyperlipoproteinemia, and increased values of serum creatine kinase. In adults with the subtype IIIa the main findings are progressive myopathy, cardiomyopathy, and sometimes altered hepatic tests [9, 10].

The number of known mutations associated with GSDIII has increased over time, with 130 mutations by the end of 2014 [11, 12].

We report on a Romanian child with a GSDIIIa phenotype, harbouring a new nonsense mutation (c.3235C>T; p.Gln1079*) in a compound heterozygote state with a previously known mutation (c.1589C>G; pSer530*). For correct segregation, molecular analysis has also been performed on the parents and the two pairs of grandparents.

2. Case Presentation

A 2.3-year-old boy was admitted to the Department of Genetic Diseases of the Emergency Hospital for Children in Cluj, Romania, for evaluation of hepatomegaly and elevated transaminases. The patient was the parents' first child, born from the second gestation, after an initial spontaneous abortion in the 8th gestational week, from apparently healthy, nonconsanguineous, and young parents (age at the child's birth: mother 24 yrs, father 27 yrs). The pregnancy was normal, with spontaneous vaginal delivery at term. The newborn appeared healthy, with a length of 56 cm (97. percentile) and weight of 3500 g (50. percentile) [13]. At the age of 1 year, hepatomegaly and highly increased transaminases were observed. A metabolic storage disorder was suspected and the patient was referred to our clinic for further investigation.

At admission to our service, the patient was in good general condition. He presented with a body height of 90.0 cm (50. percentile) and a body weight of 16.5 kg (97. percentile) [13], severe hepatomegaly, mild muscle weakness, and mild splenomegaly. On sonographic volumetric evaluation, the hepatomegaly was 4.3x the upper normal limit (UNL) and the splenomegaly was 1.3x UNL. Normal values were considered to be 2.5% of the patient's weight for the liver and 0.2% of the patient's weight for the spleen, according to published criteria [14]. Hepatic sonography showed, additionally, a slightly increased echogenic pattern.

Laboratory tests showed the following abnormalities: increased transaminases (alanine transaminase (ALT) = 760 UI/L and aspartate transaminase (AST) = 767 UI/L; normal values 20–40 UI/L) and gamma-glutamyl transferase (γGT) = 333 UI/L; normal values < 20 UI/L; viral markers for hepatitis B and hepatitis C were negative; moderately increased creatine phosphokinase (CPK) = 545 UI/L (normal values 30–200 UI/L) and lactic dehydrogenase (LDH) = 780 UI/L (normal values 120–300 UI/L), confirming muscular involvement in accordance with the clinical picture; ketotic fasting hypoglycemia (48 mg/dL) with metabolic acidosis (pH = 7.26, BE = −12.6, HCO_3^- = 12.8 mmol/L); and combined hyperlipoproteinemia, with total cholesterol = 282 mg/dL (normal values for age ≤ 170 mg/dL), triglycerides = 300 mg/dL (normal values for age ≤ 100 mg/dL).

Liver biopsy was performed before the patient's referral to our clinic. The biopsy showed enlarged hepatocytes with intracytoplasmic glycogen loading and stellate as well as periportal bridging fibrosis with incomplete nodular transformation. Cardiac ultrasound showed a hypertrophic obstructive myocardiopathy with biventricular hypertrophy on electrocardiogram (EKG).

The clinical picture and the diagnostic findings suggest a hepatic glycogenosis (type IIIa).

2.1. Genetic Testing. All of the genetic investigations performed on this patient and his family members were done after informed consent was obtained following local Institutional Review Board policies and procedures.

The genomic DNA of the index patient, isolated from peripheral blood leucocytes, was analyzed by a next generation sequencing panel (Centogene AG, Rostock, Germany), comprising the entire coding region and the highly conserved exon-intron splice junctions of the *AGL* gene (amylo-alpha-1,6-glucosidase, 4-alpha-glucanotransferase, RefSeq NM_000642.2 [variant 1], NM_000645.2 [variant 5], NM_000646.2 [variant 6]); *G6PC* (glucose-6-phosphatase, catalytic subunit, RefSeq NM_000151.3); *GBE1* (glucan (1,4-alpha), branching enzyme 1, NM_000158.3) and *SLC37A4* (solute carrier family 37 (glucose-6-phosphate transporter, member 4), RefSeq NM_001164278.1). Library preparation was based on polymerase chain reaction (PCR) amplicons and the minimal coverage was 30x.

A previously unreported heterozygous variant in exon 24 of the *AGL* gene was identified: c.3235C>T (p.Gln1079*); see Figure 1(a). This variant causes the reading frame to be interrupted by a premature stop codon and is classified, according to the American College of Medical Genetics and Genomics (ACMG) recommendations, as class 2, a sequence variation previously unreported and of the type that is expected to cause the disorder [15]. Furthermore, the mutation c.1589C>G (p.Ser*) in exon 12 of the *AGL* gene has also been detected in a heterozygous state (Figure 1(b)). This mutation has been previously described as disease-causing.

No disease-causing mutation was detected in the *G6PC*, *GBE1*, or *SLC37A4* genes.

The results were confirmed in a second independent sample at the Institute for Clinical Chemistry and Laboratory Medicine (Mainz, Germany) by conventional sequencing of exons 12 and 24 (PCR primers: ACCAGTGTTTCCTTGAAGTAATTG and AAATCAATGCTTGTGTCCAACTAG for amplification of exon 12 and TTGAAGGAAAGAAACCAAGTAAA and CTTGAGTAGCATTACAAGCTTTT for exon 24). For sequencing (Dye Terminator Cycle Sequencing Quick Start Kit, CEQ 8000 Genetic Analysis System; Beckman Coulter, Krefeld, Germany) M13/M13R tags were added to the PCR primers.

Given the autosomal recessive mode of inheritance of glycogen storage disease type III, we performed parental carrier testing to confirm the mutation phase (cis or trans). We tested the grandparents, too. The mutation analysis of family members has also been performed in the Institute for Clinical Chemistry and Laboratory Medicine (Mainz, Germany).

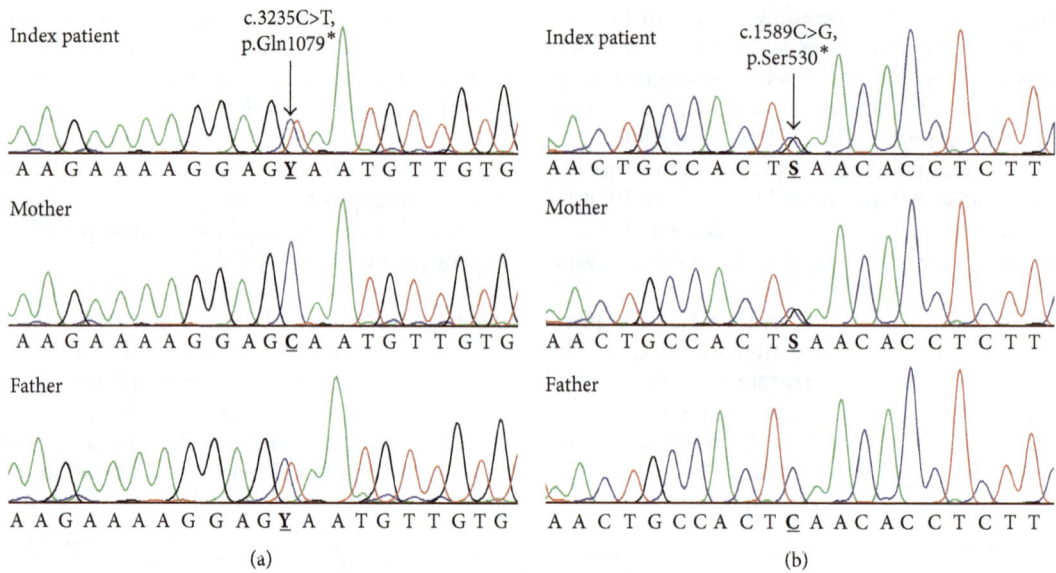

FIGURE 1: Sequence analysis of the index patient showing the novel mutation c.3235C>T, p.Gln1079* in exon 24 (a) and the known mutation c.1589C>G, p.Ser530* in exon 12 (b).

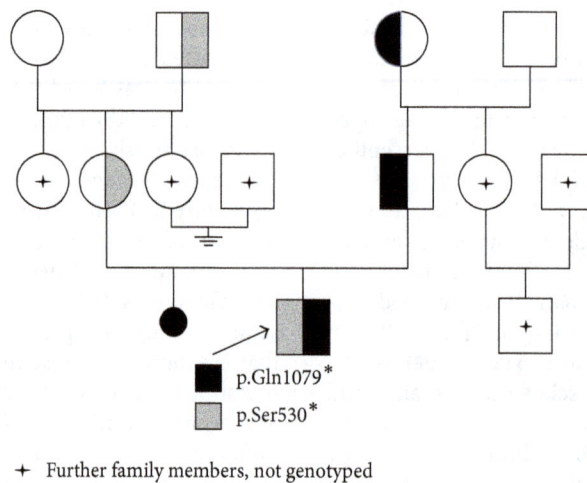

+ Further family members, not genotyped

FIGURE 2: Diagnostic sequence analysis of the AGL gene (exons 12 and 24) shows compound heterozygosity for c.1589C>G, p.Ser530* and c.3235C>T, p.Gln1079* in the index patient, and heterozygosity for either c.1589C>G, p.Ser530* or c.3235C>T, p.Gln1079* in his parents and grandparents.

The results demonstrated the inheritance of the two mutations in trans phase. The novel mutation, c.3235C>T (p.Gln1079*), was inherited from the father, who inherited it from his mother, while the known mutation c.1589C>G (p.Ser530*) was inherited from the mother, who inherited it from her father (Figure 2). Therefore, the index patient has a compound heterozygous genotype with the novel mutation c.3235C>T (p.Gln1079*) in exon 24 and the known mutation c.1589C>G (p.Ser530*) in exon 12 (Figures 1(a) and 1(b)).

2.2. Follow-Up. The therapy was according to present recommendations with a specific diet including frequent meals, high in carbohydrates; supplementation of maltodextrin

(1 g/kg/4 hrs) during the night to prevent hypoglycemia; protein enrichment during the day (up to 3 g/kg).

Six months after the start of treatment, we registered no more hypoglycemia, improvement of dyslipidemia (total cholesterol from 282 to 164 mg/dL and triglycerides from 300 to 184 mg/dL), and decrease of transaminases (ALT from 760 to 529 U/L; AST from 767 to 472 U/L) with constant values of gamma-GT.

3. Discussion

The majority of the mutations reported in the AGL gene to date are nonsense or missense mutations, small or large deletions, or insertions. Very few mutations are specific for a geographical region; most of them are private mutations [11, 12]. Three mutations (p.Arg864*, p.Arg1228*, and p.Trp680*) account for approximately 28% of the known mutations in individuals of European origin [11].

Mutations with a certain regional pattern are homozygous in affected individuals and have been described in Inuit children from the Eastern region of the Hudson bay and in Jews of North-African origin (c.4555delT) [12, 16], in inhabitants of the Faroe islands (c.1222C>T; p.R408*) [17] and in Tunisian patients: c.3216_3217delGA [18] and p.W1327* [19]. These findings are explained by a "founder effect" and are responsible for a high prevalence of the disease in these areas: 1/5,420 in North-African Jews, 1/3,600 in the inhabitants of the Faroe islands, and 1/2,500 in Inuits versus 1/100,000 in North-America [17, 18]. A higher prevalence with clustering of some mutations has been reported from Japan [20] and Korea [21].

The genetic heterogeneity due to a high number of private mutations precludes a diagnostic strategy based on screening for the most common ones. Furthermore, the heterogeneity of the clinical picture, with high phenotypic variability in patients with the same genotype, makes genotype-phenotype correlations extremely difficult [10, 11]. Heterogeneity even within a given family has been noted [9]. The only observed correlation is the association between mutations in exon 3 with GSD type IIIb [22].

The index patient reported here has a GSD type III phenotype, with a pronounced hepatic involvement (severe hepatomegaly, altered liver tests, and liver fibrosis) and a hypertrophic obstructive cardiomyopathy. The association of a mild muscular involvement suggests GSD type IIIa. The absence of a mutation in exon 3, associated with GSD type IIIb, supports the diagnosis. As shown, our patient displayed a compound heterozygous genotype c3235C>T (p.Gln1079*)/c.1589C>G (p.Ser530*). c.3235C>T (p.Gln1079*) is a novel mutation leading to a stop codon, yielding a truncated protein lacking the 3' 454 amino acids. The protein lacks exon 31, which is one glycogen binding area. The second mutation, c1589C>G, (p.Ser530*), also leads to a premature stop codon and has been described previously in a patient of Mediterranean origin, who was compound heterozygous and presented with a severe phenotype [23].

Some studies describe severe hepatopathy at older ages in patients with GSD III, such as in the second decade of life in an 18-year-old patient with the genotype c.2607_2610delATCC/c.1672dupA [24] or in the third decade in 16% of the patients reported [9]. The cardiomyopathy is also reported later, in adult life [25]. The phenotype in our patient with early hepatic and cardiac damage may be explained by the fact that both mutations generate premature stop codons, with the theoretical risk of null alleles for the development of a more severe clinical picture [9]. It is possible that further improvement will occur in time, so the severity of the phenotype will be shown in future. Nevertheless, the severe histologic damage of the liver remains a key element of concern.

4. Conclusions

We report on a new nonsense mutation (c.3235C>T; p.Gln.1079* in exon 24 of the *AGL* gene), in a compound heterozygote state with the known mutation c1589C>G (p.Ser530*) in the first genetically confirmed Romanian patient with GSDIIIa. Our observation adds to many other previous reports, pointing out to the heterogenous genetic background of the disease and the need for complete *AGL* gene sequencing in the setting of a suggestive clinical picture, in order to confirm the diagnosis, to screen further siblings and to offer correct genetic counselling in young families.

Consent

Written informed consent has been obtained.

Conflict of Interests

The authors declare that there is no conflict of interests regarding the publication of this paper.

References

[1] P. S. Kishnani, S. L. Austin, P. Arn et al., "Glycogen storage disease type III diagnosis and management guidelines," *Genetics in Medicine*, vol. 12, no. 7, pp. 446–463, 2010.

[2] W. Liu, N. B. Madsen, C. Braun, and S. G. Withers, "Reassessment of the catalytic mechanism of glycogen debranching enzyme," *Biochemistry*, vol. 30, no. 5, pp. 1419–1424, 1991.

[3] Y. Bao, T. L. Dawson Jr., and Y.-T. Chen, "Human glycogen debranching enzyme gene (AGL): complete structural organization and characterization of the 5' flanking region," *Genomics*, vol. 38, no. 2, pp. 155–165, 1996.

[4] C. B. Newgard, P. K. Hwang, and R. J. Fletterick, "The family of glycogen phosphorylases: structure and function," *Critical Reviews in Biochemistry and Molecular Biology*, vol. 24, no. 1, pp. 69–99, 1989.

[5] T. L. Yang-Feng, K. Zheng, J. Yu, B.-Z. Yang, Y.-T. Chen, and F.-T. Kao, "Assignment of the human glycogen debrancher gene to chromosome 1p21," *Genomics*, vol. 13, no. 4, pp. 931–934, 1992.

[6] Y. Bao, B.-Z. Yang, T. L. Dawson Jr., and Y.-T. Chen, "Isolation and nucleotide sequence of human liver glycogen debranching enzyme mRNA: identification of multiple tissue-specific isoforms," *Gene*, vol. 197, no. 1-2, pp. 389–398, 1997.

[7] O. N. Elpeleg, "The molecular background of glycogen metabolism disorders," *Journal of Pediatric Endocrinology and Metabolism*, vol. 12, no. 3, pp. 363–379, 1999.

[8] J.-H. Ding, T. de Barsy, B. I. Brown, R. A. Coleman, and Y.-T. Chen, "Immunoblot analyses of glycogen debranching enzyme in different subtypes of glycogen storage disease type III," *The Journal of Pediatrics*, vol. 116, no. 1, pp. 95–100, 1990.

[9] S. Lucchiari, D. Santoro, S. Pagliarani, and G. P. Comi, "Clinical, biochemical and genetic features of glycogen debranching enzyme deficiency," *Acta Myologica*, vol. 26, no. 1, pp. 72–74, 2007.

[10] C. P. Sentner, Y. J. Vos, K. N. Niezen-Koning, B. Mol, and G. P. Smit, "Mutation analysis in glycogen storage disease type III patients in the Netherlands: novel genotype-phenotype relationships and five novel mutations in the AGL gene," *JIMD Reports*, vol. 7, pp. 19–26, 2013.

[11] J. L. Goldstein, S. L. Austin, K. Boyette et al., "Molecular analysis of the AGL gene: identification of 25 novel mutations and evidence of genetic heterogeneity in patients with Glycogen Storage Disease Type III," *Genetics in Medicine*, vol. 12, no. 7, pp. 424–430, 2010.

[12] I. Rousseau-Nepton, M. Okubo, R. Grabs et al., "A founder AGL mutation causing glycogen storage disease type IIIa in Inuit identified through whole-exome sequencing: a case series," *Canadian Medical Association Journal*, vol. 187, no. 2, pp. E68–E73, 2015.

[13] A. A. Carillo and B. F. Recker, "Length for age and weight for age, boys: birth to 36 months," in *Pediatric Endocrinology*, F. Lifshitz, Ed., p. 987, Marcel Dekker, New York, NY, USA, 4th edition, 2003.

[14] N. Weinreb, J. Taylor, T. Cox, J. Yee, and S. Vom Dahl, "A benchmark analysis of the achievement of therapeutic goals for type 1 Gaucher disease patients treated with imiglucerase," *American Journal of Hematology*, vol. 83, no. 12, pp. 890–895, 2008.

[15] C. S. Richards, S. Bale, D. B. Billissimo et al., "ACMG recommendations for standards for interpretation and reporting of sequence variations: revisions 2007," *Genetics in Medicine*, vol. 10, no. 4, pp. 294–300, 2008.

[16] R. Parvari, S. Moses, J. Shen, E. Hershkovitz, A. Lerner, and Y.-T. Chen, "A single-base deletion in the 3'-coding region of glycogen-debranching enzyme is prevalent in glycogen storage disease type IIIA in a population of North African Jewish patients," *European Journal of Human Genetics*, vol. 5, no. 5, pp. 266–270, 1997.

[17] R. Santer, M. Kinner, U. Steuerwald et al., "Molecular genetic basis and prevalence of glycogen storage disease type IIIA in the Faroe Islands," *European Journal of Human Genetics*, vol. 9, no. 5, pp. 388–391, 2001.

[18] A. Mili, I. Ben Charfeddine, A. Amara et al., "A c.3216_3217delGA mutation in AGL gene in Tunisian patients with a glycogen storage disease type III: evidence of a founder effect," *Clinical Genetics*, vol. 82, no. 6, pp. 534–539, 2012.

[19] W. Cherif, F. Ben Rhouma, H. Messai et al., "High frequency of W1327X mutation in glycogen storage disease type III patients from central Tunisia," *Annales de Biologie Clinique*, vol. 70, no. 6, pp. 648–650, 2012.

[20] W.-L. Shaiu, P. S. Kishnani, J. Shen, H.-M. Liu, and Y.-T. Chen, "Genotype-phenotype correlation in two frequent mutations and mutation update in type III glycogen storage disease," *Molecular Genetics and Metabolism*, vol. 69, no. 1, pp. 16–23, 2000.

[21] J. S. Ko, J. S. Moon, J. K. Seo, H. R. Yang, J. Y. Chang, and S. S. Park, "A mutation analysis of the AGL gene in Korean patients with glycogen storage disease type III," *Journal of Human Genetics*, vol. 59, no. 1, pp. 42–45, 2014.

[22] J. Shen, Y. Bao, H.-M. Liu, P. Lee, J. V. Leonard, and Y.-T. Chen, "Mutations in exon 3 of the glycogen debranching enzyme gene are associated with glycogen storage disease type III that is differentially expressed in liver and muscle," *Journal of Clinical Investigation*, vol. 98, no. 2, pp. 352–357, 1996.

[23] S. Lucchiari, I. Fogh, A. Prelle et al., "Clinical and genetic variability of glycogen storage disease type IIIa: seven novel AGL gene mutations in the Mediterranean area," *American Journal of Medical Genetics*, vol. 109, no. 3, pp. 183–190, 2002.

[24] Y. Kondo, H. Usui, M. Ishige-Wada, T. Murase, M. Owada, and M. Okubo, "Liver cirrhosis treated by living donor liver transplantation in a patient with AGL mutation c.2607-2610delATTC and c.1672dupA," *Clinica Chimica Acta*, vol. 424, pp. 19–21, 2013.

[25] A. Ogimoto, M. Okubo, H. Okayama et al., "A Japanese patient with cardiomyopathy caused by a novel mutation R285X in the AGL gene," *Circulation Journal*, vol. 71, no. 10, pp. 1653–1656, 2007.

46

False Negative Cell-Free DNA Screening Result in a Newborn with Trisomy 13

Yang Cao,[1] Nicole L. Hoppman,[1] Sarah E. Kerr,[1] Christopher A. Sattler,[1] Kristi S. Borowski,[2] Myra J. Wick,[2] W. Edward Highsmith,[1] and Umut Aypar[1]

[1]*Department of Laboratory Medicine and Pathology, Mayo Clinic, Rochester, MN 55905, USA*
[2]*Department of Obstetrics and Gynecology, Mayo Clinic, Rochester, MN 55905, USA*

Correspondence should be addressed to Umut Aypar; aypar.umut@mayo.edu

Academic Editor: Patrick Morrison

Background. Noninvasive prenatal screening (NIPS) is revolutionizing prenatal screening as a result of its increased sensitivity, specificity. NIPS analyzes cell-free fetal DNA (cffDNA) circulating in maternal plasma to detect fetal chromosome abnormalities. However, cffDNA originates from apoptotic placental trophoblast; therefore cffDNA is not always representative of the fetus. Although the published data for NIPS testing states that the current technique ensures high sensitivity and specificity for aneuploidy detection, false positives are possible due to isolated placental mosaicism, vanishing twin or cotwin demise, and maternal chromosome abnormalities or malignancy. *Results.* We report a case of false negative cell-free DNA (cfDNA) screening due to fetoplacental mosaicism. An infant male with negative cfDNA screening result was born with multiple congenital abnormalities. Postnatal chromosome and FISH studies on a blood specimen revealed trisomy 13 in 20/20 metaphases and 100% interphase nuclei, respectively. FISH analysis on tissues collected after delivery revealed extraembryonic mosaicism. *Conclusions.* Extraembryonic tissue mosaicism is likely responsible for the false negative cfDNA screening result. This case illustrates that a negative result does not rule out the possibility of a fetus affected with a trisomy, as cffDNA is derived from the placenta and therefore may not accurately represent the fetal genetic information.

1. Background

Cell-free fetal DNA (cffDNA) circulating in maternal plasma was initially identified approximately two decades ago; however, the laboratory use of cffDNA to detect fetal chromosome abnormalities was not available until 2011 [1]. cfDNA screening (also referred to as NIPS, NIPT) analyzes cffDNA circulating in maternal plasma. Clinical utilization of cfDNA screening has been rapidly incorporated into obstetric practice, as it offers improved sensitivity, specificity, and PPV when compared to first- and second-trimester screening. However, cfDNA screening also has limitations. The cffDNA originates from apoptotic placental trophoblast cells [2]; therefore, cffDNA may not always represent the chromosomal make-up of the fetus. Although the genetic component of placental and fetal tissue is identical in the vast majority of pregnancies, false positive or false negative results may be due

to fetoplacental mosaicism. In several reported cases, follow-up amniocentesis based on positive cfDNA screening results has identified a normal karyotype, suggesting a false positive cfDNA screening result [3–8]. Even though the published data indicates high sensitivity (≥99% for trisomy 21, ≥92% for trisomy 18, and ≥87% for trisomy 13) and specificity (≥99% for trisomy 21, 18, and 13) for aneuploidy detection [9], false positive results have been reported for confined placental mosaicism, vanishing twin or cotwin demise, fetal chromosome rearrangement, and maternal chromosome abnormalities or malignancy [10–14]. Based on several reports, false negative results for fetal aneuploidy are much less common than false positive results [4–6, 15, 16]. It is generally accepted that false negative cfDNA screening results are primarily due to a low level of cffDNA fraction in maternal plasma and therefore could be overcome by technical improvement [17]. However, aside from the technical reasons, a limited number of false negative cfDNA screening cases due to fetoplacental mosaicism and/or structural chromosome rearrangement have also been reported [13, 18].

2. Case Presentation

A 19-year-old, gravida 2, para 1, female underwent obstetric ultrasound at 19 5/7 weeks of gestation, which identified multiple fetal anomalies including hypoplastic left heart, bilateral cleft lip, bilateral echogenic kidneys with hydronephrosis, echogenic bowel, and bowed right femur. Genetic consultation was provided and risks, benefits, and alternatives of further genetic evaluation, including amniocentesis and cfDNA screening, were discussed. The patient expressed concerns regarding the risks of invasive testing and opted to proceed with cfDNA screening. Limitations of cfDNA in this setting were reviewed. cfDNA screening was performed at 20 weeks of gestational age. A negative cfDNA screening result was issued for chromosomes 13, 18, 21, X, and Y. Although the fetal fraction (percentage of fetal DNA among all DNA in maternal plasma) was not included in the final report, later inquiries to the testing laboratory revealed a fetal fraction of 8.5%. Genetic counseling was provided to the patient at 24-5/7 weeks of gestation, during which amniocentesis with cytogenetic analyses was further discussed. The patient again declined invasive testing. After induction of labor due to multiple fetal anomalies, a male infant was delivered vaginally at 38-4/7 weeks of gestational age. Apgar scores were 8, 7, and 9 at one, five, and ten minutes, respectively. Physical examination revealed multiple anomalies including cutis aplasia on the scalp, cleft lip and palate, polydactyly, and cryptorchidism; postnatal echocardiogram confirmed hypoplastic left heart. The newborn also had respiratory insufficiency and was intubated due to signs of airway obstruction. A peripheral blood specimen was collected at birth and sent to the Cytogenetics Laboratory for postnatal evaluation.

Chromosome analysis was performed on 20 metaphases, which identified additional chromosome 13 in each metaphase (47, XY, +13), suggesting nonmosaic trisomy 13 (Figure 1(a)). FISH analysis was also performed, and 100% of nuclei indicated three signals of probes for chromosome 13, also consistent with nonmosaic trisomy 13 (Figure 1(b)). Unfortunately, the infant passed away four days after birth.

We proposed that the discordant cfDNA and postnatal cytogenetic results were due to fetoplacental mosaicism. To test this hypothesis, we further evaluated extraembryonic tissue samples. The placenta was of normal weight (588 grams) and gross appearances of the placenta and umbilical cord were normal for 38 weeks of gestation. The chorionic villi showed mild villous enlargement and edema with increase in Hofbauer cells, but no other morphologic abnormalities. Representative areas of the umbilical cord, amnion, villous trophoblast, villous stroma, and intermediate trophoblast were identified from placental sections for aneuploidy analysis by FISH. As shown in Figure 1(c), all five types of extraembryonic tissues demonstrated different levels of extraembryonic mosaicism of trisomy 13 (58%, 57%, 32%,

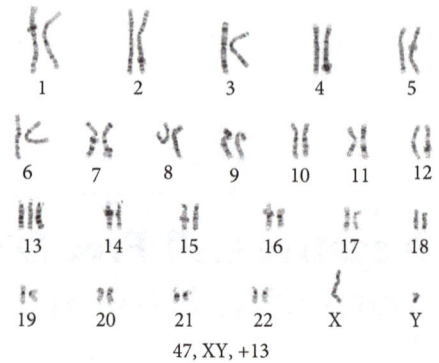

(a)

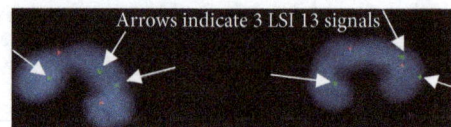

(b)

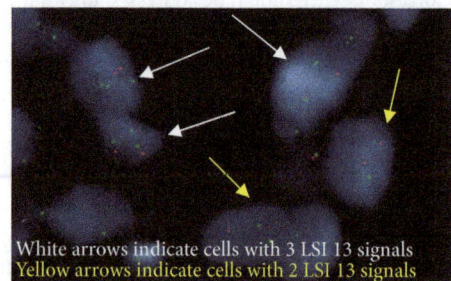

(c)

FIGURE 1: Postnatal aneuploidy detection by chromosome and FISH analysis. (a) G-banded karyotype on a blood specimen of the newborn shows trisomy 13. (b) FISH analysis on a blood specimen of the newborn shows three signals of LSI 13 (RB1) probe targeted on 13q14 (green) and two signals of LSI 21 (D21S341) probe targeted on 21q22.13-q22.2 (orange). Cells are stained with DAPI (blue) to visualize nuclei. (c) FISH analysis for aneuploidy detection in different tissue types of placental specimen shows mosaic trisomy 13. Signals of LSI 13 (RB1) probe targeted on 13q14 are shown in green. Signals of LSI 21 (D21S341) probe targeted on 21q22.13-q22.2 are shown in orange. Cells are stained with DAPI (blue) to visualize nuclei.

46%, and 64% of nuclei with trisomy 13 in umbilical cord, amnion, villous trophoblast, villous stroma, and intermediate trophoblast, resp., data listed in Table 1). These results suggest that mosaicism of the extraembryonic tissues was responsible for the false negative cfDNA screening result in this case.

3. Materials and Methods

3.1. G-Banding. Peripheral blood lymphocytes were cultured for 72 h in PB-Max plus excess thymidine and were harvested according to standard cytogenetic protocols. Metaphases were dropped in a Thermotron chamber and baked for

TABLE 1: Summary of tissue specific trisomy 13 mosaicism.

Tissue type	# of nuclei with disomy 13	# of nuclei with trisomy 13	# of total nuclei	% of nuclei with trisomy 13
Umbilical cord	21	29	50	58%
Amnion	18	24	42	57%
Intermediate trophoblast	26	46	72	64%
Villous trophoblast	28	13	41	32%
Villous stroma	23	20	43	46%

1 hour and 30 minutes at 100°C. G-banding was performed according to standard cytogenetic methods using trypsin and Leishman stain. Twenty GTL-banded metaphases were evaluated.

3.2. Fluorescence In Situ Hybridization (FISH). Initial FISH for newborn aneuploidy detection was performed on a peripheral blood sample. Additional postpartum FISH analysis for aneuploidy detection was performed on formalin fixed paraffin-embedded tissue. We used FISH probes that hybridize to the X centromere (DXZ1), Y centromere (DYZ3), 13q14 (Rb1), 13q34 (LAMP1), 18 centromere (D18Z1), and 21q22 (D21S341). Bacteria artificial chromosomes (BACs) located within the critical regions listed above were used for FISH probe development. Briefly, each BAC was extracted from *E. coli* using the Qiagen Plasmid Maxi kit according to the manufacturer's instructions and was then labeled with SpectrumOrange, SpectrumGreen, or SpectrumAqua (Abbott Molecular) using the Nick Translation Kit (Abbott Molecular) according to the manufacturer's instructions. A FISH probe working solution was made by adding 3 µL of labeled BAC to 7 µL of LSI/WCP® hybridization buffer (Abbott Molecular). Slides were pretreated according to standard cytogenetic protocols followed by application of 3 µL of probe working solution to the hybridization site. Slides were denatured at 75°C for 5 min and hybridized at 37°C for 70 h followed by washing for 2 min at 72°C with 0.4x saline-sodium citrate (SSC) and rinsed in 0.1% NP-40/2xSSC for 1 min at room temperature. 10 µL counterstain [10% 4′,6-diamidino-2-phenylindole (DAPI)] was added to the hybridization area. One hundred nuclei were scored for each specimen for aneuploidy detection.

4. Discussion

cfDNA screening is revolutionizing prenatal screening as a result of its robust test performance with increased sensitivity and specificity for the detection of common autosomal aneuploidies (trisomies 13, 18, and 21) compared to other prenatal aneuploidy screening methodologies. Since the introduction in the clinical setting, there have been several reports of cfDNA performance in high-risk population (indicated by advanced maternal age, screen positive on first- or second-trimester serum biochemical screening, the presence of a fetal abnormality on ultrasound, or a personal or family history of a chromosomal abnormality) as well as in low-risk population (general population) [4, 5, 9]. In high-risk pregnancies, cfDNA screening PPV for common autosomal

aneuploidies varies from 90.9% to 100% based on different studies, while NPV remains as 99.9%–100% [4, 5, 9]. In low-risk pregnancies, PPV for common autosomal aneuploidies has been reported as 85.3% with 99.9% NPV based on 146,958 pregnancies [4]. Thus, although clinical performance of cfDNA screening is widely accepted and desirable for screening utility, it is not appropriate for use as a diagnostic test.

Some of the reasons for false positive and negative cfDNA screening results include fetoplacental mosaicism, a vanishing twin/cotwin demise, maternal chromosome abnormality, and maternal metastatic disease. Several published reports of false positive and false negative cfDNA screening cases have implicated fetoplacental mosaicism [3, 8, 13, 18]. The most common type of fetal-placental mosaicism, confined placental mosaicism (CPM), is a conception with normal fetus and placenta mosaic for a chromosome abnormality [19]. However, false negative cfDNA screening results cannot be explained by CPM. Instead, it may be due to another type of fetoplacental mosaicism in which there is an affected (possibly nonmosaic) fetus and mosaic or normal placenta. Although false negative cfDNA screening result for trisomy 13 has been reported at least once, the causative mechanism of false negative result was not identified at that time [20]. This is the first report of a case with false negative cfDNA screening result for trisomy 13 that is caused by fetoplacental mosaicism. For trisomies 18 and 21, this mechanism has been recently described. A false negative trisomy 18 cfDNA screening result due to 48, XXX, +18 placental mosaicism and two cases with false negative trisomy 21 due to placental mosaicism have been reported [3, 13]. Potential contribution of fetoplacental mosaicism to discordant cfDNA screening results has been reported; this study suggested that the sensitivity or specificity of cfDNA screening will never reach 100% due to the nature of fetoplacental mosaicism.

This report describes a case of false negative cfDNA results for trisomy 13 due to fetoplacental mosaicism. Cytogenetics analysis demonstrated that the infant was nonmosaic for trisomy 13 with placental tissue mosaic for trisomy 13. This mosaicism was demonstrated in at least five different extraembryonic tissues including umbilical cord, amnion, villous trophoblast, villous stroma, and intermediate trophoblast. In this case, the level of trisomy 13 mosaicism in the various tissues investigated ranged from 32% to 64%. The level of fetal fraction required for robust detection of trisomies varies slightly among commercial providers but is generally in the range of 4%. In the case presented here, the proportion of the 8.5% fetal fraction that derived from trisomy 13 positive extraembryonic tissues was likely less than half, thus decreasing the functional fetal fraction to less than the level required. Similar patterns of mosaicism have been reported in cases with false negative cfDNA screening results [3, 13, 18]. This type of fetoplacental mosaicism is different from CMP, which is more commonly reported etiology for discordant cfDNA and fetal/infant cytogenetic results. Cytogenetic analyses of infant cord blood as well as physical examination suggested nonmosaic trisomy 13 for the infant. However, because our studies were limited to a single specimen type from the infant, we cannot rule out the possibility that the infant may have had mosaicism in other tissues. This case, along with other reports of discordant cfDNA screening findings, demonstrates that providers should understand and patients should be counseled regarding the limitations of cfDNA screening. In the setting of a positive cfDNA screening result, confirmatory diagnostic testing is highly recommended. This case report also underscores the importance of diagnostic testing in the setting of multiple fetal anomalies with negative cfDNA results. Pre- and posttest genetic counseling are important in such cases to educate about the benefits and limitations of cfDNA screening to ensure that patients are able to make informed decisions.

5. Conclusions

Here we report a case with negative cfDNA screening results that had a postnatal diagnostic test result of nonmosaic trisomy 13. FISH analysis on placental tissues revealed extraembryonic mosaicism of trisomy 13, which is likely responsible for the false negative cfDNA screening result. This case illustrates the limitation of cfDNA screening, as cell-free fetal DNA is derived from the placenta and therefore may not accurately represent the fetal genetic information. Therefore, in the setting of multiple fetal anomalies with negative cfDNA screening results, diagnostic testing is recommended.

Conflict of Interests

The authors declare that there is no conflict of interests regarding the publication of this paper.

References

[1] R. W. K. Chiu, R. Akolekar, Y. W. L. Zheng et al., "Non-invasive prenatal assessment of trisomy 21 by multiplexed maternal plasma DNA sequencing: large scale validity study," *British Medical Journal*, vol. 342, Article ID c7401, 2011.

[2] E. Flori, B. Doray, E. Gautier et al., "Circulating cell-free fetal DNA in maternal serum appears to originate from cyto- and syncytio-trophoblastic cells. Case report," *Human Reproduction*, vol. 19, no. 3, pp. 723–724, 2004.

[3] Y. Wang, J. Zhu, Y. Chen et al., "Two cases of placental T21 mosaicism: challenging the detection limits of non-invasive prenatal testing," *Prenatal Diagnosis*, vol. 33, no. 12, pp. 1207–1210, 2013.

[4] H. Zhang, Y. Gao, F. Jiang et al., "Noninvasive prenatal testing for trisomies 21, 18 and 13—clinical experience from 146,958 pregnancies," *Ultrasound in Obstetrics & Gynecology*, vol. 45, no. 5, pp. 530–538, 2015.

[5] P. J. Willems, H. Dierickx, E. Vandenakker et al., "The first 3,000 Non-Invasive Prenatal Tests (NIPT) with the harmony test in Belgium and the Netherlands," *Facts, Views & Vision in ObGyn*, vol. 6, no. 1, pp. 7–12, 2014.

[6] T. K. Lau, S. W. Cheung, P. S. Lo et al., "Non-invasive prenatal testing for fetal chromosomal abnormalities by low-coverage whole-genome sequencing of maternal plasma DNA: review of 1982 consecutive cases in a single center," *Ultrasound in Obstetrics & Gynecology*, vol. 43, no. 3, pp. 254–264, 1982.

[7] H. Choi, T. K. Lau, F. M. Jiang et al., "Fetal aneuploidy screening by maternal plasma DNA sequencing: 'false positive' due to confined placental mosaicism," *Prenatal Diagnosis*, vol. 33, no. 2, pp. 198–200, 2013.

[8] A. L. Hall, H. M. Drendel, J. L. Verbrugge et al., "Positive cell-free fetal DNA testing for trisomy 13 reveals confined placental mosaicism," *Genetics in Medicine*, vol. 15, no. 9, pp. 729–732, 2013.

[9] R. P. Porreco, T. J. Garite, K. Maurel et al., "Noninvasive prenatal screening for fetal trisomies 21, 18, 13 and the common sex chromosome aneuploidies from maternal blood using massively parallel genomic sequencing of DNA," *American Journal of Obstetrics and Gynecology*, vol. 211, no. 4, pp. 365.e1–365.e12, 2014.

[10] T. Futch, J. Spinosa, S. Bhatt, E. de Feo, R. P. Rava, and A. J. Sehnert, "Initial clinical laboratory experience in noninvasive prenatal testing for fetal aneuploidy from maternal plasma DNA samples," *Prenatal Diagnosis*, vol. 33, no. 6, pp. 569–574, 2013.

[11] H. Yao, L. Zhang, H. Zhang et al., "Noninvasive prenatal genetic testing for fetal aneuploidy detects maternal trisomy X," *Prenatal Diagnosis*, vol. 32, no. 11, pp. 1114–1116, 2012.

[12] C. M. Osborne, E. Hardisty, P. Devers et al., "Discordant noninvasive prenatal testing results in a patient subsequently diagnosed with metastatic disease," *Prenatal Diagnosis*, vol. 33, no. 6, pp. 609–611, 2013.

[13] Y. Gao, D. Stejskal, F. Jiang, and W. Wang, "False-negative trisomy 18 non-invasive prenatal test result due to 48,XXX,+18 placental mosaicism," *Ultrasound in Obstetrics & Gynecology*, vol. 43, no. 4, pp. 477–478, 2014.

[14] M. Pan, F. T. Li, Y. Li et al., "Discordant results between fetal karyotyping and non-invasive prenatal testing by maternal plasma sequencing in a case of uniparental disomy 21 due to trisomic rescue," *Prenatal Diagnosis*, vol. 33, no. 6, pp. 598–601, 2013.

[15] M. Smith, K. M. Lewis, A. Holmes, and J. Visootsak, "A case of false negative NIPT for down syndrome-lessons learned," *Case Reports in Genetics*, vol. 2014, Article ID 823504, 3 pages, 2014.

[16] J. C. Wang, T. Sahoo, S. Schonberg et al., "Discordant noninvasive prenatal testing and cytogenetic results: a study of 109 consecutive cases," *Genetics in Medicine*, vol. 17, no. 3, pp. 234–236, 2015.

[17] J. A. Canick, G. E. Palomaki, E. M. Kloza, G. M. Lambert-Messerlian, and J. E. Haddow, "The impact of maternal plasma DNA fetal fraction on next generation sequencing tests for common fetal aneuploidies," *Prenatal Diagnosis*, vol. 33, no. 7, pp. 667–674, 2013.

[18] Q. Pan, B. Sun, X. Huang et al., "A prenatal case with discrepant findings between non-invasive prenatal testing and fetal genetic testings," *Molecular Cytogenetics*, vol. 7, article 48, 2014.

[19] D. K. Kalousek and F. J. Dill, "Chromosomal mosaicism confined to the placenta in human conceptions," *Science*, vol. 221, no. 4611, pp. 665–667, 1983.

[20] R. Hochstenbach, G. C. Page-Christiaens, A. C. van Oppen et al., "Unexplained false negative results in noninvasive prenatal testing: two cases involving trisomies 13 and 18," *Case Reports in Genetics*, vol. 2015, Article ID 926545, 7 pages, 2015.

47

Angelman-Like Syndrome: A Genetic Approach to Diagnosis with Illustrative Cases

Ho-Ming Luk

Clinical Genetic Service, Department of Health, Kowloon, Hong Kong

Correspondence should be addressed to Ho-Ming Luk; luksite@gmail.com

Academic Editor: Christos Yapijakis

Epigenetic abnormalities in 15q11-13 imprinted region and *UBE3A* mutation are the two major mechanisms for molecularly confirmed Angelman Syndrome. However, there is 10% of clinically diagnosed Angelman Syndrome remaining test negative. With the advancement of genomic technology like array comparative genomic hybridization and next generation sequencing methods, it is found that some patients of these test negative Angelman-like Syndromes actually have alternative diagnoses. Accurate molecular diagnosis is paramount for genetic counseling and subsequent management. Despite overlapping phenotypes between Angelman and Angelman-like Syndrome, there are some subtle but distinct features which could differentiate them clinically. It would provide important clue during the diagnostic process for clinicians.

1. Introduction

Since the first description of Angelman Syndrome (AS) by Dr. Angelman in 1965 [1], there was a great advancement in understanding of its clinical features and molecular genetic mechanism. AS is characterized by distinct facial gestalt, developmental delay, absent speech, ataxic gait, seizure, and paroxysms of laughter [2]. The incidence reported was about 1/12,000 to 1/20,000 [3, 4] without racial predilection. The diagnosis of AS depends on the combination of clinical criteria and molecular and/or cytogenetic testing. The consensus criteria for clinical diagnosis of AS were proposed in 2006 [5] which included a list of core and associated features. However, the clinical manifestations of AS were highly heterogeneous that would overlap with other diseases. Methylation study on 15q11-13 imprinted region would identify 75–80% of AS that included maternal deletion, paternal uniparental disomy (UPD), and imprinting center defect. Further analysis of *UBE3A* gene would further confirm 10% of cases. However, there were still 5–10% of clinically diagnosed AS that would be rendered "test negative." With the advancement of medical genomic technology like array comparative genomic hybridization (array CGH) and next generation sequencing, it was now known that some patients of these "test negative"

Angelman-like Syndromes actually had alternative genetic diagnoses [6–8] which were important for counseling and management.

In this review, we use 4 illustrative cases to provide the overview of some Angelman-like Syndromes and highlight their difference with AS, so as to provide some guidance to clinicians on the diagnostic workup when they encounter such patients in their practice.

2. Illustrative Cases

2.1. Case 1. A 6-month-old girl was referred to genetic clinic for developmental delay. She was the second child of nonconsanguineous Chinese couple, born at full term with birth weight of 3.83 kg. The perinatal history was unremarkable. She was noted to have microcephaly (head circumference <3th percentile, body weight and body height at 75th percentile) and hypotonia at 3 months of age. Investigations including metabolic screening, muscle enzyme, and computerized tomography of brain were normal. Physical examination at 6 months of age showed microcephaly, flat occiput, right divergent squint, and hypotonia. No syndromal diagnosis could be ascertained at that time and she was

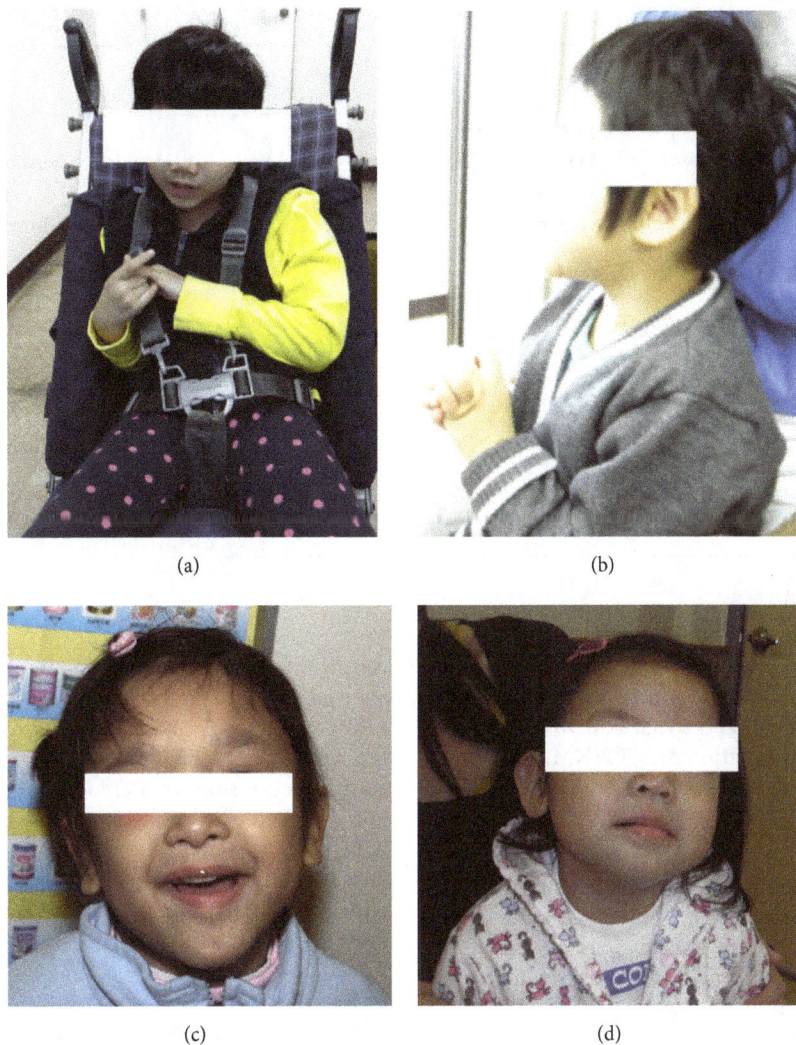

FIGURE 1: Facial features of different Angelman-like Syndromes in this series. (a) FOXG1 related disease; (b) Rett Syndrome. (c) Mowat-Wilson Syndrome; (d) Phelan-McDermid Syndrome.

regularly followed up in genetic clinic. She had epilepsy since she was 2 years of age and severe global delay at developmental assessment. EEG showed nonspecific background slowing, but no epileptiform abnormalities. Brain Magnetic Resonance Image (MRI) showed mild thinning of corpus callosum without major structural defect. There was no developmental regression, but she developed stereotypical hand movements (Figure 1), bruxism, and occasional outburst of laugher. Based on the craniofacial features like microcephaly, flat occiput, divergent squint, characteristic stereotypical hand movement, and outburst of laughter, Angelman/Rett Syndrome was suspected. However, genetic investigations including methylation-specific multiplex ligation-dependent probe amplification (MS-MLPA) for AS, UBE3A gene, MECP2 gene, and array CGH studies were negative. Based on the MRI findings and early onset of microcephaly, FOXG1 related disease was suspected. FOXG1 gene test showed a de novo frameshift pathogenic mutation FOXG1{NM_005249.3}:c.[396_397ins26];[=];

FOXG1{NP_005240.3}:p.[(Gly133Trpfs*68)];[=] which confirmed the diagnosis of FOXG1 related congenital variant of Rett Syndrome.

2.2. Case 2. A 10-month-old girl was referred to genetic clinic for global delay. She was the first child of nonconsanguineous Chinese couple, born at 38-week gestation with birth weight of 3.24 kg. Mother had gestational diabetes mellitus that required insulin therapy. She had mild grade bilateral hearing impairment and left divergent squint diagnosed at birth. On follow-up, she was noted to have microbrachycephaly and global developmental delay (Figure 1). Brain MRI, metabolic screening, and array CGH were normal. She had stereotypical handwashing movement since she was 1 year old. There was no clinical or electrical seizure. Based on the craniofacial features like microbrachycephaly, wide mouth, divergent squint, and behavioral phenotype, AS was initially suspected, but the methylation study and UBE3A

TABLE 1: Angelman-like Syndrome.

Chromatin-remodeling disorder		Synaptopathies		Unknown mechanism	
Syndrome	Genes	Syndrome	Genes	Syndrome	Genes
Rett Syndrome/MECP2 duplication syndrome	MECP2	Phelan-McDermid Syndrome/22q13.3 deletion syndrome	SHANK3	Pitt-Hopkins Syndrome	TCF4
Mowat-Wilson Syndrome	ZEB2			Christianson Syndrome	SLC9A6
Kleefstra Syndrome/9q34.3 deletion syndrome	EHMT1			HERC2 deficiency	HERC2
MBD5 haploinsufficiency/2q23.1 deletion syndrome	MBD5			Adenylosuccinase deficiency	ADSL
Koolen-de Vries Syndrome/17q23.31 deletion syndrome	KANSL1			CDKL5 syndrome	CDKL5
Congenital variant of Rett Syndrome	FOXG1			MEF2C haploinsufficiency syndrome	MEF2C
Alpha-thalassemia/intellectual disability syndrome	ATRX			Ohtahara Syndrome	STXBP1
				Methylenetetrahydrofolate deficiency	MTHFR

gene test were negative. Subsequently she had bruxism and developmental regression since she was 1 year and 6 months of age with loss of some motor and social skill. *MECP2* study showed de novo nonsense mutation *MECP2*{NM_004992.3}: c.[808C>T];[=];*MECP2* {NP_004983.1}:p.[(Arg270*)];[=] that confirmed the diagnosis of Rett Syndrome.

2.3. Case 3. A 5-year-old girl was referred to genetic clinic for AS based on the facial dysmorphism. She was the first child of nonconsanguineous Chinese couple, born at full term with birth weight of 2.9 kg. Perinatal history was unremarkable. She was noted to have dysmorphism and cardiac murmur during neonatal period. Echocardiogram showed patent ductus arteriosus and large secundum atrial septal defect. Total corrective operation was done at 1 year of age. Developmental assessment at 2 years of age showed severe grade developmental delay. Stereotypical hand movement, abnormal outburst of laughter, and ataxic gait were developed afterward. Brain MRI showed mild thinning of corpus callosum. Physical examination at genetic clinic showed head circumference at 3th percentile with body weight and body height at 10–25th percentile. There was facial dysmorphism, namely, hypertelorism, medial flared eyebrows, mild overhanging columella, pointed chin, and fleshy and uplifted earlobes (Figure 1). Based on facial gestalt, Mowat-Wilson Syndrome rather than AS was suspected. ZEB2 gene study was performed. It showed a de novo pathogenic frameshift mutation *ZEB2*{NM_014795.2}:c.[3335delACTT];[=];p.*ZEB2* {NP_055610.1}:p.[Tyr1112Cysfs*128][=]. Thus the diagnosis of Mowat-Wilson Syndrome was substantiated.

2.4. Case 4. A 2-year-old girl was referred from developmental paediatrician for developmental delay with AS phenotype, namely, flat occiput and wide mouth. She was the first child of the nonconsanguineous Chinese couple, born at full term with birth weight of 2.9 kg. The perinatal history was unremarkable. She had hypotonia and feeding difficulties during early infancy. Assessment at 1 year and 6 months showed that she had moderate to severe grade developmental delay with autistic features. Baseline investigations included brain MRI and metabolic screening was normal. There was no seizure, regression, or stereotypical hand movement. However, she had occasional abnormal outburst of laughter. The head size was normal at 10–25th percentile. Despite the fact that she had some behavioral features of AS, overall clinical profile was not typical (Figure 1). Therefore array CGH was performed, which showed a de novo arr[Hg18] 22q13.31q13.33(45,355,784-49,522,658)x1. That means that a terminal deletion in chromosome 22 at band q13.31 region with the size of 4.17 Mb included the *SHANK3* gene; thus the diagnosis of Phelan-McDermid Syndrome was substantiated.

3. Summary and Conclusion

Loss of maternal inherited *UBE3A* gene predominantly expressed in the brain was the pathomechanism of AS. Only 90% of clinically diagnosed AS would have identifiable molecular defect. The remaining 10% were labeled as test negative Angelman-like Syndrome. These Angelman-like Syndromes are actually separate disease entities that are not the variations of AS. However, due to overlapping clinical phenotype, their differentiation is sometimes challenging. Over the last decade, there were many novel AS mimic diseases being discovered and summarized in Table 1 [6–8]. The molecular basis for those AS mimic diseases could also be classified into two emerging classes, namely, the chromatin-remodeling disorder and synaptopathies [6]. However, there were still many of them with uncertain mechanism that had clinical phenotypes overlapping with AS.

The characteristic facial gestalt of AS included microcephaly, flat occiput, divergent squint, wide mouth, and widely spaced teeth. Given the phenotypic overlapping between the AS and Angelman-like Syndrome, clinical differentiation was difficult. Despite this, there were some distinct

TABLE 2: Differentiating clinical features among Angelman-like Syndromes.

	AS	Rett	MWS	FOXG1	KS	PMS	PHS	CS	CDKL5	MEF2C	ARTX
Microcephaly	+	+	+	+	+		+	+	+	+	+
Seizure	+	+	+	+	+		+	+	+	+	
Speech impairment	+	+	+	+	+	+	+	+		+	+
Ataxia	+	+					+	+		+	
Stereotypical hand movements	+/−	+		+			+		+	+	
Tremulous/jerky limb movements	+										
Happy predisposition	+	+	+				+				+
Abnormal MRI			+	+		+	+	+			
Hyperventilation/apnea episode		+					+				
Sleep disturbances	+	+		+	+	+					
Hirschsprung disease			+								
Lack of purposeful hand use		+									
Prominent jaw/chin	+		+								
Wide mouth	+		+				+				
Upturned ear lobes		+									
Genital anomalies					+						+
Congenital heart disease			+		+						+
Developmental regression		+					+	+			
Others		In female only				Mild overgrowth	Persistent finger pad Constipation	In male only			In male only HbH in blood smear

AS: Angelman Syndrome; MWS: Mowat-Wilson Syndrome; KS: Kleefstra Syndrome; PMS: Phelan-McDermid Syndrome; PHS: Pitt-Hopkins Syndrome; CS: Christianson Syndrome; ARTX: alpha-thalassemia/intellectual disability syndrome.

features that could be useful for clinical diagnosis and guided the further genetic testing. In case 1, the diagnosis was *FOXG1* related congenital variant of Rett Syndrome. It was first reported in the literature in 2011 [9]. The core clinical features of *FOXG1* related disease included early onset postnatal microcephaly, severe mental retardation, hypotonia, absent speech, dyskinesia, and corpus callosum hypogenesis [10, 11]. The other reported MRI brain abnormalities included delayed myelination and gyral simplification [11]. In this case, the early onset of postnatal microcephaly together with hypoplasia of corpus callosum was suggestive of *FOXG1* related disease. Epilepsy was also common but relatively easy to control as compared with *CDKL5* related disorder [11], another Angelman-like Syndrome. Distinct EEG pattern like high voltage slow delta activity and intermittent high-amplitude rhythmic theta activity would occasionally differentiate the AS from other Angelman-like Syndromes [8].

In case 2, the diagnosis was Rett Syndrome due to *MECP2* mutation. It was well reported that Rett Syndrome and AS have overlapping clinical features including seizures, impaired sleep pattern, inappropriate laughter, and ataxia [12]. However, normal period of development during at least first 6 months of life followed by developmental regression was quite distinctive for Rett Syndrome. Unless the epilepsy was poorly controlled, regression was unusual for AS. Although it was reported that AS had particular EEG pattern, there was also specific pattern in Rett Syndrome like generalized background slowing and/or loss of occipital dominant rhythm, with further theta and delta slowing as the developmental regression continued [12, 13].

In case 3, the diagnosis was Mowat-Wilson Syndrome due to loss of function in *ZEB2* gene on chromosome 2q22.3. The features resembling AS included moderate to severe grade intellectual disability, happy predisposition, epilepsy, and microcephaly [14]. However, congenital structural anomalies including Hirschsprung disease, congenital heart disease, and corpus callosum hypoplasia were far more common in Mowat-Wilson Syndrome than in AS. The most distinguished feature was the facial gestalt including hypertelorism, telecanthus, medial flared eyebrow, uplifted earlobes with central depression, overhanging nasal tip, low inserted columella, and prognathism [15]. It was well known that not all these facial features were present during early life and diagnosis could be missed during early childhood.

The diagnosis in case 4 was Phelan-McDermid Syndrome (PMS). It was the first microdeletion syndrome that was reported to mimic AS [16, 17]. The shared clinical features included moderate to severe grade global delay with absent speech, hypotonia, and neonatal feeding difficulties that happened in our case, but mild overgrowth with large hands, large ears, and dysplastic toenails would be the distinctive features for PMS [17, 18]. Posterior cranial fossa brain malformations were also well reported in PMS but not in AS. This case illustrated that many microdeletion/microduplication syndromes were masqueraded Angelman-like Syndrome that array CGH should be the first investigation for them.

The clinical features of selected Angelman-like Syndrome were summarized in Table 2. In terms of genetic testing for Angelman-like Syndrome, two categories of diseases based on the genetic mechanisms should be considered. These

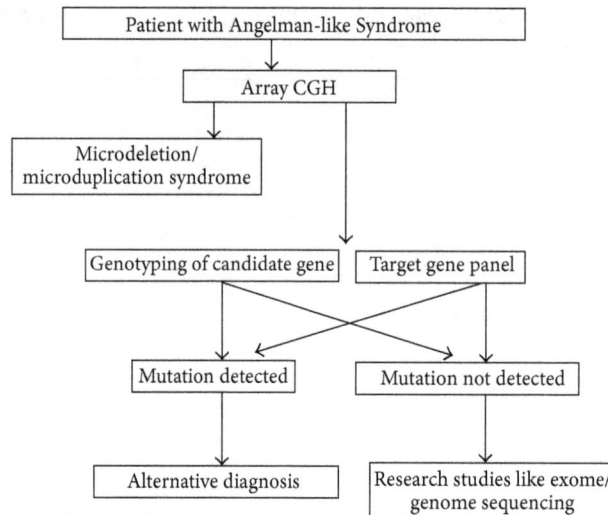

FIGURE 2: The genetic diagnostic algorithm of Angelman-like Syndrome.

included microdeletion/microduplication syndrome and single gene syndrome. Therefore, after methylation study and *UBE3A* gene analysis, the first line of investigation for Angelman-like Syndrome should be array CGH. If negative, either single gene analysis based on clinical phenotype or targeted gene panel by next generation sequencing should be pursued. The proposed diagnostic algorithm for Angelman-like Syndrome was depicted in Figure 2.

In conclusion, the Angelman-like Syndrome was not uncommon. With the advancement of genomic testing, many emerging diseases have been identified with AS mimic phenotype. Accurate diagnosis is important as the pathogenesis, potential treatment, prognosis, and mode of inheritance among them are different. Recognition of distinct features among Angelman-like Syndrome would provide useful clue in diagnostic strategies. With the jurious use of new technologies like array CGH and next generation sequencing method, it is expected that more and more test negative Angelman-like Syndromes would have definite molecular diagnosis.

Conflict of Interests

The author declares that there is no conflict of interests regarding the publication of this paper.

References

[1] H. Angelman, "'Puppet' children. A report of three cases," *Developmental Medicine & Child Neurology*, vol. 7, no. 6, pp. 681–688, 1965.

[2] J. Clayton-Smith, "Clinical research on Angelman syndrome in the United Kingdom: observations on 82 affected individuals," *American Journal of Medical Genetics*, vol. 46, no. 1, pp. 12–15, 1993.

[3] J. Clayton-Smith and M. E. Pembrey, "Angelman syndrome," *Journal of Medical Genetics*, vol. 29, no. 6, pp. 412–415, 1992.

[4] S. Steffenburg, C. L. Gillberg, U. Steffenburg, and M. Kyllerman, "Autism in Angelman syndrome: a population-based study," *Pediatric Neurology*, vol. 14, no. 2, pp. 131–136, 1996.

[5] C. A. Williams, A. L. Beaudet, J. Clayton-Smith et al., "Angelman syndrome 2005: updated consensus for diagnostic criteria," *American Journal of Medical Genetics Part A*, vol. 140, no. 5, pp. 413–418, 2006.

[6] C. A. Williams, A. Lossie, and D. Driscoll, "Angelman syndrome: mimicking conditions and phenotypes," *American Journal of Medical Genetics*, vol. 101, no. 1, pp. 59–64, 2001.

[7] C. A. Williams, "Looks like Angelman syndrome but isn't—what is in the differential?" *R.C.P.U. Newsletter*, vol. 22, no. 1, pp. 1–5, 2011.

[8] W.-H. Tan, L. M. Bird, R. L. Thibert, and C. A. Williams, "If not Angelman, what is it? A review of Angelman-like syndromes," *American Journal of Medical Genetics Part A*, vol. 164, no. 4, pp. 975–992, 2014.

[9] F. Ariani, G. Hayek, D. Rondinella et al., "*FOXG1* is responsible for the congenital variant of Rett syndrome," *The American Journal of Human Genetics*, vol. 83, no. 1, pp. 89–93, 2008.

[10] F. Kortüm, S. Das, M. Flindt et al., "The core *FOXG1* syndrome phenotype consists of postnatal microcephaly, severe mental retardation, absent language, dyskinesia, and corpus callosum hypogenesis," *Journal of Medical Genetics*, vol. 48, no. 6, pp. 396–406, 2011.

[11] C. Philippe, D. Amsallem, C. Francannet et al., "Phenotypic variability in Rett syndrome associated with *FOXG1* mutations in females," *Journal of Medical Genetics*, vol. 47, no. 1, pp. 59–65, 2010.

[12] J. L. Neul, W. E. Kaufmann, D. G. Glaze et al., "Rett syndrome: revised diagnostic criteria and nomenclature," *Annals of Neurology*, vol. 68, no. 6, pp. 944–950, 2010.

[13] E. E. J. Smeets, K. Pelc, and B. Dan, "Rett syndrome," *Molecular Syndromology*, vol. 2, no. 3–5, pp. 113–127, 2012.

[14] C. Zweier, C. T. Thiel, A. Dufke et al., "Clinical and mutational spectrum of Mowat-Wilson syndrome," *European Journal of Medical Genetics*, vol. 48, no. 2, pp. 97–111, 2005.

[15] L. Garavelli, M. Zollino, P. C. Mainardi et al., "Mowat-Wilson syndrome: facial phenotype changing with age: study of 19

Italian patients and review of the literature," *American Journal of Medical Genetics Part A*, vol. 149, no. 3, pp. 417–426, 2009.

[16] K. S. Precht, C. M. Lese, R. P. Spiro et al., "Two 22q telomere deletions serendipitously detected by FISH," *Journal of Medical Genetics*, vol. 35, no. 11, pp. 939–942, 1998.

[17] K. Phelan and H. E. McDermid, "The 22q13.3 deletion syndrome (Phelan-McDermid syndrome)," *Molecular Syndromology*, vol. 2, no. 3–5, pp. 186–201, 2012.

[18] S. U. Dhar, D. del Gaudio, J. R. German et al., "22q13.3 deletion syndrome: clinical and molecular analysis using array CGH," *American Journal of Medical Genetics Part A*, vol. 152, no. 3, pp. 573–581, 2010.

48

Clinical Report of a 17q12 Microdeletion with Additionally Unreported Clinical Features

Jennifer L. Roberts,[1] Stephanie K. Gandomi,[2] Melissa Parra,[2] Ira Lu,[2] Chia-Ling Gau,[2] Majed Dasouki,[1,3] and Merlin G. Butler[1]

[1] *The University of Kansas Medical Center, Kansas City, KS 66160, USA*
[2] *Ambry Genetics, Aliso Viejo, CA 92656, USA*
[3] *King Faisal Specialist Hospital and Research Center, Riyadh 12713, Saudi Arabia*

Correspondence should be addressed to Stephanie K. Gandomi; sgandomi@ambrygen.com

Academic Editor: Philip D. Cotter

Copy number variations involving the 17q12 region have been associated with developmental and speech delay, autism, aggression, self-injury, biting and hitting, oppositional defiance, inappropriate language, and auditory hallucinations. We present a tall-appearing 17-year-old boy with marfanoid habitus, hypermobile joints, mild scoliosis, pectus deformity, widely spaced nipples, pes cavus, autism spectrum disorder, intellectual disability, and psychiatric manifestations including physical and verbal aggression, obsessive-compulsive behaviors, and oppositional defiance. An echocardiogram showed borderline increased aortic root size. An abdominal ultrasound revealed a small pancreas, mild splenomegaly with a 1.3 cm accessory splenule, and normal kidneys and liver. A testing panel for Marfan, aneurysm, and related disorders was negative. Subsequently, a 400 K array-based comparative genomic hybridization (aCGH) + SNP analysis was performed which identified a *de novo* suspected pathogenic deletion on chromosome 17q12 encompassing 28 genes. Despite the limited number of cases described in the literature with 17q12 rearrangements, our proband's phenotypic features both overlap and expand on previously reported cases. Since syndrome-specific DNA sequencing studies failed to provide an explanation for this patient's unusual habitus, we postulate that this case represents an expansion of the 17q12 microdeletion phenotype. Further analysis of the deleted interval is recommended for new genotype-phenotype correlations.

1. Introduction

The 17q12 region contains copy number variations previously reported in association with a variety of clinical findings, most frequently renal cystic disease, maturity onset diabetes of the young type 5, pancreatic atrophy, Mullerian aplasia in females, and variable cognitive involvement [1–6]. Renal cystic disease is, perhaps, the most widely reported feature resulting from the 17q12 deletion, while cognitive impairment and autism spectrum disorder have recently been associated with this deletion [2].

Moreno-De-Luca et al. [6] propose that the 17q12 deletion is among the ten most common deletions identified by microarray analysis in children with neurodevelopmental impairments. Of 15,749 patients referred for developmental delay or autism spectrum disorder in their study, 18 patients (0.11%) were found to have a 17q12 deletion. Of these 18 patients, 9 were found to have in common a 1.4 Mb deletion [34,819,670–36,203,752 bp (hg19)]. Autism spectrum disorder was found in all six male patients studied. Other common features of these patients with 17q12 deletions included macrocephaly, mild facial dysmorphism, genitourinary tract abnormalities, renal cysts, and recurrent infections of the ear, upper respiratory system, and urinary tract.

Herein, we report a patient with the 17q12 deletion using chromosomal microarray analysis presenting with autism spectrum disorder, behavioral difficulties, cognitive impairment, and joint laxity with a remarkable marfanoid body habitus, not previously described in reported cases of pathogenic copy number variations in this chromosomal region.

2. Subjects and Methods

2.1. Proband Clinical History. The proband was a 17-year-old Caucasian male. His mother and father were 40 years old, and his mother was gravida 3, para 0 at the time of conception. The 32-week gestation was complicated by preeclampsia and maternal uterine fibroids with delivery by Cesarean section. At birth, the proband weighed 2 pounds 8 ounces (1.134 kg) (3rd centile) and measured 17.5 inches (44.45 cm) (70th centile) in length [7]. He had an 8-week NICU stay with no reported respiratory difficulties. He was released home on an apnea monitor for 8 weeks with no reported apnea spells. Our proband was nonverbal until the age of 4 years. He had significant delays in gross and fine motor and social skills. He was diagnosed with autism spectrum disorder at the age of 10 years, and neuropsychological evaluation revealed a full scale IQ of 66 using the Wechsler Intelligence Scale for Children—IV. He was found to have a limited attention span but with no history of seizures and a normal electroencephalogram at the age of 15 years. A brain CT scan at the age of 15 years was normal with focal ossification noted along the dura of the left superior sagittal sinus. Attention deficit hyperactivity disorder, obsessive compulsive disorder, and autism spectrum disorder were diagnosed by a psychiatrist. Behavioral problems included irritability, physical aggression, impulsivity, and tantrums particularly when routines were disrupted. He had decreased sensitivity to pain and normal hearing and vision. Due to marfanoid body habitus, the proband received yearly echocardiograms, and early evidence of aortic root enlargement was found. CPK and homocysteine levels were performed and were normal (49 u/L and 7.3 uM, resp.). Previous surgeries included the removal of a dermoid cyst from the bridge of his nose at the age of 2 years and a partial right medial meniscectomy following a meniscus tear. The proband had a history of mildly elevated glucose levels from the age of 12 to 17 years but insulin and hemoglobin A1C levels remained within normal limits. An abdominal ultrasound was performed, and a small but otherwise normal pancreas with mild splenomegaly and a 1.3 cm accessory splenule were found. No renal abnormalities were reported.

On physical exam at the age of 17 years, the proband had a height of 184 cm (89th centile), a weight of 60.4 kg (34th centile), and a head circumference of 57 cm (75th centile). He had a long- and narrow-appearing face, bilateral ptosis, relative hypertelorism, small chin, and a high, narrow palate (Figure 1). The nipples appeared widely spaced, and mild pectus deformity was observed (Figure 2). The arm span was equal to height, and no arachnodactyly was present although it had been reported in previous genetics evaluations at earlier ages. The proband had pes cavus, hypermobile small joints, and mild scoliosis.

Previous genetic testing included blood chromosome analysis which was normal (46, XY) and Marfan, aneurysm, and related disorders DNA panel, performed at Ambry Genetics (Aliso Viejo, CA), was normal. This panel included next generation sequencing of the following genes: *ACTA2, CBS, FBN1, FBN2, MYH11, COL3A1, SLC2A10, SMAD3, TGFBR1,* and *TGFBR2.*

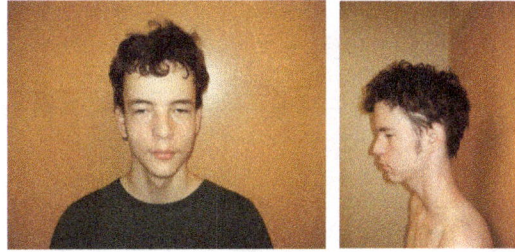

FIGURE 1: The proband presented with dysmorphic facial features, ptosis, long and narrow face, small chin, long philtrum, and high narrow palate.

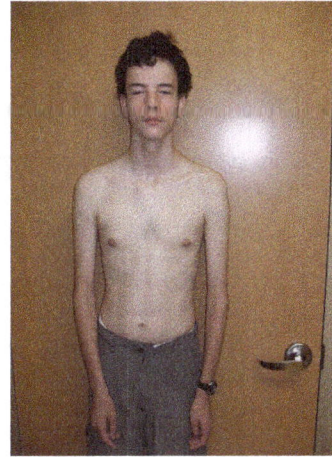

FIGURE 2: The proband presented with tall stature (90th percentile), low weight (10–25th percentile), marfanoid habitus, long fingers, hypermobile joints, mild scoliosis, and pectus deformity.

2.2. Informed Consent and Sample Collection. Informed consent to perform 400 K CGH + SNP analysis was obtained from the parent as the patient was a minor. As part of the informed consent process, the diagnostic testing process was explained to the proband and his parents and questions were appropriately answered. Informed consent to perform parental FISH studies was also obtained from each parent of the proband.

2.3. Methodology. A blood sample was collected from the proband and sent to Ambry Genetics (Aliso Viejo, CA) for 400 K CGH + SNP analysis (Agilent Technologies, Santa Clara, CA). Genomic deoxyribonucleic acid (gDNA) was isolated from the patient's specimen using a standardized Qiagen Midi kit (Valencia, CA) and quantified by agarose gel electrophoresis. The aCGH method is based on the hybridization of fluorescently labeled patient gDNA (Cy-5) with fluorescently labeled reference DNA (Cy-3) to a 400 K oligonucleotide array (Agilent Technologies, Santa Clara, CA). Patient genomic DNA relative to the reference DNA was represented as fluorescent ratios (Cy5/Cy3), further quantified by image analysis software, and interpreted with analytical software known as BioDiscovery Nexus. Quantified results indicate each targeted-DNA sequence as

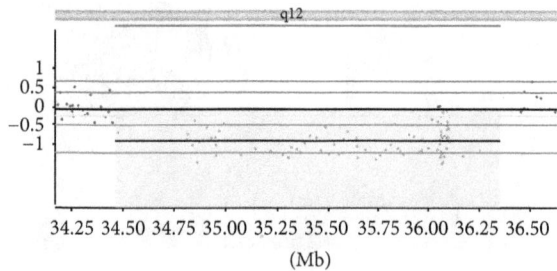

FIGURE 3: 400 K CGH + SNP array result: 17q12 (34,464,879–36,352,140) × 1. 17q12 region genes: *AATF, ACACA, C17orf78, CCL3L1, CCL3L3, CCL4L1, CCL4L2, DDX52, DHRS11, DUSP14, GGNBP2, HNF1B, LHX1, LOC284100, LOC440434, MIR2909, MIRM1, MYO19, PIGW, SYNRG, TADA2A, TBC1D3, TBC1D3B, TBC1D3C, TBC1D3F, TBC1D3G, TBC1D3H,* and *ZNHIT3.*

loss of copy number (deletion), as gain of copy number (duplication), or as a normal copy number. Regions of homozygosity/uniparental disomy (ROH/UPD) were also analyzed.

The Ambry CMA 400 K CGH + SNP array contains 400,000 probes (~300,000 CGH probes and ~100,000 SNP probes) and covers more than 400 known genetic disorders. The array includes probes for pericentromeric and subtelomeric regions with dense probe coverage spanning 10 Mb at each subtelomere. The backbone spacing of the probes is set at an average of 13 Kb throughout the entire human genome and at 5 Kb on the X chromosome.

3. Results

Results of this patient's 400 K CGH + SNP analysis identified two copy number variations of interest. The first CNV identified was a loss on 1q44 (GRCh 37/hg19: 247,185,060–247,314,022 bp) encompassing 5 genes, *C1orf229, ZNF124, ZNF669, ZNF670,* and *ZNF670–ZNF695.* A review of the literature determined that deletions in this region had not been previously described and none of the genes in this interval were known to be associated with intellectual impairment or congenital abnormalities. Therefore, its clinical significance was unknown. Subsequently, parental FISH analysis revealed that this CNV was paternal in origin, and since the proband's father was clinically unaffected, it is likely benign. The second identified CNV was a loss at 17q12 (GRCh 37/hg19: 34,464,879–36,352,140 bp) which spanned a minimum size of 1.770 Mb and a maximum size of 2.005 Mb (Figure 3). Parental FISH analysis revealed that this deletion was *de novo.* It encompassed 28 genes, including *CCL3L3, DDX52, HNF1B, LHX1, TBC1D3G,* and *ZNHIT3.* Of these genes, deletion or mutation of *HNF1B* has been associated with renal cystic disease, diabetes mellitus, and liver, pancreas, and female genital tract abnormalities [2]. *LHX1* is a candidate gene for the neurocognitive phenotype found in 17q12 deletion and is also expressed in the developing kidneys [1]. Other genes which may impact the phenotype of the proband include the following: *AATF* which is involved in regulation of gene

transcription and cell proliferation [8], *PIGW* a complex glycolipid that anchors proteins to the cell surface [9], *TADA2A* a transcriptional adaptor [10], and *CCL3L1, CCL3L3,* and *CCL4L2* which are chemokines involved in inflammatory and immunoregulatory processes [11]. Chemokines are expressed in the developing brain and increased levels of chemokines in the brain, cerebral spinal fluid, and plasma have been associated with autism spectrum disorder [12]. No regions of homozygosity (loss of heterozygosity) were identified in this proband's microarray results, confirming nonconsanguineous parents.

4. Discussion

Several reports support the association of cognitive impairment with 17q12 deletion. In a study of 4 patients with 17q12 deletion, Nagamani et al. [5] found 3 of 4 affected individuals with developmental problems ranging from speech delay to moderate or severe intellectual disability. All patients had growth failure, and 3 of 4 patients had cystic renal disease. In addition, Dixit et al. [2] reported three patients with developmental delay of varying severity and a 17q12 deletion. These patients included a 12-year-old female with a *de novo* 1.73 Mb deletion [34,569,770–36,248,889 bp (hg 19)] detected on chromosomal microarray analysis who had speech delay and dyspraxia, mild learning difficulties, and autism spectrum disorder, a 4-year-old male with a 2.07 Mb deletion [34,611,377–36,455,391 bp (hg 19)] who had speech delay, mild hypotonia, coronal hypospadias, and dysmorphic features including telecanthus, blepharophimosis, ptosis, epicanthus inversus, anteverted nares, depressed nasal bridge, long philtrum, and small ears with overfolding of the helices, and a 7-month-old male with a 1.6 Mb maternally inherited deletion [34,611,377–36,248,889 bp (hg 19)] with a head lag and inability to sit independently. All patients had renal cysts and hypercalcemia during the neonatal period [2].

Loirat et al. [4] studied 53 patients with cystic or hyperechogenic kidneys and the 17q12 deletion was found in 3 subjects (5.6%). These three children were males with autism between the ages of 3 and 9 years with *de novo* deletions ranging from 1.49 to 1.85 Mb in size, including *HNF1B* and 19 other genes. They had early onset developmental delay, social interaction difficulties, restricted and repetitive behaviors, and communication delays. All were diagnosed with renal cysts [4].

Variable features have been reported among family members with the same 17q12 deletion. George et al. [1] reported a family in which the proband was a 7-year-old female with a 1.4 Mb deletion of the 17q12 band [34,848,922–36,249,431 bp (hg19)] including the *HNF1B* and *LHX1* genes. The proband had attention deficit hyperactivity, disruptive behavior, and learning difficulty with no renal abnormalities, while her brother was found to have the same 17q12 deletion but only mild developmental delay and bilateral renal cysts. Their mother had the same deletion with learning difficulty but no renal cysts [1].

While some reports have found an association between growth retardation and 17q12 deletion, no previous reports

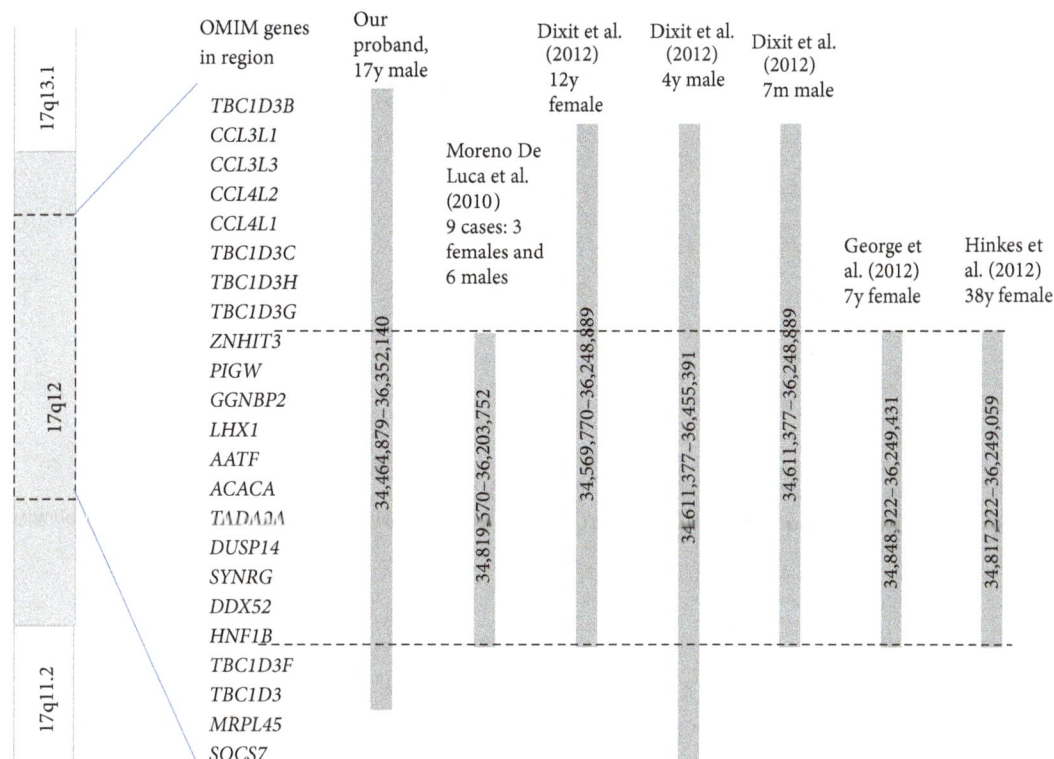

FIGURE 4: Comparison of deleted regions of 17q12. Dashed lines show the genes involved in the 17q11.2 deletion which are shared by all 7 cases. All genomic coordinates were converted to GRCh37/hg19 for comparison.

included tall stature or marfanoid body habitus. Hinkes et al. [3], however, reported a 38-year-old female with a 1.43 MB deletion at 17q12 [34,817,222–36,249,059 bp (hg19)] with features representing a connective tissue disorder including joint laxity, hypermobility of elbows, knees, and hips, and vascular hyperelasticity. This patient had no cognitive impairments but did have impaired renal function and uterine aplasia.

4.1. Implications for Clinical Practice: Expansion of the Phenotype. The HNF1B gene has been frequently reported in association with maturity onset diabetes of the young type 5 (MODY5), cystic renal disease, renal dilations, pancreatic atrophy, and liver abnormalities also seen in this deletion syndrome. Other case reports of individuals with deletions and duplications at the 17q12 critical region have included the involvement of a critical region including the AATF, ACACA, CCL3L, C17orf78, DDX52, DUSP14, DHRS11, GGNBP2, HNF1B, LHX1, LOC284100, TBC1D3G, MRM1, MYO19, PIGW, SYNRG, TADA2A, and ZNHIT3 genes [1–6] (Figure 4). Associated clinical features are developmental and speech delay, significant behavioral abnormalities including aggression, self-injury, oppositional defiance, biting, hitting, and inappropriate language, and auditory hallucinations possibly indicating their role in clinical presentation [1–6] (Table 1).

Recently, Palumbo et al. [13] described a boy with a 17q12 deletion involving the CCL4L2, TBC1D3H, TBC1D3G, ZNHIT3, MYO19, PIGW, DHRS11, MRM, LHX1, AATF,

ACACA, TADA2A, DUSP14, SYNRG, and HNF1B genes presenting with repetitive and compulsive-like behaviors, attention-deficit hyperactivity disorder, intellectual disability, language disabilities, and dysmorphic features including right posterior plagiocephaly, facial asymmetry, narrow forehead, hypotelorism, wide and fleshy auricular pavilions, protruding cheekbones, long philtrum, thin upper lip, tuft of hair on the neck, and clinodactyly of the fifth fingers [13].

The only gene contained within our proband's deletion but not within the other deletions reported in the literature prior to the recent Palumbo et al. case [13] was TBC1D3B. Other members of the TBC1 domain family including TBC1D3C, TBC1D3F, TBC1D3G, and TBC1D3H are included in our proband's deletion and in deletions described in other case reports [2, 3]. The TBC1D3 family of oncogenes has been previously shown to enhance cellular response to epidermal growth factor [14]. Deletions of TBC1D3B have not been previously reported in the literature, and members of the TBC1 domain family are not expected to be dosage sensitive [5].

In summary, deletions of 17q12 have been reported in fewer than 100 individuals, and to our knowledge none have manifested a distinctly marfanoid habitus. We propose that our proband's unique phenotype is an expansion of the described 17q12 clinical spectrum. In support of this conclusion, it is very likely that poorly understood genes involved in our proband's deletion (such as AATF, CCL3L, C17orf78, DDX52, DHRS11, GGNBP2, LHX1, LOC284100, TBC1D3G, MRM1, MYO19, SYNRG, TADA2A, and ZNHIT3)

TABLE 1: Clinical phenotype in our proband and previously reported patients with 17q12 deletion.

	Our proband	Moreno-De-Luca et al. (2010) [6]	Nagamani et al. (2010) [5]	Dixit et al. (2012) [2]	Hinkes et al. (2012) [3]	George et al. (2012) [1]	Loirat et al. (2010) [4]
Clinical findings							
Mild facial dysmorphism	+	9/9	2/9	2/3	NR	NR	NR
Ptosis	+	NR	NR	1/3	NR	NR	NR
Long philtrum	+	NR	NR	2/3	NR	NR	NR
Long, narrow face	+	NR	NR	0/3	NR	NR	NR
Pectus deformity	+	NR	NR	0/3	NR	NR	NR
Joint laxity	+	NR	NR	0/3	+	NR	NR
Marfanoid body habitus	+	0/9	0/9	0/3	NR	0/2	0/3
Short stature or failure to thrive	−	1/9	3/9	1/3	NR	0/2	0/3
Kidney cysts/anomalies	−	Most*	4/9	3/3	+	1/2	3/3
Small pancreas	+	NR	NR	0/3	NR	NR	0/3
Splenomegaly	+	NR	NR	0/3	NR	NR	NR
Behavioral and cognitive features							
Autism spectrum disorder (ASD)	+	6/9	0/9	1/3	−	0/2	3/3
Developmental delay or intellectual disability	+	8/9	8/9	3/3	−	2/2	3/3
Seizures	−	0/9	2/9	0/3	−	NR	NR
Aggression	+	2/9	2/9	NR	−	NR	NR
Anxiety/disruptive behavior	+	5/9	NR	NR	−	1/2	NR
Hyperactivity	+	2/9	NR	NR	−	1/2	NR
Laboratory testing							
Neonatal hypercalcemia	NR	NR	NR	3/3	NR	NR	NR
Diabetes mellitus	−	1/9	NR	0/3	+	0/2	NR

+: feature is present, −: feature is absent, NR: not reported.
*Most of the 9 patients had kidney cystic anomalies but no specific number is given.

may be responsible for these manifestations. Nevertheless, we also cannot rule out additional genetic phenomena such as variable expressivity, penetrance, and digenic inheritance due to the mutation of a second gene. Although clinical suspicion for the patient's microdeletion is responsible for his clinical presentation, further gene sequencing in this case, such as with whole clinical exome sequencing, is still warranted to rule out any additional contributing genetic factors. The authors encourage the reporting of other patients with this chromosome abnormality using microarray analysis to further delineate the genetic and clinical characteristics of pathogenic copy number alterations in this region.

Disclosure

Authors associated with Ambry Genetics are full-time employees of the commercial laboratory. Ambry Genetics has full control of the laboratory data associated with the aCGH testing process and agrees to allow the journal to review the data if requested.

Conflict of Interests

Authors associated with the University of Kansas Medical Center declare that there is no conflict of interest regarding the publication of this paper.

Acknowledgment

The authors are grateful to the patient and his family for their participation.

References

[1] A. M. George, D. R. Love, I. Hayes, and B. Tsang, "Recurrent transmission of a 17q12 microdeletion and a variable clinical spectrum," *Molecular Syndromology*, vol. 2, no. 2, pp. 72–75, 2012.

[2] A. Dixit, C. Patel, R. Harrison et al., "17q12 microdeletion syndrome: three patients illustrating the phenotypic spectrum," *The American Journal of Medical Genetics A*, vol. 158, no. 9, pp. 2317–2321, 2012.

[3] B. Hinkes, K. F. Hilgers, H. J. Bolz et al., "A complex microdeletion 17q12 phenotype in a patient with recurrent *de novo* membranous nephropathy," *BMC Nephrology*, vol. 13, no. 1, article 27, 2012.

[4] C. Loirat, C. Bellanné-Chantelot, I. Husson, G. Deschênes, V. Guigonis, and N. Chabane, "Autism in three patients with cystic or hyperechogenic kidneys and chromosome 17q12 deletion," *Nephrology Dialysis Transplantation*, vol. 25, no. 10, pp. 3430–3433, 2010.

[5] S. C. S. Nagamani, A. Erez, J. Shen et al., "Clinical spectrum associated with recurrent genomic rearrangements in chromosome 17q12," *European Journal of Human Genetics*, vol. 18, no. 3, pp. 278–284, 2010.

[6] D. Moreno-De-Luca, J. G. Mulle, E. B. Kaminsky et al., "Deletion 17q12 is a recurrent copy number variant that confers high risk of autism and schizophrenia," *The American Journal of Human Genetics*, vol. 87, no. 1, pp. 618–630, 2010.

[7] T. R. Fenton, "A new growth chart for preterm babies: babson and Benda's chart updated with recent data and a new format," *BMC Pediatrics*, vol. 3, article 13, 2003.

[8] World Wide Web, *Online Mendelian Inheritance in Man*, OMIM, Johns Hopkins University, Baltimore, Md, USA, 2013, http://omim.org/.

[9] Y. Murakami, U. Siripanyapinyo, Y. Hong et al., "PIG-W is critical for inositol acylation but not for flipping of glycosylphosphatidylinositol-anchor," *Molecular Biology of the Cell*, vol. 14, no. 10, pp. 4285–4295, 2003.

[10] K. C. Carter, L. Wang, B. K. Shell, I. Zamir, S. L. Berger, and P. A. Moore, "The human transcriptional adaptor genes TADA2L and GCN5L2 colocalize to chromosome 17q12-q21 and display a similar tissue expression pattern," *Genomics*, vol. 40, no. 3, pp. 497–500, 1997.

[11] K. Naruse, M. Ueno, T. Satoh et al., "A YAC contig of the human CC chemokine genes clustered on chromosome 17q11.2," *Genomics*, vol. 34, no. 2, pp. 236–240, 1996.

[12] P. Ashwood, P. Krakowiak, I. Hertz-Picciotto, R. Hansen, I. N. Pessah, and J. van de Water, "Associations of impaired behaviors with elevated plasma chemokines in autism spectrum disorders," *Journal of Neuroimmunology*, vol. 232, no. 1-2, pp. 196–199, 2011.

[13] P. Palumbo, V. Antona, O. Palumbo et al., "Variable phenotype in 17q12 microdeletions: clinical and molecular characterization of a new case," *Gene*, vol. 538, pp. 373–378, 2014.

[14] P. D. Stahl and M. J. Wainszelbaum, "Human-specific genes may offer a unique window into human cell signaling," *Science Signaling*, vol. 2, no. 89, 2009.

Permissions

All chapters in this book were first published in CRIG, by Hindawi Publishing Corporation; hereby published with permission under the Creative Commons Attribution License or equivalent. Every chapter published in this book has been scrutinized by our experts. Their significance has been extensively debated. The topics covered herein carry significant findings which will fuel the growth of the discipline. They may even be implemented as practical applications or may be referred to as a beginning point for another development.

The contributors of this book come from diverse backgrounds, making this book a truly international effort. This book will bring forth new frontiers with its revolutionizing research information and detailed analysis of the nascent developments around the world.

We would like to thank all the contributing authors for lending their expertise to make the book truly unique. They have played a crucial role in the development of this book. Without their invaluable contributions this book wouldn't have been possible. They have made vital efforts to compile up to date information on the varied aspects of this subject to make this book a valuable addition to the collection of many professionals and students.

This book was conceptualized with the vision of imparting up-to-date information and advanced data in this field. To ensure the same, a matchless editorial board was set up. Every individual on the board went through rigorous rounds of assessment to prove their worth. After which they invested a large part of their time researching and compiling the most relevant data for our readers.

The editorial board has been involved in producing this book since its inception. They have spent rigorous hours researching and exploring the diverse topics which have resulted in the successful publishing of this book. They have passed on their knowledge of decades through this book. To expedite this challenging task, the publisher supported the team at every step. A small team of assistant editors was also appointed to further simplify the editing procedure and attain best results for the readers.

Apart from the editorial board, the designing team has also invested a significant amount of their time in understanding the subject and creating the most relevant covers. They scrutinized every image to scout for the most suitable representation of the subject and create an appropriate cover for the book.

The publishing team has been an ardent support to the editorial, designing and production team. Their endless efforts to recruit the best for this project, has resulted in the accomplishment of this book. They are a veteran in the field of academics and their pool of knowledge is as vast as their experience in printing. Their expertise and guidance has proved useful at every step. Their uncompromising quality standards have made this book an exceptional effort. Their encouragement from time to time has been an inspiration for everyone.

The publisher and the editorial board hope that this book will prove to be a valuable piece of knowledge for researchers, students, practitioners and scholars across the globe.

List of Contributors

Kristen Dilzell
Department of Medical Genetics, University of Pennsylvania, Philadelphia, PA 19104, USA

Diana Darcy and Robert Wallerstein
Silicon Valley Genetics Center, Santa Clara Valley Medical Center, San Jose, CA 95128, USA

John Sum
Pediatric Neurology, Santa Clara Valley Medical Center, San Jose, CA 95128, USA

Veronica Goitia and Marcial Oquendo
Department of Pediatrics, Driscoll Children's Hospital, Corpus Christi, TX 78411, USA

Robert Stratton
Department of Medical Genetics, Driscoll Children's Hospital, Corpus Christi, TX 78411, USA

Tetsuya Kawahara
Division of Endocrinology and Metabolism, Department of Internal Medicine, Niigata Rosai Hospital, Niigata 9428502, Japan

Hiromi Watanabe
Department of Clinical Laboratory, Niigata National Hospital, Niigata 9458585, Japan

Risa Omae
Department of Pharmacy, College of Pharmaceutical Sciences, Ritsumeikan University, Shiga 5258577, Japan

Toshiyuki Yamamoto
Tokyo Women's Medical University, Institute of Integrated Medical Sciences, Tokyo 1620054, Japan

Tetsuya Inazu
Department of Pharmacy, College of Pharmaceutical Sciences, Ritsumeikan University, Shiga 5258577, Japan
Department of Clinical Research, Saigata National Hospital, Niigata 9493193, Japan

Adrian Mc Cormack, Alice M. George and Donald R. Love
Diagnostic Genetics, LabPLUS, Auckland City Hospital, P.O. Box 110031, Auckland 1148, New Zealand

Cynthia Sharpe
Department of Neuroservices, Starship Children's Health, Private Bag 92024, Auckland 1142, New Zealand

Nerine Gregersen and Ian Hayes
Genetic Health Service New Zealand-Northern Hub, Auckland City Hospital, Private Bag 92024, Auckland 1142, New Zealand

Warwick Smith
Middlemore Hospital, Private Bag 93311, Otahuhu, Auckland 1640, New Zealand

Carolina Sismani, Angelos Alexandrou and Paola Evangelidou
Department of Cytogenetics and Genomics, The Cyprus Institute of Neurology and Genetics, 6 International Airport Avenue, Ayios Dometios, 2370 Nicosia, Cyprus

Georgia Christopoulou, Jacqueline Donoghue and Voula Velissariou
Department of Genetics and Molecular Biology, General, Maternity, and Pediatric Clinic Mitera, Erythrou Stavrou 6, 15123 Athens, Greece

Anastasia E. Konstantinidou
Department of Pathology, Medical School, University of Athens, Mikras Assias 75, 11527 Athens, Greece

Marina Laplana, José Luis Royo and Joan Fibla
Human Genetic Unit, Department of Basic Medical Sciences, University of Lleida, 25198 Lleida, Catalonia, Spain
Genetics of Complex Diseases Research Group, Biomedical Research Institute of Lleida (IRBLleida), 25198 Lleida, Catalonia, Spain

Anton Aluja
Biological-Factorial Models of Personality, Department of Psychology, University of Lleida, 25001 Lleida, Catalonia, Spain

Ricard López
Human Genetic Unit, Department of Basic Medical Sciences, University of Lleida, 25198 Lleida, Catalonia, Spain
Clinical Analysis Service, Universitari Arnau de Vilanova University Hospital, 25198 Lleida, Catalonia, Spain

Damiàn Heine-Sunyer
Department of Genetics, Son Espases University Hospital, 07120 Palma de Mallorca, Spain

Patrick Lin
Department of Pediatrics, Nemours/Alfred I. duPont
Hospital for Children, Wilmington, DE 19803, USA
Thomas Jefferson University, Philadelphia, PA 19107,
USA

Sheela Raikar, Jennifer Jimenez and Katryn N. Furuya
Department of Pediatrics, Nemours/Alfred I. duPont
Hospital for Children, Wilmington, DE 19803, USA
Thomas Jefferson University, Philadelphia, PA 19107,
USA
Division of Pediatric Gastroenterology, Hepatology,
and Nutrition, Nemours/Alfred I. duPont Hospital for
Children, Wilmington, DE 19803, USA

Katrina Conard
Department of Clinical and Anatomic Pathology,
Nemours/Alfred I. duPont Hospital for Children,
Wilmington, DE 19803, USA

**Hannie Kartapradja, Nanis Sacharina Marzuki, Lita
Putri Suciati, Helena Woro Anggaratri, Debby Dwi
Ambarwati, Firman Prathama Idris, Harry Lesmana,
Chrysantine Paramayuda and Alida Roswita Harahap**
Eijkman Institute for Molecular Biology, Jl. Diponegoro
69, Jakarta 10430, Indonesia

Mark D. Pertile and David Francis
Victorian Clinical Genetics Services (VCGS), Royal
Children's Hospital, Flemington Road, Melbourne, VIC
3052, Australia

Hidayat Trimarsanto
Eijkman Institute for Molecular Biology, Jl. Diponegoro
69, Jakarta 10430, Indonesia
Agency for the Assessment and Application of Technology,
Jl. MH Thamrin 8, Jakarta 10340, Indonesia

Maria Valencia
Instituto de Investigaciones Biomédicas, Consejo Superior
de Científicas, Universidad Autónoma de Madrid,
Madrid, Spain

Lara Tabet, Khalil Charaffedine and Rebecca Badra
Department of Pathology and Laboratory Medicine,
American University of Beirut Medical Center, P.O. Box
11-0236 Riad El Solh, Beirut 1107 2020, Lebanon

Chantal Farra
Department of Pathology and Laboratory Medicine,
American University of Beirut Medical Center, P.O. Box
11-0236 Riad El Solh, Beirut 1107 2020, Lebanon
Department of Pediatrics and Adolescent Medicine,
American University of Beirut Medical Center, P.O. Box
11-0236 Riad El Solh, Beirut 1107 2020, Lebanon

Nadine Yazbeck, Alia Araj and Farah Fares
Department of Pediatrics and Adolescent Medicine,
American University of Beirut Medical Center, P.O. Box
11-0236 Riad El Solh, Beirut 1107 2020, Lebanon

Victor L. Ruiz-Perez
Instituto de Investigaciones Biomédicas, Consejo Superior
de Científicas, Universidad Autónoma de Madrid,
Madrid, Spain
Centro de Investigación Biomédica en Red de
Enfermedades Raras (CIBERER), Instituto de Salud
Carlos III (ISCIII), Madrid, Spain

Javier Sánchez
Department of Genetics, Reproduction and Fetal
Medicine, Institute of Biomedicine of Seville (IBIS),
University Hospital Virgen del Rocío/CSIC/University
of Seville, 41013 Seville, Spain

Ana Peciña, Guillermo Antiñolo and Salud Borrego
Department of Genetics, Reproduction and Fetal
Medicine, Institute of Biomedicine of Seville (IBIS),
University Hospital Virgen del Rocío/CSIC/University
of Seville, 41013 Seville, Spain
Centre of Biomedical Network Research on Rare Diseases
(CIBERER), 41013 Seville, Spain

Olga Alonso-Luengo and Antonio González-Meneses
Department of Pediatrics, University Hospital Virgen del
Rocío, Avenida Manuel Siurot s/n, 41013 Seville, Spain

Rocío Vázquez
Department of Neurophysiology, University Hospital
Virgen del Rocío, Avenida Manuel Siurot s/n, 41013
Seville, Spain

**Leah Te Weehi, Adrian Mc Cormack, Roberto Mazzaschi,
Fern Ashton, Liangtao Zhang and Alice M. George**
Diagnostic Genetics, LabPLUS, Auckland City Hospital,
P.O. Box 110031, Auckland 1148, New Zealand

RajMaikoo
Pediatrics Department, Middlemore Hospital, Private
Bag 93311, Auckland 1640, New Zealand

Donald R. Love
Diagnostic Genetics, LabPLUS, Auckland City Hospital,
P.O. Box 110031, Auckland 1148, New Zealand
School of Biological Sciences, University of Auckland,
Private Bag 92019, Auckland 1142, New Zealand

Guillaume Jedraszak
Unité de Génétique Médicale et Oncogénétique, Centre
Hospitalier Universitaire Amiens-Picardie, 80054 Amiens
Cedex, France
Laboratoire de Cytogénétique et Biologie de la
Reproduction, CECOS de Picardie, Centre Hospitalier
Universitaire Amiens-Picardie, 80054 Amiens Cedex,
France

Aline Receveur and Henri Copin
Laboratoire de Cytogénétique et Biologie de la
Reproduction, CECOS de Picardie, Centre Hospitalier
Universitaire Amiens-Picardie, 80054 Amiens Cedex,
France

Joris Andrieux
Laboratoire de Génétique Médicale, Hôpital Jeanne de Flandre, Centre Hospitalier Régional Universitaire de Lille, 59037 Lille Cedex, France

Michèle Mathieu-Dramard and Gilles Morin
Unité de Génétique Médicale et Oncogénétique, Centre Hospitalier Universitaire Amiens-Picardie, 80054 Amiens Cedex, France

R. Hochstenbach, K. D. Lichtenbelt, J. J. T. van Harssel, T. Brouwer, P. van Zon, M. Elferink, K. Kusters, O. Akkermans, J. K. Ploos van Amstel and G. H. Schuring-Blom
Department of Medical Genetics, Division of Biomedical Genetics, University Medical Centre Utrecht, P.O. Box 85090, Mail Stop KC04.084.2, 3508 AB Utrecht, Netherlands

G. C. M. L. Page-Christiaens, A. C. C. van Oppen and G. T. R. Manten
Department of Obstetrics and Gynecology, University Medical Centre Utrecht, P.O. Box 85090, Mail Stop KE04.123.1, 3508 AB Utrecht, Netherlands

Jennifer Holter Chakrabarty and Mohamad Cherry
Hematology-Oncology Section, Department of Medicine, The University of Oklahoma Health Sciences Center, Oklahoma City, OK 73104, USA

Mohamad Khawandanah
Hematology-Oncology Section, Department of Medicine, The University of Oklahoma Health Sciences Center, Oklahoma City, OK 73104, USA
University of Oklahoma Health Sciences Center, Stephenson Cancer Center, 800 NE 10th Street, Oklahoma City, OK 73102, USA

Bradley Gehrs
Department of Pathology, The University of Oklahoma Health Sciences Center, Oklahoma City, OK 73104, USA

Shibo Li
Department of Pediatrics, The University of Oklahoma Health Sciences Center, Oklahoma City, OK 73104, USA

Marta Zegre Amorim
Genetics Department, Hospital Dona Estefânia, Centro Hospitalar de Lisboa Central, 1169-045 Lisbon, Portugal

Jayne A. L. Houghton
Royal Devon and Exeter Hospital, Exeter, Devon EX2 5DW, UK

Sara Carmo
Pediatric Surgery Department, Hospital Dona Estefânia, Centro Hospitalar de Lisboa Central, 1169-045 Lisbon, Portugal

Inês Salva, Ana Pita and Luis Pereira-da-Silva
NICU, Hospital Dona Estefânia, Centro Hospitalar de Lisboa Central, 1169-045 Lisbon, Portugal

Molly B. Sheridan, Carolyn Applegate and Julie Hoover-Fong
McKusick-Nathans Institute of Genetic Medicine, Johns Hopkins University School of Medicine, Baltimore, MD 21287, USA

Elizabeth Wohler
Cytogenomics Laboratory, Johns Hopkins Hospital, Baltimore, MD 21287, USA

Denise A. S. Batista
McKusick-Nathans Institute of Genetic Medicine, Johns Hopkins University School of Medicine, Baltimore, MD 21287, USA

Cytogenomics Laboratory, Johns Hopkins Hospital, Baltimore, MD 21287, USA
Department of Pathology, Johns Hopkins University School of Medicine, Baltimore, MD 21287, USA

Leema Reddy Peddareddygari
The Neuro-Genetics Institute, 501 Elmwood Avenue, Sharon Hill, PA 19079, USA

Raji P. Grewal
Neuroscience Institute, Saint Francis Medical Center, 601 Hamilton Avenue, Trenton, NJ 08629, USA

Gulden Diniz
Neuromuscular Diseases Centre, Tepecik Research Hospital, Kibris Sehitleri Caddesi 51/11, Alsancak, 35220 Izmir, Turkey

Hulya Tosun Yildirim
Pathology Department, Dr. Behcet Uz Children's Research Hospital, 35210 İzmir, Turkey

Sarenur Gokben and Gul Serdaroglu
Pediatric Neurology Department, Faculty of Medicine, Ege University, 35100 İzmir, Turkey

Filiz Hazan
Medical Genetics Department, Dr. Behcet Uz Children's Research Hospital, 35210 Izmir, Turkey

Kanay Yararbas
Medical Genetics Department, Duzen Laboratories, Istanbul, Turkey
Medical Genetics Department, Duzen Laboratories, Ankara, Turkey

Ajlan Tukun
Medical Genetics Department, Duzen Laboratories, Istanbul, Turkey
Medical Genetics Department, Duzen Laboratories, Ankara, Turkey
Medical Genetics Department, Faculty of Medicine, Ankara University, 06100 Ankara, Turkey

Mark Johnson, Craig Richard and Robert Kidd
Bernard J. Dunn School of Pharmacy, Shenandoah University, Winchester, VA 22601, USA

Renee Bogdan
Pinnacle Health, Harrisburg, PA 17109, USA

George A. Tanteles, Elpiniki Nikolaou and Violetta Christophidou-Anastasiadou
Clinical Genetics Department, The Cyprus Institute of Neurology and Genetics and Archbishop Makarios III Medical Centre, 2370 Nicosia, Cyprus

Yiolanda Christou and Savvas S. Papacostas
Clinical Sciences Neurology Clinic B, The Cyprus Institute of Neurology and Genetics, 2370 Nicosia, Cyprus

Angelos Alexandrou, Paola Evangelidou and Carolina Sismani
Cytogenetics and Genomics Department, The Cyprus Institute of Neurology and Genetics, 2370 Nicosia, Cyprus

Kristi K. Fitzgerald, Abdul Majeed Bhat and Christian Pizarro
Nemours Cardiac Center, Nemours/Alfred I. duPont Hospital for Children, 1600 Rockland Road, Wilmington, DE 19803, USA

Katrina Conard
Department of Pathology, Nemours/Alfred I. duPont Hospital for Children, Wilmington, DE 19803, USA
Anatomy and Cell Biology, Thomas Jefferson University Hospital, Philadelphia, PA 19107, USA

James Hyland
Connective Tissue Gene Tests, Allentown, PA 18106, USA

Rolph Pfundt, Nico Leijsten, Willy Nillesen and Nicole de Leeuw
Department of Human Genetics, Radboud University Medical Center, The Netherlands Division of Human Genetics, P.O. Box 9101, 6500 HB Nijmegen, The Netherlands

Almira Zada
Department of Human Genetics, Radboud University Medical Center, The Netherlands Division of
Human Genetics, P.O. Box 9101, 6500 HB Nijmegen, The Netherlands
Center for Biomedical Research (CEBIOR), Faculty of Medicine, Diponegoro University, GSG 2nd Floor, Jl. Dr. Sutomo 14, Semarang 50244, Indonesia

Farmaditya E. P. Mundhofir and Sultana M. H. Faradz
Center for Biomedical Research (CEBIOR), Faculty of Medicine, Diponegoro University, GSG 2nd Floor, Jl. Dr. Sutomo 14, Semarang 50244, Indonesia

Jessie C. Jacobsen, Brendan Swan, Russell G. Snell and Klaus Lehnert
Centre for Brain Research and School of Biological Sciences, The University of Auckland, Auckland 1010, New Zealand

Emma Glamuzina and Callum Wilson
Adult and Paediatric National Metabolic Service, Auckland City Hospital, Auckland 1142, New Zealand

Juliet Taylor
Genetic Health Service New Zealand, Auckland City Hospital, Auckland 1142, New Zealand

Shona Handisides
Department of Radiology, Auckland City Hospital, Auckland 1142, New Zealand

Michael Fietz
Department of Diagnostic Genomics, Path West, Nedlands, WA 6009, Australia
Department of Biochemical Genetics, SA Pathology, North Adelaide, SA 5006, Australia

Tessa van Dijk and Bart Appelhof
Department of Genome Analysis, Academic Medical Centre, 1105 Amsterdam, Netherlands

Rosamund Hill
Department of Neurology, Auckland City Hospital, Auckland 1142, New Zealand

Rosemary Marks
Developmental Paediatric Service, Starship Children's Health, Auckland 1142, New Zealand

Donald R. Love
Diagnostic Genetics, LabPLUS, Auckland City Hospital, Auckland 1142, New Zealand

Stephen P. Robertson
Dunedin School of Medicine, University of Otago, Dunedin 9016, New Zealand

Sara Domingues
Pediatrics Department, Centro Hospitalar do Tâmega e Sousa, EPE, Unidade Padre Américo 4564-007 Penafiel, Portugal

Lara Isidoro, Dalila Rocha and Jorge Sales Marques
Pediatrics Department, Centro Hospitalar de Vila Nova de Gaia/Espinho, EPE, Unidade II, 4400-129 Vila Nova de Gaia, Portugal

Adrian Mc Cormack, Leah Te Weehi and Alice M. George
Diagnostic Genetics, LabPlus, Auckland City Hospital, P.O. Box 110031, Auckland 1148, New Zealand

Juliet Taylor
Genetic Health Service New Zealand-Northern Hub, Auckland City Hospital, Private Bag 92024, Auckland 1142, New Zealand

Donald R. Love
Diagnostic Genetics, LabPlus, Auckland City Hospital, P.O. Box 110031, Auckland 1148, New Zealand
School of Biological Sciences, University of Auckland, Private Bag 92019, Auckland 1142, New Zealand

Holli M. Drendel, Jason E. Pike, Katherine Schumacher, Karen Ouyang, Mary Stuy, Stephen Dlouhy and Shaochun Bai
Division of Diagnostic Genomics, Department of Medical and Molecular Genetics, Indiana University School of Medicine, 975WestWalnut Street, Indianapolis, IN 46202, USA

Jing Wang
Department of Molecular and Human Genetics, Baylor College of Medicine, One Baylor Plaza, Houston, TX 77030, USA

François Tshilombo Katombe
Department of Surgery, University Hospital, University of Lubumbashi, P.O. Box 1825, Lubumbashi, Democratic Republic of Congo

Sébastien Mbuyi-Musanzayi
Department of Surgery, University Hospital, University of Lubumbashi, P.O. Box 1825, Lubumbashi, Democratic Republic of Congo
Center for Human Genetics, Faculty of Medicine, University of Lubumbashi, P.O. Box 1825, Lubumbashi, Democratic Republic of Congo

Koenraad Devriendt
Center for Human Genetics, University Hospitals, KU Leuven, UZ Leuven, Campus Gasthuisberg, Herestraat 49, P.O. Box 602, 3000 Leuven, Belgium

Aimé Lumaka and Prosper Lukusa Tshilobo
Center for Human Genetics, University Hospitals, KU Leuven, UZ Leuven, Campus Gasthuisberg, Herestraat 49, P.O. Box 602, 3000 Leuven, Belgium
Department of Pediatrics, University Hospitals, University of Kinshasa, P.O. Box 123, Kin XI, Kinshasa, Democratic Republic of Congo

Bienvenu Yogolelo Asani
Center for Human Genetics, Faculty of Medicine, University of Lubumbashi, P.O. Box 1825, Lubumbashi, Democratic Republic of Congo
Department of Ophthalmology, University Hospital, University of Lubumbashi, P.O. Box 1825, Lubumbashi, Democratic Republic of Congo

Toni Lubala Kasole
Center for Human Genetics, Faculty of Medicine, University of Lubumbashi, P.O. Box 1825, Lubumbashi, Democratic Republic of Congo
Department of Pediatrics, University Hospital, University of Lubumbashi, P.O. Box 1825, Lubumbashi, Democratic Republic of Congo

Prosper Kalenga Muenze
Center for Human Genetics, Faculty of Medicine, University of Lubumbashi, P.O. Box 1825, Lubumbashi, Democratic Republic of Congo
Department of Gynecology, University Hospital, University of Lubumbashi, P.O. Box 1825, Lubumbashi, Democratic Republic of Congo

Shirley Lo-A-Njoe, Clementien Vermont, Louise Rafael-Croes and Vincent Keizer
Department of Pediatrics, Horacio Oduber Hospital, Oranjestad, Aruba

Lars T. van der Veken, Ron Hochstenbach, Nine Knoers and Mieke M. van Haelst
Department of Genetics, Wilhelmina Children's Hospital, UMC Utrecht, 3584 EA Utrecht, Netherlands

Trent Burgess, Mark D. Pertile, David Francis, Melissa Glass and Sara Nouri
Victorian Clinical Genetics Services, Murdoch Childrens Research Institute, Royal Children's Hospital, Parkville 3052, Melbourne, Australia

Lilian Downie and Rosalynn Pszczola
Sunshine Hospital, Western Health, Sunshine 3020, Melbourne, Australia

Sefa Resim, NazımKankılıc and Erkan Efe
Department of Urology, Kahramanmaras Sutcu Imam University, Kahramanmaras, Turkey

Faruk Kucukdurmaz
Department of Urology, Nizip State Hospital, Gaziantep, Turkey

Ozlem Altunoren
Department of Psychiatry, Kahramanmaras State Hospital, Kahramanmaras, Turkey

Can Benlioglu
Department of Urology, Adiyaman University, Adiyaman, Turkey

Sébastien Mbuyi-Musanzayi
Department of Surgery, University Hospital, University of Lubumbashi, P.O. Box 1825, Lubumbashi, Democratic Republic of the Congo
Center for Human Genetics, Faculty of Medicine, University of Lubumbashi, P.O. Box 1825, Lubumbashi, Democratic Republic of the Congo

Toni Lubala Kasole
Center for Human Genetics, Faculty of Medicine, University of Lubumbashi, P.O. Box 1825, Lubumbashi, Democratic Republic of the Congo
Department of Pediatrics, University Hospital, University of Lubumbashi, P.O. Box 1825, Lubumbashi, Democratic Republic of the Congo

Aimé Lumaka and Prosper Lukusa Tshilobo
Department of Pediatrics, University Hospital, University of Kinshasa, P.O. Box 123, Kin XI, Kinshasa, Democratic Republic of the Congo
Center for Human Genetics, University Hospital, KU Leuven, Campus Gasthuisberg, Herestraat 49, P.O. Box 602, 3000 Leuven, Belgium

Tony Kayembe Kitenge, Leon Kabamba Ngombe and Célestin Banza Lubaba Nkulu
Unit of Toxicology and Environment, School of Public Health, University Hospital, University of Lubumbashi, P.O. Box 1825, Lubumbashi, Democratic Republic of the Congo

Prosper Kalenga Muenze
Center for Human Genetics, Faculty of Medicine, University of Lubumbashi, P.O. Box 1825, Lubumbashi, Democratic Republic of the Congo
Department of Gynecology, University Hospital, University of Lubumbashi, P.O. Box 1825, Lubumbashi, Democratic Republic of the Congo

François Tshilombo Katombe
Department of Surgery, University Hospital, University of Lubumbashi, P.O. Box 1825, Lubumbashi, Democratic Republic of the Congo

Koenraad Devriendt
Center for Human Genetics, University Hospital, KU Leuven, Campus Gasthuisberg, Herestraat 49, P.O. Box 602, 3000 Leuven, Belgium

Nivedita U. Jerath, Cameron D. Crockett, Michael E. Shy, Tiffany Grider and Andrea Swenson
Department of Neurology, Carver College of Medicine, University of Iowa, Iowa City, IA 52242, USA

Steven A. Moore
Department of Neurology, Carver College of Medicine, University of Iowa, Iowa City, IA 52242, USA
Department of Pathology, Carver College of Medicine, University of Iowa, Iowa City, IA 52242, USA

Conrad C. Weihl
Department of Neurology, Washington University School of Medicine, St. Louis, MO 63110, USA

Tsui-Fen Chou
Division of Medical Genetics, Department of Pediatrics, Harbor-UCLA Medical Centre, Los Angeles Biomedical Research Institute, Torrance, CA 90502, USA

Michael A. Gonzalez and Stephan Zuchner
Dr. John T. Macdonald Foundation Department of Human Genetics and John P. Hussman Institute for Human Genomics, University of Miami Miller School of Medicine, 1501 NW 10 Avenue, Miami, FL 33136, USA

Hatice Mutlu-Albayrak and Hüseyin Çaksen
Division of Pediatric Genetics, Department of Pediatrics, Meram Medical Faculty, University of Necmettin Erbakan, Meram, 42080 Konya, Turkey

Judit Bene and Bela Melegh
Department of Medical Genetics, University of Pécs, Pécs, Hungary
Szentagothai Research Centre, University of Pécs, Pécs, Hungary

Mehmet Burhan Oflaz
Division of Pediatric Cardiology, Department of Pediatrics, Meram Medical Faculty, University of Necmettin Erbakan, Meram, 42080 Konya, Turkey

Tijen Tanyalçın
Tanyalcin Medical Laboratory, Selective Screening and Metabolism Unit, Izmir, Turkey

Rossana Molinario, Sara Palumbo, Paola Concolino, Sandro Rocchetti, Roberta Rizza, Giovanni Luca Scaglione, Angelo Minucci and Ettore Capoluongo
Laboratory of Clinical Molecular and Personalized Diagnostics, Department of Laboratory Medicine, University Hospital "A. Gemelli", 8 Largo A. Gemelli, 00168 Rome, Italy

Nivedita U. Jerath, Tiffany Grider and Michael E. Shy
Department of Neurology, Carver College of Medicine, University of Iowa, 200 Hawkins Drive, Iowa City, IA 52242, USA

Daryl Graham and Aftab Chishti
Department of Pediatrics, University of Kentucky College of Medicine, Lexington, KY 40536, USA

Megan Gooch
University of Kentucky College of Medicine, Lexington, KY 40536, USA

Zhan Ye
Department of Pathology, University of Kentucky College of Medicine, Lexington, KY 40536, USA

Edward Richer
Department of Radiology, University of Kentucky College of Medicine, Lexington, KY 40536, USA

Elizabeth Reilly
Markey Cancer Center, University of Kentucky College of Medicine, Combs Research Building, 800 Rose Street, Lexington, KY 40536-0096, USA

John D'Orazio
Department of Pediatrics, University of Kentucky College of Medicine, Lexington, KY 40536, USA
Markey Cancer Center, University of Kentucky College of Medicine, Combs Research Building, 800 Rose Street, Lexington, KY 40536-0096, USA

Ali Sami Gurbuz
Department of Obstetrics and Gynecology, Novafertil IVF Center, Meram Yeni Yol No. 75, Meram, 42090 Konya, Turkey

Ahmet Salvarci
Department of Urology, Novafertil IVF Center and Konya Hospital, Meram Yeni Yol No. 75, Meram, 42090 Konya, Turkey

Necati Ozcimen
Medicana Konya IVF Center, Medicana Konya Feritpas,a Mah., Gurz Sok. No. 1, Selc¸uklu, 42060 Konya, Turkey

Ayse Gul Zamani
Department of Medical Genetic, Meram Tip Faculty, Necmettin Erbakan University, Yunus Emre Mah., Meram, 42060 Konya, Turkey

Filipa Flor-de-Lima
Department of Pediatrics, Hospital Pediátrico Integrado, Centro Hospitalar de São João, Alameda Prof. Hernâni Monteiro, 4200-319 Porto, Portugal

Faculty of Medicine, University of Porto, Alameda Prof. Hernâni Monteiro, 4200-319 Porto, Portugal

Mafalda Sampaio
Unit of Pediatric Neurology, Hospital Pediátrico Integrado, Centro Hospitalar de São João, Alameda Prof. Hernâni Monteiro, 4200-319 Porto, Portugal

Nahid Nahavandi
Centogene AG, Schillingallee 68, 18057 Rostock, Germany

Susana Fernandes
Department of Genetics, Faculty of Medicine, University of Porto, Alameda Prof. Hernâni Monteiro, 4200-319 Porto, Portugal

Miguel Leão
Unit of Pediatric Neurology, Hospital Pediátrico Integrado, Centro Hospitalar de São João, Alameda Prof. Hernâni Monteiro, 4200-319 Porto, Portugal
Department of Genetics, Faculty of Medicine, University of Porto, Alameda Prof. Hernâni Monteiro, 4200-319 Porto, Portugal

Shaochun Bai, Anthony Lozada and Melissa Dempsey
University of Chicago, 5841 South Maryland Avenue, Chicago, IL 60637, USA

Marilyn C. Jones
University of California and Children's Hospital of San Diego, San Diego, CA 92123, USA

Harry C. Dietz
Johns Hopkins University School of Medicine and Howard Hughes Medical Institute, Baltimore, MD 21287, USA

Soma Das
University of Chicago, 5841 South Maryland Avenue, Chicago, IL 60637, USA
Department of Human Genetics, University of Chicago, 5841 South Maryland Avenue, Chicago, IL 60637, USA

M. Vavlukis, P. Zafirovska, E. Caparovska, B. Pocesta and S. Kedev
University Clinic of Cardiology, Medical Faculty, Ss. Cyril and Methodius University, Mother Teresa 17, 1000 Skopje, Macedonia

A. Eftimov and A. J. Dimovski
Faculty of Pharmacy, Ss. Cyril and Methodius University, Mother Teresa 47, 1000 Skopje, Macedonia

Ana Belén de la Hoz
Plataforma de Genética Genómica, Instituto de Investigación Sanitaria BioCruces (IIS BioCruces), Hospital Universitario Cruces, Barakaldo, 48903 Bizkaia, Spain
GCV-CIBER de Enfermedades Raras (CIBERER-ISCIII), 28029 Madrid, Spain

Hiart Maortua and María-Isabel Tejada
GCV-CIBER de Enfermedades Raras (CIBERER-ISCIII), 28029 Madrid, Spain
Laboratorio de Genética Molecular, Servicio de Genética, IIS BioCruces, Hospital Universitario Cruces, Barakaldo, 48903 Bizkaia, Spain

Ainhoa García-Rives and María Jesús Martínez-González
GCV-CIBER de Enfermedades Raras (CIBERER-ISCIII), 28029 Madrid, Spain
Sección de Neuropediatría del Servicio de Pediatría, IIS BioCruces, Hospital Universitario Cruces, Barakaldo, 48903 Bizkaia, Spain

Maitane Ezquerra
Plataforma de Genética Genómica, Instituto de Investigación Sanitaria BioCruces (IIS BioCruces), Hospital Universitario Cruces, Barakaldo, 48903 Bizkaia, Spain
Laboratorio de Genética Molecular, Servicio de Genética, IIS BioCruces, Hospital Universitario Cruces, Barakaldo, 48903 Bizkaia, Spain

F. Malvestiti, C. Agrati, S. Chinetti, A. Di Meco, B. Grimi, F. Maggi, G. Simoni and F. R. Grati
Research and Development, Cytogenetics and Molecular Biology, TOMA Advanced Biomedical Assays S.p.A., 25/27 Francesco Ferrer Street, 21052 Busto Arsizio, Varese, Italy

S. Cirrincione and M. Oggionni
Treviglio Caravaggio Hospital, 1 Pittori Cavenaghi Square, 24043 Caravaggio, Bergamo, Italy

Giorgia Mandrile and Daniela Francesca Giachino
Medical Genetics Unit, "San Luigi Gonzaga" University Hospital, University of Torino, Regione Gonzole 10, 10143 Orbassano, Italy
Department of Clinical & Biological Sciences, University of Torino, 10143 Orbassano, Italy

Eleonora Di Gregorio and Alfredo Brusco
Department of Medical Sciences, University of Torino, Via Santena 19, 10126 Torino, Italy
Medical Genetics, "Città della Salute e della Scienza" University Hospital, 10126 Torino, Italy

Alessandro Calcia and Alessandro Brussino
Department of Medical Sciences, University of Torino, Via Santena 19, 10126 Torino, Italy

Enrico Grosso and Elisa Savin
Medical Genetics, "Città della Salute e della Scienza" University Hospital, 10126 Torino, Italy

Noura Biha
Rheumatology Department, Nouakchott Military Hospital, Mauritania
Faculté de Médecine de Nouakchott, Mauritania

S. M. Ghaber
Faculté de Médecine de Nouakchott, Mauritania
Service des Laboratoires, Centre Hospitalier National de Nouakchott, Mauritania

M. M. Hacen
Service de Chirurgie Orthopédique, Hôpital Militaire de Nouakchott, Mauritania

Corinne Collet
Assistance Publique-Hôpitaux de Paris, Hôpital Lariboisière, Laboratoire de Biochimie et de Biologie Moléculaire, Paris, France

Anca Zimmermann
Department of Endocrinology and Metabolic Diseases, 1st Clinic of Internal Medicine, University of Mainz, Langenbeckstrasse 1, 55131 Mainz, Germany

Heidi Rossmann
Institute for Clinical Chemistry and Laboratory Medicine, University of Mainz, Langenbeckstrasse 1, 55131 Mainz, Germany

Simona Bucerzan and Paula Grigorescu-Sido
Center of Genetic Diseases, Emergency Children's Hospital, University of Medicine and Pharmacy, Motilor Street 68, 400370 Cluj, Romania

Yang Cao, Nicole L. Hoppman, Sarah E. Kerr, Christopher A. Sattler, W. Edward Highsmith and Umut Aypar
Department of Laboratory Medicine and Pathology, Mayo Clinic, Rochester, MN 55905, USA

Kristi S. Borowski and Myra J. Wick
Department of Obstetrics and Gynecology, Mayo Clinic, Rochester, MN 55905, USA

Ho-Ming Luk
Clinical Genetic Service, Department of Health, Kowloon, Hong Kong

Jennifer L. Roberts and Merlin G. Butler
The University of Kansas Medical Center, Kansas City, KS 66160, USA

Stephanie K. Gandomi, Melissa Parra, Ira Lu and Chia-Ling Gau
Ambry Genetics, Aliso Viejo, CA 92656, USA

Majed Dasouki
The University of Kansas Medical Center, Kansas City, KS 66160, USA
King Faisal Specialist Hospital and Research Center, Riyadh 12713, Saudi Arabia

www.ingramcontent.com/pod-product-compliance
Lightning Source LLC
Chambersburg PA
CBHW080502200326
41458CB00012B/4057